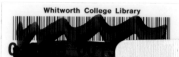

WOMEN OF COLOR
Integrating Ethnic and Gender Identities
in Psychotherapy

WOMEN OF COLOR
Integrating Ethnic and Gender Identities in Psychotherapy

Edited by
LILLIAN COMAS-DÍAZ
BEVERLY GREENE

Forewords by
Jean Baker Miller
Elaine Pinderhughes

THE GUILFORD PRESS / New York & London

© 1994 The Guilford Press
A Division of Guilford Publications, Inc.
72 Spring Street, New York, NY 10012

Printed in the United States of America

This book is printed on acid-free paper.

Last digit is print number: 9   8   7   6   5   4   3   2

Library of Congress Cataloging-in-Publication Data

Women of color : integrating ethnic and gender identities in
    psychotherapy / edited by Lillian Comas-Díaz, Beverly Greene.
        p.   cm.
    Includes bibliographical references and index.
    ISBN 0-89862-371-5
    1. Minority women—Mental health.   2. Minority women—Mental
health services.   3. Psychotherapy—Social aspects.   I. Comas-
Díaz, Lillian.   II. Greene, Beverly.
    [DNLM: 1. Psychotherapy—methods.   2. Women—psychology.
3. Women's Health.   4. Cross-Cultural Comparison.   WM 460.5.W6
1994]
RC451.4.M58W66   1994
616.89'14'08693—dc20
DNLM/DLC
for Library of Congress   94-10840
                                                                      CIP

To my family of origin, who encouraged my dreams, and to my present family, who transformed them

L. C.-D.

To my mother and father, for their love, wisdom and many sacrifices; my sister and brothers, for the preciousness of their friendship; and Robert and Jennifer, with my hopes for their future

B. G.

Contributors

JOAN SAKS BERMAN, PhD, Clinical Psychologist, Mental Health Department, Albuquerque Indian Hospital, New Mexico

NANCY BOYD-FRANKLIN, PhD, Professor, Graduate School of Applied and Professional Psychology, Rutgers University, Pisctaway, NJ; Consultant, Children's Hospital AIDS Program and National Pediatric HIV Resource Center, Newark, NJ

CARLA BRADSHAW, PhD, Clinical Psychologist, private practice, Kirkland, WA

JANET BRICE-BAKER, PhD, Assistant Professor, Ferkauf Graduate School of Psychology, Yeshiva University Bronx, NY; private practice, Somerset, NJ

JEAN LAU CHIN, EdD, Executive Director, South Cove Community Health Center, Boston, MA

LILLIAN COMAS-DÍAZ, PhD, Executive Director, Transcultural Mental Health Institute, Washington, DC

OLIVA M. ESPÍN, PhD, Professor, Department of Women's Studies, San Diego State University, CA; Core Faculty, California School of Professional Psychology, San Diego

NYDIA GARCÍA-PRETO, MSW, Clinical Director, Family Institute of New Jersey, Metuchen

BEVERLY GREENE, PHD, Associate Professor, Department of Psychology, St. John's University, Jamaica, NY; Clinical Psychologist, private practice, Brooklyn, NY

VALLI KANUHA, MSW, Deputy Director for Programs, Hunter College Center on AIDS, Drugs and Community Health, New York, NY

FREDERICK M. JACOBSEN, MD, MPH, Medical Director, Transcultural Mental Health Institute, Washington, DC; Guest Researcher, Laboratory of Clinical Science, National Institutes of Mental Health, Bethesda, MD; Associate Clinical Professor of Psychiatry, George Washington University School of Medicine and Georgetown University School of Medicine, Washington, DC

KUSHALATA JAYAKAR, MD, private practice, New York, NY; Medical Director, Outpatient Treatment Program, Long Island Jewish Medical Center, New York, NY

TERESA D. LAFROMBOISE, PHD, Associate Professor, Department of Counseling Psychology, University of Wisconsin, Madison; Associate Professor, School of Education, Stanford University, Stanford, CA

SANDRA LEWIS, PSYD, Assistant Professor, Clinical Psychiatry and Pediatrics, University of Medicine and Dentistry of New Jersey–New Jersey Medical School, National Pediatric HIV Resource Center, Newark

MARIA P. P. ROOT, PHD, Clinical Psychologist, private practice, Seattle, WA; Clinical Associate Professor of Psychology, University of Washington, Seattle

BALVINDAR K. SOHI, MA, MSSW, doctoral candidate, Department of Counseling Psychology, University of Wisconsin, Madison

LIANG TIEN, PSYD, Assistant Professor, Asian American Studies Program, Department of American Ethnic Studies, University of Washington, Seattle; Clinical Psychologist, private practice, Seattle, WA

MELBA J. T. VASQUEZ, PHD, ABPP, private practice, Austin, TX

Foreword

Jean Baker Miller

I am very pleased to be able to celebrate the publication of this book with you. The editors have made a valuable contribution by bringing together these chapters on the life experiences of women of many different cultures and then adding chapters on what different forms of therapy have to offer women of color. They have also included chapters on certain specific groupings of women of color, such as mixed-race women and lesbians.

For some years now, women of color have had to make the crucial point that psychology's discussion of women has been based largely on the experiences of White middle-class women, and that White middle-class women should not presume to speak for all women. Indeed, if they do, they are liable to fall into the same position for which they have criticized men, that is, generalizing about all people when they really only speak from their own experience. Men have neglected or misperceived women's experience, and because they misperceive women's experience they run the risk of missing or misperceiving the total human experience.

To select just one example, until women began to speak of their experience and thereby began to expose the vast amount of sexual and physical abuse that occurs in this society, men did not "know" that men, too, have often been abused as children. The proportion of boys abused is significant even if it is still much less than that of girls; some current estimates say that 33% of girls and 5–7% of boys have been sexually abused before age 18. The cited figures probably still underestimate the true rates for boys and perhaps for girls as well.

More fundamentally, the expansion of the dialogue to include the voices of women is forcing men to think about what it means for men (and women) to develop within a society that allows and often encourages such widespread violence. Could this violence perhaps have to do with the fact that we live in a social system that is basically oppressive to half the human race? Living with such a myopic perspective has to skew the possibilities of psychological development. Therefore, people developing in the dominant group, with this built-in bias, are not going to produce very accurate or comprehensive theories of human psychological development.

Similarly, as several of the writers in this book suggest, White women have lived in and benefited from a social system that has oppressed women and men of other racial and ethnic groups through the practices of racism and colonialism. Not only can White women not speak for women of color, it is not likely that White women will be able to develop a satisfactory understanding of the psychology of women that validly reflects the general experience of women.

This book, then, is extremely important. It is important because it brings together the voices of women of many racial and ethnic groups who describe their mutual experience as women of color as well as the variety of experience within each group. As the authors here emphasize, all women in a specific racial group are not the same. There are many different African American women or Chinese American women with many differing life experiences.

This book extends its portrayal to include the lives of women who are oppressed for additional reasons, such as class or sexual orientation, which are intertwined with racism. It also articulates the distinctions between different forms of destructive experience and their implications, as in Lillian Comas-Díaz's discussion of oppression on the basis of sex, age, or disability compared to that based on social, cultural, and economic colonization.

The mental health field, in general, has not had an understanding of the lives of women of many different cultures, nor an understanding of how specific forms of racism or colonialism affect particular groups of women. In recent years, a number of women of color have made major contributions to right this wrong. Certainly a central task in our time is the fuller and deeper carrying out of this work. This book takes us a major step forward on that path.

Jean Baker Miller
The Stone Center
Wellesley College

Boston University
School of Medicine

Foreword

Elaine Pinderhughes

Women of color, living as they do in a racist social system that is also patriarchal, are a "double minority." Along with the men of their cultural groups, they are trapped in roles that maintain the equilibrium of the larger social system. These dynamics operate through a societal projection process, which encourages the dominant group in society to perceive and treat subordinate groups as inferior and incompetent, and thereby to benefit from the continued exploitation of these groups (Bowen, 1978).

Being victimized by the societal projection process and serving as systems balancers and anxiety reducers for the larger social system has had profound consequences for people of color in their individual, family, and group functioning. It has also had profound consequences for the beneficiaries of this process, creating high vulnerability to an intolerance for cultural differences, an unrealistic sense of entitlement, poor reality testing, and unsound judgment of self and others (Pinderhughes, 1989) These are issues that remain largely out of the dominant group's awareness, and unexamined by them.

Whether a woman of color is considered a member of an oppressed cultural group and it is her subordinate sex-role status that must be understood, or whether she is considered a member of an oppressed sex group and it is her subordinate cultural identity that must be understood, her circumstances are unique. In belonging to two groups whose positions are determined by oppression, her experience differs from that of her fellow victims, the man of color and the White woman, because her reality involves the dynamics of both racism and sexism. Not only must she cope with the confusion and contraction inherent in her position as a member of a minority cultural group that functions at the boundary of society, but she must also cope with expectations related to her role of nurturer and supporter of others. This role pushes her to fulfill the role of provider and protector from which men of color have been blocked. At the same time it is expected that she will nurture men in her life and cope with their reactive anger as well as nurture and support their children's attempts to thrive in a hostile environment.

Women are generally expected to relieve tension and reduce anxiety within their families, but this expectation for the woman of color must be realized with fewer resources and societal supports than are available to White women.

The woman of color is called upon to compensate for the costly consequences of her family's and cultural group's role as balancer in the larger social system. In so doing, she herself becomes a balancing mechanism within her family and cultural group. Such a role places her at a nodal point in the overall functioning of a society.

Viewed then via stereotypes that too often have determined societal treatment of her; confined by the dynamics of the societal projection process to low-paying, low-status work; with a weakened or absent extended family and few alternate forms of support to buffer her interface with a nonsupportive, frequently racist, external world; and blamed for consequent family conflict and breakdown, the woman of color finds her nodal role a formidable one.

Mental health intervention with women of color requires an understanding of this nodal societal role, the dynamics that maintain it as a significant contextual factor in the problems of women of color and those of their families, the solutions they might seek, and even the intervention process itself. Empowerment of these women so that they can cope effectively with the consequences of their societal entrapment becomes a fundamental goal in the work. Clinicians, if they are beneficiaries of this unjust social system, are, like their minority women clients, nevertheless trapped in it. They may find their ability to help compromised by the automatic benefits inherent to their beneficiary status, making them susceptible to the perpetuation of their clients' victim status. A volume such as this can help them to anticipate this susceptibility, clarifying as it does the realities of minority women and the many ways in which their needs are unique, and making clear how and in what ways their responses to societal entrapment must be enhanced for their empowerment efforts to succeed.

In particular, the emphasis in this book on the strengths of women of color will promote respect in practitioners for culturally different worldviews and practices, as well as the survival mechanisms they have devised that demonstrate their resilience and crystallize the broader perspective needed for effective practice. Emphasis on the heterogeneity among groups of women of color, the diversity within a given cultural group, and especially on subpopulations of the larger groups goes still further in creating a context for the complex issues that must be comprehended for clinical work to be effective. This comprehensive presentation highlights the way in which flexible thinking and behavior on the part of mental health clinicians is critical. It is a volume that will become an invaluable resource for all clinicians, irrespective of discipline, and a landmark publication in the field of mental health—its long overdue appearance is welcomed enthusiastically.

Elaine Pinderhughes
Boston College
Graduate School of Social Work

REFERENCES

Bowen, M. (1978). *Family therapy in clinical practice.* New York: Jason Aronson.
Pinderhughes, E. (1989). *Understanding race, ethnicity and power: Key to efficacy in clinical practice.* New York: Free Press.

Preface

As therapists and scholars, we need to reconstruct our psychological knowledge of women by incorporating a more inclusive thinking into our approaches to psychotherapy. When scholarship relevant to women of color infuses our psychological paradigms, it challenges both our traditional definitions of womanhood and our conceptualizations of mental health. This informed context necessitates a revision of the assumptions made about normalcy and deviance, adaptive and maladaptive (dysfunctional) behavior, and psychotherapeutic success or failure. Race, gender, class, and sexual orientation are examples of variables that may profoundly affect women's lives. The importance of these variables makes it essential to recognize the significance of racism, sexism, and heterosexism; oppression and domination; and power and powerlessness as critical and often ignored realities in the lives of women of color.

The dominant mainstream culture places expectations on women of color that are often a mass of contradictions and a series of paradoxes: They find themselves in circumstances that require them to be strong, resilient, instrumental, and self-affirming in order to survive, yet cultural norms frequently define "normal" women as weak, fragile, vulnerable, submissive, and oppressed. Many women of color have spent so little time focusing on their own needs rather than others' that in mental health treatment they are often unaware of what their needs even are. When they seek clinical services they bear the additional burden of determining whether the practitioner will be familiar with the worldviews of their cultures. In addition, traditional mental health treatment has been an institutional voice that tends to invest White middle-class values with the legitimacy of psychological normalcy. Hence, when White middle-class women seek mental health services they often correctly presume that the treatment and the clinician incorporate their worldviews in some way. This is not the case for women of color.

This book addresses the mental health status of women of color and presents an integration of culturally relevant and gender-sensitive guidelines for clinical practice. Understanding the realistic mental health needs of hyphenated women of color—African American, Asian American, Latina/ Hispanic American, East Indian American, and Native American—requires an appreciation of the contexts of their psychological realities. Women of color have unique strengths and vulnerabilities that warrant special consideration in psychotherapy. Their realities are marked by the convergence of both gender and ethnicity and the complex interactions between them. A thoughtful consideration of the unique interaction of these variables is conspicuously absent from the mental health and psychotherapy literature, rendering women of color marginal and their needs invisible.

This volume has been conceived and developed in response to the absence of scholarly inquiry into the interaction of gender and ethnicity in mental health treatment. We explore the effects of these previously neglected variables on one another and on the psychological and psychosocial development of women of color, and the consequent delivery of mental health services to them. The exclusion of a formal consideration of the mental health needs of women of color provided the impetus for our collaboration. We invited the contributions of experts on gender issues within specific ethnic groups as well as those of experts on the efficacy of varying therapeutic approaches with women of color. Contributors to this volume are scholars and practitioners whose work acknowledges and explores the impact of multiple overlapping parameters of gender and ethnicity in the lives of women of color and thus in conducting mental health treatment with them.

The book was developed with the goal of advancing gender-sensitive and ethnoculturally relevant mental health treatments. The heterogeneity of women of color, their unique contextual experiences, and their intragroup diversity inform our clinical approaches. With the aforementioned factors in mind we have developed this volume around three working paradigms and organized sections of the book accordingly.

Part I, "Women of Color: A Portrait of Hetereogeneity," validates the specific realities of women of color. In this section, contributors illustrate the effectiveness of gender-aware and culturally relevant treatment by reviewing major clinical issues with specific ethnoracial groups of women of color. Contributors were asked to conform to a common format in order to contrast the similarities and differences in the presented groups. This format includes a brief historical overview, sociocultural issues, family relations, gender roles, and developmental issues. The application of mental health treatment with women in each group as well as case examples are presented.

Part II, "Theoretical and Applied Frameworks," provides a critical examination of the applicability of a range of existing treatment orientations. Different therapeutic perspectives and their applicability to women of color are reviewed. In examining the applicability of divergent therapeutic models, contributors cover similar areas in all of the presented therapeutic orientations. The principles of each theoretical orientation are reviewed, in addition to its gender and cultural sensitivity, and specific applicability to women of color. Guidelines for the use of each therapeutic orientation are aided by clinical illustrations.

Part III, "The Labyrinth of Diversity: Special Populations of Women of Color," provides an explication of the unique needs of special subpopulations of women of color in mental health treatment. Guidelines are presented on the treatment of women of color from special subcultures and clinical groups. Some of these groups include women with professional status, lesbians, mixed-race women, battered women, and refugee women.

This volume represents a significant step in advancing multicultural frameworks for the treatment of women in the mental health profession. Emphasizing both theoretical evolution and clinical applications, it provides accessible tools for seasoned clinicians as well as novices. Similarly, both the academician and the practitioner will find this resourceful account of the mental health of women of color useful. Intended for all types of mental health professionals, this volume was constructed from an interdisciplinary perspective. Contributors represent many different disciplines and theoretical perspectives and have extensive clinical experience with the specific ethnic groups and/or the issues that they address. We hope that this volume provides a foundation for the clinical understanding and sensitive integration of the confluence of racial, gender, and ethnocultural factors in the psychotherapeutic treatment of women of color.

Lillian Comas-Díaz
Beverly Greene

Acknowledgments

This book has been inspired by our work with clients, colleagues, practitioners, and trainees. Our mutual collaboration has mothered, nurtured, and refined the conceptualization and applications of the mental health constructs presented in this book. While we have received help from many different individuals, we would like to acknowledge publicly our special gratitude to those whose direct participation was crucial to the completion of this work. Our thanks and deep appreciation go to Laura S. Brown, who as a reviewer midwifed the entire volume; to Sharon Panulla, our Guilford editor who acted as the book's godmother; and to the volume's contributors, whose labor of love, patience, and wisdom is evidenced in this volume.

I, Lillian, have been very fortunate in having both female and male mentors. However, I wish to acknowledge here the special mentorship that I have received from minority women and women of color. These female mentors imparted to me the unique gift of negotiating complex realities as a woman, as a woman of color, as an outsider, and as a denizen of different worlds. My deep gratitude goes to all of them. Bonnie R. Strickland, Ph.D., chairperson of my doctoral dissertation, masterfully managed my transition from student to colleague to friend. Laura Leticia Herrans, Ph.D., created new visions for Latinas, and encouraged me to become a psychologist. Always believing in me, Raquel Marrero, Ph.D., showed me how transplanted flowers survive and blossom. As a peer mentor and as an African American woman, Joan W. Duncan, Ph.D., inspired me to explore alien seas while building bridges and remaining grounded in my own reality. As a friend and as a sister, Julia Ramos Grenier, Ph.D., tenderly taught me games my mother never taught me. Luz M. Ramos, poet and teacher, was my Virgil during Dantean years. Finally, I would like to acknowledge Francesca Xavier Cabrini, immigrant and healer, for giving me my voice. To all of them: mil gracias.

I, Beverly, wish to acknowledge publicly a few of my most important mentors. First, I must express my gratitude to Dorothy Gartner, Ph.D., for tangibly and actively nurturing my contribution to this volume and for facilitating my earliest career efforts to develop scholarship on cultural diversity in the delivery of psychological services. Her active mentoring and support were essential ingredients in the unfolding of much that was to follow. Nancy Boyd-Franklin, Ph.D., as a contemporary psychologist and African American woman, was one of my earliest and most enduring peer mentors. Our mutual collaboration and friendship has enriched and supported the development of my work and I am pleased to acknowledge formally her generous contributions. William "Bill" Johnson, Ph.D., was one of my precious few African American psychologist mentors who taught me early in my career how to view traditional psychotherapy approaches through many diverse cultural lenses. At that time, his was a lone voice in a wildnerness; I am most grateful to have been within earshot. My most important female mentors and role models are neither professional, nor well known to others. Florence Cook Brown, Lucy Turk, and Rose Robinson epitomize the notion of grace and determination under fire and in the midst of disappointment. They are among the earliest and most profound influences in my professional development and life as an African American woman. Finally, it is with great affection that I thank Dorith Brodbar, M.S.Ed., and Peter W. Carmel, M.D., for reasons that are known to them.

Contents

Part II
THEORETICAL AND APPLIED FRAMEWORKS

Part III
THE LABYRINTH OF DIVERSITY:
SPECIAL POPULATIONS
OF WOMEN OF COLOR

WOMEN OF COLOR
Integrating Ethnic and Gender Identities
in Psychotherapy

I

WOMEN OF COLOR: A PORTRAIT OF HETEROGENEITY

Overview: An Ethnocultural Mosaic

Lillian Comas-Díaz
Beverly Greene

People of color constitute the fastest growing population in the United States. The percentage of African Americans/Blacks is estimated as being 12.4%; Hispanic/Latinos as 8.1%; Asian American/Pacific Islanders as 3%; and American Indians/Alaska Natives as .7% (U.S. Bureau of the Census, 1991). It is predicted that if current trends in immigration and birth rates persist, the Hispanic/Latino presence will have further increased an estimated 21%, the Asian population about 22%, African Americans almost 12%, while that of Whites only about 2% (Henry, 1990). By the year 2056, the United States will be a demographic mosaic, and the typical resident will trace his or her descent to Africa, Asia, the Latin American world, the Pacific Islands, Arabia—almost anywhere but White Europe (Henry, 1990).

These demographic changes are affecting the fabric of North American society; cultural pluralism appears to be emerging as a distinct feature of the United States. Such demographic trends and the ascendancy of cultural pluralism need to be reflected in the delivery of mental health services. As our society becomes increasingly multicultural, the ability to address multicultural and gender-informed contexts competently may well become a mandatory skill for clinicians. The persistence of racial and ethnic group identity results in a sociological kaleidoscope: Its parts relate to each other in constantly changing ways, producing fresh shapes and new patterns (Fuchs, 1990). Women of color play a central role in this sociological kaleidoscope, constituting a pivotal force within their own communities (Boyd-Franklin, 1991; McGoldrick, García-Preto, Hines, & Lee, 1989) as well as in the larger society. The strengths that have made them so pivotal

3

notwithstanding women of color have needs that require a closer examination and urge a special focus in the delivery of mental health treatment.

Women of color are culturally and emotionally distinct from mainstream White women and thus should not be marginalized when they do not conform to the mainstream group norm (Wright, 1972). The mythical uniformity of sisterhood has led to the homogenization of women's diverse cultures, languages, ethnicities, classes, and sexualities (Andersen & Collins, 1991; Cole, 1986). Gender, race, and culture are important determinants of an individual's identity. Age, socioeconomic level, ethnicity, education, religion, sexual orientation, geographic location, degree of assimilation or acculturation, history of immigration, and citizen status also constitute some of the many factors that need to be considered when addressing the mental health needs and treatment of women of color. However, it is important to recognize that while a woman is shaped by different human dimensions, each woman is an individual unique in her needs, strengths, and limitations.

The heterogeneous groups that comprise women of color have woven an ethnocultural and racial tapestry in the United States. These groups encompass those who define themselves as women of color and those whose experiences of oppression, social status, plus phenotypical and racial characteristics differ from women of the White dominant group—differences usually regarded as denoting deficiency and/or inferiority. The definitions of women of color are not static; they are dynamic, changing according to context. The heteeogeneous populations of women of color presented in this volume are not exhaustive nor entirely inclusive. They correspond to current sociopolitical and geopolitical designations including American Indians/Alaska natives; women of African descent, namely African Americans, West Indians, and African Caribbeans; women of Asian descent, such as Asians, Asian Americans, Pacific Islanders, and East Indians (women from India); as well as Latinas/Hispanic women.

COMMONALITIES AND DISPARITIES: WOMEN OF COLOR, WHITE WOMEN, AND MEN OF COLOR

Women of color tend to have different life experiences from those of White women. Skin color is a determinant variable in the life experiences of persons of color in the United States. Race and color tend to differentiate the status of women of color from those immigrants of European and White extraction. Regardless of when their ancestors came here women of color are perceived as women of color, while European and other White immigrants become mainstream Americans as early as the second generation. Another major difference is the choice between racial or gender alliances that women of color must make, that White women do not face (Reid, 1988). For instance, due to the pervasive effects of racism and the concomitant need for people of color to bond together, women of color experience conflicting loyalties in which racial solidarity often transcends gender and sexual orientation solidarity (Kanuha, 1990). Another important difference between women of color and White women is the greater level of social acceptability White women receive compared to women of color, due in part to the fact that White women are necessary to the continued existence of White men, while women of color are not (Reid, 1988).

Women of color are not only exposed to oppression within the dominant group, but also experience sexism and oppression within their own ethnic and racial communities as well. For example, Lorde (1984) asserts that due to racism African American women have been manipulated by the power structure in such a way that their (relative) success in the work place over African American men may cause those men to be resentful of them. This often creates underlying antagonism between women and men of color, which is frequently translated into sexist reactions by men of color. Consequently, for many women of color, it has been a strain to separate the need to accommodate the oppressor from their own legitimate conflicts within their communities. Lorde (1984) argues that this situation does not exist among women from the dominant group, who may be seduced into joining the oppressor under the pretense of sharing power.

Women and men of color share common life experiences. Both groups are exposed to racial and ethnic discrimination. Their salient identification with ethnicity and race is strong, due to the common oppression experienced by all individuals in the group regardless of gender (Almquist, 1989; Espín & Gawelek, 1992). The experiences of racism, identity conflict, oppression, colonialism, and cultural adaptation, as well as the stressful and hostile environments in which people of color very often live, tend to create a tenacious bond between men and women of color—a bond crucial to their survival. For example, Hines and Boyd-Franklin (1982) argue that African American women may feel empathy for their male partner's frustration within a racist society and may have difficulty holding him responsible for his behavior. Similarly, some Latinas may sustain their male partners' macho behaviors as compensating for the emasculation of minority males in an oppressive society (Comas-Díaz, 1989). These conflicts often evolve into the struggle that women of color have with the devaluation of their realities and, sometimes, with the internalization of such experiences in negative self-images.

WOMEN OF COLOR: HETEROGENEITY AND CONNECTEDNESS

Regardless of their heterogeneity, as a group many women of color share common bonds. The combined and independent effects of racism, sexism, oppression, classism, and colonization (external and internal) often act as a common denominator for women of color (Comas-Díaz, 1991). An illustration of this common denominator is presented in the report on the special populations subpanel on women of the President's Commission on Mental Health (1978), which stated that the societal inequalities faced by women of color result from both gender and ethnoracial discrimination and oppression.

The common denominator of gender and ethnic oppression facilitates connectedness among women of color. The racial, gender, and cultural legacies of women of color often emphasize interconnectedness as well as collective and contextual self-definitions (Comas-Díaz, Chapter 11, this volume). Many women define themselves within the context of family, group, and community of color. Both gender and racial factors are central to their self-definition (Barret, 1990). Consequently, women of color tend to have multiple sources of identity. Ethnocultural and gender roles also tend to be interconnected with the well-being of their ethnic group (Almquist, 1989). This attention to both group and individual needs may appear alien and complex to members of the dominant group (Boyd, 1990).

Although the experiences of women of color have strong commonalities, they also have significant differences. Their experiences are differentiated by intricate factors. Some of these factors include the experience of ethnocultural translocation. For example, due to imperialism and racism American Indians have been made emigrants in their own land (Attneave, 1982). This historical and sociopolitical context has made survival, both at a cultural and a physical level, the central issue for Native American Indian women (Allen, 1986). Many Latina, Asian, West Indian, and East Indian women have a personal or generational history of immigration, while some African American women have a history of immigration and others a history of migration around the United States. Similarly, the degree of acculturation and transculturation to the mainstream society is another variable pointing to the heterogeneity among women of color. Other factors include skin color and racial features; English language proficiency; socioeconomic class; a patrimony of American political colonization, as in the case of Filipinas and Puerto Rican women; and a legacy of slavery, as in women of African descent such as African Americans, West Indians, and African Caribbeans. The differences among women of color are also extended to each ethnoracial group's structure, coping style within hostile environments, negotiation of differences, adjustment to changes, problem solving, and response to mental health treatment (Ho, 1987), among many others.

The tradition of gender roles also tends to differ among the heterogeneous ethnoracial groups. Some groups are relatively egalitarian, as in the case of African Americans and some American Indians, while others are more rigidly demarcated, as in the case of Hispanics/Latinas and Asian Americans. However, the diversity of gender roles within ethnic groups is illustrated by the Asian American group, where Filipinas have a history of more egalitarian gender roles than other Asian groups (Bradshaw, Chapter 3, this volume). Furthermore, women of color who cope with oppression by assimilation and compliance may respond differently to gender role norms than women from families where differences are given positive salience by ethnocultural identification or separation from the mainstream culture (Brown, 1986).

Since women of color comprise highly heterogeneous populations, they are individuals who make diverse choices in coping, functioning, and empowering or disempowering themselves. For example, some women of color may not turn to their ethnic and cultural traditions for emotional support. However, many women of color will look at some level to a source of comfort and/or nurturing that only their community or family of origin can offer (Boyd, 1990). Indeed, there is no monolithic concept of women of color. What applies to an African American woman does not necessarily apply to a Hispanic/Latina. Similarly, differences exist among women from the same ethnic and racial group. For instance, what applies to a Chinese American woman does not necessarily apply to a Japanese American woman. The differences also extend to individuals' preferences for self-designation. As an illustration, the majority of Mexican Americans, Puerto Ricans, and Cubans chose the name of their national origin as self-designation instead of general rubric of Hispanics and/or Latino (García, cited in Duke, 1991). Even the generic terms "Hispanic" and "Latina" are not uniformly used in this very volume, for instance, Boyd-Franklin and García-Preto use "Hispanic" while Vasquez prefers "Latina." Similarly, Asian American groups may prefer their national origin as self-designation instead of the generic term Asian Americans.

PREAMBLE TO A PORTRAIT OF HETEROGENEITY

This section of the book, "Women of Color: A Portrait of Heterogeneity," constitutes a fledgling step in addressing the exclusion, marginality, and invisibility of women of color in the mental health literature. Specifically, it presents the unique characteristics of six groups of women of color. These include chapters by Beverly Greene on African Americans, by Teresa LaFromboise, Joan Saks Berman, and Balvindar Sohi on American Indians, by Carla Bradshaw on Asian Americans/Pacific Islanders, by Melba Vasquez on Hispanics/Latinas, by Kushalata Jayakar on women from India, and by Janet Brice-Baker on Jamaican women. Unfortunately, we were unable to present all groups of women of color. This omission is due to practical limitations, and does not imply a judgment of irrelevancy or a lack of interest in other groups of women of color. The omission, however, underscores the need to pay more attention to all groups of women of color. As an illustration, one of the missing groups is women of Arabic ancestry. Arab Americans are beginning to be recognized in the mental health literature as an ethnic/racial group requiring special attention (Budman, Lipson, & Meleis, 1992). Although Arab American women may not be highly visible, they are often victims of prejudice, discrimination, and oppression. In addition to the rigidity in their gender roles, Arab American women often cope with special issues such as bicultural and multicultural backgrounds and the struggle for individual and group self-definition and determination (Friedman & Pines, 1992).

The contributors in this section examine the six aforementioned ethnic female groups, providing a cultural, racial, and gender context for the mental health needs and treatment of women of color. This section also illustrates the effectiveness of gender and culturally informed mental health treatment by presenting ethnocultural and clinical issues with specific groups of women of color. Additionally, the contributors discuss mental health issues, including help-seeking behavior, assessment and diagnosis, and clinical issues special to each population of women. Clinical case examples enrich the discussions by illustrating the issues presented in each chapter, and clinical guidelines for the treatment of these populations are suggested.

REFERENCES

Allen, P. G. (1986). *The sacred hoop: Recovering the feminism in American Indian traditions.* Boston: Beacon Press.

Almquist, E. (1989). The experience of minority women in the United Stated. In J. Freeman (Ed.), *Women: A feminist perspective* (4th ed., pp. 414–445). Mountain View, CA: Mayfield.

Andersen, M. L., & Collins, P. H. (Eds.). (1991). *Race, class and gender: An anthology.* Belmont, CA: Wadsworth.

Attneave, C. (1982). American Indians and Alaskan Native families: Emigrants in their own homeland. In M. McGoldrick, J. K. Pearce, & J. Giordano (Eds.), *Ethnicity and family therapy* (pp. 55–83). New York: Guilford Press.

Barret, S. E. (1990). Paths toward diversity: An intrapsychic perspective. *Women and Therapy, 9,* 41–52.

Boyd, J. A. (1990). Ethnic and cultural diversity: Keys to power. *Women and Therapy, 9,* 151–167.

Boyd-Franklin, N. (1991). Recurrent themes in the treatment of African Americans. *Women and Therapy, 11,* 25–40.

Brown, L. S. (1986). Gender-role analysis: A neglected component of psychological assessment. *Psychotherapy, 23,* 243–248.

Budman, C. L., Lipson, J. G., & Meleis, A. I. (1992). The cultural consultant in mental health care: The case of an Arab adolescent. *American Journal of Orthopsychiatry, 62,* 359–370.

Cole, J. B. (1986). Commonalities and differences. In J. B. Cole (Ed.), *All American women: Lines that divide, ties that bind* (pp. 1–30). New York: Free Press.

Comas-Díaz, L. (1989). Culturally relevant issues and treatment implications for Hispanics. In D. R. Koslow & E. Salett (Eds.), *Crossing cultures in mental health* (pp. 31–48). Washington, DC: Society for International Education Training and Research.

Comas-Díaz, L. (1991). Feminism and diversity in psychology: The case of women of color. *Psychology of Women Quarterly, 15*, 597–609.

Duke, L. (1991, August 30). Latinos identify themselves as politically conservative. *Washington Post*, pp. A19–A20.

Espín, O. M., & Gawalek, M. A. (1992). Women's diversity: Ethnicity, race, class and gender in theories of feminist psychology. In L. Brown & M. Ballou (Eds.), *Personality and psychopathology: Feminist reappraisals* (pp. 88–107). New York: Guilford Press.

Fuchs, L. H. (1990). *The American kaleidoscope: Race, ethnicity, and the civic culture.* Middletown, CT: Wesleyan University Press.

Friedman, A., & Pines A. (1992). Increase in Arab women's perceived power in second half of life. *Sex Roles: A Journal of Research, 26*, 1–9.

Henry, W. A. (1990, April 9). Beyond the melting pot. *Time, 135*(15), 28–31.

Hines, P. M., & Boyd-Franklin, N. (1982). Black families. In M. McGoldrick, J. K. Pearce, & J. Giordano (Eds.), *Ethnicity and family therapy* (pp. 84–107). New York: Guilford Press.

Ho, M. K. (1987). *Family therapy with ethnic minorities.* Newbury Park, CA: Sage.

Kanuha, V. (1990). Compounding the triple jeopardy: Battering in lesbian of color relationships. *Women and Therapy, 9*, 169–184.

Lorde, A. (1984). *Sister outsider: Essays and speeches.* New York: Cross Press.

McGoldrick, M., García-Preto, N., Hines, P. M., & Lee, E. (1989). Ethnicity and women. In M. McGoldrick, C. M. Anderson, & F. Walsh (Eds.), *Women in families: A framework for family therapy* (pp. 169–199). New York: Norton.

President's Commission on Mental Health. (1978). *Report of the Special Populations Subpanel on Women* (Task Force Reports, Vol. III). Washington, DC: U.S. Government Printing Office.

Reid, P. T. (1988). Racism and sexism: Comparisons and conflicts. In P. A. Katz & D. A. Taylor (Eds.), *Eliminating racism* (pp. 203–221). New York: Plenum.

U.S. Bureau of the Census. (1991). *Statistical abstract of 1991* (11th ed.). Washington, DC: Author.

Wright, M. (1972). I want the right to be black and me. In G. Lerner (Ed.), *Black women in white America.* New York: Pantheon.

1

African American Women

Beverly Greene

African American women are born into a social environment that is rich but also treacherous. Their lives are inextricably linked to a history of racist and sexist oppression that institutionalizes the devaluation of African American women as it idealizes their White counterparts. (This legacy is further complicated for African American lesbians by pervasive heterosexism, giving rise to a dilemma explored in Chapter 14 in greater detail.) The interrelationship between racism and sexism must be appreciated for its complexity and for its effect on the social and psychological realities of African American women. This chapter explores the cultural history of African American women in the United States, its effect on the development of their psychological resilience and vulnerability, and psychotherapeutic interventions that take into account their unique constellation of attributes and conditions.

HISTORICAL OVERVIEW

African Americans are one of the oldest and largest groups of persons of color within the United States. At the time of the first census in 1790, African Americans numbered 760,000 (Brown, 1990). In 1860, their numbers had reached 4.4 million, and of that number all but 488,000 were slaves. By 1990 that number had grown over 30 million—with females outnumbering males—is expected to grow an additional 6.6 million by the year 2000 (Henry, 1990).

In 1910, 90% of African Americans lived in the rural South (Ruiz, 1990). In the 1940s a great migration took place, with over one million African Americans moving from the South to northern and midwestern cities (Ruiz, 1990). Seeking better job opportunities in industrialized urban areas, they became competitors for jobs with Whites. Currently over 60% of African Americans live in urban areas (Ruiz, 1990).

African Americans are descendants of the people of the tribes of the West African coast, who were the primary objects of the U.S. slave trade. Many African Americans also have partial Native American and European ancestry. Unlike other immigrants, who came to the United States seeking and often finding a more advantageous political climate or working conditions, African slaves entered the United States unwillingly, as pieces of property with no legal or human rights. Rather than improving their circumstances, the removal of West Africans from Africa resulted in countless deaths and loss of community, original language, and freedom itself for those who survived. The institutional racism that followed the abolition of slavery has continued the oppression of African Americans with over a century of legal racial discrimination and a legacy of discrimination that still must be overcome.

As slaves, African Americans were to provide free labor and were sold like any other saleable commodity. African American women had a special role in this because they bore children who became saleable commodities as well. A concrete example of the connection between an African American woman's value as a slave and her breeding capacity was the price she would bring on the auction block. The greater her childbearing capacity, the greater the price she would fetch (Berry & Blassingame, 1982). Her children were routinely conceived as a result of forced sexual relations with both African male slaves and white slavemasters. Her maternal attachment to those children was just as routinely ignored; they were taken from her, sold, and often never seen again.

From the outset, an African American woman's role in American society was synonymous with labor outside the home. This distinguished her from her White counterparts. For the most part in American society, traditional gender-role stereotypes resulted in social conventions that prohibited females from many forms of labor that were routine for males. This courteous protection of femininity was not, however, extended to African American women. By definition, one could not achieve the status of "woman" in society without first achieving the status of "person," and this was a status that African slave women conspicuously lacked. For the most part they worked in fields alongside African American males or performed any other manual labor required by slavemasters. Fox-Genovese (1988), in her discussion of life in plantation households, notes that under slavery African American women were somehow exempt from the observance of traditional gender roles accorded their White counterparts (hooks, 1981; Lerner, 1972; Robinson, 1983). This has remained consistent throughout their history in the United States.

PSYCHOLOGICAL REALITIES OF AFRICAN AMERICAN WOMEN

African American women face a range of cultural imperatives and psychological realities that may challenge, facilitate, or undermine their development and adaptive functioning. There is a cultural imperative to maintain and integrate aspects of the West African cultures that can constitute an important and adaptive part of their heritage. This task is compromised by the hostility with which non-Western cultures and models are viewed in the United States, as well as by the history of distortions in Western cultures of African civilizations and their peoples.

Another important task involves both the integration and the mitigation of the influence of aspects of the dominant culture. The institutions of the dominant culture have historically denigrated and exploited African peoples, justifying that exploitation by means of a web of pernicious myths about the inferiority of African Americans when compared to their White counterparts (Berry & Blassingame, 1982; Friedman, 1966; Nobles, 1974). This can make it difficult for African American women to make use of beneficial aspects of the dominant culture because they must avoid internalizing its insidious devaluation of persons of African descent. Specifically, there are powerful and pervasive stereotypes that African Americans lack emotional control or are impulsive, lack sexual restraint, are of lower intelligence than their White counterparts, and harbor violent tendencies (Friedman, 1966; Thomas & Sillen, 1972). Such devaluation of persons of African descent complicates the formation of a positive ethnic identity. The development of adaptive mechanisms required to combat the routine reality of such devaluation is an additional stressor.

African American women must address the daily, mundane life stressors that all women face, in addition to the stressors of racism. Like anyone else they bring their own complex constellations of family history and individual biological, social, intellectual, emotional, and characterological determinants to any task. These determinants must be understood in the context of their interaction with the environment, with each shaping the other.

Jones (1985) has suggested viewing these realities as separate spheres that overlap in varying points in the presenting problem or symptom. The point or points of overlap and the relative importance of one sphere to the other will vary from time to time in treatment, as they will vary during different developmental periods of a client's life. They will also most certainly vary from client to client. The clinician's task is to determine the most important area of focus at a particular time.

African Cultural Characteristics

Derivatives of African cultural characteristics in African Americans do not appear as they might have 300 years ago. Certainly African Americans have been socialized within the dominant culture as well as within their own, and have absorbed some of the latter's values. Hence their practices reflect a combination of both value systems.

Akbar (1985) writes that derivatives of African worldviews may be observed in the statement, "I am because we are," rather than the Cartesian view captured in the proposition, "I think, therefore I am." The former concept underscores an important value of tribe over individual, with emphasis on interdependence and collective responsibility. Individuals are encouraged to look beyond their own personal needs to consider what is in the greater interest of the group. This may conflict with the Western value of rugged individualism. Every member of the tribe is presumed to have something to contribute and is expected to do so. This expectation may be a causative factor in the observed flexibility of gender roles in African American families. While such flexibility is a function of the need to adapt to the effects of discrimination in the workplace against African American males, it has important cultural roots in the less stratified gender roles of many African tribes.

Boykin (1985) has noted that African cultures respond to the spirit rather than the letter of the law. From this perspective, laws, rules, or social structures do not exist as abstract entities with a life of their own. They are created as tools that may be modified or discarded when they no longer serve their purpose. Boykin goes on to elaborate on cultural characteristics of African Americans. Personal style and attributes are valued rather than status or office in the dominant culture. This is not uncommon in cultures where formal status or legitimized power is not available to members of a group because of institutional discrimination, economic impoverishment, or both. The valuing of personal attibutes over material accoutrements also reflects African cultural roots. The appreciation of personal distinctiveness can be seen in the styles of Black music and dance, which highlight improvisation and originality.

Boykin (1985) and Hale-Benson (1986) observe a heightened sensitivity to nonverbal communications. This may also be a function of living in a hostile environment, where attention to subtle cues can mean the difference between life and death. The history of African people reflects a preference for oral or auditory, as opposed to written, communications. Akbar (1985), Boykin (1985), and Levine (1977) suggest that spoken words may convey deep textural meaning and affect in ways that may be lost in attempts to reconstruct them grammatically.

Unlike many of their White counterparts, African American women are not socialized to expect marriage to relieve them of the need for employment. Their financial contribution to the household is usually presumed necessary. The role of mother is an important one for many African American women, but is accompanied by tasks that are not required of their White counterparts (Boyd-Franklin, 1989; Joseph & Lewis, 1981). In precolonial Africa, the roles of childbearer and child rearer were highly valued, a philosophical orientation that places a special value on children as representing the continuity of life (Bell, 1971; Ladner, 1971; Nobles, 1974).

In African American culture, family is defined as an extended kinship network rather than as the nuclear unit central to White cultural values. In this network, non-blood relations who have close affectional ties with family members may be treated and experienced as family. Hence, African American children frequently have many people involved in their upbringing, who may not be natural parents. While motherhood is an important role for African American women, this concept is not limited to biological mothers. Many women in families play major roles in the raising of children who are not their biological children, but are the children of "kin." Boyd-Franklin (1989) observes that strong kinship bonds are perhaps the most enduring legacy of African heritage. Children are viewed as part of a communal network that extends beyond a child's natural parents. This may serve many adaptive purposes. The kinship network within African American families can provide children with alternative role models, both mothers and children with emotional safety valves, and mothers with respites from child care (Hill, 1971; Stack, 1974; Troester, 1984). The presence of grandmothers is a significant one in child rearing, and it is not uncommon for grandmothers to raise their grandchildren or live in multiple generational households (Boyd-Franklin, 1989). Because their importance and status in the family is enhanced with age, African American women may encounter fewer "crises" related to the loss of youth than their White counterparts (Freudiger & Almquist, 1980). In contemporary environments the absence of kinship networks may be keenly felt and if so, reestablishing them becomes an important aspect of the therapeutic work. Boyd-Franklin and García-Preto cover this more extensively in their discussion of family therapy (Chapter 9, this volume).

Despite its much maligned status, the African American family is a crucial barrier against the racism of the dominant culture. African American mothers are charged with the task of teaching their children mechanisms of mastery over racism. They must determine how to warn their children successfully about racial barriers in ways that do not minimize the challenge they pose, but do not overwhelm the children either. Family constitutes an important survival mechanism for African American women. Hill (1971) describes what he considers to be the major strengths and characteristics of African American families. He posits that these characteristics reflect both the derivatives of African cultural roots and the slowly evolved adaptations to a racist environment. As Boyd-Franklin (1989) has noted previously, Hill (1971) reaffirms the presence and importance of strong kinship bonds, a strong achievement motivation, a strong religious and spiritual orientation, and a strong work orientation or ethnic in African American families.

Cultural Characteristics Specific to African American Women

Despite flexibility in gender roles, African American women are clearly socialized to expect to be caretakers. Female children are given responsibility for child care and develop an early motherhood identification (Hale-Benson, 1986). This is observed less in the socialization of African American males, although their participation in child care is more frequent than that observed in cultures in which gender roles are more rigidly stratified. Conflicts may occur in African American couples as a function of both racism and sexism within the African American community. There is no evidence that African American couples divorce or separate more than their White counterparts, but their relationships operate under considerable pressure.

Traditionally, African American women have been blamed for family ills and problems that are really a result of institutionalized racism. The pervasive deficit approach to research with African American families has measured them against idealized rather than realistic concepts of their White counterparts. Despite this, African American women have demonstrated that they are competent mother figures in antagonistic environments.

In the dominant culture, the practice of subordinating women is associated with establishing a man's masculinity. When this value is internalized by the African American woman, she may be predisposed to forgive, or even feel she deserves, mistreatment. This is particularly salient for African American women, because their partners' frustrations with racism are so legitimate. For example, a client of mine lamented that although her live-in boyfriend was intermittently abusive to her, "He gets abused by White people all day . . . he doesn't deserve trouble from me too. . . ." Many women in these situations also observe that if they report an abusive spouse, he will be treated more harshly by law enforcement officials because he is Black. The sense of a conflict of loyalty between their own needs and the needs of others is a common problem presented by African American women in my clinical experience. Although there is doubtless some truth to the client's observation regarding law enforcement, the therapist must be sensitive to her feelings while assisting her both in protecting herself and in understanding that she is not to blame for the racial barriers her mate encounters, barriers that she encounters as well.

Another issue that surfaces for many African American heterosexual women is that of man-sharing. Many clients express considerable distress at what they perceive to be a paucity of available African American men and their consequent difficulty finding mates. Some complain of their partner's infidelity but suggest, "I guess I have to share him 'cause there're just not enough [African American males] to go around . . . if I don't there will be other women who will." While it is important that the therapist not underestimate the realistic aspects of the client's dilemma, it is equally important to determine whether or not her solution is a pragmatic one, consistent with her own values, or whether it reflects the client's low self-esteem.

Low self-esteem is an issue that arises routinely in my practice and is articulated by women from a wide range of socioeconomic and educational backgrounds. Professional and educated African American women tend to view this problem as a consequence of their level of education. These women may be particularly vulnerable to the charge that their status contributes to the oppression of Black males. For some, the requirement that a mate be of the same educational level, regardless of other factors, can indicate problems with intimacy. They effectively avoid relationships by creating a list of characteristics that significant numbers of African American males have not had sufficient opportunity to develop. In this case, these clients fulfill their own prophecy of being alone or of being unworthy.

Influential Characteristics of the Dominant Culture

A major element of psychological reality for African American women involves integrating the influences of the majority culture without internalizing the accompanying devaluing messages that are a result of its racism and sexism. This leaves African American women with the challenge of developing coping mechanisms in response to racism and sexism, negotiating the discriminatory barriers that result from institutional racism and sexism, and addressing the full range of life's normal and catastrophic stressors.

Sexist Imagery Resulting from Racism

Racism is an ongoing part of routine life for African American women. It does not occur only in sporadic events in specific settings; rather, it surfaces in the most benign settings, with or without warning. Because of its ongoing nature, and its association with an unalterable, unconcealable physical characteristic, it can be considered a chronic stressor that requires ongoing management. Race operates as a powerful social variable that can intensify other social variables, such as class and education (Ladner, 1971). Therefore, the history of racism in the United States affects the experience of gender and may intensify the effects of sexism for African American women.

Coming down from the time of slavery there has been a range of stereotypes that suggests that African American women are sexually promiscuous, sexually aggressive, morally loose, independent, strong, and assertive when compared to their White counterparts (Christian, 1985; Collins, 1990; hooks, 1981). There was also a companion image for African American women which was just the opposite: She is depicted as sexually neutered, reflected in the image of the mammy. The mammy was usually represented as obese, pitch black in color, unkempt, and dirty (in comparison to White maids), the opposite of the dominant culture's beauty standards, her sexuality could be denied (Christian, 1985; Fox-Genovese, 1988; hooks, 1981). The latter image took her supposed flaw as a woman, her innate assertiveness and strength, and rendered it safe as long as it was used to defend fiercely the interests of the plantation household (Collins, 1990; Fox-Genovese, 1988; hooks, 1981). Both images cast her as the repository of the features and characteristics that the dominant culture in the United States and patriarchal cultures in general would view as abnormal for women. Their only redeeming feature is that these characteristics could be harnessed for a display of loyalty to the White upholders of the status quo.

These stereotyped images of African American women as the opposites of their genteel White counterparts did not evolve in a vacuum. Carby (1987) writes that the purpose of stereotypes is not to reflect reality accurately but to serve as a disguise for societal reality. The breeding practices of slaveowners could not have been maintained in a society founded on Christian and democratic principles had they been accurately depicted as the sexual exploitation of African American women by White males. Instead, blame was assigned to the victims, preserving the image of White planters as morally superior to Africans, especially in their capacity for sexual restraint (Greene, 1993). This disguise for societal reality served many purposes. It soothed the conscience of a society whose espoused ideals were blatantly contradicted by the behavior of its members. These stereotypical images of African American women further served to support the maintenance of social power in which African American men and women were subordinate to Whites, and women were subordinate to men.

Economic Subordination

It is fair to state that African American women occupy social and economic positions that are subordinate to their White counterparts and to their African American male counterparts, reflected in less access to positions of power and authority in the United States (Davis, 1981; Epstein, 1973; hooks, 1981; Joseph & Lewis, 1981; Myers, 1980; Robinson, 1983).

It should be noted that African American women maintained significant presence in the workplace long after the end of slavery and well into the contemporary era, despite the dominant cultural norm of women remaining in the house and men working in the outside world. Racism in the workplace made it difficult and at times impossible for African American men to find employment that would be deemed suitable for a male. Employment suitable for women, however, such as domestic work and child care, was more available. Hence, African American men were unable to assume the dominant culture's male ideal of the sole breadwinner in the household. African American women are still often required to bring essential rather than supplementary income into the family, although when they do so, they confront a legacy of both racism and sexism in the treatment of their success as workers, as proof of their inferiority as African Americans and as women. These realities make rigid gender-role stratification somewhat impractical for African American families.

Moynihan (1965) legitimized the stereotype of African American women as assertive and sexually aggressive and their continued economic role in the family with the contention that African American families are matriarchal and that family ills could be attributed to the fact that African American families did not measure up to the patriarchal ideal (cf. Christian, 1985). It is important to note that the Western use of the term "matriarchies" refers to social systems in many different cultures that are, matrilineal and more egalitarian than patriarchal systems. They are *not* the mirror image of the patriarchal society—women assuming the financial burdens of households and men inhibited from participating equally in the broader society. Rather, they facilitate the contributions of all members of the group, based on the best interests of the group and its survival. Nonetheless, the stereotyped depiction of African Americans as matriarchal fueled the already distorted images of African American women. When internalized, these myths and distortions can have pernicious effects on the psychological development of African American women.

Reaction to Negative Imagery

African American women in both individual and group psychotherapies report concerns about the adequacy of their hair texture, skin color, body shape and size, and size of facial features (Boyd-Franklin, 1989; Greene, 1985, 1990; Neal & Wilson, 1989; Okazawa-Rey, Robinson, & Ward, 1987). These concerns are not pervasive in all African American women, but there are few who do not report experiencing some degree of emotion regarding physical self-image, from mild dissatisfaction to shame. Physical attractiveness is an important social variable for women, and for some is a measure of their femininity and worth. The dominant culture in the United States idealizes the physical characteristics of White women and measures women of color against this arbitrary standard (Mays, 1985; Neal & Wilson, 1989). When compared to the White female ideal as the norm, traditional African features, darker skin, eye, and hair colors, broad or thick facial features, and kinky hair textures are deemed unattractive and inferior by the dominant culture (Collins, 1990; Neal & Wilson, 1989; Okazawa-Rey et al., 1987). Hence there is pressure to approximate the ideal. To be womanly and feminine in American culture is to be White. This is problematic in African American women who have internalized this ideal, one which they can rarely approximate.

Because of the connection between physical attractiveness and feelings of self-worth in many women, discussing this connection constitutes an essential aspect of therapeutic inquiry. It is important to ask the client who was or was not considered beautiful in her family and why. It may also be helpful to determine whether she has childhood memories of a parent or parenting figure encouraging her to alter her physical appearance, as well as the kinds of messages she was given about its adequacy. This can give the therapist a sense of the extent to which family members internalized the dominant culture's standard, as well as how family members were treated regarding their own physical appearance. It would be a mistake to assume that the cultural movement that asserted that "Black is beautiful" eradicated the centuries-old effects of these negative messages. A cursory review of media images and advertisements, particularly those targeting African American consumers, continues to advertise products that offer the promise of altering African American women's physical characteristics.

In a social climate where skin color becomes an important social variable it is predictable that skin color variations in African American families can be a source of conflict between family members. Skin colors within an African American nuclear family can vary from extremely dark to light. Because these physical characteristics are highly visible, they lend themselves to being used when disputes in families occur. It is important therefore to inquire about the skin color variations within the family, particularly those of family members about whom there are intense feelings. These variations may intensify a normal range of interfamilial and sibling rivalries. Some clients may have been idealized or scapegoated in their families based on skin color or other physical features. Many women may be left with a sense of shame or even guilt, reinforced or cultivated by the preoccupations and perceptions of family members about the relative "goodness" of physical characteristics of White women and the "badness" of those features more characteristic of African American women (Boyd-Franklin, 1991; Greene, 1992; Neal & Wilson, 1989).

The therapist should not assume that the presence or absence of certain kinds of hairstyles or dress are automatic indicators of a client's feelings about these issues, although for some clients they may be reflected in these choices. Furthermore, just as darker skinned African American women are devalued for failing to live up to the American standard of beauty of light skin, long straight hair and keen rather than broad facial features, lighter skinned African American women may be similarly devalued by family members or peers for "looking" or "trying to look White." Many African American women who are clients in psychotherapy, who have lighter skin and straighter hair textures, report being treated either like a curiosity or a traitor, who is never quite "Black enough." This is often intensified for African American women who are biracial; issues facing these women are discussed in greater detail in Chapter 16. Feelings of anger, shame, resentment, and guilt may emerge during inquiries around this material, which must be sensitively explored.

PSYCHOLOGICAL RESOURCES AND VULNERABILITIES

African American women, who have had to make psychological sense out of their historical and contemporary predicaments if they were to survive, continue to strive for fair treatment and to maintain hope, often in the face of hopeless conditions. If African Americans as a group are to survive, they and their families have to teach their children to do the same.

Internalized Racism

Internalized racism is observed in African American women when they internalize both the negative stereotypes about African Americans and their cultural origins and the idealization of White persons and their cultural imperatives, negatively affecting their sense of self (Butts, 1971; Friedman, 1966; Gardiner, 1971).

Clinical manifestations of internalized racism may be observed in many forms and are likely to have multiple determinants. The client may harbor the fear that expressing any behavior that is associated with negative stereotypes of African American women proves that the stereotypes are valid. In this case, acting or attempting to act against or disprove the stereotype may be reflected in the client's inhibition, repression, or emotional constriction. This behavior clearly reflects the level of shame the client experiences for characteristics that she believes define her.

A corollary of acting *against* the stereotype is represented by the acting *out* of stereotypes. This compulsion may reflect the need to expose a feared part of the self that corresponds to the caricature of the way the client believes other people expect her to behave. This may leave her with a (false) sense that she controls when she is "discovered" or "found out." In either response the therapist must address the client's misperceptions about herself and other African Americans, as well as exploring the significance of the more complex dynamics of her plight.

Another example of internalized racism may be reflected clinically in the tendency for the client to express a sense of distance and/or disdain for other African Americans. Expressions of this sentiment in clients may range from their openly disparaging all Black people as a group to using derogatory racial epithets to describe or label certain types of African Americans when referring to them. Pinderhughes (1989) suggests that although this may represent a need for specialness or elitism within a group, it is nonetheless a distancing defense mechanism. Women who display this behavior may actually believe the negative stereotypes associated with African Americans, but of course they cannot deny their group membership. Hence they see themselves as essentially different from the group in salient ways, the exception to the negative rule. Clients who engage in this behavior may fear that they harbor the characteristics that they reject in African Americans as a group, and are thus simultaneously rejecting a part of themselves. By distancing themselves, however, they run the risk of isolation as well as being unable to correct distortions in their perceptions.

A combination of internalized racism and sexism may be observed in the "impostor phenomenon." Clance and Imes (1978) conceptualize this phenomenon as an internal sense of intellectual phoniness or of generally feeling like a fraud or failure, despite repeated successes. It is frequently observed in African American women, as a result of early family dynamics and the internalization of the dominant culture's gender-role and racial stereotyping. Francis Trotman (1984) observes that the client may be unable to appreciate her realistic accomplishments or activities despite evidence of her ability. She may express (1) a preoccupation with failure or the potential of failure, (2) her perceived flaws or worthlessness, (3) a readiness to accept the negative perceptions that others hold of her (with a conspicuous resistance to accepting positive feedback), (4) the perception that her successes are fraudulent and are the result of "fooling" or "tricking" others, or (5) a persistent sense of dread that she will be caught or found out when presented with the next challenge.

— Many African American women internalize the stereotype of the ubiquitous strong matriarch: In the tradition of the mammy, she acknowledges no personal pain, can bear all burdens, and will take care of everyone. Consequently, many African American women feel deficient if their burdens are too heavy, and will resist asking for help. On entering therapy these women express great reluctance at the prospect of "wasting time" talking about their problems when they have "so much to do." When questioned about their reluctance even to enter therapy, a common response is that it will mean that they are "weak" or "couldn't take it." The therapist may in fact find that the client has endured some very stressful events or has assumed the role of caretaker for numerous family members over an extended period of time. When asked why they have finally considered a solution that they consider extreme (therapy), some common responses are "I'm having a nervous breakdown," or "I had a break." In psychodiagnostic parlance a "break" or "nervous breakdown" usually implies the presence of serious psychopathology. Such pathology is marked by seriously impaired reality testing as well as an inability to function. For these women, the nature of their "breakdown" is not the same. (Descriptions of their "breakdown" include variations on the theme of "I cried" or "I just cried and cried and couldn't stop.") The clinician who does not inquire about what the client means when using this and other terms may misunderstand and incorrectly diagnose the client's condition. This reasoning reflects the level at which many African American women do not feel entitled to be cared for or even to take care of themselves, but rather see their self-worth as rooted in being a caretaker. This may also be reflected in behavior in which these women make it difficult for others to care for them, leaving them in a cycle of frustration, exhaustion and anger. It is important to address these issues with clients, particularly its connection to the internalization of a convergence of stereotypes about African American women.

Many women express additional concerns that therapy will make them "dependent" and will somehow control them. Given their history of being taken advantage of and being denied the luxury of dependence on benign or helpful figures, such concerns are understandable. These concerns, however, may mask African American women's difficulty in requesting and accepting help, thereby prolonging their involvement in situations that are routinely stressful or overwhelming.

Any specific client will likely present one or many of the aforementioned dilemmas. Other manifestations in African American women in professional occupations or in training for such may be expressed in unrealistic levels of anxiety or panic at the prospect of board, bar, or licensing examinations, promotions or the possibility of any new challenge. Some clients may consistently delay or procrastinate at critical career stages to avoid their feared discovery as a fraud.

Another example of internalized racism may be expressed in the client's unconscious assumption of responsibility for the discomfort that may be present when interacting with her White counterparts. In this case the client may attempt to engage in behavior designed to make herself appear as nonthreatening as possible. This behavior qualitatively goes beyond being socially engaged and pleasant; rather, it includes the client's inappropriate and often unconscious assumption of blame if White counterparts experience discomfort in the interaction. The client may engage in this behavior if she assumes—even when the assumption is accurate—that as an African American female she elicits fear, and if she thus maintains an illusion of control in a situation where there is potential for victimization. The therapeutic goal in working with such a client involves assisting her to examine both the assumptions that would lead someone to fear her and the validity of such assumptions. Clients who engage in this behavior may use it with the therapist as well. The therapist must therefore be careful not to encourage this behavior by inadvertently communicating his or her own anxiety about race to the client, or by accepting overly compliant behavior too readily.

Internalized racism can be understood as a maladaptive result of the need to develop coping mechanisms in response to racism. To understand this as a major piece of psychological work in the lives of African American women, the therapist must acknowledge that African American women are forced to be aware of themselves racially in ways that their White counterparts are not. The need to learn how to manage the anxieties and prejudices of the dominant culture is an important aspect of their socialization, an ongoing aspect of their reality. Clinical manifestations of this phenomenon must be addressed as a part of the therapeutic work.

Adaptive Strategies

Problematic adjustments to racism are prevalent, but they are only a part of the story. Despite the ubiquitous realities of racism, African American women should not be understood as passively reacting to racism and its sequelae or as blindly accepting the dominant culture's values or views of them. There is ample evidence of a variety of adaptive and resourceful strategies utilized by African American women throughout their history.

Each generation of African Americans, usually but not exclusively parenting figures or family members, prepares the next generation for the challenge of being African American in a society that devalues them. African American mothers face a range of unique challenges in socializing their daughters to make psychological sense out of the racist and sexist messages they receive on a routine basis. Despite having to function in environments where there may be little if any physical or emotional safety, African American women have made healthy adjustments that are neither deniable nor accidental. Their psychological flexibility is often a reflection of an active socialization process that takes place within their families and communities to prepare its members to confront institutional barriers. Adaptive responses to coping with racism may be observed in the processes of "armoring" (Faulkner, 1983; Sears, 1987), "healthy cultural paranoia" (Grier & Cobbs, 1968), and "racial socialization" (Greene, 1992b).

Sears (1987) and Faulkner (1983) use the term "armoring" to describe behavioral and cognitive skills used by African Americans and other persons of color to decrease their psychological vulnerability in encounters where there is a potential for racism. It is important that therapists understand the need for such behavior and do not regard as pathological the complex attitudes that give rise to wariness and the interpersonal reserve that may accompany it.

The sensitivity of many African Americans to the potential for maltreatment and exploitation by Whites has been referred to by Grier and Cobbs (1968) as "cultural paranoia." This term, despite the use of the word "paranoia," encompasses an appropriate level of vigilance. Like armoring, it might be better understood as a physiological or psychological predisposition, perhaps based on past direct experiences or observations, to perceive a wider range of environmental stimuli as potentially dangerous and/or stressful and to react to them accordingly.

Racial socialization is a complex process that has three major components. The first phase is that of learning to label racism accurately and to acknowledge its extent. This includes identifying it correctly when it occurs. This phase makes major use of cognitive skills in the identification and accurate labeling of the phenomena (Greene, 1992a). A second phase involves the presence of role models or demonstrators in a young woman's life, usually adults. By their actions, adult figures—often but not exclusively mothers—can model appropriate responses to situations and demonstrate the importance of self-advocacy. The third phase encompasses understanding the experience, which may be fraught with feelings of difference, rejection, and confusion. The provision of emotional support for the predictable feelings of anger and impotence that often emerge when anyone experiences direct or subtle confrontations with racism and sexism is a critical component at this stage of this process.

When working with a client, the therapist should assist her in accepting such feelings and validate the client's appropriate response to this reality. Finally, if the client is a parent, she should be assisted in understanding the legacy of negative images that her children will encounter in the world. It will be incumbent on her to take an active role in mitigating the effect of those stereotypes by means of positive images, rather than reinforcing them (Greene, 1992c).

These maneuvers represent a few those that African American women use to make sense out of their institutionally disadvantaged position and to negotiate and deflect the hostility of a racist and sexist culture in healthy and adaptive ways. There is a noteworthy paucity of information in the psychological literature about how these adaptive phenomena work and how they might be utilized in psychotherapies to assist persons who experience difficulty coping with both personal and institutional barriers. Comer (1988) observes that understanding the strategies and strengths of survivors will tell us more about obstacles and their circumvention than will the traditional exclusive focus on the victims.

THERAPEUTIC INTERVENTIONS WITH AFRICAN AMERICAN WOMEN

In psychotherapy with African American women it may be helpful to assist them in identifying the conscious and unconscious methods they employ in confronting and responding to racial as well as other personal difficulties. This process cannot take place if the therapist believes that problems that result from racism are of minimal importance or that they are limited to African American women in the lower economic and or educational strata. One may then compare the client's strategies with a range of available options, helping the client make conscious and active choices, compatible with her own personal and cultural values and goals (Greene, 1992b).

Therapy may also be useful in helping the client set priorities regarding which conflicts and issues to respond to, when it is most important to respond to them, and how to do so. In a racist and sexist culture, an African American woman who feels compelled to respond actively to every suggestion, potential incidence, or actual episode of racist behavior will have little energy available to address other life issues.

Introducing or responding to the issue of race within the treatment situation presents therapists with a dilemma that training has often ignored. While our culture has always and still continues to make important distinctions between people on the basis of race and ethnicity, it is often considered impolite or inappropriate to discuss those distinctions openly. In this context it is not unusual for a client to assume that she will offend, alienate, or make the therapist anxious if she initiates an inquiry. This underscores the importance of the therapist taking the responsibility for raising the issue of race if the client does not do so. It is important that the therapist communicate to the African American woman that she or he recognizes the extent to which race and racism may play a significant role in her life, and that she does not have to protect the therapist from her experiences or feelings about it.

It may be appropriate to ask an African American woman if she feels that a White (or African American) therapist can understand her, and to determine the reasons for this feeling. While such questions may appear to be of obvious importance when the therapist is White, it remains important when the therapist is African American. An African American therapist cannot assume that an African American woman necessarily prefers having a therapist of the same race. Similarly, African American therapists, when preferred or requested, cannot presume that they know why they are preferred without exploring the issue with clients. The therapist must take care not to patronize an African American woman by questioning whether race is an important issue if the therapist has not seriously thought through its relevance. Therapists who do not feel that race is an important area of scrutiny should utilize peer and other forms of supervision to explore racial issues before raising them with the client.

The client's choice or preference for the race of the therapist should always be accepted, but must be understood as well. Such a choice may represent the hope for or the avoidance of a certain kind of relationship, fantasized about or realistic, arising from expectations or images. It is reasonable to assume that the preference may always have more personal meaning, which should be explored regardless of the race of the therapist.

Because of the pressure to deny racial identity and difficulties encountered in the face of racism, many African American women may deny the significance of race even when asked directly. The therapist should not assume that such a denial means that there are no conflicts present. It is helpful to listen for metaphors about lightness, whiteness, darkness, and blackness in the client's communications, particularly in dreams. Black and White figures may appear as polar opposites with respect to their status, roles, feelings, impulses, or behavior. Furthermore, Black or White figures may serve as repositories for the client's unwanted or unacceptable feelings or impulses. Metaphorically, White persons may represent the client's grandiose self and African American persons may represent or be associated with the client's self-loathing or shameful self. When the issue of race is conspicuously absent, the therapist should consider whether or not such material is being avoided, and if so assist the client in understanding her need to avoid it (Greene, 1992b).

The therapist should not use social class as an excuse for failing to consider seriously the impact of race in African American women's lives. It can be suggested that, just as poverty interacts with racism and affects its victims in particular ways, middle-class and educated status among African American women also interacts with racism in particular and equally problematic ways. The notion of privileged status must be reexamined. Money and education, privileges that normally enhance one's chances in life, may not do so for African American women in the ways that they may for White women, and for African American and White men. Well-educated and middle-class African American women may be confronted with situations in which few or no African American women preceded them and in which they remain unwelcome. These women may face tremendous isolation and despair at the same time that they are told that they have somehow "made it." In addition to these issues, African American women who have been successful financially are often among the minority in their families. In African American families, there is frequently a clear and explicit expectation that those who have some measure of success will help to "bring others along." This may impinge on a woman's financial resources in a way that it does not for her White counterparts. There may also be issues of ambivalence or regret about leaving others behind.

High income or position should not obscure for the therapist the extent to which many of these women feel and in fact are devalued as African American persons and their achievements disparaged on a daily basis, while they are simultaneously depended on by many of their families to share whatever resources they may have. Many of these women will require assistance in setting priorities regarding the demands of their own lives, the demands of their extended families, and the maintenance of a sense of connectedness with their families. It is predictable that such women will have feelings about these matters that should be respectfully explored.

It is essential to remember that we live in a society that still maintains double standards based on racial identity in judging the same phenomena. Middle-class status for African American persons has always been based on levels of income that are significantly lower than incomes for middle-class Whites. Furthermore, those income levels are often based on one income in White families, as opposed to two incomes in African American families.

It may be difficult for therapists to distinguish between legitimate racial anger, race used in the service of resistance, and race as a metaphor for intrapsychic conflict. Certain aspects of an African American woman's racial heritage and experiences with racism may be superimposed on or interact with structural and characterological dynamics and defenses in particular ways. It is therefore important that the therapist listen for the intensification of characterological conflicts that may be triggered by racial realities. If the therapist can be sensitive to what precedes the initiation of a focus on race, it should be helpful to decide whether or not there is a pattern to this initiation. In this situation, the identification of a pattern can help determine whether or not race becomes easier for the client to discuss than issues that may be even more painful, and whether or not race is used to avoid exploration of other issues.

Families are of cultural significance and importance to most African American women. Assisting them in identifying and understanding the racial tradition in their families and how they carry on or do not carry on that tradition may be helpful as well. This may be understood as a generational issue. The therapist may want to raise the client's curiosity about what her family members instructed her to do when confronting racism, how to determine if it was present, and what she can recall about how her family actually behaved in such situations. It is important to be attuned to discrepancies between the woman's parents' actual behavior and what they instructed their daughter to do. Further exploration of the client's extended family and her relationships with them should be explored as well (Greene, 1992b, 1993a).

Managing racism is one of many issues whose importance will vary from client to client and will be a function of the multiple factors that help shape the client's psyche. Many environmental factors contribute to molding the psyche of African American women on many levels, but those factors always interact with characterological aspects of who she is. Early life experiences, familial relationships, and biological factors are among those that contribute to the shaping of her core self. Individual factors, societal stressors, and cultural contexts all help determine what resources or vulnerabilities any woman brings to her situation. The therapist must avoid the temptation of using racial oppression to explain all of a client's problems. To do so can prevent her from understanding any role she may play in her own dilemma, and limit her options for making changes. Simultaneously, therapists must be careful not to romanticize her successful struggles to overcome oppression without an awareness of the costs (Greene, 1992b, 1993a).

While African American women share many group characteristics, an individual will attempt to cope with racial life stressors with the same characterological and defensive structures she uses to respond to other life stressors. This does not mean that African American women are to blame for their victimization or its legacy. Rather, it is suggested that the requirement to routinely manage racism for African American women, particularly in the context of a racist society, is a dimension, that can make life more difficult. Her ethnic heritage, on the other hand, can be a source of support and enrichment central to her life. Therefore, both the difficulty of coping with racism and the richness of a woman's ethnic identity should be a routine part of treatment considerations.

REFERENCES

Akbar, N. (1985). Our destiny, authors of a scientific revolution. In H. McAdoo & J. McAdoo (Eds.), *Black children* (pp. 17–31). Newbury Park, CA: Sage.

Bell, R. L. (1971). The relative importance of mother and wife roles among Negro lower class women. In R. Staples (Ed.), *The Black family: Essays and studies*. Belmont, CA: Wadsworth.

Berry, M. F., & Blassingame, J. (1982). *Long memory: The Black experience in America*. New York: Oxford University Press.

Boyd-Franklin, N. (1989). *Black families in therapy: A multisystems approach*. New York: Guilford Press.

Boyd-Franklin, N. (1991). Recurrent themes in the treatment of African American women in group psychotherapy. *Women and Therapy, 11*, 25–40.

Boykin, A. W. (1985). Black child socialization: A conceptual framework. In H. McAdoo & J. McAdoo (Eds.), *Black children* (pp. 33–51). Newbury Park, CA: Sage.

Brown, D. R. (1990). Depression among Blacks: An epidemiological perspective. In D. S. Ruiz (Ed.), *Handbook of mental health and mental disorder among Black Americans* (pp. 71–93). New York: Greenwood Press.

Butts, H. F. (1971). Psychoanalysis and unconscious racism. *Journal of Contemporary Psychotherapy, 3*, 67–81.

Carby, H. (1987). *Reconstructing womanhood: The emergence of the African American woman novelist*. New York: Oxford University Press.

Christian, B. (1985). *Black feminist criticism: Perspectives on Black women writers*. New York: Pergamon.

Clance, P. R., & Imes, S. A. (1978). The impostor phenomenon in high achieving women: Dynamics and therapeutic intervention. *Psychotherapy, 15*, 241–247.

Collins, P. H. (1990). *Black feminist thought*. Boston: Unwin Hyman.

Comer, J. (1988). *Maggies American dream: The life and times of a Black family*. New York: New American Library.

Davis, A. (1981). *Women, race and class*. New York: Vintage Books.

Epstein, C. F. (1973). Positive effects of the multiple negative: Explaining the success of Black professional women. *American Journal of Sociology, 78*, 912–935.

Faulkner, J. (1983). Women in interracial relationships. *Women and Therapy, 2*, 193–203.

Fox-Genovese, E. (1988). *Within the plantation household: Black and white women of the old South*. Chapel Hill, NC: University of North Carolina Press.

Freudiger, P., & Almquist, E. M. (1980). *Sources of life satisfaction: The different worlds of Black and White women*. Paper presented at the annual meeting of the Southwestern Sociological Association, Houston.

Friedman, N. (1966). James Baldwin and psychotherapy. *Psychotherapy, 3*, 177–183.

Gardiner, L. (1971). The therapeutic relationship under varying conditions of race. *Psychotherapy, 8*, 78–87.

Greene, B. (1985). Considerations in the treatment of Black patients by white therapists. *Psychotherapy, 22S*, 389–393.

Greene, B. (1990). Sturdy bridges: The role of African American mothers in the socialization of African American children. *Women and Therapy, 10*, 205–225.

Greene, B. (1992a). Black feminist psychotherapy. In E. Wright (Ed.), *Feminism and psychoanalysis*. Oxford, England: Blackwell.

Greene, B. (1992b). Still here: A perspective on psychotherapy with African American women. In J. Chrisler & D. Howard (Eds.), *New directions in feminist psychology* (pp. 13–25). New York: Springer.

Greene, B. A. (1992c). Racial socialization: A tool in psychotherapy with African American children. In L. Vargas & J. Koss-Chioino (Eds.), *Working with culture: Psychotherapeutic interventions with ethnic minority youth* (pp. 63–81). San Francisco: Jossey Bass.

Greene, B. A. (1993). Psychotherapy with African American women: Integrating feminist and psychodynamic models. *Journal of Training and Practice in Professional Psychology*, 7(1), 49–66.

Grier, W. H., & Cobbs, P. (1968). *Black rage*. New York: Basic Books.

Hale-Benson, J. (1986). *Black children: Their roots, culture and learning styles*. Baltimore: Johns Hopkins University Press.

Henry, W. A. (1990, April 9). Beyond the melting pot. *Time*, p. 135.

Hill, R. (1971). *The strengths of Black families*. New York: National Urban League.

hooks, b. (1981). *Black women and feminism*. Boston: South End Press.

Jones, A. (1985). Psychological functioning in Black Americans: A conceptual guide for use in psychotherapy. *Psychotherapy*, 22, 363–369.

Joseph, G., & Lewis, J. (1981). *Common differences: Conflicts in black and white feminimist perspectives*. New York: Doubleday.

Ladner, J. (1971). *Tomorrow's tomorrow: The Black woman*. Garden City, NY: Doubleday.

Lerner, G. (1972). *Black women in white America: A documentary history*. New York: Vintage.

Levine, L. (1977). *Black culture and Black consciousness*. New York: Oxford University Press.

Mays, V. M. (1985). The Black American and psychotherapy: The dilemma. *Psychotherapy*, 22, 379–388.

Moynihan, D. P. (1965). *The negro family: The case for national action*. Washington, DC: U.S. Department of Labor.

Myers, L. J. (1980). *Black women: Do they cope better?* Englewood Cliffs, NJ: Prentice Hall.

Neal, A., & Wilson, M. (1989). The role of skin color and features in the Black community: Implications for Black women in therapy. *Clinical Psychology Review*, 9, 323–333.

Nobles, W. (1974). African root and American fruit: The Black family. *Journal of Social and Behavioral Sciences*, 20, 52–64.

Okazawa-Rey, M., Robinson, T., & Ward, J. V. (1987). Black women and the politics of skin color and hair. *Women and Therapy*, 6, 89–102.

Pinderhughes, E. (1989). *Understanding race, ethnicity and power: The key to efficacy in clinical practice*. New York: Free Press.

Robinson, C. R. (1983). Black women: A tradition of self reliant strength. *Women and Therapy*, 2, 135–144.

Ruiz, D. S. (1990). Social and economic profile of Black Americans, 1989. In D. S. Ruiz (Ed.), *Handbook of mental health and mental disorder among Black Americans* (pp. 3–15). New York: Greenwood Press.

Sears, V. L. (1987). *Cross cultural ethnic relationships*. Unpublished manuscript.

Stack, C. (1974). *All our kin: Strategies for survival in a Black community*. New York: Harper & Row.

Thomas, A., & Sillen, S. (1972). *Racism and psychiatry*. New York: Brunner/Mazel.

Troester, R. (1984). Turbulence and tenderness: Mothers, daughters and "othermothers" in Paule Marshall's *Brown Girl, Brownstones*. *Sage: A Scholarly Journal on Black Women*, 1, 13–16.

Trotman, F. (1984). Psychotherapy with Black women and the dual effects of racism and sexism. In C. Brody (Ed.), *Women therapists working with women* (pp. 96–108). New York: Springer.

2

American Indian Women

Teresa D. LaFromboise
Joan Saks Berman
Balvindar K. Sohi

Finding a suitable form or style of therapy for a population as intertribally diverse as American Indian[1] women is a monumental task. American Indians defy easy description and analysis. Nonetheless, in this chapter we have attempted to offer clinicians a general appreciation for American Indian ways by outlining the historical background, general statistics about health and well-being, traditional and sociocultural issues, spiritual beliefs, and family structures of contemporary Indian life. In addition, the gender roles salient in Indian society, as well as the marriage customs and various developmental stages Indian women go through are described in order that clinicians may better understand the social context that contributes to the origin and persistence of problems.

In the mental health treatment section, assessment and diagnostic methods are delineated, as are expectations about therapy and special clinical issues salient to American Indian women. Studies describing the community values and practices of the different tribes are also reviewed along with research that supports indigenous healing prevention and treatment practices such as the talking circle and community prayer ceremonies. Finally, two case vignettes are included with details regarding the use of conventional psychotherapeutic practices and culturally specific interventions.

HISTORICAL OVERVIEW

The American Indian population, currently estimated at more than 1.9 million generally can be characterized as rapidly growing, increasingly more urbanized, and culturally diverse. Consequently, each of the 587

Indian tribal entities and Alaska Native villages[2] to which American Indian women belong (P. Zell, personal communication, August 8, 1991) maintains customs, social organizations, and ecological relationships distinct from other tribes. Further, tribal cultures and customs existing before European contact have undergone significant changes in the past 500 years. Finally, while almost every tribe was subjected to forced removal from its ancestral homeland, brutal colonization and confinement to reservations, and great pressure for acculturation into European American society, each experienced different direct and indirect levels of European domination. Thus, despite having similar experiences and fundamental values, American Indians reflect immense diversity, so that tremendous differences exist among Indian women who come from distinct tribal heritages.

Statistically the median age of Indians is 22.6 years (U.S. All Races [USAR] median is 30 years), with 32% of the population under the age of 15 (USAR 23%) (U.S. Bureau of the Census, 1983). In the last decade, the Indian population has grown by 538,834 people (U.S. Bureau of the Census, 1991). This rise may be due to a combination of factors: the increased number of people who publicly acknowledge their Indian identity, interracial marriages, and a birth rate 79% greater than the USAR rate (Sandefur & McKinnell, 1986; U.S. Department of Health and Human Services, 1989). And Indian families, averaging 4.6 members, are larger than those of any other U.S. ethnic group. Women head 45% of Indian households, many of whom have never married and 42% of whom had their first child as a teenager (USAR 24%) (Snipp & Aytac, 1990).

Within the past two decades, socioeconomic growth among Indians has been very uneven. Many Indian women work primarily in federal and local government jobs. Others are employed in unconventional roles such as artists, poets, university instructors, heavy equipment operators, truck drivers, and small farmers. In all 49% of Indian women in their 20s and 55% in their 30s are employed. Nevertheless, a number of women, especially those 40 and older, are very likely to be unemployed (Snipp & Aytac, 1990).

More than half of all Indian women live in urban areas (U.S. Bureau of Census, 1991), which undermines the strength of their community and tribal affiliations and complicates family and clan support systems. In cities, as on reservations, the majority of Indian communities are disadvantaged by poverty, substandard living conditions, frequent relocation, and pervasive unemployment.[3] Further, those who place themselves in greater contact with the majority culture by increasing their interactions with outsiders, migrating to cities, working in professional jobs, or attending boarding schools and universities may face considerable acculturation stress (Ablon, 1964; Berry, Wintrob, Sindell, & Mawhinney, 1982; LaFromboise, 1988b), which makes them even more vulnerable to developing psychological problems.

Indian women show unusually high mortality rates due to violence, alcoholism, treatable/preventable diseases such as diabetes and tuberculosis, and suicide. They also have lower life expectancy rates compared with the rest of the U.S. population (U.S. Department of Health and Human Services, 1989). Physical, sexual, and emotional abuse of Indian women and children is a serious problem within Indian communities today. This harsh reality contradicts traditional Indian ideals, which teach respect for women and recognition of children as cherished gifts of life. Nevertheless, in the past two decades Indian women have begun to make innovative use of traditional coping mechanisms and transcultural exchanges to facilitate their effectiveness in tribal communities and U.S. society at large. Some seek psychotherapy for understanding and support during periods of individual and social change, most others seek therapy for immediate assistance once their efforts at coping with their own as well as their family's stresses have been expended.

SOCIOCULTURAL ISSUES

There are approximately 200 indigenous languages spoken by American Indians today (Leap, 1981), despite past measures to eradicate them in Indian boarding schools. In 1893, Tlingit Indians requested baptism into the Eastern Orthodox Christian church so that they could worship in their own language and thereby make their communication with the Great Spirit a more personal experience (Father M. Oleska, personal communication, August 5, 1990). Fortunately, tribes who have not retained active use of their respective languages are now beginning to revitalize them. At present, those who are fluent in their native language are held in high esteem.

American Indians view life as continuous and reciprocal, in which relationships are interdependent and patterns repeat themselves. In order to foster a natural progression of events, emphasis is placed on the present and awareness of the past predominates over concern for the future. As might be expected, this outlook conflicts with the contemporary American emphasis on what people are striving to become rather than what they are continuing to be (Shangreaux, Pleskac, & Freeman, 1987).

According to Indian beliefs animals, plants, and humans make up the spirit world (Locust, 1985). A Navajo myth talks about a monster called He-Who-Kills-With-His-Eyes and teaches Navajo children to avert their eyes to avoid bringing harm to others (Moss & Goldstein, 1973). Interestingly, direct eye contact also signifies disrespect and hostility in some tribes (Allen, 1973).

Research in sociolinguistics documents other characteristic Indian nonverbal behaviors such as differences in "pause time response." The time between an Indian person finishing a statement in a conversation and another person beginning to speak is often perceived as protracted from a non-Indian point of view (Tafoya, 1989). Indians often use rhetorical embellishment to emphasize a point and are accustomed to talking without interruption until they have stated what they feel needs to be said. According to Hall (1973), time for the traditional Navajo is like space. Many native languages do not measure time in standard units. The Sioux language has no translatable equivalents for words like late, waiting, or time. The term "Indian time," often interpreted as being late, in fact refers to doing something when "it [the time] is right" (Tafoya, 1989).

Indians value wisdom, intelligence, poise, tranquility, cooperation, unselfishness, responsibility, kindness, and protectiveness toward all forms of life (Trimble, 1981). Elders are venerated as the keepers of traditions and guides to traditional culture (Sullivan, 1983). Indian spirituality is very different from Christian belief systems in that many Indian people still seek assistance from medicine men and women and solace from the spirit world. Although most medicine persons are males, women are not barred from learning or performing healing ceremonies, but most do not refine their skills in this area until after their childbearing years (Allen, 1991; Lake, 1991). The causes of illness are sometimes attributed to an imbalance in one's body, mind, or spirit, to the breaking of taboos, or to witchcraft (Topper, 1987).

Traditional tribal lifestyles are quite diverse, and the relative power and esteem women enjoy within the community varies across tribes. However, distinct representations of female spiritual beings exists in Indian tradition. White Buffalo Calf Woman, a life-giving figure, brought the sacred pipe to the Sioux people. Changing Woman, one of the principle holy people in Navajo mythology, was involved in the creation of the Earth Surface People, forming the first four clans from parts of her body. Spider Woman, who demonstrates weaving to the Hopi and the Navajo, has divine powers and unlimited wisdom. Clay Woman, a pan-Pueblo figure from New Mexico, teaches people to make pottery. The Wintu of Northern California have two important spiritual beings: Mem Loimis, who controls the world's water supply, and Norwan, the goddess of light. The Tagish and the Inland Tlingit of the Canadian Yukon and the Tahltan of Northern British Columbia share the myth of the Animal Mother, who gives birth to all game animals. Other respected spiritual women from the Northwest Coast include Tide Woman, Salmon Woman, and Healing Woman. Finally, the Tagish look to Wealth Woman for the transformation of certain objects into gold (Zak, 1984). These examples of language use and beliefs are but a few concrete particulars further documenting the rich and varied nature of tribal cultures. These and other sociocultural issues influence Indian women and their families in unique ways and must be considered in psychotherapy.

FAMILY RELATIONS

To be poor in the Indian world is to be without relatives (Primeaux, 1977); the extended family is an integral part of Native American life. Family networks may include several households consisting of many relatives along both vertical and horizontal lines. In addition, a complex system of clan relationships (Red Horse, Lewis, Feit, & Decker, 1978) may further influence family relations. Finally, relatives are expected to teach young people life skills, and grandparents often share in child-rearing responsibilities (Red Horse, 1981).

Some tribes, like the Hopi, practice matrilineal descent and matrilocal residence, wherein the daughters live close to their mother's home after marriage. Children within this structure belong to the woman's clan (Queen & Habenstein, 1967). Among Navajos, incest taboos prohibit marriages between clan members, although the relationship may be so distant that a young couple meeting at school may not be aware that they are related in this way. Family problems may arise when parents, discovering that a daughter's boyfriend is a clan relative, try to break up the relationship. This may result in suicide attempts by the daughter.

Traditionally, divorce was an option in most tribes, although it was sometimes more difficult for women than for men. Common grounds for divorce included sterility, adultery, laziness, bad temper, and cruelty. On the other hand, an Indian woman's parents or in-laws could pressure her to stay in a bad marriage "for the sake of the children." Even today this creates a serious problem where physical or verbal abuse is recurrent. Also, battered Indian women usually manifest the helplessness, hopelessness, and self-blame seen in such victims in the mainstream population, and experience shame, which prevents them from reaching out to other family members or potentially supportive services. In-laws may blame the wife for marital problems, including the husband's alcoholism, and if the woman is a Christian, social pressure to remain married may also be increased through the church. Nonetheless, some extended families may accept a battered wife for a prolonged visit, allowing her time and space to consider more clearly her options. Attitudes and customs regarding divorce changed drastically after massive numbers of Indians converted to Roman Catholicism. In some conservative pueblos, divorce is not sanctioned even when obtained in state courts, and this may be due to the influence of the Catholic church. However, divorce is increasing among Alaska Natives, despite the conservative influence of missionaries (T. Devlin, personal communication, September 5, 1990).

The dissolution of intertribal marriages can be quite complicated. For example, a woman might be unable to persuade her ex-husband to move out of the house because it belongs to him through his family. After many years of residence in the husband's tribal community, she may still be considered an outsider. An Indian woman in this situation is often reluctant to move to a nearby town or another community until her children reach the age of majority, so that they do not lose their hereditary claims within the tribe or their home. This hampers her employment opportunities and may make it necessary for her to commute great distances to work in order to support her family.

These are but a few issues associated with the interactive patterns in Indian family relations. Many questions concerning how the changing family structure contributes to the problems of Indian women remain unanswered. Those estranged from their families, or taxed by excessive role demands and complex family relations, often experience overwhelming emotional concerns.

GENDER ROLES

A woman's identity in traditional Indian life is firmly rooted in her spirituality, extended family, and tribe (Green, 1980; Jaimes, 1982; Welch, 1987). Indian women see themselves in harmony with the biological, spiritual, and social worlds. Biologically, they value being mothers and raising healthy families; spiritually, they are considered to be extensions of the Spirit Mother and keys to the continuation of their people (Allen, 1986; Jenks, 1986); socially, they serve as transmitters of cultural knowledge and caretakers of children and relatives (Niethammer, 1977).

While both Indian men and women suffer the consequences of societal dislocation and the denial of basic human rights, women's lives have been particularly affected by the pressing effects of acculturation into the dominant society. Although tribes differed in terms of the specific roles and behavior expected of women, most Indian women experienced greater flexibility and power than did women in European societies. Consequently, the federal boarding school system was introduced as a primary mechanism for indoctrinating non-Indian values. Indian children were forcibly separated or "kidnapped" from the "savage" influence of their families and placed in boarding schools to become "civilized" (Tafoya, 1989; Udall, 1977). They were taken to schools a great distance from their homes, where church attendance was mandatory and traditional beliefs were regarded as being "dangerously pagan and shameful." Girls received much less classroom instruction than boys and were held responsible for the maintenance and cleaning of school facilities. Their devaluation in the educational arena transferred into the family household. Research conducted during the 1970s indicates that Indian women who attended boarding schools experienced anxiety while parenting due to limited opportunities to bond with loved ones or witness ongoing parenting practices as they were growing up (Metcalf, 1976). European American acculturation further established sex-differentiated activities within Indian communities and attempted to limit Indian women's freedom and participation in community power sharing.

Women's roles and power within tribes today vary among Indian communities and according to clan and family structure (LaFromboise, Heyle, & Ozer, 1990). Before European contact, women sometimes obtained formal governing authority based on a belief in their spiritual power. The head of the Women's Council of the Cherokee was believed to speak the words of the Great Spirit (Allen, 1986). The flexibility in role and behavior of Cherokee women was unmatched by tribes in the surrounding area and arose from beliefs associated with the "harmony ethic," which treated Cherokees of both sexes equally (French, 1976). Other characteristics of this ethic included obligatory hospitality and generosity with kinfolk, unwillingness to contradict others publicly, lack of importance placed on formal greetings and exchanges, and a hesitancy to give others directives.

At the present time, Indian women's power is significant and on the rise in many communities. Cherokee women continue to wield considerable domestic and political authority. It is the woman who decides the size of the family and whether or not to terminate a pregnancy (French, 1976). Oglala Sioux women, who are occupying an increasing number of positions as tribal council members, judges, and decision-makers, count their traditional family skills and experiences as important factors in their leadership ability. Although Oglala women of all ages have become politically involved, and many have led or participated in protests for treaty rights, only a few would consider themselves activists, rather seeing themselves as people fulfilling vital tribal needs (Powers, 1986). Similarly, Northern Paiute women's long-term concerns for community issues, along with their kinship connections and experience in coordinating social and community goals, contribute to their effectiveness as leaders (Lynch, 1986). In a study of ten tribal councils on Nevada reservations, Lynch (1986) reported that women constituted the vast majority of membership on local committees and service clubs, and only one tribal council did not have female members.

These examples of extending traditional caretaking and cultural transmission roles vital to the continuity of Indian communities have been labeled "retraditionalization." According to Green (1983), these efforts by Indian women represent a major current attempt to integrate traditional and contemporary role demands in a positive, culturally consistent manner. "Retraditionalized" Indian women rely on the use of cultural beliefs, customs, and ritual and egalitarian relationships with Indian men to improve the quality of Indian life.

The Canadian Blackfeet validated institutionalized roles for postmenopausal women, called "manly-hearted women," who were aggressive, independent, ambitious, bold, and sexually active (Lewis, 1941). They sponsored ceremonials and also had the ability to dominate others. Even today there are numerous examples of Indian women, including married women and some with children, who assume male tasks in everyday life and ceremonies, sometimes because of economic necessity, or in response to traditional upbringing.

A cross-gender tradition existed in over one hundred North American tribal groups (Blackwood, 1984; Roscoe, 1991). This tradition is described as the *berdache* tradition,[4] which involved a complete shift to the social and occupational behavior of the opposite gender. Here, dress and occupation, rather than sexual object choice, determined gender definition. Two *berdache* never formed a couple. According to Whitehead (1981), gender was seen as a social attribute, distinct from sex. In Whitehead's analysis, the anatomical component of gender was more important for women because of their reproductive capacities. In the Southwest, where almost all reported cases for cross-gender identity were found, there was a mystique surrounding claims of anatomical change for these women. Cross-gender women seldom married men because they chose not to perform traditional female-specific tasks. In order to gain the household and kinship benefits of marriage, they married women and fulfilled a man's household, community, and ritual obligations. There is substantial support for the view that successful cross-gender role activity was respected and rewarded. But European American intolerance toward variation in sexual and gender behavior, and Native American acquisition of hostile attitudes from the dominant culture (e.g., by Indian veterans of World War II) suppressed the *berdache* tradition (Roscoe, 1991).

Changing gender roles affect both Indian women and men. While traditional roles have remained relatively intact for Indian women, many traditional gender roles for Indian men (e.g., warriors, hunters) are no longer operable. Indian women generally attribute the rage and violence directed toward them by Indian men as manifestations of their anger and pain associated with the loss of these respected male roles.

DEVELOPMENTAL STAGES

Many American Indians view development as being circular in nature, having no beginning and no end. They believe that prior to birth they existed as spirit beings with the Supreme Creator, and that their spirit beings will return to the Creator after death (Locust, 1985). The following discussion of the developmental stages of infancy, youth, maturity, and the transition stage will be presented in light of the belief in a spirit life preceding birth and following death.

Infancy

Specific ceremonies and rituals often mark stages of life development. Rituals unique to each tribe celebrate the birth and developmental milestones (first smile, first step, etc.) of Indian children. No particular age is designated for completion of these stages. A child's name-giving occurs at infancy and again at later stages in life. In tribes where a person receives the name of another, the recipient is expected to assume the attributes of the person whose name she or he has received (Morey & Gilliam, 1972). Conversely, the one whose name is given to a child assumes important child guidance responsibilities and an obligation to care for the child should illness or hard times befall the parents (Red Horse, 1980).

Youth

Nowadays in certain tribes, including the Hopi, childhood socialization teaches community values without stressing sex differences. Native American girls participate in active sports like swimming, horse racing, and snow sledding. However, in traditional times the focus of girls' education at puberty shifted to domestic tasks and responsibilities (Schlegal, 1973), and the girls prepared themselves for motherhood by taking care of younger children.

Disciplinary practices and the use of physical punishment in caring for children vary substantially among tribes (Everett, Proctor, & Cartmell, 1983). Tribes such as the Tohono O'odham (Papago), Quinault, Fox, and Winnebago are very gentle with children. Within their social networks, adults indulge infants and children, and serious punishment for them usually involves depriving the child of a meal or a desired object. Similarly, the Cheyenne and other Plains groups do not scold or slap youngsters to insure obedience, but isolate children whose behavior is unacceptable. As much as possible, adults show children the "right" way to behave, in order to enable them to choose their actions more appropriately. In traditional times, when a child faced punishment it was not inflicted by parents but by other adult members of the tribe. For example, the Crow designated "teasing cousins" who shamed children in public. These formalized, nonparental castigation methods were based on the belief that punishment meted out directly by parents would breed resentment within the child–parent relationship.

Maturity

In Indian communities, the transition from youth to adult roles occurs through gender-specific rites of passage rather than gradually through adolescent development (French, 1989). For example, traditionally a series of critically important puberty rites marked a young woman's menarche. Much of the girl's future depended upon her accurate performance of these rituals. In nearly all tribes, pubescent girls were isolated from the rest of the community and particularly required to stay away from men during menstruation, so that they would not bring harm to others through their sacred power. During this time of isolation, girls were instructed about their responsibilities as women and the virtue of hard work. Today a joyous public or private celebration marks the Indian female's change of status from girl to woman.[5]

Courtship customs, past and present, differ greatly across tribes. The ideal of premarital chastity, which is part of some Indian cultures, is often not realized. Traditionally, many tribes arranged the marriages of women upon the onset of puberty to avoid the chastity issue and potential problems of premarital sex, but others allowed women time to mature and be courted by village men. The Apache, probably the most sexually strict North American tribe, would ridicule overt displays of affection between boys and girls, and publicly whipped any girl who had engaged in premarital sex. Among other tribes an unwed mother's status was diminished, and she and her parents "lost face." However, in the Southwestern pueblos bearing children outside of wedlock usually is not considered sinful or degrading (Niethammer, 1977).

Indian women, like women in general, typically make decisions regarding when, where, and what type of work to pursue within the framework of family obligations. Most Indian women are employed in their peak childbearing years. Thus, despite the extended family support system, these women find that child care responsibilities interfere substantially with work. This raises the question as to whether the extended family network, particularly in urban areas, can effectively contribute to alleviating the role conflicts and child care difficulties that working Indian women experience (Snipp & Aytac, 1990).

In contrast to non-Indian culture, Indian women's status increases with motherhood and advancing age. Those unable to have their own children often choose to care for them within the extended family through informal or formal adoption, or foster care. Still, an increasing number of Indian women choose not to raise children and use contraceptives for family planning. As mentioned, older Indian people enjoy a high status within Native American societies, their prestige being determined by their longevity and the quality of their experiences during functional adult years. As a result, older women's age and wisdom are revered, and their opinions regarding tribal history, herbal medicines, and sacred matters are valued (Lurie, 1972; Metoyer, 1979). Menopausal women are considered to be, as the Winnebagos put it, "just like a man" (Witt, 1974). The self-esteem of an older woman depends on her continued contribution to her community; she often cares for children and instills in them traditional wisdom and values.

Despite the fact that now more than one third of elderly Native American women live in poverty, many of those 60 years or older report generally positive experiences in old age. Most Southwestern Indian women participating in the cross-ethnic research conducted by Harris, Begay, and Page (1989) reported several advantages to "life after 60," including increased freedom, independence, close feelings toward their family, and enjoyment derived from spending time with family members. More than two thirds of these women live within 5 miles of other family members, and more than 50% regularly care for children (compared with 14% for White Americans; 32% for Latinos). The Native American women in this study indicated more satisfaction with their lives and greater enjoyment in spending time with old people than did the European American respondents. However, when substance abuse and family dysfunction exist the stress experienced by elderly Indian women assuming parenting responsibilities should not be overlooked.

Transition

American Indians characterize death as a transition from earthly life into the spirit world. The death of any relative, except for a newborn infant, or in some tribes a very old person, is observed through ritual mourning. Women play a prominent role in annual mourning ceremonies to honor the dead. A recent widow is expected to be utterly grief-stricken, or at least able to perform the requisite for expressing sorrow. Among the Plains tribes, some women still cut their hair to signify that they are in mourning. The Plains Indian woman mourns for approximately one year, during which time she gives away all of her husband's property. Sometimes women consciously participate in planning their own funerals, saving food for the funeral feast, or waiting to die until certain family members come home.

The custom of announcing dreams that predict that an individual is soon to be reborn demonstrates the belief in reincarnation found among numerous tribes (Slobodin, 1970). Birthmarks corresponding to the wounds of a deceased person with whom a child is identified, memories regarded as being of a previous life, and perceived behavioral similarity between a certain child and a deceased person also indicate a belief in reincarnation (Stevenson, 1975). Further, Indians experiencing grief or major depression often share accounts of having heard voices of deceased relatives (Matchett, 1972).

Some tribes believe that those who have passed away remain in contact with the living and retain concern, benevolent or otherwise, for them (McCone, 1968). Again, in some tribes mediation and "bartering" between the living and dead illustrate a belief in the continuation of the spirit as an integral part of the community after death (Slobodin, 1970). Many Indian women associate personal misfortune, disease, or death with direct or indirect retaliation by evil spirits, or traditional enemies of the deceased or the family of the deceased. Customs still practiced today include discarding the possessions of the deceased, refraining from using his or her name, and avoiding locations associated with his or her death. Among the Navajo, contact with the dead, including entering the house in which a death has occurred, is prohibited. After four days of mourning, it is not acceptable to mention the dead by name. These examples demonstrate Indians' considerable efforts to maintain good relations with the dead by acknowledging respect for the power of the spirit world (Brown, 1953; Opler, 1946).

In summary, Indian women do not regard individuation as a fundamental developmental issue. Family relationship and attachment in earthly and spiritual realms are more vital than separation. In some tribes, each aspect of a woman's development affects her ability to join others as a welcomed member of either her or her partner's family of origin. Each contact she has with others (e.g., her therapist) provides her a unique opportunity for further connection in the task of overcoming adversity.

MENTAL HEALTH AND TREATMENT

Pre-therapy Expectations

From the Native American point of view, wellness represents a balance and harmony in spirit, mind, and body. A woman will not become ill or have negative things happen to her if the spiritual energy around her is strong (Locust, 1985). On the other hand, disharmony creates unwellness and should be avoided. One's violation of a sacred or tribal taboo causes unwellness, and someone in the extended family, such as a child or an elder, could become ill just as easily as the person breaking a taboo (Tafoya, 1989). Avoiding such violations often brings Indians into conflict with behavior expected by non-Indian institutions. For instance, values may conflict in an educational setting where a female student may opt to fail physical education rather than dress and shower in a locker room and thereby commit the sacrilegious act of exposing her body to others.

Also, the misuse of spiritual power causes unwellness, and the activity of individuals who choose to walk with malevolent spirits brings harm to others. The English word "witchcraft" has been applied loosely to this set of phenomena (Locust, 1987). Navajo, Zuni, Yaqui, Hopi, Apache, and Rio Grande Pueblo people use the term "witchcraft." Other tribes use descriptors such as one's being affected by "bad medicine" or being "bear walked." Depression, irrational thinking, unusual behavior, accidents, or sudden physical illness may reveal evidence of the misuse of spiritual power. The belief in witchcraft is a powerful method of social control. Many Indian clients attribute all types of misfortune to witchcraft, including fires that destroy homes and uncontrolled violence perpetrated by husbands upon their wives. Finally, the belief in witchcraft emphasizes external causation, natural or supernatural, rather than personal responsibility (Berman, 1989).

An Indian woman's faith in a medicine person, tribal prophecies, or tribal traditions may have substantial healing power in therapy. Medicine men and women help others to heal themselves or dissolve the negative energy of witchcraft around them. These "warriors for light" are endowed with supernatural power, they understand the problem, and they know how to treat it. Traditional healing ceremonies such as sweat lodge ceremonies, Navajo sings,[6] and peyote meetings treat and prevent psychological and physical illnesses, and strengthen family and community commitment (LaFromboise, Trimble, & Mohatt, 1990).

Bicultural demands often require Indian women to fulfill multiple and perhaps conflicting social roles. Professional or academic pressures and time constraints may prevent them from observing culturally valued practices or tribal responsibilities. If the process of integrating these roles conflicts with achieving harmony in spirit, mind, and body, one's psychological well-being may suffer.

Help-Seeking Behavior

Native Americans are generally reluctant to seek professional therapeutic help, perhaps because of the cultural emphasis on endurance and noninterference or mistrust toward non-Indian service providers (Ho, 1987). Lewis (1984) observed that Native Americans of all lifestyles first contact the extended family network, spiritual leaders, and tribal community elders for help, and then as a last resort, the mainstream health care system. Thus, individuals from traditional families are less likely to seek help from a psychotherapist because they adhere to culturally defined patterns of behavior.

An American Psychological Association site visit report to the Indian Health Service (IHS) service units within the Bemidji area states that, as a rule, "Indian people are tolerant of others' behaviors, no matter how extreme" (Jacobs, Dauphinais, Gross, & Guzman, 1991, p. 5). As a result, when disruptive negative behaviors occur within family units, Indians tend not to refer family members to an external source, or seek assistance as victims to deal with their own pain and suffering. For example, the elderly may tolerate someone taking over their living quarters rather than complain, parents may overindulge a child exhibiting extreme negative behaviors, and young mothers may give AFDC monies to absent and nonsupportive fathers. Thus, unless an Indian community has an alert and well-organized health care delivery system, support for a family with problems may be wanting, and community residents may avoid referring troubled family members for necessary help (Jacobs et al., 1991).

However, reports of mental health service utilization rates in reservation settings show some progress in this area. Kahn, Lejero, Antone, Francisco, and Manuel (1988) note a reduction among Indian people in the stigma attached to mental health treatment and increased acceptance of mental health services. Increasing caseloads, and individual and agency referrals to indigenous community mental health services support these claims. This could be related to greater Indian involvement in traditional and contemporary health care.

Further, the bicultural or nontraditional Indian client is more receptive to mental health services (LaFromboise, Trimble, & Mohatt, 1990). The O'Sullivan, Peterson, Cox, and Kirkeby (1989) replication of the Sue,

Allen, and Conaway (1978) study in the Seattle area found that the "failure to return" rates for American Indians have decreased and are not very different from that of Caucasians. They concluded that the variability in return rates among American Indians, Asian Americans, African Americans, and Latino Americans was more strongly related to the client's level of functioning than to minority status.

The typical client seeking help from IHS service units, on or off reservations, is depressed or anxious due to situational crises such as domestic violence, disruption, victimization, and exposure to alcohol use, and has been or is now using drugs or alcohol (Jacobs et al., 1991). A 1982 study of mental disorders among Indian children found that Indian girls have a much higher rate of outpatient psychiatric treatment after the age of 14 than do Indian boys or USAR girls and boys (Beiser & Attneave, 1982). In 1988, the Social and Mental Health Services of the IHS reported the percentages of Indian women patients seen in the following problem categories: alcohol misuse in the family (82%), adult–child relationships (78%), grief reactions (77%), depression (76%), child management or abuse (72%), and marital conflict (72%) (IHS, 1988). The percentage of women seeking IHS treatment for violent behavior (e.g., incest, battery, rape or sexual assault) is 38% (Old Dog Cross, 1982).

Like males in the general population, Indian males seek help for problems associated with alcohol abuse and antisocial personalities (e.g., violent behavior and parole violations) (IHS, 1988). Unfortunately, these problem categories do not reflect the diagnostic categories of the third revised edition of the *Diagnostic and Statistical Manual of Mental Disorders* (DSM-III-R; American Psychiatric Association, 1987). At the time covered by the report, mental health professionals in the IHS used DSM terminology and paraprofessionals did not.

As many as 50% of American Indian students attending colleges report seeking mental health services, in part because of their desire for psychological support in competitive educational settings. A recent survey of Indian women college students indicates that they rely most heavily on social support when under stress. Again, those living near their home communities are likely to first seek support from family members. Other strategies include cognitive methods such as self-talk, or recall of personal and cultural spiritual beliefs, and behavioral actions such as working harder, or exercising to relieve tension. Of the students interviewed 17% sought help from formal support systems such as counseling services, Alcoholics Anonymous, or university programs providing financial or academic aid (LaFromboise, 1988b). Unfortunately, data on the problems of Indian women utilizing private or nonreservation community mental health services, or health maintenance organizations, is unavailable.

The cultural values and lifestyle alternatives discussed thus far, along with the beliefs about wellness and problems inherent in seeking psychological services, should aid therapists in ascertaining how Indian women percieve mental health services. A strong outreach campaign conducted by influential community gatekeepers and targeted at the clinical needs and expectations of Indian women could further facilitate their help-seeking efforts.

ASSESSMENT AND DIAGNOSIS

Early in the diagnostic process, culturally naive service providers may interpret the expression of cultural and spiritual beliefs and practices as symptoms of mental illness, or maladaptive behavior. Also, standard diagnostic instruments may be unsuitable for assessing American Indians and Alaska Natives (Manson, Walker, & Kivlahan, 1987). Dana (1986) has written extensively about the cultural impropriety of personality assessment instruments, presenting an alternate assessment framework that includes components of cultural knowledge, preferred assessor characteristics, relationship style, and assessment techniques. Also, Chance (1962) found a number of items in the Cornell Medical Index to be invalid for Eskimos. In particular, he cited the finding that Eskimo women, some of whom seem to take a passive role in decision making, might not be expressing feelings of inadequacy, but rather adhering to the cooperative decision making when they answer "yes" to the question, "Do you always feel like you need someone to help you make up your mind?" Other investigators found problems, for example, in differentiating between terms such as "usually" and "always." Clearly, translations between cultures can be misleading.

Even though the process of developing the Minnesota Multiphasic Personality Inventory (MMPI) included small numbers of American Indians, research investigating the relevance or validity of the MMPI with Indians is sparse. In 1980, Pollack and Shore reported significant elevations in the Validity score, Psychopathic Deviate Scale, and the Schizophrenia Scale across a diverse sample of Indian mental health patients seen at IHS clinics in the Portland area. Cultural factors may mask psychopathological variation among Native Americans, as suggested by the difference in performance on the MMPI between Indian and non-Indian psychiatric patients. The number of Native Americans in the normative sample of the MMPI-2 has been increased to 3.3%. Given the high level of diversity among Indians, as evidenced throughout this chapter, the interpretation of an individual profile of an Indian woman, raised in areas of the country not included in the normative sample, is questionable. The MMPI-2, like its predecessor, is more effective as a screening tool than a diagnostic instrument with this population.

In a review of studies estimating depression among Indian adolescents (U.S. Congress, 1990), self-report screen methods resulted in 50%

or more of the adolescents reporting serious depressive symptoms. The Beck Depression Inventory (BDI) is one of several self-rating scales used in studies assessing Indian depression. Spero Manson (personal communication, October 11, 1990) contends that the BDI yields excessive false positives for depression among Native Americans and suggests that more restrictive diagnostic criteria be used for diagnosing clinical depression. Local norms and validation studies are necessary adjuncts to any diagnostic tool with culturally distinct populations. Nevertheless, the large number of depressive symptoms reported by Indian women and men are cause for concern. When Goldwasser and Badger (1989) used the General Health Questionnaire (GHQ) as a psychiatric screen at the Chinle Indian Hospital general medicine clinics on the Navajo reservation, they found a significant difference between the way women and men answered the questions. Women reported somatic complaints more frequently than did men. They also found that unemployed women, or those having large families, had significantly higher GHQ scores. In contrast, employed Indian men scored higher on the GHQ than those who were unemployed.

Given the difficulties with standard assessment instruments, culturally sensitive interviews are essential. Guilmet and Whited (1987) recommend that the intake interview be longer and involve personally supportive conversations centered around client needs rather than direct questioning. They recommend that the "generational history" of a client be explored to determine traditional background and cultural commitment to Indian and non-Indian ways, as well as to define the client's social network. Information obtained should also include the client's history of physical and sexual abuse, other victimization experiences, eating disorders, drug, caffeine, and alcohol use including alcohol abuse by other family members, sleep or appetite disturbance, recent and significant relationship disruptions, educational background, and suicide ideation and history. It is especially important to determine whether or not a client is considered to be mentally ill by her community (Fleming, 1989). A naive therapist may think that an Indian client suffers from extreme looseness of association when she includes many apparently unnecessary details in her accounts (Bergman, 1974). This lack of continuity may be puzzling, but in time the logic and connectedness of things presented by either the therapist or the client will become apparent to an attentive listener.

Recent advances in the ethnocultural assessment of a client's identity and historical background provide useful alternatives to conventional diagnostic procedures. With a cautionary use of standardized assessment tools and an honest exploration of potential personal bias, therapists can make informed decisions about the selection of intervention approaches. Before discussing the basic premise and practice of the psychotherapeutic forms that have been effectively used with American Indian women, a number of special clinical issues must be considered.

SPECIAL CLINICAL ISSUES

A recent consensus statement on Indian women's health care identified a number of health and mental health problems from which Indian women suffer disproportionately (IHS, 1991). Indian women face incredible dilemmas that increase the risk of psychological disturbance. The lifestyle-related clinical issues presented in this section shed further light on the complex and multifaceted problems of Indian women.

Depression

Depression, coupled with racism from the surrounding community, seriously affects the mental well-being of Indian women. As stated earlier, 76% of women using IHS mental health services are suffering from depression (IHS, 1988). The prevalence of depression within select Indian communities may be four to six times higher than previous estimates (Manson, Shore, & Bloom, 1985). Clare Brant, a Canadian Native psychiatrist, estimates that 44% of depressed Indian clients are suffering from grief reactions (Timpson et al., 1988). Manson et al. (1985) found that female boarding school students were more prone to depression than male students. Diagnoses of cyclothymic personality was more frequent among women than men when the American Indian Depression Schedule was used. Far fewer men (22%) than women (78%) were diagnosed as having experienced primary depression (Manson, Shore, Bloom, Keepers, & Neligh, 1987). The Keller, Labori, Endicott, Coryell, and Klerman (1983) study found that 50% of the clinical group experienced concurrent chronic and major depression.

A number of theories on the prevalence of depression among Native Americans have been proposed over the years. Timpson et al. (1988) connected depression with spiritual illness and shame, relating it to the complex issues confronting a colonized minority group in an industrialized world. Guilmet and Whited (1987) and Jilek (1978, 1982) linked depression to subjective feelings of rejection and discrimination, the inability to acquire upward mobility in American society, guilt stemming from collective and personal denial of one's heritage, and moral disorientation due to the fragmentation of traditional cosmological systems. Manson and his colleagues (1985) attribute a high incidence of chronic depression to the substantially greater number of personal losses Native Americans suffer such as sudden accidental deaths of relatives or friends and acculturative pressures that threaten personal identity. They suggest that the greater frequency of depression among Indian women may be related to the demands their families make on them in attempting to cope with the psychosocial stressors associated with cultural change.

Alcohol and Fetal Alcohol Syndrome

Alcoholism and its multigenerational effects are the most critical mental and physical health problem plaguing American Indians today (French,

1989). A number of authors (e.g., Heath, 1983; Kahn, 1982; May, 1982; Oetting, Edwards, Goldstein, & Mason, 1980; Thomas, 1981) have suggested that the extensive use of alcohol and drugs by American Indians may be a response to the stress of cultural disruption and exploitation that they have suffered for generations. Studies offering a sociocultural explanation for Indian alcoholism indicate that excessive substance abuse also may be a response to the demands for integration into and identification with the dominant culture. May, Hymbaugh, Aase, and Samet (1983), Powers (1986), and White and Cornely (1981) assert that in Indian communities drugs and alcohol contribute to a high incidence of accidental deaths, homicide, suicide, sexual violence, child abuse and neglect, and fetal alcohol syndrome, and although it is declining, the death rate due to alcoholism among American Indian women is alarmingly high.

Indian women have a much higher alcoholism rate than women in the general U.S. population. A recent study by Manson, Shore, Baron, Ackerson, and Neligh (1992) indicating that the alcoholism rates for Indian women are the same as those for Indian men contrasts with previous reports that alcoholism rates for Indian females are lower than rates for Indian males (Ozer, 1986). The alcohol/substance abuse death rate of young Indian women 15 to 24 years of age exceeds that of Indian men by 40% (IHS, 1991). The rates of alcoholism, particularly among women, do vary from tribe to tribe, and in some tribes only a small proportion of Indian women have serious alcohol abuse problems (Hill, 1989). For example, surveys among the Navajo and Plains tribes show that only 13–55% of women drink at all (Levy & Kunitz, 1974; Longclaws, Barnes, Grieve, & Dumoff, 1980; Whittaker, 1962, 1982), while national surveys indicate that 60% of all U.S. women consume some alcohol (National Institute on Alcohol Abuse and Alcoholism, 1981). Because some tribes are at higher risk than others, more culturally specific treatment approaches need to be developed for these tribes.

According to Ozer (1986), Native American men are twice as likely as non-Native Americans to be in treatment for drug-related problems. Indian women are reluctant to go into inpatient drug treatment programs because of child-care responsibilities. The existing child welfare and foster care placement system is not designed to meet the needs of women entering treatment, and the history of forced removal of Indian children from their families is grim. When chemical dependency is ongoing throughout the family system, the extended family may not be a viable alternative for support (Fleming & Manson, 1990).

Recent studies indicate a high rate of fetal alcohol syndrome (FAS) and fetal alcohol effect (FAE) among the children of Indian women (May et al., 1983; Whittaker, 1982). The incidence of FAS among southwest Indian tribes is highly variable but increasing. May and his colleagues (1983) reported a range of 10.3 per 1,000 births (1 per 97) for the Plains tribes to 1.3 per 1,000 births (1 per 749) for Navajos.[7] They also reported a Pueblo rate of 1 per 495, which, while lower than the Plains rate, is higher than those for the other Southwestern populations they studied (26 reservations in New Mexico, Southern Colorado, Southern Utah, and Northern Arizona). This research also found an unexpectedly high occurrence of mothers having two or more alcohol-damaged children. One explanation offered by May et al. (1983) for the higher FAS rate among Plains tribes is their greater tolerance for socially deviant behavior given their loose tribal social integration. Finally, a majority of female substance abusers in Indian substance abuse treatment programs are survivors of childhood sexual abuse (Dixon, 1989).

Child Abuse and Neglect

There is wide variation in incidence and reporting of child abuse and neglect from one tribe to the next. And child protection workers unfamiliar with cultural practices have misunderstood Indian child-rearing practices. For example, a study by Gray and Cosgrove (1985) characterized Blackfeet child-rearing practices as neglectful and emotionally abusive, since children are watched but not told how to behave, not given any public displays of affection after age 10, and school truancy is tolerated. Researchers Lujan, DeBruyn, May, and Bird, who were familiar with the cultures under study, documented the intergenerational perpetuation of child abuse and neglect in a 1989 study. They found the following rate of abuse among 11 Pueblo tribes and one Apache tribe: over 87% of the adults (biological parents, stepparents, grandparents and some great-grandparents of children who were abused) grew up in homes with either their natural parents or stepparents as primary caretakers, and many who grew up in alcohol abusive homes were neglected or abused as children. In addition, 76% of these adults were exposed to, or victims of, domestic violence. Young girls moved from home to home were most likely to be abused. Similarly, a study among the Navajo conducted by White (1977) found a high percentage of cases (neglect, 80%; abuse, 50%) that were alcohol-related.

Sexual Abuse

A paucity of data surrounds the issue of Indian sexual assault and sexual abuse. Lujan et al. (1989) stated that their data, experiences, and verbal reports by mental health staff strongly suggest that incidents of sexual abuse are vastly underreported, as is the case in European American culture. Incestuous relationships in particular are seldom reported, which makes it difficult to obtain accurate information on the extent of sexual abuse in Indian communities. A victim's loyalty to an offender through clan and extended family membership causes additional resistance to coming forward and prosecuting (D. Willis, personal communication, March 29, 1990).

Indian girls indicated on the Indian Health Survey that they were six times more likely to be physically and sexually abused than Indian boys (U.S. Congress, 1990). In another recent survey of over 13,900 Indian adolescents, 20% of the respondents reported that they had been sexually abused (Meyer, 1991). Wischlacz, Lane, and Kempe (1978) found child sexual abuse among the Cheyenne River Sioux to be less frequent than in U.S. averages, but when it did occur it was much more violent, frequently resulting in the death of the child. A survey of Indian women clients at a regional psychiatric center revealed that at least 80% had experienced sexual assault (Old Dog Cross, 1982). The *Navajo Times* in 1982 reported that rape was the most prevalent crime on the Navajo reservation and described a trend of organized gang rape in which a group of adolescent males would take premeditated revenge on a particular woman (Old Dog Cross, 1982). Cases of Indian women being raped, particularly when those women have been drinking, are often not taken seriously by law enforcement (IHS, 1991).

Data from Alaska suggest that the incidence of incest is higher among Eskimo and Indian groups than among non-Native groups (Fischer, 1983). Although Navajo incest taboos are broader in scope than those among non-Indians, incest still exists. The known perpetrators of incest are usually uncles or stepfathers. Reports of sexual abuse by a natural father are rare (among Indians, as well as in the general population, this may in part be due to underreporting). Among the Navajo, an additional restrictive factor may be the traditional association of father–daughter incest with witchcraft (Reichard, 1950). When incest is revealed, some non-Indian clinicians have been known to belittle its importance as a problem in Indian groups because they believe, quite incorrectly, that it is culturally acceptable (A. Yoder, personal communication, August 27, 1990). Indian leaders, on the other hand, cite this problem as evidence of the breakdown in traditional cultural values.

When the family's main residence is in a city and incest occurs, the Indian Child Welfare Act requires that the tribe be contacted and given the choice of assuming jurisdiction. Often, the tribe declines, leaving the case in the state's jurisdiction. On the other hand, if the family lives on a reservation, the process will be governed by tribal regulations, which vary from tribe to tribe. When the state has jurisdiction, if the mother seems to be denying the occurrence of the sexual abuse, or for some other reason is seen as unable to protect the child from the abuser (e.g., if she refuses treatment, or is unwilling to support the child by rejecting a husband or boyfriend), the child is placed with a local foster family, which is rarely an Indian family (Porter & Berman, 1988).

The emotional problems commonly experienced by Indian sexual abuse victims are similar to those found in the non-Indian population. These include a difficulty in developing trusting personal relationships, expressing anger in effective and appropriate ways, and an inability to overcome the stress related to withholding feelings associated with victimization and betrayal (Ashby, Gilchrist, & Miramontez, 1987).

Eating Disorders

America's obsession with the size of women's bodies has permeated Native American cultures. In a survey of 85 Chippewa (Ojibwa) girls and women in Michigan, three fourths of them were trying to lose weight. Of the dieters, 75% were using potentially hazardous techniques, and 24% included purging behaviors (Rosen et al., 1988). Snow and Harris (1989), in their study of Pueblo Indian and Hispanic girls, concluded that the rural subjects they studied, who were probably of lower socioeconomic status (SES) than those in most other groups in which eating disorders have been studied, expressed excessive concerns about weight and had disordered eating patterns similar to those found in urban, well-educated young women. These survey results are contrary to the assumption that ethnic minority group members are more resigned to being overweight than members of the majority non-Indian culture (Massara & Stunkard, 1979).

The Secretary's Task Force on Black and Minority Health (U.S. Department of Health and Human Services, 1986) reported that both American Indians and Hispanics are at increased risk for obesity and diabetes. Snow and Harris (1989) conclude that biological and cultural factors, such as patterns of food preparation and periods of limited food availability, may also contribute to this problem. Feasting connected with traditional religious and social events may also contribute to the high incidence of obesity in Indian women.

Suicide

The statistics on suicide among American Indians and Alaska Natives indicate a preponderance of completed suicides in 15- to 24-year-old men (Lester & Lester, 1971; Massey, 1967). The age-adjusted suicide completion rate for American Indian and Alaska Native women is 5/100,000 (for Indian men the rate is 24/100,000), while the rate for women in the U.S. population as a whole is 6/100,000 (Group for the Advancement of Psychiatry, 1989). Again, there is great variability in suicidal behavior among tribes. Levy and Kunitz (1974) caution against using national statistics as a standard for comparison with particular tribes.

Suicide attempts by adolescent Indian women are more frequent, but less lethal than those of adolescent Indian men. Generally, it is thought that sex differences in Indian adolescent suicide attempts are not as striking as in the general U.S. or African American populations (Biernoff, 1969; Manson, Beals, Dick, & Duclos, 1989). However, a recent study of suicide attempts and suicide ideation among 84 Zuni freshmen revealed that 39% of the females and 16% of the males had attempted suicide (Howard-

Pitney, LaFromboise, Basil, September, & Johnson, 1992). These current findings point to the need to consider gender differences as important variables in the study of tribe specific factors associated with suicidal behavior. Of the many suicide attempts and gestures among Native American females, overdoses of aspirin, or whatever happens to be in the medicine cabinet, sometimes in combination with alcohol intoxication, is common. Depressive symptomatology, alcohol use, and a perceived lack of family support are also strongly related to suicide attempts.

Suicidal behavior, or even suicidal thoughts, are taboo in some tribes. Among the Tohono O'odham (Papago), suicide is considered sinful, evil, or a sign of possession by bad spirits. Among the Zuni, even thoughts of taking one's life are taboo (LaFromboise & Howard-Pitney, 1994). Directly mentioning death is taboo for the Navajo, and to think of death is to invite it. Therefore a Navajo woman willing to respond positively to questions about suicidal ideation on the General Health Questionnaire is in actuality seeking help (Goldwasser & Badger, 1989). Because of the implied taint on the family, referrals for assistance to those who later complete suicide are few (Kahn et al., 1988).

Given the harsh realities of Indian life reiterated throughout this enumeration of clinical issues, therapists are challenged to be able to identify and mobilize cultural beliefs and lifestyle factors that enhance Indian wellness. In the next section, a number of intervention approaches are presented that could serve as prototypes in the further development, delivery, and evaluation of culturally sensitive and innovative approaches aimed at helping Indian women overcome multiple and often conflicting concerns.

INTERVENTION APPROACHES

Unfortunately, treatment approaches with American Indians do not have a long history of theoretical development and supporting research. The Mental Health Program of the IHS was not established until the mid-1960s when a pilot project was set up in Pine Ridge, South Dakota (the Sioux reservation that includes the site of the Wounded Knee massacre). This program consisted primarily of Mental Health Technicians (MHTs), indigenous people fluent in their own language and familiar with their community, who served as paraprofessional counselors as well as interpreters for predominantly non-Indian psychiatrists and psychologists.

Since that time it has remained evident that a therapist effective with Native Americans must be aware of the attitudes and customs particular to her (or his) own ethnic and cultural heritage and be knowledgeable about alternatives in a client's background, both self-disclosed and those from sources other than the client. In this regard, the therapist's goal is to uncover, respect, and learn to understand differences in culture, community, and past and present experience (Lerman & Porter, 1990).

Bennett recently explored the question of the importance of therapist–client ethnic similarity among Indian adults and adolescents, utilizing a methodology that compares preference for ethnic similarity with preference for other therapist attributes. Indian female clients ranked the importance of the therapist having a similar personality higher than Indian male clients, and both women and men ranked the therapist being of the same sex as quite important (Bennett, 1991). With American Indian college students, ethnicity was ranked below similar attitudes, more education, and similar personality as a desirable therapist attribute (Bennett & Big-Foot-Sipes, 1991). In a similar study with American Indian adolescents, BigFoot-Sipes, Dauphinais, LaFromboise, Bennett, and Rowe (1992) found that Indian females expressed a strong preference for talking with a female Indian counselor, particularly when discussing personal problems. The authors suggest that since American Indian women counselors are not in great supply, somewhat older Indian female peer counselors might be considered. It appears that the role of Indian female MHTs is validated.

A female therapist working with a tribal group different from her own (including those of Indian descent) can involve herself in community activities and meetings to learn about tribal culture and how it affects the lives of her clients. Such behavior demonstrates an interest in the lives of the residents and enables the therapist to learn more about the life and problems of the area (Berman, 1990).

The therapist who by choice or chance finds herself working with American Indian clients must recognize the distinctive cultural differences in psychosocial development and life experiences that do exist, as well as the similarities between Indians and individuals from other ethnic groups. Also, she must respect the distinctive personal culture each Indian woman brings to therapy. The Ethnic Validity Model (Tyler, Sussewell, & Williams-McCoy, 1985) acknowledges the relevance and importance of working with racial and ethnic variables rather than focusing primarily upon personal/individual factors. This model can be helpful for a therapist unaccustomed to exploring a client's cultural history. These occasional conflicts between individual uniqueness and the way in which individuals are affected by their cultural history are important issues in the process of therapy (Ivey, 1991).

Individual Therapy

It is important that the therapist balance the needs for establishing trust and the desire for effecting change. Some Indian women may expect immediate results and, therefore, be frustrated by a slow rate of change, or the reluctance of a therapist to supply answers. Single session therapy that helps bolster client's strengths, restore autonomy and confidence, and explore solutions for immediate implementation as detailed by Talmon (1991), may in fact be the treatment of choice in these situations. Likewise, Sue and Zane (1987) suggest that the direct benefits of therapy should be demonstrated as soon as possible in therapy. Depending upon the client and situation, these could include alleviation and reduction of negative emotional states (in the case of depression and anxiety), or cognitive clarity as a means of better understanding chaotic experiences (in a state of crisis and confusion). When appropriate, clients can be helped to realize that their thoughts, feelings, or appearance are shared by others. By emphasizing that other women have encountered similar experiences, clients may place their concerns in a more realistic context.

When working through an interpreter in bilingual conversations, one must recognize the additional complexities of a three-person relationship in therapy. Once the therapist finds an interpreter with translation skills and some counseling knowledge (preferably of the same tribe, sex, and age as the client), it is helpful for her to decide beforehand what questions to ask and what information is important (Bergman, 1974). In a workshop by Wong, Comas-Díaz, Kennedy, LaFromboise, and Miyahira (1987), Wong recommended that the therapist and the interpreter meet in a pre-interview session to build a relationship of trust and plan the objectives of the interview, topics to be covered (including the background and concerns of the client), estimated time the interview might require, preferred translation format (e.g., word for word, summarizing, or cultural interpretation translation), and discuss the interpreter's past experience with clients having problems like those of the client.

If brief or ongoing therapy is planned, asking Indian women early in therapy to keep behavior logs, or to solicit help from the extended family, may actively engage them and allow immediate insight into the nature of the problem (LaFromboise & Low, 1989). Early in therapy, the client may feel more comfortable if the therapist uses self-disclosure and demonstrates cultural sensitivity before asking personal questions (LaFromboise & Dixon, 1981; LaFromboise, Coleman, & Hernandez, 1991).

In rural areas, it is often useful to make home visits to facilitate follow-up on clients who may not have regular transportation to a clinic office and to familarize therapists with the real living situations of their clients. Further, it may provide the opportunity for a home-based family therapy session, which might not be possible in an office visit (Schacht, Tafoya, & Mirabla, 1989). Guilmet and Whited (1987) found that during treatment a high level of involvement with outside agencies may also be necessary because of the extent of dysfunction a client's family may experience. Other outreach activities may include going to court with clients, coordinating with other treatment programs and schools, and becoming involved in interagency meetings.

A number of conventional treatment techniques can be used appropriately with American Indian women. With clients who have an adequate education level and English fluency, one can recommend bibliotherapy. For example, since many clients are sexual abuse survivors, clinicians frequently recommend that they read books such as *Courage to Heal* (Bass & Davis, 1988) to stimulate thinking about the various issues related to abuse. They also recommend completing the writing exercises presented in the accompanying workbook (Davis, 1990). For those finding it difficult to begin this threatening task, one can suggest that they first read the stories of heroic survivors, like the one by a Native American woman at the back of the same book.

Stress reduction techniques can be very useful to individuals experiencing a personal crisis or exerting extensive coping efforts to deal with the stress. Muscle relaxation and guided imagery exercises should be adapted to be more representative of Indian cultural and environmental contexts. For example, when asking a client to imagine a peaceful place, one must avoid the incongruity of proposing a beach scene to someone living in a mountain area or desert. Instead, one might evoke images of a sanctuary adorned with works of art, pottery, or beadwork, birds and other wildlife, or the pleasing colors of the rainbow (LaFromboise, 1991).

Art therapy techniques also may be useful with American Indian women, especially when language differences exist between therapist and client. When interpreting drawings, one must again consider the cultural context (Lofgren, 1981). For example, adolescent girls may not indicate significant differences between male and female figures in their drawings if jeans, T-shirts, boots, and long hair are typical styles of dress for both boys and girls, men and women. Also, the themes and symbols in Native American drawings are likely to differ from those of European American culture.

Group Therapy

According to Edwards and Edwards (1984), group work is becoming the treatment of choice for a number of agencies with programs serving American Indians. Many who have participated in cultural group activities transfer positive feelings to therapeutic groups. However, professionals with clients in other agency or school settings may have difficulty promoting participation in therapy groups because of client fears about confidentiality, given the gossip and rumors that are often passed along in close-knit Indian communities. In one case, a group for women structured along the lines of a consciousness-raising group disbanded after others in the community criticized the members of the group. Although the group was open to all women in this small Pueblo community, the only ones who consistently attended were those who worked in tribal offices. But they were criticized for using up resources (i.e., the services of the mental health professional facilitating the group) that could be better allocated to individuals more in need. Other members of the community became uncomfortable about what might have developed from this group's discussions about, among other things, the exclusion of women from the governing council of their male-dominated community.

It is often useful to structure a group as a time-limited experiential class, or workshop, around a theme such as "Self-Esteem for Women," or "Women in Transition." Many Indian groups have grown out of community attempts to deal with crises. For instance, when the Hopi faced the horror of more than one hundred boys having been sexually abused by a teacher ("Assault on the Peaceful," 1988), meetings of concerned parents turned into therapy sessions where adults, for the first time, revealed their own childhood experiences of abuse. A similar process is shown in the film, "Circle of Healing," which describes the use of community groups in the Alkali Lake Community of Canada (Canadian Broadcasting Company, 1989). Since Indian women come from a tradition of self-sufficiency and are taught at puberty to care for themselves and their children (Landes, 1971), educational programs such as those providing information on FAS could be important preventative interventions. A program conducted on the Navajo reservation, in Tuba City, Arizona, is currently attempting to reduce the rate of FAS by 25%. The counselors in this program are called prevention workers, so as to encourage the cooperation of women reluctant to admit they are alcohol abusers but motivated to prevent birth defects in their children. The program targets women in their childbearing years and screens pregnant women for alcohol use in a prenatal clinic (Roberts, 1989). By clearly emphasizing how the amount of alcohol consumed over time determines blood alcohol levels and, consequently, the amount of alcohol delivered to the fetus, women can make their own decisions about the amount of alcohol that is safe to drink during pregnancy. This approach contrasts with recent punitive tribal court decisions attempting to incarcerate women, on the grounds of fetal abuse, for the duration of their pregnancy to prevent them from drinking.

Manson, Walker, and Kivlahan (1987), and Fleming (1989) suggest two American Indian group treatment strategies based on traditional healing practices: the "four circles" and the "talking circle." The four circles structures group exploration around issues related to individuals within each of the four increasingly larger concentric circles representing the Creator at the center, one's partner or spouse at the next level, one's immediate or "blended" family, and in the outermost circle, one's extended family, co-workers or classmates, and community and tribal members.

The talking circle is a form of group therapy that includes elements of ritual and prayer, but does not depend on interaction between the participants. L. Carole (personal communication, September 14, 1990) described talking/healing circles that were led by native Alaskan women for their 3- and 4-year-old grandchildren, teaching them to talk about their feelings through role playing and modeling. Ashby et al. (1987) found that their participants selected the talking circle as the most helpful and useful activity in a program addressing sexual abuse.

Network therapy, a form of family therapy created by Carolyn Attneave, a Delaware Indian, involves recreating the clan network to mobilize a family's kin and social system to help a client (LaFromboise & Fleming, 1990). This approach has proved to be a viable approach for preventing and dealing with psychiatric problems in communities (Schoenfeld, Halevy-Martini, Hemley-Van der Velden, & Ruhf, 1985), and has been applied in various situations and settings with Indians and non-Indians alike (Rueveni, 1984). The sessions are conducted in the home and involve considerable numbers of people, including members of the intervention team, the extended family, and others unrelated but known to the family. To be effective, the therapists and members of the family need to be able to review the family problem, facilitate community meetings, and develop strategies of engaging the system in rebuilding connections and healing relationships to help solve the problem. Network therapy has been used not only in crisis intervention, but also in establishing support systems of elders in rural communities, in reviving traditional healing systems of clients, and in dealing with natural and human disasters (Speck & Speck, 1984).

Clinicians have also found group social skills training to be effective with Indian women in reducing unplanned pregnancies, drinking behavior (Carpenter, Lyons, & Miller, 1985; Schinke, 1982; Schinke et al., 1988) and tobacco use (Holden, Botvin, & Orlandi, 1989; Schinke, Schilling, Gilchrist, Ashby, & Kitjima, 1987), in dealing with sexual abuse (Ashby et al., 1987), and in increasing their assertion skills (LaFromboise, 1989; LaFromboise & Rowe, 1983). In general, social skills training should not replace traditional Indian behaviors, or therapeutic processes, but serve both as a prevention effort and as an adjunct to therapy that empowers Indian women by expanding their repertoire of behaviors. Schools, job training programs, and community colleges offer ready sites for blending skills training with educational advising.

Increased Indian involvement in skills- or theme-focused groups and therapy attests to the usefulness of group treatment modalities with Indian women. A therapist working with Indian women, individually or in a group, must be culturally sensitive and maintain a flexible agenda. A number of group and individual interventions could easily be blended with health service delivery systems to elevate the mental health status of Indian women. Two case studies are presented below to further illustrate the potential responsiveness of reservation and urban Indian women to therapy. Personal information for each client was altered to insure confidentiality.

CASE ILLUSTRATIONS

Case 1: Ms. Shimasani (Ms. S.)

Ms. S. was referred to a non-Indian IHS therapist by the New Mexico Human Services Department (HSD) as part of the treatment plan.[8] She was a 49-year-old Navajo woman wanting her two granddaughters returned to her home and care. They had been placed in a non-Indian foster home after one of the girls revealed to a school counselor that their uncle, Ms. S.'s son, had been sexually abusing them. The girls started therapy at another agency that specialized in the treatment of children. Other family members' offers to become foster parents were disregarded, despite the HSD policy to place children in substitute care with relatives. It seems that HSD assumed the pathology extended to all members of the family. Ethnic prejudice is suspected here, since in this case HSD did not follow its own policy.

Ms. S. had a history of being battered by her husband, leaving that relationship and eventually marrying another man. Her own children, who were born on the reservation, had several fathers. One son was killed. Ms. S. divorced her last husband because of his repeated infidelity and moved her family, which included her mentally retarded oldest daughter and disabled mother, to a city to support them better.

Ms. S. had her son arrested after he threatened her with a knife and raped her. He justified his behavior by saying that he was too drunk to know what he was doing. When he pleaded with his mother to have the authorities release him, she agreed to drop the charges. Seven months later, he was accused of sexually abusing her two granddaughters, ages 5 and 7, which he had apparently been doing since before the rape. An investigative visit was made to Ms. S.'s home after the school counselor reported the abuse to Child Protective Services. Both girls were placed in protective custody. The girl's mother, divorced from their father, moved out of the family home because her current boyfriend also was accused of abuse. Ms. S.'s other grown children moved out of the family home, fearing that they also would be accused of molesting the children. This put an additional strain on the family, since they were no longer available to share financial and child care responsibilities.

The court ordered an evaluation of Ms. S., since she had been acting as her granddaughters' primary parent, to assess her mental status and level of functioning, and to determine her ability to provide a safe and stable environment for her granddaughters. Ms. S. had never been to school, and her primary language was Navajo. Although services were available at the IHS hospital in her home city she was referred to the psychologist at the Indian hospital in Gallup, 150 miles from home, presumably to provide culturally sensitive services such as the aid of a Navajo language interpreter. Her mental status exam and psychosocial history revealed that she appeared to be functioning at a very concrete reasoning level. A culture-fair instrument such as the Leiter was recommended to obtain a more accurate profile of her intellectual functioning. She showed signs of depression. She was upset by the removal of the grandchildren from her home and still suffered from unresolved grief over the death of one of her own children a few years earlier.

Ms. S. was referred for therapy to help her regain custody of the children. The focus of the HSD treatment plan was to help her overcome her depression and enable her to "regain self-control, particularly with regard to defending herself from her son." She also felt abused and disempowered by the state social service and legal systems. Her family life had been completely disrupted by her son's behavior, its discovery by a foreign agency (HSD), and the interventions imposed by a hostile and alien system.

The first therapy session, 6 months after the children were taken into custody, focused on Ms. S. wanting to get the children back. She felt deceived because she had been told that the children were being taken for only a short time. The first task of the therapist was to gain her trust and convince her that she would be her advocate, not her enemy. This involved communicating respect for her cultural heritage and customs.

Throughout the therapy process the IHS staff interpreter attended whenever possible. The woman interpreting for the HSD turned out to be a family relative, and at times complicated the process by leaking information to them which was both inaccurate and in violation of confidentiality.

In this family, denial was a significant issue. Ms. S. has been denying the abuse of the girls, saying that since she didn't see it she couldn't believe it. The interpreter said that because the Navajo language doesn't distinguish between rape and sexual abuse, it was necessary to describe the molestation more graphically. Still Ms. S. insisted that she didn't know how it could have happened, and she couldn't accept it.

She said that her son had behaved inappropriately because he was witched, and that he had a sing to neutralize the witchcraft. The therapist asked her whether she had ever seen witchcraft performed or seen its effects directly, and she tried to make it clear that she was not being accused of being a witch, and that her beliefs were taken seriously. Ms. S. said she did not need to see witchcraft in order to believe in it. The therapist asked if she could believe the girls were molested just because they said so, even if she didn't see it. At this point, she said she could. This analogy applied in the cultural context seemed to be an effective intervention.

During a therapy session, she spoke about her distress that the girls' foster mother had cut their hair without obtaining her consent. One of the issues for her seemed to be a loss of parental control. She said that she had been planning to have the girls' portrait taken in traditional Navajo dress, with their hair styled in the traditional bun wrapped with yarn. Further, she wanted to restore them to harmony by having a sing done for them and had been told by the crystal gazer, a traditional diagnostician of medical, psychological, or spiritual maladies in the context of Navajo beliefs, that it would have to be postponed until after their hair grew back. These explanations did not seem to sufficiently account for the intensity of feelings she was expressing until the therapist remembered that Navajos always dispose of hair and nail clippings carefully to prevent them from falling into the hands of a witch and being used to cast a spell against them (Kluckhohn & Leighton, 1962). It became clear that the client felt the non-Indian foster mother and case worker disregarded her culturally based concerns, as was evidenced by a perceived lack of respect for her specifically and Native Americans in general.

Ms. S. was also referred to the mother's group at Programs for Children. The group included women of diverse racial and ethnic backgrounds, which probably helped her develop trust faster than when in individual therapy with the non-Indian therapist. In the group, Ms. S. was finally able to come to grips with the actuality of the children's sexual abuse after viewing tapes of the granddaughters' therapy sessions. The group also effectively promoted the parent–daughter relationship. For example, one of the activities involved the mothers teaching their daughters the names of parts of their bodies, including the genitals. Given the extent of modesty within the traditional Navajo culture, this was difficult for Ms. S., but by this time she was willing to make a greater effort for the sake of the girls.

By now it was obvious that more family members needed to be included in the treatment plan, especially since other family members continued to distrust the actions of the legal and social service systems. Therapists for all involved parties, the children, the grandmother, and the group were involved in the initial stage of Ms. S.'s family therapy. They listened carefully to the issues raised by the family. The HSD case worker also attended the family therapy sessions to answer family's questions about HSD procedures and the girls' treatment. After these sessions, the therapists felt they could start working on issues tailored to the needs of the family.

Ms. S.'s struggle to keep her family together meant that at times she was not available to her children during their adolescent years. In therapy, the family dealt with the need for greater communication between Ms. S. and her daughters, their grief over the loss of their father, and the recent expulsion of the son who had raped his mother and his two nieces. When the daughter who was the mother of these girls decided to stay with her boyfriend and give up her parental rights, Ms. S. decided to adopt the children legally. It is not uncommon in Navajo families for the grandmother, or another relative, to bond closely with the children and raise them. The adoption process was another issue requiring a great deal of sensitivity and cultural awareness. The HSD case worker attended the hearing in which the mother relinquished her parental rights to the state, a necessity for legalizing the adoption, and she saw this as a routine legal procedure, thinking it unnecessary to invite the grandmother to attend. However, the grandmother felt excluded and still suspected the motives of this alien legal system. It seemed to her that the state might once again be stealing the children. The caseworker did not understand that in Navajo custom, the mother would simply give her child directly to the adopting relative, without the intervention of third parties outside of the family.

Not only the American legal system, but the therapy process itself differed from and conflicted with Navajo customs and values. A conventional therapist expects that the client will talk about traumatic events that occurred in the past in order to resolve present conflicts and initiate changes in attitudes and behavior. The Navajo solution is more likely to involve a sing performed by a traditional healer who neutralizes the effects of possible witchcraft, any damage done by external forces, or the harmful consequences of violating a taboo, thus proscribing further focus on past events.

In summary, this collaborative attempt at therapy included working across agencies, so that both the children and the parental figure were represented by therapist/advocates. A modified network approach included other members of the extended family, as well as relevant social service personnel, and incorporated extensive use of an interpreter. Here the role of the therapist involved balancing issues she saw as important with Ms. S.'s sense of how they should be done, and interpreting the Navajo culture to personnel from the legal and social systems working with the case.

Case 2: Roberta

Roberta was a 42-year-old Apache woman referred to the therapist by her male psychiatrist. At the time of initial contact, she had been hospitalized for the third time with symptoms of bipolar depression and suicidal ideation. (Hospital records indicate that no formal assessment procedures beyond the clinical interview were used with Roberta.) Her treating psychiatrist felt that she could better resolve her issues centered around identity confusion with a Native American therapist. The psychiatrist continued to supervise her medications, which included lithium carbonate and tricyclic antidepressants. Roberta attended sessions with her therapist once a week for 16 months.

At the time of initial contact, Roberta's presenting problem was discouragement over her major recurrent depression. She had two teenage sons from two different husbands, and since her divorce 15 years ago she lived with both the sons and her sister. Her brother lived out of the country. Her younger son had a learning disability and was emotionally disturbed. He was violent, destructive, and had recently been released from a juvenile detention center. Her older son did not seem to have substantial problems. Roberta was raised by an Apache mother and a White father. As she was growing up, her father discouraged her mother and the children from identifying with their tribal culture. Her family moved from place to place, due to the nature of her father's job, so she had not lived on the reservation since early childhood and was unable to participate in her tribal culture during formative years.

Roberta's mother had had several successive miscarriages and a history of abusing prescription drugs, which she obtained from her husband, a health care professional who was also a gambler and an unfaithful husband. She had little energy after the miscarriages and had been hospitalized once following a suicide attempt for an extensive period of time. At that time Roberta and her siblings were placed in the care of distant relatives. After Roberta's parents divorced, her father lived a great distance away from the family and had minimal contact with them. Her mother had recently suffered a stroke and was placed in a nursing home because of her deteriorating condition. Roberta expressed strong feelings of guilt and sadness because she could not care for her mother at home.

Roberta's second marriage was to a foreign national who had married her to obtain a work permit. Her employment form showed that she had adopted his nationality and did not indicate that she was American Indian. She had been working for 5 years as a bookkeeper in the administrative building of a major university until she was unexpectedly fired from her job for what she perceived as unfair reasons (sexual jealousy). At the time of therapy, Roberta received Social Security, Supplementary Social Security, and Medicare due to her physical and mental problems. She had high blood pressure, chronic depression, limited concentration ability, and short-term memory loss. In addition, she had attempted suicide by drug overdose four times. Despite having undertaken vocational training to keep up with her accounting and computer skills, she panicked every time she anticipated applying for a job. One of the goals of therapy was to encourage her to volunteer for work to build confidence around issues of acquiring and maintaining employment.

Roberta had a history of alcohol and marijuana abuse. She attended Alcoholics Anonymous (AA) meetings, but she could not relate to the AA testimonial process and the rigidity of the 12-step program. She was uncomfortable with the strong Christian overtones and having to seek forgiveness from people she had supposedly wronged. She liked the dual diagnosis group she was in because the leaders of this group emphasized controlled, responsible drinking rather than total abstinence. Also, this group was smaller than the AA groups, and this made it more personal.

The focus of therapy was to help Roberta resolve her identity and self-esteem issues, keep her depression under control, and develop her career. She appeared to open up as the therapist shared stories about how she herself and other Indian people dealt with problems similar to Roberta's. She reported that she felt the therapist could understand her, since she herself was Indian. Issues of jealousy directed toward the therapist did emerge, and Roberta indicated that she felt the therapist expected her to always be strong, fearing that if she couldn't show strength and resilience the therapist might become judgmental about her. At times she felt the therapist was pressuring her. When that happened, she became less involved in sessions, and the therapist accordingly backed away from addressing career issues. The therapist encouraged her to interact more with members of the intertribal Indian community close to where she lived by attending community events and becoming involved in activities to the extent she found comfortable. Interventions for her depression and anxiety associated with job-seeking included the cognitive and behavioral interventions of relaxation training, identification and increased involvement in pleasant events, cognitive restructuring of negative thoughts, and communication, problem solving, and social skills training.

Roberta's mother died 6 months into therapy. Her brother returned home and immediately moved in with them, and problems with her troubled son escalated. Her brother did not identify himself as part Apache and in fact had acquired a British accent during his sojourn abroad. He presented himself as a European American to others. Further, his value system was quite different from that of his sisters. His reentry into the family happened at a time when both sisters were becoming more comfortable asserting their Apache identity. Also, his employment at a liquor store accelerated the drinking at home, since he brought home a steady supply of alcohol, thus making it increasingly difficult for Roberta to refrain from alcohol consumption at a time when she was seeking sobriety.

In the year following her mother's death, there was a lot of tension between the sisters regarding the proper burial of their mother's remains. Their mother had been cremated according to her wishes and Roberta's sister wished to keep her ashes in a wooden box displayed on a shelf in their living room. Roberta wanted to follow the traditional practice of returning the ashes to the earth.[9] During this phase of therapy the therapist disclosed information about her own tribal beliefs associated with death and grief and showed how these had influenced her own reactions to her mother's death.

On the first anniversary of Roberta's mother's death, the therapist was in the process of terminating therapy because she was moving out of the area, and thus referred the client to another therapist. Roberta's medications continued to be supervised by the referring psychiatrist. During this time, one of the local tribes was having a major ceremony. The therapist encouraged Roberta to attend this gathering and even accompanied the client and her family to the event. At the close of the night dances, Roberta and her sister encountered a medicine woman who seemed to have a profound impact on all present, as she prayed for them and told them to "let her go," implying that they had grieved long enough for their mother. As the sisters shared accounts of the experience with various

Indian people, it became clear to them that their mother's spirit would not be free as long as they kept her ashes in the manner in which they were stored. Shortly thereafter, the sisters disposed of the ashes appropriately and held a feast in their mother's honor. A Navajo friend blessed their home to counteract the negative effect of having kept the ashes in the household.[10]

In Roberta's perception, things appeared to change for the better after this episode. Her son moved out of her house and caused less trouble. Relations among her sister, her brother, and herself improved remarkably, and the alcohol abuse substantially diminished. During a 1-year follow-up visit, Roberta reported that she had graduated from a vocational training program and was beginning college course work toward a bachelor's degree.

CONCLUSION

Throughout this chapter we have provided a substantial amount of information about personal, cultural, social, and environmental factors influencing the mental health of Indian women today. Our main intention was to draw attention to the role that culture and gender play in the etiology, effects, and treatment of psychological problems of Indian women. These problems are likely to continue well into the future unless appropriate and adequate interventions aimed at the health promotion of Indian women and their children are employed.

We suggest that therapists learn to appreciate the strengths (e.g., long-term coping mechanisms of victimized women) and adaptations of Indian women. Many of the points raised in this chapter emphasize the importance of tradition and ritual in therapy and hint at the need for reexamination of the subtle dynamics of sex bias and sex-role and cultural stereotyping in therapy with Indian women. We do believe, however, that much can be accomplished by increasing the number of existing community care givers to better address women's needs.

In addition to progress in clinical practice and outreach, further research on the link between mental health and role conflict related to the family and the community is necessary. Given the extent to which Indian women are victims of physical and sexual violence, further research on anxiety disorders and posttraumatic stress disorder is also deemed appropriate. We also need to understand better the factors that contribute to depression and increase the relevance of diagnostic instruments with Indian women. Finally, we hope that this basic overview can serve as a guide for clinicians keenly interested in working with this population.

ACKNOWLEDGMENTS

We thank Winona Simms Shilling, Candace Fleming, Jean LaCourt, Linda Dyer, Phyllis Hersh, Junella Haynes, Lynn Mitchell, Emily Ozer, and Doug Johnson for their help in preparing this chapter. *Migwetch!*

NOTES

1. The designator "American Indian" refers to all North American native people, including Indians, Alaska Natives, Aleut, Eskimos, Metis, or mixed bloods. Throughout this chapter, the terms "American Indian," "Indian," and "Native American" are used interchangeably to denote these varied peoples from distinctive and diverse tribes.

2. The Indian Health Service (IHS) uses a statistical code list which includes over 900 tribes, bands, and Alaska Native villages.

3. See LaFromboise (1988) for information on Indian family and per capita income, educational attainment, and related problems; and Snipp and Aytac (1990) for further information on the labor force participation on Indian women.

4. A *berdache*, according to Roscoe (1991) is a female or male American Indian who engages in cross-dressing and fulfills an alternative gender role in tribal societies.

5. See Ryan (1988) for a description of a recent Navajo Kinaalda ceremony.

6. A sing is a group of prayers and rituals engaged in to remove or neutralize the cause of disharmony and return harmony. A sing may include curing chants, dry paintings, massage and heat treatments, sweatbaths, ceremonial baths in yucca suds, public dances, and other procedures, depending upon the ailment and its cause (Kluckhohn & Leighton, 1962).

7. According to May et al. (1983), the rate for the Navajo tribe is comparable to that reported by the city of Seattle, Washington (1 per 750) and lower than the rates for Roubaix, France (1 per 700) and Gateberg, Sweden (1 per 600).

8. The case of Ms. Shimasani was previously presented in Porter and Berman (1988) and Berman (1989). Shimasani is the Navajo word for grandmother and is also used as a term of respect and affection for an older woman.

9. Before the missionaries came to the Southwest, the Chiricahua Apache buried their dead, though some bodies were cremated and the ashes buried or hidden away in pottery (National Parks Service, Tumacacori National Monument, Visitors Center Exhibit, 1989).

10. Traditionally, the Navajo "believed that most of the dead may return as ghosts, to the burial place or former dwelling, especially if the dead were not buried properly" (Nagel, 1988, p. 35). These ghosts were believed to be "especially malevolent towards their own relatives" (Leighton & Kluckhohn, 1948, p. 91).

REFERENCES

Ablon, G. (1964). Relocated American Indians in the San Francisco Bay area: Social interaction and Indian identity. *Human Organization, 23,* 296–304.

Allen, J. R. (1973). Psychosocial tasks of the Plains Indians of western Oklahoma. *American Journal of Orthopsychiatry, 43,* 368–375.

Allen, P. G. (1986). *The sacred hoop.* Boston: Beacon Press.

Allen, P. G. (1991). *Grandmothers of the light: A medicine woman's sourcebook.* Boston: Beacon Press.

American Psychiatric Association. (1987). *Diagnostic and statistical manual of mental disorders* (3rd ed., rev.). Washington, DC: Author.

Ashby, M. R., Gilchrist, L. D., & Miramontez, A. (1987). Group treatment for sexually abused American Indian adolescents. *Social Work with Groups, 10,* 21–32.

Assault on the peaceful: Indian child abuse. (1988, December 26). *Newsweek,* p. 31.

Bass, E., & Davis, L. (1988). *Courage to heal: A guide for women survivors of child sexual abuse.* New York: Harper & Row.

Beiser, M., & Attneave, C. (1982). Mental disorders among Native American children: Rates and risk periods for entering treatment. *American Journal of Psychiatry, 139*(2), 193–198.

Bennett, S.K. (1991). *American Indian client preferences for counselor characteristics.* Unpublished dissertation, University of Oklahoma, Norman, OK.

Bennett, S. K., & BigFoot-Sipes, D. S. (1991). American Indian and White college student preference for counselor characteristics. *Journal of Counseling Psychology, 38,* 440–445.

Bergman, R. L. (1974). Paraprofessionals in Indian mental health programs. *Psychiatric Annals, 4,* 76–84.

Berman, J. R. S. (1989). A view from rainbow bridge: Feminist therapy meets Changing Woman. *Women and Therapy, 8*(4), 65–78.

Berman, J. R. S. (1990). Problems of overlapping relationships in the political community. In H. Lerman & N. Porter (Eds.), *Feminist ethics in psychotherapy* (pp. 106–110). New York: Springer.

Berry, J. W., Wintrob, R. M., Sindell, P. S., & Mawhinney, T. A. (1982). Psychological adaptation to culture change among the James Bay Cree. *Naturaliste Canadian, 109,* 965–975.

Biernoff, M. A. (1969). *Report on Pueblo Indian suicide.* Unpublished manuscript, Indian Health Service, Albuquerque, NM.

BigFoot-Sipes, D., Dauphinais, P., LaFromboise, T., Bennett, S., & Rowe, W. (1992). American Indian secondary school students' preference for counselors. *Journal of Multicultural Counseling and Development, 20,* 113–122.

Blackwood, E. (1984). Sexuality and gender in certain Native American tribes: The case of the cross gender females. *Signs: Journal of Women in Culture and Society, 10,* 27–42.

Brown, J. E. (1953). *The sacred pipe.* Norman, OK: University of Oklahoma Press.

Canadian Broadcasting Company (Producer). (1990). *Circle of healing* [Film]. (Available from CBC Enterprises, Education Sales, Box 500, Station A, Toronto, Ontario M5W1FC.)

Carpenter, A., Lyons, C., & Miller, W. (1985). Peer-managed self-control program for prevention of alcohol abuse in American Indian high school students: A pilot evaluation study. *International Journal of the Addictions, 20,* 299–310.

Chance, N. (1962). Conceptual and methodological problems in cross-cultural health research. *American Journal of Public Health, 52,* 410–417.

Dana, R. H. (1986). Personality assessment and Native Americans. *Journal of Personality Assessment, 50,* 480–500.

Davis, L. (1990). *Courage to heal workbook: For men and women survivors of child sexual abuse.* New York: Harper & Row.

Dixon, J. K. (1989). *Group treatment for Native American women survivors of incest.* Billings, MT: Indian Health Service and Mental Health Program.

Edwards, E. D., & Edwards, M. E. (1984). Group work practice with American Indians. *Social Work with Groups, 7,* 7–21.

Everett, F., Proctor, N., & Cartmell, B. (1983). Providing psychological services to American Indian children and families. *Professional Psychology: Research and Practice, 14,* 588–603.

Fischer, M. (1983). Adolescent adjustment after incest. *School Psychology International, 4,* 217–222.

Fleming, C. (1989, August). *Mental health treatment of American Indian women.* Paper presented at the meeting of the American Psychological Association, New Orleans, LA.

Fleming, C., & Manson, S. (1990). Native American women. In R. Engs (Ed.), *Women: Alcohol and other drugs* (pp. 143–148). Dubuque, IA: Kendall/Hunt.

French, L. A. (1976). Social problems among Cherokee females: A study of cultural ambivalence and role identity. *American Journal of Psychoanalysis, 36,* 163–169.

French, L. A. (1989). Native American alcoholism: A transcultural counseling perspective. *Counseling Psychology Quarterly, 2,* 153–166.

Goldwasser, H. D., & Badger, L. W. (1989). Utility of the psychiatric screen among the Navajo of Chinle: A fourth-year clerkship experience. *American Indian and Alaska Native Mental Health Research, 3*(1), 6–15.

Gray, E., & Cosgrove, J. (1985). Ethnocentric perception of childrearing practices in protective services. *Child Abuse and Neglect, 9,* 389–396.

Green, R. (1980). Native American women. *Signs: Journal of Women in Culture and Society, 6,* 248–267.

Green, R. (1983). *Native American women: A contextual bibliography.* Bloomington: Indiana University Press.

Group for the Advancement of Psychiatry. (1989). *Suicide and ethnicity in the United States.* New York: Brunner/Mazel.

Guilmet, G. M., & Whited, D. L. (1987). Cultural lessons for clinical mental health practice the Puyallup tribal community. *American Indian and Alaska Native Mental Health Research, 1*(2), 32–49.

Hall, E. T. (1973). *The silent language.* New York: Anchor Books.

Harris, M. B., Begay, C., & Page, P. (1989). Activities, family relationships and feelings about aging in a multicultural elderly sample. *International Journal of Aging and Human Development, 29,* 103–117.

Heath, D. B. (1983). Alcohol use among North American Indians: A cross-cultural survey of patterns and problems. In R. G. Smart & F. B. Glasner (Eds.), *Research advances in alcohol and drug problems* (pp. 343–396). New York: Plenum Press.

Hill, A. (1989). Treatment and prevention of alcoholism in the Native American family. In *Alcoholism and substance abuse in special populations* (pp. 247–265). Rockville, MD: Aspen.

Ho, M. K. (1987). Family therapy with American Indians and Alaska natives. In *Family therapy with ethnic minorities* (pp. 69–122). Newbury Park, CA: Sage.

Holden, G. W., Botvin, G. J., & Orlandi, M. A. (1989). American Indian youth and substance abuse: Tobacco use problems, risk factors and preventive interventions. *Health Education Research, Theory and Practice, 4,* 137–144.

Howard-Pitney, B., LaFromboise, T., Basil, M., September, B., & Johnson, M. (1992). Psychological and social indicators of suicide ideation and suicide attempts in Zuni adolescents. *Journal of Consulting and Clinical Psychology, 60,* 473–476.

Indian Health Service. (1988). *A progress report on Indian alcoholism activities.* Rockville, MD: U.S. Department of Health and Human Services, Public Health Service.

Indian Health Service. (1991). *Indian women's health care: Consensus statement.* Rockville, MD: U.S. Department of Health and Human Services, Public Health Service.

Ivey, A. E. (1991). *Developmental strategies for helpers.* Pacific Grove, CA: Brooks/Cole.

Jacobs, G., Dauphinais, P., Gross, S., & Guzman, L. (1991). *American Psychological Association site visitation report.* Washington, DC: American Psychological Association.

Jaimes, M. A. (1982). Towards a new image of American Indian women. *Journal of American Indian Education, 22*(1), 18–32.

Jenks, K. (1986). "Changing woman": The Navajo therapist goddess. *Psychological Perspectives, 17*(2), 202–221.

Jilek, W. G. (1978). Native renaissance: The survival and revival of indigenous therapeutic ceremonials among North American Indians. *Transcultural Psychiatric Research Review, 15*, 117–147.

Jilek, W. G. (1982). *Indian healing: Shamanistic ceremonialism in the Pacific Northwest today.* Baline, WA: Hancock House.

Kahn, M. W. (1982). Cultural clash and psychopathology in three aboriginal cultures. *Academic Psychology Bulletin, 4*, 553–561.

Kahn, M. W., Lejero, L., Antone, M., Francisco, D., & Manuel, J. (1988). An indigenous community mental health service on the Tohono O'odham (Papago) Indian reservation: Seventeen years later. *American Journal of Community Psychology, 16*, 369–379.

Keller, M. B., Labori, P. W., Endicott, J., Coryell, W., & Klerman, C. L. (1983). "Double depression": Two year follow-up. *American Journal of Psychiatry, 140*(6), 689–694.

Kluckhohn, C., & Leighton, D. C. (1962). *The Navaho* (rev. ed.). Garden City, NY: Anchor.

LaFromboise, T. D. (1988a). American Indian mental health policy. *American Psychologist, 43*, 388–397.

LaFromboise, T. D. (1988b). *Cultural and cognitive considerations in the coping of American Indian women in higher education.* Unpublished manuscript, School of Education, Stanford University, Stanford, CA.

LaFromboise, T. D. (1989). *Circles of women: Professionalization training for American Indian women.* Newton, MA: Women's Educational Equity Act Press.

LaFromboise, T. D. (1991). *American Indian life skills development curriculum.* Palo Alto, CA: Stanford Center for Research in Disease Prevention.

LaFromboise, T. D., Coleman, H., & Hernandez, A. (1991). Development and factor structure of the Cross-Cultural Counseling Inventory—Revised. *Professional Psychology: Research and Practice, 22*, 380–388.

LaFromboise, T. D., & Dixon, D. N. (1981). American Indian perception of trustworthiness in a counseling interview. *Journal of Counseling Psychology, 28*, 135–139.

LaFromboise, T., & Fleming, C. (1990). Keeper of the fire: A profile of Carolyn Attneave. *Journal of Counseling and Development, 68*, 537–547.

LaFromboise, T. D., Heyle, A. M., & Ozer, E. J. (1990). Changing and diverse roles of women in American Indian cultures. *Sex Roles, 22*, 455–476.

LaFromboise, T. D., & Howard-Pitney, B. (1994). The Zuni life skills development curriculum: A collaborative approach to curriculum development. *Journal of the National Center Monograph Series*, 4(4), 98–121.

LaFromboise, T. D., & Low, K. G. (1989). American Indian children and adolescents. In J. Gibbs, & L. Hwang (Eds.), *Children of color* (pp. 114–147). San
Francisco: Jossey-Bass.

LaFromboise, T., & Rowe, W. (1983). Skills training for bicultural competence:
Rationale and application. *Journal of Counseling Psychology*, 30, 589–595.

LaFromboise, T., Trimble, J., & Mohatt, G. (1990). Counseling intervention and
American Indian tradition: An integrative approach. *Counseling Psychologist*,
18, 628–654.

Lake, M. G. (1991). *Native healer: Initiation into an ancient art*. Wheaton, IL:
Quest Books.

Landes, R. (1971). *The Ojibwa woman*. New York: W. W. Norton.

Leap, W. L. (1981). American Indian language maintenance. *Annual Review of
Anthropology*, 10, 271–280.

Leighton, D., & Kluckhohn, C. (1948). *Children of the people*. Cambridge, MA:
Harvard University Press.

Lerman, H., & Porter, N. (Eds.). (1990). *Feminist ethics in psychotherapy*. New
York: Springer.

Lester, G., & Lester, D. (1971). *Suicide: The gamble with death*. Englewood Cliffs,
NJ: Prentice-Hall.

Levy, J. E., & Kunitz, S. J. (1974). *Indian drinking: Navajo practices and Anglo
American theories*. New York: Wiley.

Lewis, O. (1941). Manly-hearted women among the Northern Piegan. *American
Anthropologist*, 43, 173–187.

Lewis, R. (1984). *The strengths of Indian families: Proceedings of the Indian Child Abuse
Conference*. Tulsa, OK: National Indian Child Abuse Center.

Locust, C. S. (1985). American Indian beliefs concerning health and unwellness.
Monograph of the Native American Research and Training Center. Tucson: University of Arizona.

Locust, C. S. (1987). *Hopi beliefs about unwellness and handicaps* (Monograph of
the Native American Research and Training Center). Tucson: University
of Arizona.

Lofgren, D. E. (1981). Art therapy and cultural difference. *American Journal of Art
Therapy*, 21(1), 25–30.

Longclaws, L. C., Barnes, C., Grieve, L., & Dumoff, R. (1980). Alcohol and
drug use among the Brokenbend Ojibwa. *Journal of Studies on Alcohol*,
41, 21–36.

Lujan, C., DeBruyn, L. M., May, P. A., & Bird, M. E. (1989). Profile of abused
and neglected American Indian children in the Southwest. *Child Abuse and
Neglect*, 13, 449–461.

Lurie, N. O. (1972). Indian women: A legacy of freedom. In R. L. Lacopi & B. L.
Fontana (Eds.), *Look to the mountaintop* (pp. 29–36). San Jose, CA: Gousha.

Lynch, R. (1986). Women in Northern Paiute politics. *Signs: Journal of Women in
Culture and Society*, 11, 352–366.

Manson, S. M., Beals, J., Dick, R. W., & Duclos, C. (1989). Risk factors for
suicide among Indian adolescents at a boarding school. *Public Health Reports*,
104, 609–614.

Manson, S., Shore, J., Baron, A., Ackerson, L., & Neligh, G. (1992). Alcohol abuse and dependence among American Indians. In J. E. Helzer & G. J. Canino (Eds.), *Alcoholism in North America, Europe, and Asia* (pp. 113–130). Oxford, England: Oxford University Press.

Manson, S., Shore, J., & Bloom, J. (1985). The depressive experience in American Indian communities: A challenge for psychiatric theory and diagnosis. In A. Klienman & B. Goods (Eds.), *Culture and depression* (pp. 331–368). Berkeley: University of California Press.

Manson, S., Shore, J., Bloom, J., Keepers, G., & Neligh, G. (1987). Alcohol abuse and major affective disorders: Advances in epidemiologic research among American Indians. In D. Spiegler, D. Tate, S. Aitken, & C. Christian (Eds.), *Alcohol use and abuse among ethnic minorities* (Research Monograph No. 18, pp. 291–300, DHHS Publication No. ADM 89-1435). Rockville, MD: National Institute on Alcohol Abuse and Alcoholism.

Manson, S. M., Walker, R. D., & Kivlahan, D. R. (1987). Psychiatric assessment and treatment of American Indians and Alaska Natives. *Hospital and Community Psychiatry, 38*, 165–173.

Massara, E. B., & Stunkard, A. S. (1979). A method of quantifying cultural ideals of beauty and the obese. *International Journal of Obesity, 3*, 149–152.

Massey, J. T. (1967). *Suicide in the United States, 1950–1964: Vital and health statistics* (National Center for Health Statistics, Ser. 20, No. 5). Washington, DC: U.S. Government Printing Office.

Matchett, W. F. (1972). Repeated hallucinatory experiences as a part of the mourning process among Hopi Indian women. *Psychiatry, 35*, 185–194.

May, P. A. (1982). Substance abuse and American Indians: Prevalence and susceptibility. *International Journal of Addictions, 17*, 1185–1209.

May, P. A., Hymbaugh, K. J., Aase, J. M., & Samet, J. M. (1983). Epidemiology of fetal alcohol syndrome among American Indians of the Southwest. *Social Biology, 30*, 374–387.

McCone, R. C. (1968). Death and the persistence of basic personality structure among the Lakota. *Plains Anthropologist, 13*, 305–309.

Metcalf, A. (1976). From schoolgirl to mother: The effects of education on Navajo women. *Social Problems, 23*, 535–544.

Metoyer, C. (1979). The Native American woman. In E. Snyder (Ed.), *The study of women: Enlarging perspectives on social reality* (pp. 329–335). New York: Harper & Row.

Meyer, D. J. (1991). The medical evaluation of child sex abuse. *The IHS Primary Care Provider, 16*(2), 17–25.

Morey, S. M., & Gilliam, O. J. (Eds.). (1972). *Respect for life.* New York: Waldorf Press.

Moss, R. N., & Goldstien, G. S. (1973). An encounter experience among the Navajo. *Social Change: Ideas and Applications, 3*(1), 3–6.

Nagel, J. K. (1988). Unresolved grief and mourning in Navajo women. *American Indian and Alaska Native Mental Health Research, 2*(2), 32–40.

National Institute on Alcohol Abuse and Alcoholism. (1981). *Alcohol and health* (4th ed.). Washington, DC: U.S. Government Printing Office.

Niethammer, C. (1977). *Daughters of the earth.* New York: Macmillan.

Oetting, E. R., Edwards, B. A., Goldstein, G. S., & Mason, V. G. (1980). Drug use among adolescents of five southwestern Native American tribes. *International Journal of Addictions, 15*, 439–445.

Old Dog Cross, P. (1982). Sexual abuse: A new threat to the Native American woman: An overview. *Listening Post, 6*(2), 18.

Opler, M. E. (1946). The creative role of Shamanism in Mescalero Apache mythology. *Journal of American Folklore, 59,* 268–281.

O'Sullivan, M. J., Peterson, P. D., Cox, G. B., & Kirkeby, J. (1989). Ethnic populations: Community mental health services ten years later. *American Journal of Community Psychology, 17,* 17–30.

Ozer, E. (1986). *Health status of minority women* (A summary and response to the DHHS report of the Secretary's Task Force on Black and Minority Health). Washington, DC: American Psychological Association.

Porter, N., & Berman, J. R. S. (1988, May). *Incest and Native Americans: Rebuilding the family.* Paper presented at the University of New Mexico conference on Psychotherapeutic Interventions with Hispanic and Native American Children and Families, Albuquerque.

Powers, M. (1986). *Oglala women: Myth, ritual, and reality.* Chicago: University of Chicago Press.

Primeaux, M. H. (1977). American Indian health care practices: A cross cultural perspective. *Nursing Clinics of North America, 12,* 55–65.

Queen, S. A., & Habenstein, R. W. (1967). *The family in various cultures.* Philadelphia: J. B. Lippincott.

Red Horse, J. G. (1980). American Indian elders: Unifiers of Indian families. *Social Casework, 61,* 490–493.

Red Horse, J. G. (1981). American Indian families: Research perspectives. In F. Hoffman (Ed.), *American Indian family: Strengths and stressors* (pp. 1–11). Isleta, NM: American Indian Social Research and Development Associates.

Red Horse, J. G., Lewis, R., Feit, M., & Decker, J. (1978). Family behavior of urban American Indians. *Social Casework, 59,* 67–72.

Reichard, G. A. (1950). *Navajo religion: A study of symbolism* (Bollinger Series XVIII). New York: Pantheon.

Rhinehart, L. M., & Engelhorn, P. (1984). The full rainbow: Symbol of individuation. *Arts in Psychotherapy, 11*(1), 37–42.

Roberts, S. S. (1989). Indians battle fetal alcohol syndrome. *Journal of the National Institute of Health Research, 1,* 32–36.

Roscoe, W. (1991). *The Zuni man–woman..* Albuquerque: University of New Mexico Press.

Rosen, L. W., Shafer, C. L., Dummer, G. M., Cross, L. K., Deuman, G. W., & Malmberg, S. R. (1988). Prevalence of pathogenic weight-control behaviors among Native American women and girls. *International Journal of Eating Disorders, 7,* 807–811.

Rueveni, U. (1984). Network intervention for crisis resolution: An introduction. *Family Therapy, 6*(2), 65–67.

Ryan, B. (1988). Kinaalda: The pathway to Navajo womanhood. *Winds of Change, 3*(3), 74–77.

Sandefur, G. D., & McKinnell, T. (1986). American Indian intermarriage. *Social Science Research, 15,* 347–371.

Schacht, A. J., Tafoya, N., & Mirabla, K. (1989). Home-based therapy with American Indian families. *American Indian and Alaska Native Mental Health Research, 3*(2), 27–42.

Schinke, S. P. (1982). A school based model for teenage pregnancy prevention. *Social Work in Education, 4*(2), 34–52.

Schinke, S. P., Orlandi, M. A., Botvin, G. J., Gilchrist, L. D., Trimble, J. E., & Locklear, V. S. (1988). Preventing substance abuse among American Indian adolescents: A bicultural competence skills approach. *Journal of Counseling Psychology*, *35*, 87–90.

Schinke, S. P., Schilling, R. F., Gilchrist, L. D., Ashby, M. R., & Kitajima, E. (1987). Pacific Northwest American youth and smokeless tobacco use. *International Journal of Addiction*, *22*, 881–884.

Schlegal, A. (1973). The adolescent socialization of the Hopi girl. *Ethnology*, *12*, 449–462.

Schoenfeld, P., Halevy-Martini, J., Hemley-Van der Velden, E., & Ruhf, L. (1985). Network therapy: An outcome study of twelve social networks. *Journal of Community Psychology*, *13*, 281–287.

Shangreaux, V., Pleskac, D., & Freeman, W. (1987). *Strengthening Native American families: A family systems model curriculum.* Unpublished manuscript, Native American Adolescent Research Project, Lincoln Indian Center, Lincoln, NE.

Slobodin, R. (1970). Kutchin concepts of reincarnation. *Western Canadian Journal of Anthropology*, *2*, 67–79.

Snipp, C. M., & Aytac, I. A. (1990). The labor force participation of American Indian women. *Research in Human Capital and Development*, *6*, 189–211.

Snow, J. T., & Harris, M. B. (1989). Disordered eating in Southwestern Pueblo Indians and Hispanics. *Journal of Adolescence*, *12*, 329–336.

Speck, R. V., & Speck, J. L. (1984). Family networking in the 1980s: A postscript. *Family Therapy*, *6*(2), 136–137.

Stevenson, I. (1975). The belief and cases related to reincarnation among the Haida. *Journal of Anthropological Research*, *31*, 364–375.

Sue, S., Allen, D., & Conaway, L. (1978). The responsiveness and equality of mental health care of Chicanos and Native Americans. *American Journal of Community Psychology*, *6*, 137–145.

Sue, S., & Zane, N. (1987). The role of culture and cultural technique in psychotherapy: A critique and reformulation. *American Psychologist*, *42*, 37–45.

Sullivan, T. (1983). Native children in treatment: Clinical, social and cultural issues. *Journal of Child Care*, *1*, 75–94.

Tafoya, T. (1989). Circles and cedar: Native Americans and family therapy. *Minorities and family therapy* (pp. 71–96). Binghamton, NY: Haworth House.

Talmon, M. (1991). *Single session therapy.* San Francisco: Jossey-Bass.

Thomas, R. K. (1981). The history of North American Indian alcohol use as a community based phenomenon. *Journal of Studies on Alcohol*, *9*, 29–39.

Timpson, J., McKay, S., Kakegamic, S., Roundhead, D., Cohen, C., & Matewapit, G. (1988). Depression in a Native Canadian in Northwestern Ontario: Sadness, grief or spiritual illness? *Canada's Mental Health*, *36*(2–3), 5–8.

Topper, M. D. (1987). The traditional Navajo medicine man: Therapist, counselor, and community leader. *Journal of Psychoanalytic Anthropology*, *10*, 217–249.

Trimble, J. E. (1981). Value differentials and their importance in counseling American Indians. In P. Pedersen, J. Draguns, W. Lonner, & J. Trimble (Eds.), *Counseling across cultures* (pp. 203–226). Honolulu: University Press of Hawaii.

Tyler, F. B., Sussewell, D. R., & Williams-McCoy, J. (1985). Ethnic validity in psychotherapy. *Psychotherapy*, *22*, 311–320.

Udall, L. (1977). *Me and mine: The life story of Helen Sekequaptewa.* Tucson: University of Arizona Press.

U.S. Bureau of the Census. (1983). *1980 census of the population: Characteristics of the population* (Ser. PC80-1-B1). Washington, DC: U.S. Government Printing Office.

U.S. Bureau of the Census. (1991, March 11). Census bureau completes distribution of 1990 redistricting tabulations to states. *United States Department of Commerce News.* Washington, DC: Author.

U.S. Congress, Office of Technology and Assessment. (1990). *Indian adolescent mental health* (OTA-H-446). Washington, DC: U.S. Government Printing Office.

U.S. Department of Health and Human Services. (1985). *Report of the Secretary's Task Force on Black and Minority Health.* Washington, DC: U.S. Government Printing Office.

U.S. Department of Health and Human Services. (1989). *Indian Health Service trends in Indian health.* Washington, DC: U.S. Government Printing Office.

Welch, D. (1987). American Indian women: Reaching beyond the myth. In C. Calloway (Ed.), *New directions in American Indian history* (pp. 31–48). Norman: University of Oklahoma Press.

White, R. (1977). *Child abuse and neglect study.* Baltimore: Department of Maternal and Child Health, John Hopkins University.

White, R., & Cornely, D. (1981). Navajo child abuse and neglect study: A comparison group examination of abuse and neglect of Navajo children. *Child Abuse and Neglect, 5,* 9–17.

Whitehead, H. (1981). The bow and burden strap. In S. Ortner & H. Whitehead (Eds.), *Sexual meanings: The cultural construction of gender and sexuality* (pp. 80–115). Cambridge, England: Cambridge University Press.

Whittaker, J. O. (1962). Alcohol and the Standing Rock Sioux tribe. *Quarterly Journal of Studies on Alcohol, 23,* 80–90.

Whittaker, J. O. (1982). Alcohol and the Standing Rock Sioux tribe: A twenty-year follow-up study. *Journal of Studies on Alcohol, 43,* 191–200.

Wischlaz, C., Lane, J., & Kempe, C. H. (1978). Indian child welfare: A community team approach to protective services. *Child Abuse and Neglect, 2,* 29–35.

Witt, S. H. (1974). Native women today: Sexism and the Indian woman. *Civil Rights Digest, 6*(3), 29–35.

Wong, H., Comas-Díaz, L., Kennedy, C., LaFromboise, T., & Miyahira, S. (1987, August). *Psychotherapy with ethnic minority clients: Cross-cultural communications and understanding.* Workshop conducted at the annual meeting of the American Psychological Association, New York, NY.

Zak, N. (1984). Sacred and legendary women of native America. *Wildfire, 1*(1), 12–15.

3

Asian and Asian American Women: Historical and Political Considerations in Psychotherapy

Carla K. Bradshaw

Asian and Asian American women residing in the United States are a highly diverse group comprising individuals who differ in ethnicity, cultural background, socioeconomic status, acculturation, education, marital status, and the generation of immigrants to which they belong. In this chapter I seek to provide readers with a greater understanding of these women's lives, which involves an appreciation of the subtle as well as the overt political, economic, and social pressures that emanate from their particular Asian culture as it exists in the United States, as well as those imposed on them by the majority culture of the United States.

Although the subject of this chapter is women of Asian background living in the United States, out of respect for some immigrants, especially recent immigrants, who do not identify themselves as American, I sometimes use the term "Asian" in addition to the term "Asian American." I also want to acknowledge the problem of overinclusively referring to people from very diverse cultural backgrounds using only one category: Asian Americans.

The term "Asian" as a racial category encompasses vast and diverse populations, cultures, and extensive geographic territories. In addition to the peoples of China, Japan, Korea, India, Southeast Asia, and South Asia, "Asian" also refers to Pacific Islanders, which include the culturally heterogeneous peoples of Micronesia, Melanesia, Polynesia, and the U.S. Hawaiian Islands. Essentially, "Asian," as a descriptive term, is grossly overinclusive and, for purposes of cultural understanding, meaningless. The conceptual simplicity and economy of language achieved by using a single racial category to reference such diverse peoples, cultures, and ethnic variations betrays true appreciation for the substantial differences among these peoples.

Highlighting the Eurocentric use of the term "Asian" illustrates two points: the irrational nature of racial categories and the ignorance it encourages. Spickard (1989) points out that there is more homogeneity between races on dimensions of physical attributes than within races. Therefore, racial designations based on phenotype alone are irrational. Given the vast geographic regions designated as "Asian," clearly the designation is not made on the basis of cultural similarity. If the term "Asian" lacks both physical or cultural homogeneity, it is essentially meaningless. How, then, can these people be characterized meaningfully? By clearly defining at the outset the particular geographic region or culture addressed, it is possible to gain clarity while accurately depicting similarities across ethnicities. In order to do justice to this heterogeneity, the temptation to reduce culturally significant themes to manageable proportions by oversimplification and overinclusiveness must be transcended. True cultural understanding and multicultural psychotherapy requires tolerance of the messiness inherent in complexity.

In this chapter I present information about several areas that affect the psychology of Asian American women. The most important factors are (1) the cultural values, beliefs, and tendencies immigrants bring with them from their former homes in Asia and the ways these are passed down through the generations and (2) the way Asian immigrants interact with the culture they face once they arrive: how they are treated, and how they feel about their new culture and former culture. Because Asians have been immigrating to the United States for close to 150 years there is already a history of the interaction of these two factors; therefore I begin this chapter by outlining the history of the immigration of Asians, and Asian women in particular, to this country.

Being part of an ethnic minority in the United States, Asian women must somehow consolidate their old culture with their new one. The "Society and Family" section of this chapter outlines the cultures from which Asian women come. Their culture of origin then affects the way they cope. Unfortunately, in the United States, Asians often face negative ethnic stereotyping, a history of economic exploitation, and a powerful pressure that encourages them to forsake their culture and assimilate, which can lead to conflict with their families. A mental health professional who works with Asian American women will need to understand the interactions of these factors in their lives in order be truly helpful.

IMMIGRATION

Demographics

Who are the "Asians" in America? Because of the removal of certain legal restrictions, the Asian population is one of the fastest growing minority groups in the United States, having increased 143% in the decade between 1970 and 1980 (Takaki, 1989). Half of all immigrants entering the United States each year are Asian (Takaki, 1989). In 1985, the Asian population, over five million and representing 2.1% of the population included 1,079,000 Chinese, 1,052,000 Filipinos, 766,000 Japanese, 634,000 Vietnamese, 542,000 Koreans, 526,000 Asian Indians, 161,000 Cambodians, 70,000 Laotians, 60,000 Hmong, 10,000 Mien, and 169,000 other Asians (Gardner, Robey, & Smith, 1985). The perception that Asians in the United States are either Chinese, Japanese, Filipino, or Korean is no longer true, as these statistics illustrate. Other Asian populations are now resident here, although they may remain less visible to much of mainstream America. The new immigrant groups, which have not received much academic attention or media coverage, include Southeast Asians (Indonesians, Vietnamese, Cambodian Khmer, Laotians, Thais, and Malaysians) and South Asians, who include among others those from India, Pakistan, and Bangladesh. (See Jayakar, Chapter 6, this volume, and Tien, Chapter 17, this volume, for discussions of Indian women and Southeast Asian refugee women in the United States.)

Early Immigration History

The presence of Asians in American history dates back to about 1848 when the first wave of voluntary immigration occurred among Chinese seeking fortunes in gold. Subsequent importation of Chinese laborers to the United States was recommended by the U.S. government for the establishment of a transcontinental railroad and to cultivate lands in California, which had been newly acquired from war with Mexico. The economic necessity to cultivate and to industrialize the western United States, the ready availability of cheap Asian laborers, and the racist views of the Asian as inferior yet diligent and passive functioned to fuel the demand for Asian workers. This in turn dictated a foreign policy and a domestic agenda that encouraged immigration.

The use of Asian workforces to support the dreams of capitalism engendered the problems of controlling and suppressing the workforce in order to keep labor costs from rising. The technique of importing diverse groups of Asians could be used to control the immigrant Asian workforce, and these groups could also be pitted against the immigrant White work force in the manner of an "industrial reserve army" (Takaki, 1989). The presence of intraracial competition among the diverse Asian cultures in the United States and the interracial discord between White and Asian immigrants has its roots in basic economic and corporate strategies intended to suppress labor costs: competition in an atmosphere intentionally hostile to creating comfort or permanence. Similarly, the various immigration laws and naturalization laws also functioned to protect the economic interests of the prevailing Eurocentric interests. These various forms of oppression have ramifications for Asian women immigrants because they faced the problems of sexism within their own cultures and also the racism and sexism of the dominant White culture.

Early Immigration of Women

Over 90% of the initial Asian immigrants were men (Kim & Otani, 1983), because of legal restrictions and a cultural tendency for women to remain at home; therefore immigration of women increased slowly and only substantially after 1965 (i.e., after the new Immigration Act). The combination of exclusion and antimiscegenation laws acted to suppress the presence of Asian women in the United States to such a degree that the imbalance in the gender ratio was still high as recently as 1970 (Kim & Otani, 1983). The 1980 census on Asian American women indicated that half of Asian immigrants were women, and many of these women were highly educated and seeking social conditions more conducive to realizing personal achievement and escape from repressive regimes. However, these data likely do not adequately recognize the educational and economic conditions of the illegal Asian immigrant women and Southeast Asian refugee women who are also immigrating in larger numbers.

Legal restrictions on the immigration of Asian women, laws that revoked citizenship for any U.S. woman who married an "alien ineligible for citizenship" (the 1922 Cable Act), and the artificial community of single Asian men created by these laws influenced to a great degree both the status and the role of Asian women when they finally did arrive. Many of the earliest Chinese and Japanese women in the United States were prostitutes, who had been lured or sold into sexual servitude (Kim & Otani, 1983). Chinese women were sometimes sold by relatives to raise money to pay debts or to secure the price of a bride for sons who, in the Confucian ethic, were more valuable than daughters for the patrilinial perpetuation of the family. When they could not be purchased outright, women and girls were lured by tales of marriage and wealth, or simply kidnapped.

In the United States, these Chinese prostitutes were regarded as daughters who, out of loyalty and filial piety, were sacrificing their bodies in order to provide for the security of their parents and brothers (Kim & Otani, 1983). The moral opprobrium with which prostitution is generally regarded today was mitigated by the economic context in which it existed. Prostitutes were typically indentured for four to five years without wages, after which they generally turned to employment as seamstresses, domestic servants, laundresses, cooks, laborers, miners, and rooming house operators (Yung, 1986). The transition from sexual object to worker illustrates one possible origin for the stereotyped view of the Asian as either highly erotic or sexless (M. P. P. Root, personal communication, April, 1991).

Unlike Chinese women, most Japanese women had been brought to America by Japanese men (Kim & Otani, 1983), lured by myths, sold by husbands for profit or to resolve debts, or intentionally for use as prostitutes. The relative lucrativeness of sexual labor in comparison to agricultural work provided incentive. However, for the Japanese, the enactment of strict measures by the Japanese government to end emigration of prostitutes out of Japan and the phenomenon of Japanese "picture brides" between 1907 and 1924, which encouraged the growth of family communities in the United States, reduced reliance on prostitution.

The procurement of "picture brides" was an extension of the tradition of arranged marriages, and involved the exchange of photographs. If the marriage was approved by both families, the woman emigrated from Japan, already the man's legal wife. Unfortunately for these women, they were often lured by false promises of wealth. Even the images of their prospective spouses were at times falsified by the men, who would use old pictures or pictures of better-looking relatives or friends. However, the immigrants' ability to establish families played an integral role in stemming prostitution because the presence of Asian communities created a feeling of permanence and a context in which to revive traditional values and relationships. The artificial bachelor communities would not have maintained traditional values and cultural practices without the influence of women and families. The relative economic strength of Japan at the time in comparison to China, the Philippines, or Korea provided for an ability to influence immigration policies in the United States (Takaki, 1989). Thus while other Asian groups suffered under forced separation from family and the inability to create communities, the Japanese government effected provisions for "nonlaborers" to immigrate. Korea was annexed by Japan in 1909 and immigrants from Korea were classified by U.S. immigration officials as "Japanese." Korean women, therefore, could also immigrate as "picture brides" before 1924.

Although the early Filipino immigrants were single young men, the conditions that restricted the influx of women were somewhat different than those for Chinese and Japanese women. Filipinas were systematically excluded from importation because of the requirement that they perform hard physical labor, because of moral and cultural mores prohibiting travel by unchaperoned women, and because most married men chose not to emigrate with their wives. As "wards" of the United States, Filipinos were classified as "American nationals" and thus given status not awarded to other Asian immigrants, though not citizenship (Takaki, 1989). The men were able to invite their wives to join them if they wished. Consequently, the conditions that encouraged prostitution among the Chinese and to a lesser extent the Japanese women were not as operative for the Filipina immigrants. The Filipinas' traditional role as the managers of domestic finances and family responsibility enhanced their value because they increased the security of their families under conditions of impoverishment. Their ability to earn money through domestic work contributed to their importance (Kim & Otani, 1983).

The relative absence of prostitution in the history of Filipina immigration may also have been influenced heavily by Spanish Catholicism. While the indigenous beliefs of Philippine culture elevated women and women's influence above that generally prescribed for women in Confucian-based societies, with the coming of White men and the Catholic faith, female virtues of chastity, obedience, and self-sacrifice were emphasized. Similarly, the more repressive attitudes toward sexuality were enforced. Though the restrictions on women were likely increased as a result of these influences, ironically these very values may have proscribed the use of female sexual labor for economic gain during the early years of immigration.

The large-scale immigration of Korean women did not begin until about 1910 and 1924 when the first wave of immigrant Korean women was followed by 1,200 "picture brides." By 1940, several hundred more immigrants arrived, among them some women, most of whom returned to Korea. As with the other immigrant groups, the initial years were characterized by a critical shortage of women, which was to some degree addressed by the coming of the "picture brides." With prohibitions against interracial marriage, and with no substantial immigration of Korean women after 1940, the Korean community in the United States remained small. It was not until the Korean War that the population grew precipitously.

After the Korean War, from 1950 to 1965, women married to U.S. servicemen were the main immigrants. Unlike their predecessors, these were largely uneducated women for whom the transition was extremely difficult, resulting in culture shock, impoverishment, isolation, alienation, physical abuse, mental health problems, a high divorce rate, and poor occupational skills (Kim, 1977). Often brought to the United States by their American husbands, isolated from their own social supports and the Korean American community, these women were especially vulnerable to the psychological effects of displacement.

Since the 1950s, adoption of Korean children has become a major route of immigration. Female children far outnumber the male children adopted, with an estimated 60 boys for every 100 girls under the age of 5 (U.S. Bureau of the Census, 1980). It is likely that the cultural preference for sons created a larger population of girls available for adoption, though Yu (1987) offers an alternative suggestion: that American families preferred female adoptees, suggesting strongly the effect of gender stereotypes predicting that daughters will be less demanding on the parents. Though the research about development and maturation are yet scarce, some data indicate that outcomes have been favorable for these adoptees (Kim, 1977).

Special Populations of Immigrants

Wives of U.S. Military Men

Kim and Otani (1983) cite the statistics for the immigration of Asian wives of U.S. military personnel. Between the years 1947 and 1977, nearly 70,000 Asian women—predominantly Japanese—married to American military personnel came to the United States. The second large influx began in the

1950s, resulting in 63,241 Filipinas living in the United States two decades later. Currently, Asian wives of U.S. military men are mostly Filipina and Korean, with increasing numbers of Indochinese women immigrating since 1960. Clearly, the changes in the demographics correspond to U.S. military involvements in the Pacific. Since the majority of these women immigrate as a result of wartime experiences, they are subject to the overwhelming challenges of language and cultural adjustment, social isolation, racism, and the psychological sequalae of war trauma such as posttraumatic stress disorder (PTSD). Additional problems arising out of struggles to acculturate include depression, unemployment, and rejection by others of their nationality in response to their interracial partnerships. Despite these substantial difficulties, reports indicate that many of the interracial marriages meet these challenges adaptively (Kim & Otani, 1983).

Pacific Islanders

Although over several hundred years the Pacific Islands (South Sea Islands) have been invaded and inundated with European explorations and colonization, little information of substance has emerged that does not depend on a Eurocentric bias in reporting and interpreting cultures (Munoz, 1983). Colonization by various European powers including France, Germany, and Spain left a legacy of varying political and religious ideologies among the islands. The description that follows applies primarily to American Samoa, Guam, the Commonwealth of the Northern Marinas, and the U.S. Trust Territories of the Pacific.

Immigrants from the South Pacific islands have been brought by the tourist trade, entertainment industry, the military draft, and marriage. Many who have immigrated did so seeking better economic circumstances and educational opportunities. The concentration of the population in the United States remains close to the port of entry along the West Coast. While Hawaiians, Guamanians, and American Samoans are considered residents of U.S. territories and U.S. citizens, they do not have full voting rights or government representation. One familiar pattern cited by Munoz (1983) for Guamanians is that the first person who comes to the United States is usually a member of the military. Often immediate and extended family follow and tend to concentrate geographically near one another. Older Guamanians tend to marry other Guamanians, while subsequent generations are more likely to marry into other ethnic groups. Although there is some contact between family members living on the mainland and those on the island, by the third generation the original nuclear family is usually living on the mainland in close proximity to each other.

Recent Patterns of Immigration

Since the 1965 immigration law, which abolished the national origins quotas, a second wave of Asian immigration has ensued, producing both a large increase in the U.S. Asian population but also a change in its proportional composition (Gardner et al., 1985). The second wave has consisted of proportionately fewer Japanese and greater numbers of Chinese, Filipinos, Koreans, Asian Indians, and Southeast Asian refugees (Takaki, 1989). These new Asian immigrants have been generally better educated, tend to be urban rather than rural inhabitants, have included a significant number of professionals, and have immigrated as families rather than as single men (Takaki, 1989). Kim and Otani (1983) cite that the majority of Filipinos and Koreans in the United States today have less than 15 years of residence here. Many Filipinas migrate upon having completed extensive higher education, often in medical careers. Filipinos are more likely than any other ethnic group, including European Americans, to have specialization in a medical field (Almquist, 1989). Additionally, Filipinas statistically may have the highest level of education of all Asian groups in the United States, except perhaps Asian Indian women (Gardner et al., 1985).

The Indochinese, Taiwanese, South Koreans, Filipinos, and those from Hong Kong all have histories of colonization by various European powers, the withdrawal of which has had profound implications for employment, economy, security, and retention of wealth. Takaki notes that the effect of imperialism and colonization has been to create labor havens for foreign investors in the Pacific and Asian Pacific rim countries, which has resulted in wealthy, educated Asians leaving for more favorable business and political climates. Therefore, unlike their predecessors, the new wave of Asian immigrants are more likely to be professionals or technically trained persons of economic means rather than laborers. Half of the new immigrants are women, a large number of whom are wives of U.S. citizens. The current policies do not restrict the immigration of families to the extent experienced in the past. However, the character of the immigrating population continues to be affected greatly by the laws of immigration.

Woo (1989) cites census statistics showing that the Chinese population in the United States is the largest Asian group in the country and the Filipino population the second largest group. The majority of Chinese and Filipino women are foreign born. Many of these immigrants arrive with professional education—66% of Asians with doctorates in the United States have been trained abroad. Of foreign-educated health professionals most experience downward mobility in employment due to restrictive practices in the United States that exclude foreign training. The majority of these professionally trained immigrants are employed as menial laborers, in clerical jobs, or as technical auxiliaries.

Summary

The history of the immigration of Asian women illustrates the vast economic and political forces that were at work, both in their countries of origin as well as in their destination, the United States. These forces contributed to very differing conditions for the immigrant women, with important implications for subsequent acculturation experiences and psychological conditions. The various conditions, consequences, and demographics of the immigrating women also show that cultural identity, as internalized by the women themselves and ascribed by the majority culture, was highly relevant to subsequent economic success and community building. Additionally, mainstream attitudes toward particular groups of Asians fluctuated in response to international politics, as well as to internal economic forces. The changing attitudes toward the different Asian groups exerted an influence on both the opportunities for success and on the pressure acculturate and assimilate. The immigration history of the individual Asian woman is likely to have a great impact on the context and meaning of personal struggles, and therefore also on the perceived options for resolution of those struggles. The mental health professional who ignores or remains ignorant of the historical context will fail to understand the subtle internal conflicts that may contribute to the need for therapy, the values that guide the client's acceptance of various interventions, and important family of origin experiences, which take on extra importance as a result of acculturation processes subsequent to initial immigration. The historical context also informs the underlying gender-role expectations, which vary across Asian subgroups, which are influenced by family history, which may be in transition as a function of acculturation, and which may be at odds with traditional or family expectations.

DEVELOPMENT OF ETHNIC MINORITY IDENTITY

One of the most important and difficult tasks facing the racial minority is the consolidation of identity in a multicultural environment. In some cases, achieving a sense of racial and cultural pride, as well as connection to the culture of origin, is hindered by racism in the majority culture. For Asian American women specifically, identity development is further complicated by the dual forces of sexism and racism, both in the culture of origin and in the majority culture.

Atkinson, Morten, and Sue (1979) propose a stage theory to account for minority identity development. Briefly, they posit five developmental stages which describe the gradual process whereby an individual's minority identity crystalizes within a majority culture. Two stages in their schema, if applied indiscriminately to Asian women, risk introducing a sexist bias that may not account for the Asian woman's experience of multiple oppression. The *resistance and immersion* phase of minority identity development happens when dominant group values are rejected and a return to an appreciation of the minority culture and immersion in it theoretically occurs. However, this may evoke ambivalence in some Asian women. The Asian woman who seeks increased freedom and opportunities for personal achievement may not necessarily find acceptance of this in her culture of origin. For these women, White social ideals may represent hope for opportunities clearly denied her in her culture of origin. By necessity, such a woman will have to embark on a process that may involve alternatives that expose the woman to rejection and alienation on many levels: (1) she may repress or relinquish her desire for personal achievement in favor of reducing conflict with her culture of origin; (2) she may achieve assimilation to the majority culture on this issue; (3) she may attempt to change her own culture; or (4) she may attempt to transcend both cultures. Therefore this stage of minority identity development fails to account for the absence of opportunities for female achievement within many Asian traditions and also fails to account for how this affects Asian female identity development. In a dual cultural environment in which the majority culture, at least rhetorically, offers opportunities for women's actualization, reconciliation with a minority culture that persists in repression of women will be difficult for some women to accept.

Additionally, the final stage, *synergetic articulation and awareness*, is described as the ability to appreciate oneself, appreciate others of the same minority as well as others of different minorities, and selectively appreciate members of the majority group (Atkinson et al., 1979). Again, in the context of female oppression exacerbated by the frustrations of racism in most minority communities in the United States, appreciation of one's own minority culture as well as other minorities may be coupled with ambivalence. The minority woman who seeks to transcend traditional values that endorse suppression of female achievement and aspirations will experience the conflicts of minority identity formation in a way that men of the same minority culture will not. This is true to the extent that men typically face fewer cultural prohibitions against ambitions, and minority identity consolidation for minority women will be more complicated. Clearly the mental health professional who attempts to apply the minority identity model without specifically considering the dual oppression that minority women typically face will reinforce an androcentric and sexist bias in the treatment.

Despite the fact that the ethnic identity model of Atkinson et al. is not entirely satisfactory for women, it is necessary for there to be an acceptance of, and a celebration of one's culture of origin. Central to the culture of origin of Asian Americans is a deep level of concern for community (society) and family.

SOCIETY AND FAMILY

Sociocultural Philosophies

To comprehend fully the diversity in Asian social structure and family structure requires an appreciation of some of the principal forces that shaped the cultural philosophies underlying many Asian social systems. One important conceptual division is that some Asian societies are based in Confucian social ethics and some are not (Tien, personal communication, 1991). Another is the influence of colonization and imperialism, primarily but not exclusively, by European countries in the Asian Pacific region. A third issue involves the interaction of sociocultural philosophies and religion. Thorough understanding of these forces requires a scholarship and breadth of understanding that is beyond the scope of this chapter. However, a cursory inventory will address two distinct Asian sociocultural systems represented in the United States that have significant implications for family construction, gender-role expectations, power balance between genders, and female identity.

Confucian Social Philosophy

Confucius was deeply concerned with the moral character of men, exclusively. He spoke indifferently or disparagingly of women or largely ignored them. Though Confucius' precepts underwent change over several hundred years of their observance, it seems likely that current Confucian proscriptions for women had their origins in principle, if not in edicts, with Confucius himself (see Jaspers, 1957).

Confucian precepts dominated the cultures of China, Japan, and Korea and continue to characterize the cultural fabric of these societies. Very superficially, Confucian dictates were patriarchal in power distribution, and the maintenance of power was transmitted patrimonially. Female indoctrination on a superficial level consisted of the "Three Obediences"—to father at home, to husband after marriage, and to sons at old age. The "Four Virtues" of women were chastity, reticence, a pleasing manner, and domestic skills. A girl's "lack of talent" intellectually or physically was considered a virtue, which fostered the attitude of deference to men and boys.

Birth order conferred clear role expectation for both men and women; although the overall subjugation of women in Confucian society relegated women regardless of birth order to subservient roles. The eldest daughter was handmaid to her mother, responsible for domestic chores and the tending of younger siblings. She was inferior in status and therefore power to her brothers, but especially to the oldest son, regardless of his age relative to hers. The daughter exercised no influence in the selection of her mate, and was in fact often barred from meeting the prospective spouse until the wedding night (Yung, 1986). Woman's stature as sexual property and object was demonstrated by "aesthetic" practices in China that eroticized female disability and symbols of her subservience such as the crippled feet that resulted from binding.

Confucian social order is the cultural philosophy most often identified with Asians. However, many Asian cultures do not subscribe to these doctrines either in their countries of origin or after immigration. Among succeeding generations of Asians in the United States, the departure from traditional values emerges both as a source of emancipation for Asian women and a source of family crisis.

Buddhism

The basic teachings of Buddhism, the Middle Path of salvation, asserts that all existence is suffering, that immersion in the path will lead to knowledge about the truth of suffering, and release from suffering is achieved through a state of nondesire. In practice, Buddhism was primarily a male pursuit, given the cultural constraints against female literacy, education, and the mobility to gain access to Buddha's teachings. The spread and transformation of Buddhist thought affected China, Japan, Tibet, Mongolia, Siberia, and Indochina, for example, but ironically has nearly disappeared in India itself, where Hinduism remains preeminent.

In principle, Buddha's teachings related to religious and spiritual concerns that by definition regard society and its pursuits as distractions from enlightenment. Confucius, on the contrary, believed it necessary for spiritual thought to concern itself with the lives of *men* in order that *men* should strive to become superior beings. In this way, Confucius contradicted his predecessors, notably Lao-tzu, who prescribed asceticism for spiritual attainment (Jaspers, 1957). Thus, while Confucianism seems to have provided a basis for social order as opposed to spiritual concerns, Buddhism appears to belong more to the realm of religious thought, more occupied with matters of the spirit than social order.

Such differentiations are, however, less clear cut than one might expect. Buddhism as a religion forms the basis for Japanese society, leading to distinctive beliefs that affect fundamental aspects of daily life. These effects are sometimes profound, such as the nonlinear view of life events, which circumvents the importance of causality (DeVos, 1980) and underlies the passive acceptance of events that characterizes some Japanese. Nevertheless, while Buddhism affects social structures such as the role and organization of the family, it cannot be said to dictate social rules directly. Confucianism, in contrast, explicitly comments on the proper place and conduct required of men and suggests spiritual bases for its structural recommendations. Therefore, Confucianism exists both as a social system and as a religious doctrine. Where Confucianism exists within a context of another or other primary religious system(s), it may still exert an influence on social philosophy and transactions.

Other Indigenous Social Philosophies

While in both China and Japan female archetypes are deeply rooted in the indigenous cultures (Doi, 1973; Kingston, 1976), the power of the female and the feminine was diminished, probably as a result of the rise of Confucianism. The Pacific Islands, Philippines, and parts of Indochina, which also have a rich tradition of shamanism and matriarchal values, retained these values more consciously. This in turn appears to have contributed to the elevation of the status of women relative to that found in Confucian, Hindu, or Moslem societies. The richness of indigenous social philosophies cannot be justly characterized or even adequately synopsized in this short section. Therefore, this particular discussion will be limited to some of the effects and implications of colonization and imperialism, which have in some cases decimated indigenous cultures and in other cases strongly suppressed them. An understanding of Pacific Island cultures depends on the appreciation of the fact that colonization has enforced or encouraged adoption of religious and social values that have their origin in European culture, as do those of the European American population in the United States.

The societies of the Pacific Islands, which were largely colonized by French, Spanish, and German forces, can now be characterized as heavily influenced by Christian religious doctrines, which in turn have influenced social mores. However, the realities of island life such as confinement to a typically small land mass, the abundance of food, and a temperate climate exert an influence on the people's psychology and social patterns, making them distinctive. Munoz (1983) describes Pacific Island peoples as commonly friendly, hospitable, and generous, in part as a function of the necessity for interrelatedness and need for social harmony. Munoz states that extended intergenerational families and child adoption among relatives is more common and typical among island peoples than among other Asian American minority groups. Describing the differences between extended family networks and intergenerational ones, she points out that intergenerational families may have any combination of relatives and generations living under one roof. The flexibility of family structure is demonstrated by the practice of adopting infants among relatives, and the absence of any stigma associated with this type of adoption. Children, like the land and its resources, are considered precious and a shared responsibility. The ethic of sharing or exchange of children between families provides social, economic, and psychological security for both the child and child rearers. The child is given an enriched opportunity for family contact and belonging while the child rearers as "parents" are offered the potential of being cared for in later life. This practice often benefits the biological parents as well, who may not have the financial resources to support the child. The elevated view of children in the South Sea Island societies is reflected in the language which lacks pejorative or negative referents for children (Munoz, 1983). When terms such as "illegitimate" are used, the origin of the word is usually traceable to European influences.

The traditional social structure of the Pacific Islanders was characterized by the importance of the family or clan. The family served as the primary socializing and disciplinary force and thus as the organizing principle for the society. This stands in some degree of contrast to the United States, in which the principle organizing force tends to be government, as a result of a national ethic based on individuality. Interactions and interdependency among Pacific Islanders are transacted primarily within this large network of family, thereby reducing the need for friends as conceived in American social networks. Mothers occupy a powerful position as the manager of the household, the finances, and the overseer of children even after their marriages. Often fathers share these responsibilities, but management is primarily expected of the mother. The primacy of the family, with the mother as the designated head of the household, creates a gender-role that is the exact inverse of the position of women in Confucian-based societies. Women are important, to some extent revered as extensions of earth the provider, and vital to the social structure. With increasing Western imperialistic influences and the financial crises generated by the dissolution of bartering and interfacial sharing in favor of using currency as the standard for exchange, the social structure has been strained fundamentally. The influence of women has eroded, becoming consistent with Western practices of gender dominance.

From this brief description of South Sea Island societies, it is clear that the family and social structures among Asian societies vary with regard to the role and importance of women. The Philippines, colonized early by Spain, briefly by Japan, and lastly by the United States, exists as a complex amalgam of Catholic, Moslem, and indigenous values and beliefs that share some but not all of the repressions of women characterizing the Confucian-based societies with which most Westerners are more familiar. Most importantly, many of the Pacific Islands—the Philippines and Hawaii, for example—have strong matriarchal values, which have served as a buffer against the oppression of women, since these values arise from a history of reverence for the feminine, and by extension, the female. The male bias in these societies is a result of imperialist destruction of indigenous traditions, literature, and religious leaders, paving the way for the devaluation of women. But lest Europe shoulder all of the blame, Japanese and Chinese imperialism with its attendant cultural disregard for women, have also participated in the destruction of indigenous, often pagan, religious and social structures.

Individual versus Group Dependency

While the subordinate role of women may not constitute a uniform dimension for generalizing about Asian cultures, the sociopolitical philosophy of individualism versus group dependency does seem to differentiate Asian cultures from European or North American ones. Asian cultures vary regarding the degrees and expressions of individualism they will tolerate among their members, but relative to the United States' European American social norms, Asian cultures on the whole promote the group as the proper focus of aspirations. Several sources point to the historical origins of social philosophies, hypothesizing that in the United States the importance of personal freedom underlies the emphasis on individualism (Doi, 1973; DeVos, 1980). Asian societies are predicated not on the ideology of personal freedom, but on that of group harmony.

The emphasis on community and family as the organizing social structure exerts fundamental pressure on the individual to subordinate rather than elevate personal need. The sense of belonging and obligation to the family extends throughout the family network, as well as forward to posterity and backward to ancestors (Shon & Ja, 1982). The sense of personal responsibility for honorable action is a matter of duty to the past, present, and future of the family. These characteristics of Chinese, Japanese, and Korean families and societies, for example, have received ample attention in the literature (Akiyama, Antonucci, & Campbell, 1987; Shon & Ja, 1982). The concern for harmony at all levels of human relationships also underlies the passivity, fatalism (the absence of a belief in the efficacy of personal action in changing future events), deference to authority, and conformity often observed in Asian people. However, given a different ideological context, these behaviors have significantly different implications and purposes, which is not readily apparent to the outside observer.

For the Asian woman this concern for harmony on all the many levels exerts strong cultural pressure to maintain the status quo. Where the subordinate role of women is culturally prescribed, the emphasis on social harmony exerts both an internal and an external pressure against changing the status of women. Internally, these values create conflict, which discourages the desire for change. Externally, efforts to elevate the position of women are resisted by social institutions based on cultural proscriptions against disruptions and conflict. As such, the emphasis on social harmony, while promoting social cohesion, may also function in complex ways to maintain oppression of women.

The emphasis on harmony naturally does not eliminate conflict; rather, it prescribes how it is expressed and resolved. As codified in Confucian doctrine, the resolutions frequently rely on hierarchy. Status and levels of obligation determines who may be confronted, under what circumstances, and in what manner. However, social rules for behavior also depend on whether the interaction takes place publicly or privately, and whether it involves outsiders. The definition of public, private, insider, and outsider are complex, such that, for example, public can at times mean in front of children or extended family, or it may mean in front of nonfamily or clan. Similarly, the definition of insider versus that of outsider, is dependent on context; there are varying degrees of outsidership, with foreigners (non-Asians) occupying the farthest extreme.

The literature on Asian society is replete with references to obligation. It is paramount to understand that the Asian feeling which, in English, has been translated as "obligation" is not well understood. This is because English, lacking a full lexicon for discussing dependency in its various forms, also lacks words for describing the feelings that underlie obligations to others (Bradshaw, 1990). For more complete discussions of these issues in Japanese, Chinese, and Filipino cultures, the reader is referred to Doi (1973), Chan (1963), and Marcelino (1990), respectively.

In summary, the range in social and family practices among Asian cultures can be roughly differentiated by the sociocultural systems on which they are based. The reader is urged not to rely on stereotyped descriptions of Asian families, but to investigate the specific culture or ethnicity for relevant information. The hierarchical structure of Confucian-based cultures discussed in preceding sections of this chapter has been treated with excellent descriptions of traditional East Asian family structure in Sue and Morishima (1982) and Shon and Ja (1982). Discussions that differentiate several Asian cultural orientations toward family and effects on child development appear in Powell (1983).

OPPRESSIVE FORCES ASIAN AMERICANS FACE IN THE UNITED STATES

As the preceding section has shown, Asian cultural values have quite a different emphasis from those of the White majority in the United States. Even over generations, Asian immigrants may retain both overt and subtle cultural values that deviate from the cultural norms of the majority. The achievement of belonging—involving identity formation, creation of minority communities, and access to social privileges such as education and financial success—is complicated by deliberate insensitivity on the part of U.S. society to their needs and rights. The forms of this insensitivity that I will explore are negative stereotypes of Asians and Asian Americans and the pressure to assimilate, which often involves an unreasonable and painful expectation that the minority group forsake its original culture.

Stereotyping

The reductionist process of ignoring cultural differences and ethnic variation among the Asian groups in the United States, in the service of conceptual parsimony, has been pervasive in both in the mainstream culture and in academic disciplines. Even those Asian groups that are presumably better understood given their longer history of residence in the United States, are still relegated to stereotyped treatment. The newer Asian arrivals have in turn received scant recognition and are subsumed into familiar Asian stereotypes. More recent writings have begun to cry out against the monolithic view of Asian populations in the United States in favor of addressing their cultural and ethnic heterogeneity. However, this is a vast task, which challenges many of the basic assumptions and even semantic traditions that characterize the body of literature on Asian Americans.

Socioeconomic Stereotyping

The influence of socioeconomic privileges on cultural values is poorly analyzed and understood. Comparatively little attention is devoted to understanding the affluent peoples of Asian ethnic populations. While economic privileges may insulate them from problems that arise directly or secondarily from financial necessity, the need for access to culturally appropriate social support and services remains. Mainstream images of Asians and Asian Americans are dichotomous with regard to affluence, depicting them either as highly affluent or destitute. Both images serve to maintain "otherness" in the eyes of the majority. Underrepresentation of affluent Asians and Asian Americans supports images of inferiority, yet, when affluence is depicted the images often encourage disdain. Asian affluence may be associated with immorality (e.g., Imelda Marcos), and may tend to capitalize on mainstream fears of being overrun by outsiders (e.g., Japan bashing). These stereotypes have several important consequences for Asians and Asian Americans. First, these images do not distinguish between those whose families have resided in the United States for generations and more recent arrivals who vary on several important dimensions. Second, these stereotypes preserve the "otherness" of long-time Asian U.S. residents who identify their loyalties and allegiance first to their American citizenship (e.g., Japanese internment) and secondarily to their ethnicity or race. Third, these stereotypes encourage fears that affluence among new Asian arrivals necessarily constitutes a threat to American ways of life or White American job security and serve to justify further racism or exclusionary practices.

Gender and Racial Stereotyping

Gender stereotypes combined with racial stereotypes challenge Asian and Asian American women with the compounded difficulties of dual oppression. To the extent that traits ascribed to the "feminine" are perceived as weak or inferior in Western culture, and Asians are caricatured consistent with these traits, Asians are relegated to inferior status. The self-perpetuating nature of stereotypes, and thus their insidious danger to the minority person, is that they are often confirmed in selective observation. For an individual of the majority culture, it is possible to have only limited contacts with minority persons. Typically, the context of the interaction favors the majority. In such contexts, Asians as well as other minority people are more likely to act in passive, deferential ways. Unfortunately, these are the expected characteristics of Asians, and thus confirm racially stereotyped expectations. Stereotyped expectations imposed by the majority culture create highly dehumanizing identities which may be especially crippling to the development and maintenance of healthy self-image for Asian American women.

Asian American women are also subjected to conflicting gender stereotypes that characterize them as exotic, shy, submissive, demure, erotic, and eager to please on the one hand or wily, manipulative, inscrutable, and untrustworthy on the other. The prevalence of these stereotypes is supported by the paucity of realistic representations of Asian women. Images of sexual objectification have been perpetuated by war experiences of male soldiers, sexual commerce encouraged by the U.S. military presence in Asian Pacific rim countries, tourist and commercial activities involving importation of Asian women for sexual labor, and stereotyped popular media representations (e.g., Suzie Wong, the geisha girl, and the dragon lady). Diametrically opposed to the sexualized view, Asian women are also stereotyped as the asexual, unattractive, impersonal yet efficient worker (worker bee). This image portrays Asian woman workers as androgynous beings, grouped in undifferentiated masses. This image fuels the use of a divisive rhetoric that elevates democracy and individualism by disparaging other social systems and equating them with the absence of identity or beauty. The third popular image is of the Asian as domestic servant. Asian women and Asian American women are damaged by these images because they obscure their individuality, prevent the expression of their aspirations and dreams, and oppress opportunities for self-actualization.

Many, though not all, Asian cultures themselves impose devaluing sanctions against their women, which reinforce the majority view of Asian women as inferior and submissive. Asian cultures built on the social philosophies of Confucius are particularly oppressive toward women. In these Asian societies, women in particular are subjected to the collective control exerted by family, community, and the patriarchs. She is likely to have been indoctrinated to embody deference, acceptance of suffering, and personal sacrifice, all of which are consistent with the prevailing stereotypes. Under these conditions, she is bound by both her own cultural demands and by projections of the majority culture. This particular stereotyped view of the Asian woman is likely very familiar to most readers. It is one that obscures the fact that not all Asian cultures subscribe to Confucian doctrines. One notable example of an Asian group not so influenced is Filipinas, whose indigenous culture ascribes to a more egalitarian distribution of power between males and females. Even among the Confucian-based societies, pressures to modernize and industrialize for economic gain have to some degree mitigated proscriptions against women.

Acculturation of Asian males to American values exerts an added pressure on the self- and sexual identity of the Asian woman. American culture values and publicizes a highly sexualized image of White women, which has become the standard for beauty in this country. Even though mixed-race people are depicted with increasing frequency as standards for attractiveness, overall, the primary image remains White. Minority and majority women aspire to this image, an aspiration often hopeless and injurious to the self-images of Asian women and girls. Yi (1989) reported a relationship between degree and type of acculturation among Japanese, Korean, and Chinese American females and diagnosis for bulimia. Their preoccupation with mainstream ideals for thinness suggested that in combination with maturational and developmental factors, acculturation to American standards for beauty can have destructive effects. Cosmetic or aesthetic surgeries such as breast enhancements or eyelid alterations may also be used among Asian girls who aspire to White physical characteristics. Asian men and boys are influenced and attracted by the White standard for beauty and the implied power that may be conferred by association with such women. Some Asian men thus prefer White women to Asian women, a preference, if communicated, that is additionally harmful to the self-image of the Asian woman.

Asians in the United States constitute a diverse population poorly served by the use of overinclusive stereotypes and semantic categories. The reduction of ethnic richness to a single and limited image is a form of racism, which provides simplistic answers to complex issues. Asian women are damaged by the perpetuation of racial and gender stereotypes in ways particular to their ethnic context, caught in the cross fire of conflicting and dehumanizing images, most of which are pejorative in the hierarchy of Western ideals. New models for Asian women are needed to encourage a sense of power, beauty, and belonging in American society.

The Pressure to Assimilate

Ethnic stereotyping is a form of oppression that inhibits or injures the development of healthy self-esteem for Asians in general and for Asian women in particular. In the subsequent sections two additional pressures, those of acculturation and assimilation, which result from exposure to cultural differences, are considered. Implicitly, minority cultures are expected to take on the prevailing (majority) values, much as a guest would observe the rules of the host. Yet, the former immigrants and subsequent generations are no longer guests; nor are they renters. They are residents. This permanence confers certain rights, which in turn exert an influence on both cultures. The process of reciprocal influence is mediated by politics and economy such that the burden of change lies primarily with the newcomer. This demand to change is largely an implicit expectation of the majority culture and has important ramifications for the identity development and self-concept of the minority resident. This process of *acculturation* is one by which members of one sociocultural background, usually the minority, incorporate the sociocultural values of another, usually the majority, through social contact (Chow, 1985). Though the terms acculturation and assimilation are often used synonymously, Chow's (1985) discussion on the adaptation of Asian American women into American society suggests a subtle difference between the two processes. Whereas acculturation may refer to the selective acquisition of another group's traits, *assimilation* implies a process of melding into the majority culture by denying or forfeiting conflicting foreign values held by the minority culture. Though full assimilation is often viewed as favorable from the majority perspective, growing minority politics and perspectives view it as pejorative.

Acculturation

Chow (1985) observes that the standards for acculturation in the United States are typically based on middle-class, White male values for behavior, achievement, and even "permissible social pathology." She concludes that an implicit hierarchy is established with a White male prototype to which both White women and minorities are supposed to aspire. The Asian woman, as a minority and as a woman, occupies the farthest extreme in this hierarchy; her struggles are compounded by her status as a minority in a majority White culture, by her status as a woman in a male dominated majority culture, and likely by her similarly oppressed status as a woman in an androcentric Asian American culture. The economic and political realities created by immigration has created androcentrism even when gender differences may have been more balanced in the culture of origin. From a minority perspective, adherence to the White standard may not be desirable nor healthy. Given the multiple levels of oppression this would be particularly true for the Asian woman. Even the adoption of feminist values, since they still tend to conform to White middle-class ethics, may be attractive but also may pose fundamental obstacles to full self-actualization for many Asian women.

Given the diametric opposition in value orientation between White American culture and many Asian values, "cultural self-determination" typically involves either a rejection of one culture in favor of the other or an amalgamation of the two. The third alternative of transcending both cultures demands certain access to privileges and support that as yet most Asian women do not have, although these may be forthcoming as more achieve positions of power and visibility. Since the tenets of feminism or women's liberation, in order to maximize personal achievement, tend to support a lifestyle base on White middle-class values, adopting them means repressing or violating basic Asian socialization and attitudes that conflict with personal goals. Furthermore, by violating these edicts in favor of personal gain, the Asian woman, like many White women, risks rejection by significant people in her life. The minority woman risks more, however, because when she loses her family or community, there is often little else to which she can turn for belonging and acceptance. In a general cultural milieu oppressive to minorities and women, she also loses the protection afforded to her by her community and family. Whatever the path for resolution the challenge exists to find a home or sense of belonging.

Assimilation

Asians are frequently touted as the "model minorities" due to apparent upward mobility and socioeconomic success in comparison to other American minority groups. Various explanations have been advanced to account for this "fact," ranging from claims that Asians have been more successful at assimilating White cultural norms and expectations (Peterson, 1971; Feagin & Fujitake, 1972; Montero, 1982); that Asian cultural values are more compatible with American values (Connor, 1976); or that retention of basic Asian values enhances achievement (Kuo & Lin, 1977). Several problems emerge regarding both the assertion of Asian success and the explanations put forth to explain it. First, the "Asians" as a whole have not enjoyed such success. Some groups suffer high unemployment and poverty conditions, while other more established groups such as the Japanese, Chinese, Koreans, and Filipinos do experience some affluence, but although these groups are no longer unemployed overall, they are underemployed (Wong, 1983; Wong & Hayashi, 1989). Second, the "success" is relative to other minority groups and not relative to privileges enjoyed by the White mainstream population. Third, even when successful groups are specifically identified, sex differences are not examined (Chow, 1985).

The stereotype of "Asian success" distorts the reality in the lives of Asian American women who, for the large part, have not attained the same advantages ascribed to their male counterparts. This is because the Asian American woman has few role models for choosing alternatives to traditional Asian cultural proscriptions, may experience resistance from both cultures against adopting more self-actualizing behavior, and must reconcile her identity and sense of belonging were she to choose cultural values different from her own. Research on acculturation of Asian American professional women by Chow (1982) suggested that these women recognize the possibilities for greater freedom as Americans even if not fully actualized. The problem may lie with American feminism as well as with Asian cultural proscriptions.

The Role of Feminism

Revealing a feminist identity is often more dangerous and conflictual for women of color generally. External and internal conditions inhibit full participation among women of color in feminist activities, even though on the surface of it feminist goals appear consistent with the needs of oppressed women of color. In practice, feminism on the whole has failed to educate either its own constituents or the general population about the dual oppression of racism and sexism whenever issues of sexism have gained attention. Yamada (1983) observes that the continuing insistence on the part of many White majority women to be educated about the "plight" of women of color by women of color as opposed to educating themselves perpetuates the hierarchical notion that minorities must prove their importance or earn the attention. Yamada also asserts that embedded in the request to be educated lies a double bind; the unspoken request that women of color only speak what is acceptable and not criticize the dominant values of their White sisters. She states that criticism by an "out group" is perceived as an expression of personal anger not based in ideological concerns that are taken seriously. Furthermore, criticism of the dominant society by minorities is often viewed as ingratitude.

Specific to Asian women, expressions of anger per se are often viewed as contrary to expected attitudes of deference and meekness. On this basis, an individual Asian woman expressing anger may be perceived by members of the dominant culture as abnormal, unrepresentative of her culture, expressing personal circumstances that can be dismissed. Thus, subtle forms of racism operate within social forces as well as within some feminist groups to perpetuate the perception of "otherness," acting to oppress the participation of women of color and specifically Asian and Asian American women. These pressures to maintain stereotypes of polite acceptance or polite dissent also contribute to producing internal barriers to Asian and Asian American women's participation in the feminist movement.

Asian female interests—which may include focus on family rather than self, fatalism, obedience, inhibition, passivity, self-restraint, and adaptiveness—are all positions that are often rejected and criticized as negative role types by White middle-class feminist formulations on sexist oppression. These attributes are also implicitly used by some feminists to differentiate feminists from nonfeminists or to hierarchically classify "feminist consciousness" among women. The absence of a transcendent vision of feminism that is inclusive of greater diversity prevents acceptance of women of color whose cultural backgrounds clash with feminist rhetoric, and prevents women of color from feeling acceptable to White feminists.

Other impediments to participation in feminism by Asian and Asian American women include the pervasive patriarchy within and without Asian communities. Within Asian communities and families, especially among ethnicities based on Confucian values, internal oppression includes prevailing values that overvalue men and boys, inhibition of female achievement in favor of male achievement, and pressures to restrict political participation outside of one's own ethnic group. Underemployment and differential pay substantially compromises the freedom of the working-class Asian and Asian American woman, who must also manage multiple domestic responsibilities. As a worker, these factors restrict her ability to engage in activism. In the absence of financial comfort for the family and children, focus on the individual freedom or plight of the Asian woman would seem self-indulgent.

The identity of the Asian woman in the United States is influenced by the various forces of acculturation, assimilation, gender politics, and cultural conflicts. The Asian women, for whom cultural prescriptions for behavior parallel traits considered repressive or negative for White American women, are caught in a particularly painful conflict between retaining loyalty to the minority culture while seeking the freedoms apparently enjoyed by women in the majority culture. Understanding the absence of Asian women in feminist activities requires a knowledge of psychological as well as environmental pressures with which Asian women must cope (Chow, 1989).

The Stress on Family Structure

Negative stereotypes and the pressure to assimilate also have effects on family practices. Because of certain negative consequences of being Asian in the United States, such as with the internment of Japanese Americans during World War II—based on racial prejudice and the xenophobic idea that Japanese would be more loyal to Japan than to the United States—some Asian Americans want to assimilate as quickly and completely as possible. This can create conflict in families because such a person's family members can see the person as disloyal to her or his heritage.

Internment Experience

The internment of 112,000 Japanese Americans living on the West Coast in 1942 had far reaching consequences for the future of the Japanese American community and family (Yung, 1989). Prior to internment the Japanese father, as protector and provider for the family, occupied an undisputed position in the family hierarchy. The massive disruption caused by the incarceration altered family dynamics and lessened the father's capacity to influence his children or direct the course of his family's future. Many families relied on the government for survival and subsistence while they were interned, and the father's power was therefore somewhat eroded (Kim & Otani, 1983). First-generation women gained autonomy and power during this time, since the economic structure of camp life elevated the value of women's labor to equal that of men's. Many families attempted to shed any identification with Japan that might cause them to become suspect as traitors or sympathizers. As a result, fragmentation of the traditional Japanese ways began. For the American-born children, the fragmentation of the traditional Japanese family system provided the opportunity for assimilation into larger American society. For second-generation women, the opportunity to function autonomously in society arose. One effect of this new-found autonomy was to assimilate and identify more strongly with American social values.

Generational Issues

Almquist (1989), primarily discussing the experiences of Japanese, Chinese, and Filipino women in the United States, notes the sharp differences between the older and younger generations of these women on several dimensions. Regarding employment status, while older women are typically employed in service jobs or factory jobs, especially the garment business, women of the younger generation resemble European American women in occupational distribution (Glenn, 1986). Though second- and third-generation Asian American women are often well educated, racial and sexual discrimination continue to be obstacles to promotion and higher professional achievement.

Differences in personal values and lifestyles contribute to substantial family discord when the often more traditional parents and grandparents are both appalled and disappointed by their daughter's departure from traditional expectations. The content of these concerns vary with the particular Asian cultural background.

Members of the newer generation of daughters have recorded their experiences (often in fictionalized form, perhaps to protect the family's honor), communicating the struggles of growing acculturation and gender-role transitions. Monica Sone, in *Nisei Daughter* (1953), gives an autobiographical account describing struggles for identity in a cultural environment far different from that experienced by her immigrant parents, removed from "real Japanese," and struggling with her own resentment about her Japanese blood. While many Issei (first-generation) Japanese without the benefits of citizenship struggled to achieve recognition, Nisei (second-generation) beneficiaries of that struggle resented being Japanese because it prevented complete access to American life. Sansei (third-generation) Japanese struggle again with integrating minority identity and majority values, attempting a personal reconciliation of multiple cultures, values, and traditions. Similarly, generational issues and mother–daughter relationships among Chinese American women are richly described by Tan (1989) and Wong (1989).

Interracial Marriages

Historically and presently the United States has proscribed—culturally if not legally—the intermixing of races by marriage. Legal, political, cultural, and familial pressures have existed in various degrees over time to discourage crossing racial boundaries. For example, antimiscegenation has only recently been declared unconstitutional by the Supreme Court, in the 1967 Loving case in Virginia (Sickels, 1972). Despite the national rhetoric of democracy and pluralism and the lifting of legal restraints, strong taboos remain regarding interracial marriage and relationships. However, some data indicate that exogamous marriages (out marriages) among Asian

Americans are increasing (Kikumura & Kitano, 1973), and that, depending on geographical location in the United States, Asian American women intermarry at higher rates than Asian American men and both primarily marry White people (Shinagawa & Pang, 1988). This appears to be a general trend among Asian American youth. Why do Asian American women so frequently marry White men?

Two theories are most often advanced to explain *outmarrying*: assimilation and hypergamy. Very briefly, assimilation theory hypotheses that *outmarriage* indicates growing acceptance of a minority group by the majority group such that race, as a boundary discouraging social contact, is diminished (Kitano, 1984). Alternatively, hypergamy theory suggests that outmarriage occurs so as to maximize the status of each marital partner. For example, a majority-race male of high socioeconomic status (SES) may marry a minority female of low SES for her other attributes, such as beauty or intelligence, to their mutual benefit. Alternatively, racial minority males with higher socioeconomic standing may gain access to privileges blocked by racial boundaries via marriage to a majority-race female. Social exchange theory has been advanced as additional support for the hypergamy model; data presented by Shinagawa & Pang (1988) appear to support the model.

Though hypergamy theory appears to account to some degree for the gender difference observed in the tendency toward outmarrying, there are some troubling consequences to viewing the phenomenon solely from the perspective of status maximization. Hypergamy theory perpetuates familiar stereotypes, casting minority women as low in social status, high in physical attributes, and opportunistic about status improvement. The charge that this theory perpetuates sexist and racist stereotypes is not addressed by its theorists. However, the demeaning implications for both Asian American males and females of such stereotypes should be recognized for the force of the negative image projected, depicting minorities as covetous of majority privilege, willing to "trade" for increased power presumably unavailable among their own racial group.

It is unlikely that either assimilation or hypergamy theory alone adequately accounts for the complex phenomenon. Tien (personal communication, April 1991) hypothesizes that culture clash may also exert an effect, such that some Asian American men may to some extent avoid Asian American women in a way that they do not avoid first-generation immigrant women. She suggests that Asian American men from traditional families may be encouraged by their families to find partners who are more likely than Asian American women to uphold traditional family roles. Women new to the United States may be more likely to obey the traditional rules of subservience to the man's mother, who has devoted her life to her son bolstered by her anticipation of being cared for eventually by her son's wife. Tien found some support for this hypothesis among Asian American college students. It implies that more acculturated views of Asian American women may work against their finding acceptance by traditional Asian

American families and men. However, stereotypes about Asian women encourage partnering of Asian American women with White men, who themselves may offer more egalitarian relationships or freedom from extended family obligations.

Interracial marriage is still considered unacceptable or even disgraceful by many traditional Asian families. Although the incidence of interracial marriage among younger generations of Asian Americans appears to be increasing, social supports are few. There is little cultural education available for interracial couples that facilitates an understanding of how differences in cultural background affect relationship dynamics, expectations of one another, relationships with their respective families, relationship role behavior, or dealing with negative social responses to an interracial union. Often the combination of adolescent or young-adult rebellion against family expectations, in conjunction with rebellion against cultural expectations, results in attempts to deny or repress awareness of important issues in service of an appearance of autonomy. Under these conditions, problems are likely to emerge in the relationship as the inevitable negotiations begin among conflicting expectations and the pressure of social censure. Therapy with such couples often involves cultural education for both partners, about their own backgrounds as well as that of their partner's. Within the context of such education, examination of both subtle and overt expectations regarding the relationship is likely to develop.

A clinical example of one such hidden agenda occurred in the therapy of Carol and Russell, a young interracial couple who came to therapy when crises emerged around the time of their decision to become engaged. All identifying data have been changed for confidentiality reasons.

Carol was a junior at a local university, attending school far away from her family. She was a third-generation Japanese American woman who had met Russell approximately 2 years earlier through mutual friends. Though her family quietly disapproved of the relationship, they had expressed no overt objection. She was an outstanding student, though somewhat isolated socially. Russell, a White man, was several years older than Carol, established in his work, also living some distance from his family of origin.

The couple sought psychotherapy from a private practice therapist at Carol's insistence, when they couldn't resolve differences related to Carol's desire for graduate education, the relocation that aspiration might have required, and negotiating the compromises concerning what they each expected from the relationship.

Carol, who was very fluent in English, was not bilingual, having come from relatively affluent Japanese parents who socialized both in the majority culture as well as in the Japanese American community. She had sought psychotherapy previously from a private practice clinician for adjustment difficulties when she first began college. Though she had been an excellent student throughout her educational career, she had felt different and conspicuous in a new environment in which there were few Asians, and feared her past success would not be enough to insure her success in college. She reported that her psychotherapy had proceeded well, and had similar expectations for this experience.

Russell had not engaged in psychotherapy previously, and felt uncomfortable and somewhat suspicious of the therapy process, which he feared would be long, expensive, and drawn-out and would lead to the blaming of somebody. Progress in therapy revealed that Russell, himself rather traditional regarding male role behavior, had expected that Carol would be supportive of his career by not requesting of him changes to his well-established and comfortable life. Though he was receptive and willing to challenge both his sexist views and uncommunicated expectations, he did not consider himself racist and had considerable difficulty challenging his racial and sexual stereotype of Carol.

During the initial year of their courtship, Carol had acted in very agreeable and supportive ways toward Russell's needs and expectations, leading him to assume that she would not move in personal directions that would jeopardize his setting and lifestyle. However, over time, Carol in his view had become increasingly feminist and had begun to "demand" things from him that he found surprising. Carol agreed that she had been quite deferential toward Russell during the initial phase of their courtship, but denied that her "feminism" had changed substantially over time. She had been surprised to find his values "so traditional" and wondered why she had not seen this before. Each partner felt betrayed and misled, and therefore doubted the basis for the relationship.

Therapy with this couple revealed that Carol, despite her highly acculturated stance, which departed sharply from traditional Japanese values, had nonetheless internalized some of what she later identified as her mother's ways of being in a marriage. In her self-identification as being primarily American, she was not aware of the ways she acted that reinforced the stereotype held by Russell of the passive, agreeable Asian woman. She herself had expected Russell to embody feminist attitudes and to promote her freedom and equality, which she felt most Asian men were unwilling or unable to do because of family pressures. The interaction of both Asian female stereotype and European American male stereotype had gone undisclosed and operated insidiously in the relationship, only emerging as the couple contemplated marriage and long-range plans for their future. Therapy acted to help Carol understand and cherish the legacy of Japanese values transmitted through her family. Rather than seeing them as liabilities in her pursuit of her career and personal goals, she was helped to see them as important enhancements to her identity and aspirations. Russell was similarly helped in his understanding of Japanese culture and therefore of Carol. The level of Carol's acculturation had aided his denial of her difference from him, in that he perceived her as Asian but the same as he in every other respect. He was also challenged to acknowledge the subtle ways in which he demonstrated his expectation that she would defer to him. Carol's own attempts to disinherit her culture aided in his misperception.

Interracial marriages in a social environment that still holds antimiscegenist values and biases incur special stresses involving complex explicit and subtle forces that challenge their right to perpetuation. These forces apply to minorities who have established lives in the United States, but they are especially difficult for the immigrant woman, the refugee woman, or the wife of the U.S. military man who is brought to the United States without the benefit of family or community support and is thus wholly dependent on her husband for her cultural education, cultural understanding, and livelihood.

MENTAL HEALTH AND PSYCHOTHERAPY

The Cultural Contexts of Psychotherapy

Seeking Help

Asian and Asian American women on the whole struggle with multiple forces in order to achieve belonging in a multicultural environment. These struggles can have significant emotional sequelae that are appropriate for psychotherapeutic attention. However, the treatment literature on Asian Americans indicates that psychotherapy is not sought as often as it is probably needed or useful (Homma-True, 1990; Root, Ho, & Sue, 1986; Tsai, Teng, & Sue, 1980). The reasons for this are complex. How emotional distress is expressed and from whom intervention is sought depends on a number of factors such as gender, socioeconomic standing, length of residency in the United States, place of birth, and education. Earlier literature suggested that the underutilization of mental health services by Asian Americans derived from several sources. These included reluctance to admit psychological disorders and tendencies to use alternative sources of mental health care (Root, Ho, & Sue, 1986; Sue & McKinney, 1975; Sue & Sue, 1974); beliefs that emotional distress results from a lapse in willpower, so that they would try to strengthen will rather than seek help; the desire to avoid social stigma and shame (Tsui, 1985; Sue & McKinney, 1975; Sue & Sue, 1974); conformity to the cultural mandate to suffer in silence; and tendencies to somatize emotional distress (Lin, Kleinman, & Lin, 1980; Sue & Morishima, 1982). Sue and Morishima (1982) have suggested that when Asian Americans finally do seek mental health treatment, it is often after exhausting other means of intervention and the relative severity of problems seen therefore is greater than it might be for other populations.

One study surveyed adult residents of San Francisco's Chinatown in an attempt to evaluate some of these conjectures (Loo, Tong, & True, 1989). Results revealed an extremely low rate of utilization (5%), consistent with earlier reports, roughly comparable to the rate of utilization for the general American population 30 years ago (Loo et al., 1989, p. 293). However, contrary to suggestions that expressions of emotional distress are inhibited, Loo et al. found that reported psychological disorders in the community were prevalent, with a sizable proportion of respondents admitting to emotional tension, depression, loneliness, and psychological–physiological symptoms. The researchers concluded that underutilization results not from inhibitions about admitting psychological distress or use of alternative resources, but rather lack of knowledge of available services, belief that mental disorders cannot be prevented, lack of awareness that psychological problems can be treated, and low priority for seeking professional help for depression. As Loo et al. observed, respondents were Chinatown residents, who are more likely to be low-income immigrants, with limited education, having low occupational prestige, and limited resources. Conditions of poverty, immigration difficulties, aging, and life pressures represent real pressures, and coping with them is differentiated from "craziness," thus inclining these respondents to admit to difficulties regarded as normal and unavoidable.

Regarding more severe psychopathology, stigmatization may still occur. It appears that at least for Chinese Americans in this sample, education about available resources, causes of psychological distress, and its prevention and treatment would help to increase the use of mental health services. It is not clear that these results are generalizable to other populations of Asians or Chinese who do not live in Chinatowns. Additionally, there is growing awareness that socioeconomic status, regardless of immigration status, significantly affects help-seeking behavior. Among the better educated and more affluent, there is often a corresponding familiarity with Western ideas about mental health, greater bilingual capabilities, and increased likelihood of seeking independent practitioners for psychotherapy (Tien, personal communication, April 1991). The need for more detailed investigations is clear, as is the need to investigate assumptions about cultural proscriptions to mental health treatment. It may be that the frequent reference to the function of shame and stigmatization in inhibiting participation in psychological treatment is overgeneralized.

Homma-True (1990) cites that nearly 50% of the Asian American clients seen at a San Francisco Community Mental Health Center in 1987 were women. Due to the lack of other surveys, it is not clear how generalizable her data may be. However, Homma-True reports that this pattern is consistent with the impressions of a number of Asian therapists. These reports are not surprising, in light of the multiple pressures Asian and Asian American women face. Explanations for the higher rates of use by Asian American women are not given. Homma-True (1990) suggests that rates of affective disorders among Asian women are greater than among Asian men, paralleling the problems of White American women. Women are more vulnerable to multiple oppressions with which they must cope: sexism that favors men in getting dependency needs met in the family, for example, and lack of resources for dealing with or escaping dangerous or oppressive conditions. Extrapolating further, it appears that Asian and Asian American women are more likely to seek mental health intervention due to the lack of other resources that recognize their problems within their own communities. Intentional efforts to seek an authority who will support changes that the family or community may be unwilling or unable to support, desperation, or perhaps a tendency to acculturate to Western views more flexibly are possible explanations for Homma-True's findings. These hypotheses are suggested for clinical consideration, although they have not been empirically validated.

Pre-therapy Expectations

Many, though not all, Asian and Asian American clients will have had little or no previous experience in psychotherapy. Familiarity with psychotherapy is also mediated by the length of time since a person's immigration, with successive generations being more likely to have experience with it. Therefore, one of the first tasks in establishing the therapeutic alliance will be to educate oneself about client expectations and to educate the client about therapeutic process and behavior. Sue (1981) and Sue and Morishima (1982) are widely cited for their suggestions regarding the value conflicts that may arise for Asians engaged in standard Western psychotherapy. Some of these include: that Western thought draws a distinction between the mind and the body, whereas Asians may think of the two realms as highly interconnected if not synonymous; that verbal expression and communication, especially of criticism or dissatisfaction may be indirect and restrained, whereas Western socialization encourages verbal expressiveness as a sign of honesty; that silence in the Asian tradition may reflect respect instead of resistance or repression; that Asian clients may expect that therapy will enhance their willpower to withstand morbid or ill thoughts, and on this basis may misunderstand the therapist's nondirectiveness when a client-centered or psychodynamic approach is taken; and last, that the Western psychotherapeutic orientation toward self-examination or self-actualization will run contrary to some Asian cultural practices and potentially drive clients from therapy.

Mrs. F. was a 36-year-old interracially married native Japanese woman who immigrated to the United States with her White husband. The family, which consisted of their three children, herself, and her husband, lived in an affluent, White suburb in the Northeast. Her husband, a hard-working executive was supportive but most often unavailable regarding domestic responsibilities and childrearing. Over the course of her marriage she experienced many years of moderate depression, which escalated, eventually resulting in an episode of acute paranoid psychosis. She was briefly hospitalized and referred for outpatient psychotherapy with a White male psychiatrist, who initiated traditional psychodynamic insight-oriented psychotherapy. Over the course of six sessions he encouraged self-expression, after which she terminated psychotherapy. She explained that she was determined not to succumb to depression again for the sake of her children, for whom she felt total responsibility. She regarded psychotherapy as an unnecessary expenditure of time and money that encouraged being self-centered and self-pitying; rather, she thought that she should straighten herself out, avoid "stupid" thoughts, and attend to her duties. She viewed the episode as a lapse in her ability to be selfless, which resulted in her indulging temporarily in selfishness and self-pity. Her husband's high level of affluence afforded her access to domestic privileges, but she had not taken them because she regarded the use of domestic help and accessories as a waste of financial resources, which could be retained for the children's future benefit if she would simply meet her domestic responsibilities. Although she was bilingual and had been substantially acculturated, having immigrated 10–15 years previously, she retained traditional Asian values with respect to her role in the family while following Western family practices and raising her children in the Western style.

Specifically, the Asian or Asian American woman is likely to have a range of pre-therapy expectations that need specific evaluation. The suggestions in the literature pertaining to psychotherapeutic concerns for Asians (Homma-True, 1990; Root et al., 1986; Root, 1985; Shon & Ja, 1982; Sue, Sue, & Sue, 1983; Sue, 1981; Sue & Morishima, 1982; Tsai, Teng, & Sue, 1980) in general apply to Asian women as well. Furthermore, it is my opinion as well as that of Homma-True (1990), Ho (1990), and Chow (1989) that therapy with Asian women differs from therapy with Asian men in that there is an implicit need to respond in a way that is politically and culturally activist in order to challenge the multiple oppressions that are causing or exacerbating emotional distress or mental illness. Therapy concerns that distinguish treatment with Asian and Asian American women from more general culturally sensitive treatment for Asians involves the therapeutic understanding and treatment of these women in light of the interactive effects of gender and race discussed earlier in this chapter. The need for more Asian women professionals to act visibly toward this expanded perspective is imperative. Role models are few who are able to demonstrate that changes toward more egalitarian cultural rules can be adopted without threatening the basic fabric of Asian cultural identity. Women of color in the mental health professions are in a particularly potent position to support such changes both among women of their own ethnicity, and also in their community at large.

Assessment and Diagnosis

Kleinman, Eisenberg, and Good (1978) (cf. Root, 1985) state that proper assessment of psychological functioning, dysfunction, and guidelines for healthy functioning must take into account the individual's culture, level of acculturation, and existing community standards for a particular behavior. As the influences of cultural assimilation increase, the effect of the minority values may decrease, but as in the case cited above, they nonetheless influence behavior in subtle ways. Context is crucial to the understanding of the presenting problem. As Root (1985) states, "The influences of ethnicity are powerful and cross-generational," (p. 352) such that the individual's current involvement with his or her family of origin may not be indicative of its influence or the influence of cultural values and expectations.

Attention to nativity (place of birth), length of time since immigration, language capability, the generation since immigration, level of acculturation or assimilation, adherence to traditional values and beliefs, beliefs about expression of feeling, beliefs about prevention and treatment of mental disorders, minority identity development, socioeconomic status, current social context, and contact with family of origin and extended family are some of the issues that will be critical to the assessment and diagnostic process. Thorough evaluation of these issues on an individual basis, in an attempt to put aside monolithic, homogeneous stereotypes about Asians, will yield rich information that will quite naturally illuminate treatment goals.

In the case of Mrs. F., the failure to recognize cultural differences regarding self-importance versus self-sacrifice led to the sense on Mrs. F.'s part that the therapy was promoting more of what had made her ill. She resolved to repress morbid thoughts in a culturally consistent response. Several years later, she was again seen in psychotherapy when adolescent misbehavior on the part of her child resulted in referral. After careful assessment of the previous incident, it was learned that she had been considering divorce, but could not justify her feelings in the absence of overt abuse on the part of her husband. Conjoint counseling was initiated with positive results.

Psychotherapy Modes and Orientations

Western Psychotherapeutic Approaches

Attempts to provide a comprehensive review of the current psychotherapeutic approaches for minority women are essentially lacking in the literature. The field appears still preoccupied with minority- and culture-sensitive treatment, without extending these conclusions to the gender by race or ethnicity interaction (Homma-True, 1990). In an initial effort to address this need, Homma-True briefly surveyed several of the major schools of therapy and their application to the treatment of Asian American women. It is, however, this author's opinion that efforts to evaluate the efficacy of Western modes of psychotherapy for minorities will not yield data pertinent to minority group individuals. The research on Western psychotherapy gives only moderate indication that specific techniques constitute the potent variables accounting for psychotherapeutic effectiveness (Smith, Glass, & Miller, 1980; Strupp & Binder, 1984). Rather, Strupp and Binder suggest that psychotherapy works best "if patients desire change of their own accord and are motivated to work toward it; if the environment in which they live tolerates the possibility of change; and if the inner obstacles to learning (defenses and rigidities of character) are not insurmountable" (p. 269). It is evident that goals for therapy will meet with fundamental resistance and failure from clients whose environments (external) and personal beliefs (internal) fail to sustain and validate the values therapy promotes. To the extent that most Western psychotherapies have as a goal individuation of the client, Asians whose ideological assumptions conflict with this goal will be poorly served. Psychotherapeutic techniques must be altered to accommodate the Asian client's particular values. Culturally sensitive techniques will help identify and surmount barriers to psychological access and change; community advocacy about mental health functioning and women's issues will help establish external supports for these changes.

If we accept this conclusion, what then are the curative or efficacious factors of which we need to be aware in order to discern how to alter what we know, as Western trained therapists, in order to help non-Western clients? What must be altered or reconsidered in therapy with minorities and, for our purpose specifically, Asian and Asian American women? Again, the literature on psychotherapy research can help. Though it still seems unclear what specific factors of psychotherapy exert specific effects on outcome, some nonspecific factors seem to contribute reliably to positive outcomes: when clients feel accepted, understood, and liked by the therapist; when the client's active participation and collaboration is fostered; when there is respect for the client's freedom and autonomy to influence the goals and process of therapy and these are clear goals declared at the onset of treatment; when the treatment meets the needs of the individual client; when negative transferences are actively confronted, when therapeutic experiences lead to increments in self-acceptance and self-respect; and when the therapist takes an interest in the client as a person, avoiding creation of a caricature of good human relationships by persisting without basic interest and commitment (Strupp & Binder, 1984). It is very likely that these essential ingredients may also operate in the psychotherapy of the Asian client. The purpose of the literature on culturally sensitive therapy is to delineate differences in cultural values, how these differences may be expressed, and how different values may be misconstrued and misinterpreted. Awareness on these levels is crucial for facilitating a genuine understanding and affection between the therapist and client who are culturally different.

Indigenous Psychotherapies

Another route for understanding the effective ingredients for psychotherapy with cultural minorities is to examine the indigenous psychotherapies of the culture in question. Reynolds (1980) offers descriptions of five forms of therapy indigenous to Japan, that is, interventions built on basic Japanese social precepts, reflecting Japanese attitudes toward life and living. These are Morita (named after its founder), Naikan (*nai* meaning inner, *kan* meaning observation), Shadan (isolation), Seiza (*sei* meaning quiet, *za* meaning sitting), and Zen (derived from the Chinese *ch'an* meaning meditation) therapies. Reynolds, attempting to synthesize the common aspects of these therapies, states that these therapies treat the flux in emotional and physical being. They treat the flow of awareness directly, accept suffering as a integral part of life to be accommodated rather than eliminated, they do not recognize the Western distinction between mind and body, and they are based on a Buddhist premise that people are basically good; they are only in need of education to achieve a better state of mind. Reynolds further describes that happiness is not a goal for Japanese therapy, contrary to the American obsession with it, the right to the pursuit of which is even guaranteed in the U.S. Constitution (Reynolds, 1980, p. 104). These therapies seek to resocialize unhappiness, which is viewed as obsession with self-centered concerns, in favor of behaving as a mature adult who is more loving and giving. The vehicle for resocialization is isolation, not talk, which hones inner focus and acceptance by releasing the grip of resentment over "what ought to be but isn't" or "what might have been but wasn't." In many of these therapies the theme of obligation also serves as the resocializing cognitive content.

DeVos (1980), in his afterward to Reynolds' book, notes that these therapies are predicated to some degree on the expression of gratitude. He suggests that American society's overemphasis on the individual produces alienation in its youth, resentment about family dysfunction or inadequacy, and resistance to self-discipline. The Japanese therapies attempt to capitalize on the important role of gratitude and shame through self-discipline. These therapies attempt to reconcile the individual to the "legitimate functioning of parents" based on the belief that resentment occurs when one is unable to release any feeling of gratitude toward another person. DeVos observes that in contrast, many Western therapies are predicated on rejecting or challenging the functioning of parents and their competence. He conjectures that Japanese will continue to reject psychoanalysis because delving into the unconscious and making connection with rage at unmet needs and incompetence in parents will threaten family cohesion. By the same token, Japanese therapies may be poorly suited for American clients, who seek to change their lot in life and do not want reconciliation with occupational or family roles.

The brief comparison of indigenous Japanese therapies and Western therapeutic models illustrates some fundamental differences in treatment technique that necessarily emanate from social philosophy. Precisely because therapy is a socializing agent that takes its direction from societal values, it in turn fosters change that the cultural environment will tolerate and accept. In the case of Asian women, this function of indigenous forms of therapy is disastrous. Focusing on gratitude and fate in life likely serves social harmony at the expense of women's emotional health. The Buddhist ethic on this matter appears to neglect that a great portion of female suffering is not in the nature of life, but in the nature of male domination. As such, is this aspect of women's suffering still legitimate? In cultural systems, both Asian and Western—that advocate and perpetuate suppression of women, women will not be healthy. Yet, acknowledging the value of healthy women will demand a change in society such that the contribution of women be seen as equal to that of men. In this sense, the Western goal of individuation may be to some extent appropriate and necessary. However, encouraging this type of social change will have to be accomplished deftly. Other Asian societies likely have interventions aimed at alleviating what we as Westerners identify as emotional distress. Examination of these indigenous practices will likely help illuminate who is oppressed, how, and the route for change.

Special Topics in Psychotherapy for Asian American Women

Domestic Violence

Asian Americans have a reputation for low rates of domestic violence. Several authors have remarked on this reputation, speculating that while rates of reporting are low, the correspondence to actual occurrence is unknown. This may be a result of the underutilization of public services by Asian Americans, inadequate access to mental health services, inadequacy of available mental health services, or other culturally related factors (Ho, 1990; Rimonte 1989; Eng, 1986; Root et al., 1986).

A number of factors affect both the occurrence of domestic violence and individual and cultural perspectives on it. Sexism in the culture, power differentials between men and women, women's access to alternatives and self-sufficiency, cultural views of physical violence, racism extant in the culture, attitudes toward marriage or partnership, as well as a host of other variables too numerous to discuss fully here constitute some of these factors. However, the cultural context in which the domestic violence occurs should not become cause for mental health professionals to determine that it is unwise to intervene. Though violence against women is tolerated to different degrees across cultures, I advocate intervention in violent situations against women or children, regardless of cultural norms. Rather, cultural context is important to understanding the proper routes for intervention that may not be apparent from the perspective of the cultural stranger.

To illustrate examples of cultural variation regarding use of physical violence, Ho's (1990) research on four populations of Southeast Asian refugees in the United States will be summarized. Her data show how certain cultural consistencies may be expressed differently across ethnicities. Using a culturally sensitive method and allowing expression in the respondents' native language, she found that among the Laotians, Khmers, Vietnamese, and Southeast Asian Chinese, male domination over females prevailed across all four groups even though the degree to which men may exercise this power varied across groups. Regarding power balance between men and women, the Chinese men reported giving wives the illusion of some influence by agreeing with them, but in actuality the final authority remained with the men. While the Chinese respondents reported instances of subtle exercise of male domination, Vietnamese men described a more overt sense of ownership about their wives and their domination was more overt. Ho cited examples of male prerogative such as intolerance of wives refusing sexual overtures and expectations that wives would tolerate their extramarital sexual activity. By comparison to Vietnamese women, Laotian and Khmer women were dominated to an even greater extent, as illustrated by a word in Khmer meaning that women "stay in the shadows and in the home" (Ho, 1990, p. 141). Laotian women reported similar proscriptions for behavior and both groups reported that males enforce a cultural intolerance for refusal of sex to a husband for any reason.

Attitudes toward physical violence are often evident in the power dynamics between men and women, as well as in the expression of discipline toward children. Ho (1990) investigated this correspondence in her study, finding that all four groups endorsed physical punishment as an acceptable form of discipline. All groups had clear definitions of locations on the child's body that were acceptable sites for hitting, and clear senses of whether implements for hitting were appropriate, at what level of disobedience hitting was appropriate, and the role of anger in hitting. Variations emerged across groups however: Ho suggested that physical punishment appeared less acceptable among the Southeast Chinese than among the other groups. Nevertheless, she was careful to point out that this attitude may not reduce the occurrence of physical punishment in actual practice.

Regarding violence against wives, Chinese men and women reported attitudes least tolerant of domestic violence yet estimated that 20% to 30% of marriages resulted in some form of male violence toward wives. Vietnamese women and men were reported to be more tolerant of physical violence, citing occasional hitting or hitting when out of control as expectable. In contrast, Khmer and Laotians expressed the highest tolerance, reporting that domestic violence is common. In view of even these few examples, it is hard to believe that in a general context of Asian cultural tolerance for spousal violence, under the especially stressful conditions of immigration, or under the different yet substantial stresses of minority life, that domestic violence is as infrequent as public statistics imply.

Several populations of Asian and Asian American women are at particular risk for domestic violence, including women who are immigrants or refugees. The losses these women are forced to confront compound the struggle to respond to unfamiliar demands and expectations (Rimonte, 1989). When these women are subjected to rejection in the new community, their cultural training facilitates feelings of personal failure and social incompetence. Depression is therefore a primary liability for these women, and often their indigenous culture has no acceptable label or explanation for these feelings. Refugee women are at risk both within their cultural contexts, and especially in the context of their displacement as refugees. Similarly, Asian wives of U.S. military men are at special risk because of their displaced status, lack of familiarity with American norms, and their isolation from other members of their cultural or ethnic group.

Interventions: Techniques and Considerations

Rimonte (1989) outlines the need for intervention to help the battered Asian woman see herself as a victim, learn to speak, and learn to act. Due to the cultural acceptance of domestic violence, in combination with cultural expectations and socialization that women learn to suffer with dignity, the battered Asian woman may not perceive herself as a victim. Her culture (e.g., Confucian values) may even encourage the acceptance of battering, as fate to be tolerated rather than changed. Yet, without some understanding of herself as a victim, there will be little impetus for creating change or understanding that change is possible. The counselor, as the agent of change, is likely to have little power if her family cannot be mobilized as advocates for her. Learning to speak (give voice to complaint) is, again, culturally proscribed; in fact, in some Asian cultures, silence is a specific way of communicating, especially of pain or anger. Through silence, these feelings are communicated without jeopardizing the family or its harmony. Yet, in domestically violent families the sanctity of the family must be challenged, and this cannot be done without breaking the code of silence. Learning to act on rights and legal privileges requires information, emotional support, and a level of assertiveness that likely surpasses much of what has been required or allowed the woman in the past. Choosing independence from the batterer has serious consequences for the minority woman. The mental health counselor should prepare the woman for these eventualities. Though there is no research on the occurrence of battered woman's syndrome (BWS) and how it is expressed in minority cultures, it seems that the symptom complex identified as BWS is very consistent with culturally prescribed behavior for many Asian women under many circumstances. Because of this similarity, BWS in Asian and Asian American women may be hard to detect.

In addition to the individual orientation that must be established in order for an intervention to occur, Ho (1990) suggests using the community, family, and social pressure as potent forces aiding intervention. Ho advocates capitalizing on Asian values concerning obedience to authority and hierarchy. Use of police intervention is reportedly very effective (Dao, 1988) and the general respect conferred on law and order facilitates compliance to court-mandated treatment and education. Ho (1990) also suggests that by mobilizing the process of shaming by family elders and community, the batterer may be confronted and the cultural imperative that the battered woman have loyalty to her husband can be superseded. Use of translators in treatment may be advised, but caution is recommended because of situations in which translators have editorialized on the communication, interjecting their own opinions about domestic violence, which are not necessarily helpful to the treatment (Ho, 1990; Dao, 1988; Kanuha, Chapter 15, this volume).

Similar to domestic violence, rape and incest occur but may not be interpreted as victimization, may be subsumed under male prerogative, and reporting may be inhibited by Asian values concerning shame and personal failure. Many of the intervention strategies outlined above may also apply to situations in which rape or incest must be addressed. Asian women most likely to have experienced sexual victimization are recent refugees of war, recent immigrants, and wives of servicemen. Although there is much more that can be said on this topic, the literature is sparse. There is probably a great deal to be learned from individual women, and thus these culturally taboo questions must be raised in treatment, thoroughly assessed, and culturally appropriate interventions must be attempted.

Lesbians

The topic of lesbians of color deserves special attention because the belief commonly held, as a result of sexist stereotypes and efforts by most communities of color to deny their existence, is that there are no lesbian women of color. Kanuha (1990) observes that lesbians' relative invisibility, which continues to characterize communities of color, relates to the adherence by communities of color to the use of sexism as a force for ensuring the control of women. She states that visibility of lesbians in their respective communities of color threatens the institutionalization of male domination, and that lesbians are perceived as betrayers of the community because of their perceived nonparticipation in the perpetuation of the race. The "triple jeopardy" of racism, sexism, and homophobia that faces lesbians of color essentially means there is no safe place, no place to belong, whether in the majority or minority community. Often as a result of this condition, violence occurs, further complicating the feelings of shame, guilt, and fear. For a complete analysis of the multiple oppressions lesbians of color face, Kanuha (1990) provides a feminist conceptualization as well as recommendations for intervention for abusers and victims of lesbian battering. Pamela H. (1989) deals more specifically with Asian lesbians, speaking more broadly about issues related to acceptance of self and by community. Both provide perspectives on the effects of cultural rejection by both the minority and the majority community.

CONCLUSIONS

The aim of this chapter has been to continue the trend, only recently begun, to break down monolithic treatment of Asians and Asian Americans as a single racial and ethnic group. In attempting to encourage a heterogeneous perspective that reflects the richness and complexity of Asian cultures both abroad and in the United States, the enormity of the task became apparent. Consequently, there is much in the chapter that has been neglected. The hope is to stir an awakening for the need to research more diligently and specifically the individual context with which we are faced when we deal with Asian and Asian American women. The second aim is to face the task of speaking directly to the needs and conditions of Asian women in a way that enhances what little has already been done, and in a way that encourages more analysis and experience. Asian women, if they are to be viewed in their true contexts, would virtually fill volumes.

ACKNOWLEDGMENTS

I would like to acknowledge Liang Tien, Psy.D., who provided several critical conceptualizations that aided my own understanding of this topic and who gave editorial help in preparing this manuscript. Additional acknowledgements are due to Maria P. P. Root, Ph.D., who provided invaluable emotional support and critical feedback on the manuscript, who shared her resources and above all her friendship. Thanks also to clients and other Asian women who taught me through sharing their experiences.

REFERENCES

Akiyama, H., Antonucci, T. C., & Campbell, R. (1987). Rules of social support exchange: The U.S. and Japan. *Asian American Psychological Association Journal*, *12*(1), 34–37.

Almquist, E. M. (1989). The experiences of minority women in the United States: Intersections of race, gender, and class. In J. Freeman (Ed.), *Women: A feminist perspective* (4th ed., pp. 414–445). Mountain View, CA: Mayfield.

Atkinson, D., Morten, G., & Sue, D.W. (1979). *Counseling American minorities: A cross-cultural perspective*. Dubuque, IA: Brown.

Bradshaw, C. (1990). A Japanese view of dependency: What can Amae psychology contribute to feminist theory and therapy? In L. Brown & M. P. P. Root (Eds.), *Diversity and complexity in feminist therapy and theory* (pp. 67–86). New York: Haworth Press.

Chan, W. T. (1963). *A source book in Chinese philosophy*. Princeton, NJ: Princeton University Press.

Chow, E. N.-L. (1982). *Acculturation of Asian American professional women*. Washington, DC: National Institute of Mental Health, Department of Health and Human Services.

Chow, E. N.-L. (1985). The acculturation experience of Asian American women. In A. Sargeant (Ed.), *Beyond sex roles* (2nd ed., pp. 238–251). St. Paul, MN: West.

Chow, E. N.-L. (1989). The feminist movement: Where are all the Asian American women? In Asian Women United of California (Ed.), *Making waves: An anthology of writings by and about Asian American women* (pp. 362–377). Boston: Beacon Press.

Connor, J. W. (1976). Joge Kanei: A key concept for an understanding of Japanese American Achievement. *Psychiatry, 39*, 266–279.

Dao, H. (1988, July). *The battered Southeast Asian woman: Who is she?* Paper presented at the fourth national conference of the National Coalition on Domestic Violence, Seattle, WA.

DeVos, G. (1980). In D. K. Reynolds (Ed.), *The quiet therapies: Japanese pathways to personal growth.* Honolulu: University of Hawaii Press.

Doi, T. (1973). *The anatomy of dependence.*Tokyo: Kodansha International.

Eng. (1986, October 10). Shelter: Offers help to battered Asian wives. *Los Angeles Times*, pp. 2, 30, 31.

Feagin, J. R., & Fujitaki, N. (1972). On the assimilation of Japanese Americans. *Amerasia Journal, 1*, 13–30.

Gardner, R., W., Robey, B., & Smith, P. C. (1985). Asian Americans: growth, change, and diversity, *Population Reference Bureau, 40*(4), 5.

Glenn, E. N. (1986). *Issei, nisei, war bride: Three generations of Japanese American women in domestic service.* Philadelphia, PA: Temple University Press.

Ho, C. K. (1990). An analysis of domestic violence in Asian American communities: A multicultural approach to counseling. In L. Brown & M. P. P. Root (Eds.), *Diversity and complexity in feminist therapy and theory* (pp. 129–150). New York: Haworth Press.

Homma-True, R. (1990). Psychotherapeutic issues with Asian American women. *Sex Roles, 22*(7/8), 477–486.

Jaspers, K. (1957). *The great philosophers.* New York: Harcourt, Brace, & World.

Kanuha, V. (1990). Compounding the triple jeopardy: Battering in lesbian of color relationships. In L. Brown & M. P. P. Root (Eds.), *Diversity and complexity in feminist therapy and theory* (pp. 169–184), New York: Haworth Press.

Kikimura, A., & Kitano, H. H. L. (1973). Interracial marriage: A picture of the Japanese Americans. *Journal of Social Issues, 29*(2), 67–81.

Kim, B.-L. C. (1977). Asian wives of U.S. servicemen: Women in shadows. *Amerasia, 4*, 91–115.

Kim, E. H. , & Otani, J. (1983). Asian women in America. In E. H. Kim (Ed.), *With silk wings: Asian American women at work.* Oakland, CA: Asian Women United of California.

Kingston, M. H. (1976). *The woman warrior.* New York: Knopf.

Kitano, H. H. (1984). Asian American interracial marriage. *Journal of Marriage and the Family, 46*(1), 179–190.

Kleinman, A. M., Eisenberg, L., & Good, B. (1978). Culture, illness, and care: Clinical lessons from anthropologic and cross-cultural research. *Annals of Internal Medicine, 88*, 251–258.

Kuo, W. H., & Lin, N. (1977). Assimilation of Chinese Americans in Washington, D.C. *Sociological Quarterly, 18*, 340–352.

Lin, K. M., Kleinman, A. M., & Lin T. Y. (1980). Overview of mental disorders in Chinese cultures: Review of epidemiological and clinical studies. In A. M.

Kleinman & T. Y. Lin (Eds.), *Normal and deviant behavior in Chinese culture.* Dorderecht, Germany: D. Reidel.

Loo, C., Tong, B., & True, R. (1989). A bitter bean: Mental health status and attitudes in Chinatown. *Journal of Community Psychology, 17,* 283–296.

Marcelino, E. P. (1990). Towards understanding the psychology of the Filipino. In L. Brown & M. P. P. Root (Eds.), *Diversity and complexity in feminist therapy* (pp. 105–128). New York: Haworth Press.

Montero, D. (1982). The Japanese Americans. *American Sociological Review, 46,* 826–839.

Munoz, F. U. (1983). Family life patterns of Pacific Islanders: The insidious displacement of culture. In G. Powell (Ed.), *The psychosocial development of minority group children* (pp. 248–257). New York: Brunner/Mazel.

Pamela, H. (1989). Asian American lesbians: An emerging voice in the Asian American community. In Asian Women United of California (Ed.), *Making waves: An anthology of writings by and about Asian American women* (pp. 282–290). Boston: Beacon Press.

Peterson, W. (1971). *Japanese Americans: Oppression and success.* New York: Random House.

Powell, G. J. (Ed.). (1983). *The psychosocial development of minority group children.* New York: Brunner/Mazel.

Reynolds, D. K. (1980). *The quiet therapies: Japanese pathways to personal growth.* Honolulu: University of Hawaii Press.

Rimonte, N. (1989). Domestic violence among Pacific Asians. In Asian Women United of California (Ed.), *Making waves: An anthology of writings by and about Asian American women* (pp. 327–337). Boston: Beacon Press.

Root, M. P. P. (1985). Guidelines for facilitating therapy with Asian American clients. *Psychotherapy: Theory Research, and Practice, 22,* 349–356.

Root, M. P. P., Ho, C. K., & Sue S. (1986). Issues in the training of counselors for Asian Americans. In H. P. Letley & P. B. Pedersen (Eds.), *Cross-cultural training for mental health professionals* (pp. 199–209). Springfield, IL: C. Thomas.

Shinagawa, L. H., & Pang, G. Y. (1988). Intraethnic, interethnic, and interracial marriages among Asian Americans in California. *Berkeley Journal of Sociology, 33,* 95–114.

Shon, S. P., & Ja, D. Y. (1982). Asian families. In M. McGoldrick, J. K. Pearce, & J. Giordano (Eds.), *Ethnicity and family therapy* (pp. 208–228). New York: Guilford Press.

Sickels, R. J. (1972). *Race, marriage, and the law.* Albuquerque, NM: University of New Mexico Press.

Smith, M. L., Glass, G. V., & Miller, T. I. (1980). *The benefits of psychotherapy.* Baltimore, MD: Johns Hopkins Press.

Sone, M. (1953). *Nisei daughter.* Seattle: University of Washington Press.

Spickard, P. R. (1989). *Mixed blood: Intermarriage and ethnic identity in twentieth-century America.* Madison, WI: University of Wisconsin Press.

Strupp, H., & Binder, J. (1984). *Psychotherapy in a new key: A guide to time-limited dynamic psychotherapy.* New York: Basic Books.

Sue, D. (1981). *Counseling the culturally different: Therapy and practice.* New York: Wiley.

Sue, S., & McKinney, H. (1975). Asian Americans in the community mental health care system. *American Journal of Orthopsychiatry, 45,* 111–118.

Sue, S., & Morishima, J. (1982). *The mental health of Asian Americans: Contemporary issues in identifying and treating mental problems.* San Francisco: Jossey-Bass.

Sue, S., & Sue, D. (1974). MMPI comparisons between Asian American and non-Asian students utilizing a student health psychiatric clinic. *Journal of Counseling Psychology, 21,* 423–427.

Sue, D., Sue, D., & Sue, S. (1983). Psychological development of Chinese American children. In G. J. Powell, J. Yamamoto, A. Romero, & A. Morales (Eds.), *The psychosocial development of minority group children* (pp. 159–166). New York: Brunner/Mazel.

Takaki, R. (1989). *Strangers from a different shore.* New York: Penguin Books.

Tan, A. (1989). *The joy luck club.* New York: G. P. Putnam's Sons.

Tsui, A. M. (1985). Psychotherapeutic considerations in sexual counseling for Asian immigrants. *Psychotherapy: Theory, Research, and Practice, 22,* 357–362.

U.S. Bureau of the Census. (1980). *Census of population* (PC 80-1-D1-A, Table 255). Washington, DC: U.S. Government Printing Office.

Wong, D. Y.-M. (1983). Asian/Pacific American women: Legal issues. In *Civil rights issues of Asian and Pacific Americans: Myths and realities* (pp. 153–164). Washington, DC: U.S. Government Printing Office.

Wong, D. Y., & Hayashi, D. (1989). Behind unmarked doors: Developments in the garment industry. In Asian Women United of California (Ed.), *Making waves: An anthology of writings by and about Asian American women* (pp. 159–171). Boston: Beacon Press.

Wong, J. S. (1989). *Fifth Chinese daughter.* Seattle: University of Washington Press.

Woo, D. (1989). The gap between striving and achieving: The cases of Asian American women. In Asian Women United of California (Ed.), *Making waves: An anthology of writings by and about Asian American women* (pp. 185–194). Boston: Beacon Press.

Yamada, M. (1983). Asian Pacific American women and feminism. In C. Moraga & G. Anzaldira (Eds.), *This bridge called my back: Writings by radical women of color.* New York: Kitchen Table–Women of Color Press.

Yi, K. Y. (1989, April). Symptoms of eating disorders among Asian-American college female students as a function of acculturation. *Dissertation Abstracts International, 50,* 10.

Yu, E.-Y. (1987). Korean-American women: Demographic profiles and family roles. In Yu, & E. H. Phillips (Eds.), *Korean women in transition: At home and abroad.* Los Angeles: Center for Korean American and Korean Studies, California State University.

Yung, J. (1986). *Chinese women of America: A pictorial history.* Seattle: University of Washington Press.

Yung, J. (1989). A chronology of Asian American History. In Asian Women United of California (Ed.), *Making waves: An anthology of writings by and about Asian American women* (pp. 423–431). Boston: Beacon Press.

4

Latinas

Melba J. T. Vasquez

Understanding the conditions that make for Latinas' mental health requires both an awareness of factors specific to Hispanic culture and a sensitivity to individual variation. We must become adequately informed and respectful of the Latinas' relevant individual, sociocultural, and environmental influences if we are to provide her competent, ethical, and responsible services. Mental health practitioners who ignore cultural values, attitudes, behaviors, and experiences different from their own deprive themselves of crucial information. From that ignorance comes a tendency to impose their own worldviews and assumptions upon clients in a erroneous and destructive manner. On the other hand, clinicians must avoid making simplistic, unfounded assumptions on the basis of one's ethnicity and gender. Many clinicians, sometimes even well-meaning ones, apply ethnic stereotypes, rather than carefully assessing a particular Latina woman's experience. Knowledge about cultural and socioeconomic contexts is best used as the basis for informed inquiry, rather than as blanket group characteristics with which to stereotype the client.

This chapter will present a clinical/counseling framework (Casas & Vasquez, 1989) for the competent and ethical treatment of Latina women. The framework comprises three categories. The first category identifies personal and professional attitudes, beliefs, and knowledge of the therapist. The second identifies individual, sociocultural, and environmental experiences of Latina women that must be understood and addressed in psychotherapy. The third category describes therapeutic approaches to counseling Latinas, including the importance of empowering clients through acknowledgement of the positive aspects of their culture. Critical issues in the delivery of both individual and group psychotherapy will be described. The terms "Latino" and "Latina" are growing in preference over the term "Hispanic" (Chapa & Valencia, 1993), and will thus be used throughout the chapter.

THE CLINICIAN

Language and cultural differences, as well as personal and professional biases, can serve as barriers to the delivery of mental health services to Latinas. Pope (Pope & Vasquez, 1991) interviewed several prominent therapists with expertise in identifying and responding to suicidal risk, among them Ricardo Munoz, Ph.D., a principal investigator in National Institute of Mental Health (NIMH) depression prevention research involving English-, Spanish-, and Chinese-speaking populations. Dr. Munoz presented a worst-possible scenario that could evolve from lack of language compatibility:

> Recently, a Spanish-speaking woman, suicidal, came to the emergency room talking of pills. The physician, who spoke limited Spanish, obtained what he thought was her promise not to attempt suicide and sent her back to her halfway house. It was later discovered that she'd been saying that she'd already taken a lethal dose of pills and was trying to get help. (p. 167)

A study (Wampold, Casas, & Atkinson, 1981) investigating the attitudes of practicing psychotherapists toward African Americans, Chinese Americans, Japanese Americans, Jews, and Mexican Americans found that of all the responses provided by the therapists, 79.2% indicated the presence of subtle stereotypic attitudes, and 22.6% demonstrated blatant stereotypic attitudes. The stereotypes most frequently ascribed to Latinos tended to be negative (lazy, dumb, dirty, overemotional). Other research also supports the reality that therapists are personally and professionally biased. Furthermore, the risk of miscommunication in psychotherapy is thought to be highest when the client is an ethnic minority female and the therapist is an Anglo American male (Wilkinson, 1980).

Therapists face many challenges in identifying, understanding, and transcending differences between therapist and Latina client. Each of us must accept the reality that we are indeed influenced by our socialization, which includes assumptions, values, attitudes, biases, and stereotypes. We must remain constantly vigilant and engage in ongoing professional training to free us from our personal and professional biases.

Perhaps the therapist's biggest challenge is to work to prevent in the therapeutic relationship replication of various inequities of opportunity and other prejudices that the client encounters in society. To do so, therapists must recognize the personal and professional assumptions that determine and direct their interactions with clients. A healthy clinical relationship is difficult, perhaps impossible, if the counselor is unaware of his or her own perceptions of and attitudes about particular differences, such as gender, race, ethnicity, skin color, socioeconomic status, nationality, and sexual orientation. Without awareness, the exploration that should occur regarding these issues cannot take place honestly and openly in the therapeutic relationship (Casas & Vasquez, 1989; Pinderhughes, 1989).

A fundamental set of cultural values forms the core of the therapeutic profession, regardless of therapeutic orientation. Those values reflect the majority culture: rugged individualism, autonomy, competition, action orientation, the Protestant work ethic, progress and future orientation, the scientific method of inquiry, the nuclear family structure, assertiveness, and rigid timetables. These are *not* universal values. A Latina woman who strongly identifies with traditional Latino culture may hold values in sharp contrast to some of them. She may emphasize family and group achievement over individual achievement; value extended family as well as nuclear family; lack the "proper" amount of assertiveness; or reveal a less rigid, present-focused time orientation. If so, she displays some traditional Latino values that may conflict with those of her counselor. Alternately, a highly acculturated Latina may espouse values, attitudes, and beliefs more similar to the White majority culture, varying only in manner and degree.

Yet, some therapists ascribe blind and unquestioning importance to those cultural factors, perceiving them as universal (Casas & Vasquez, 1989). Imposing one's culture-specific values and/or assuming pathology in the absence of those values is prejudicial and destructive, however well-meaning one's intent. Often, our treatment process intrudes our prejudicial attitudes in both the assessment and the treatment of culturally different individuals (Goodyear & Sinnet, 1984). Quite simply, without awareness of one's biases, a therapist is incapable of providing ethical and competent services for culturally different clients.

Several writers (Casas & Vasquez, 1989; Corvin & Wiggins, 1989; Katz & Ivey, 1977) have challenged psychotherapists to explore their own racism. They believe avoidance of this process allows mental health providers the luxury of denying responsibility for or connection with the racist system that oppresses others. In truth, too many mental health providers continue to view culturally different populations as inherently inferior and White American as superior to all existing cultures. We too often fail to realize that racism is not the result of cultural differences, but the consequence of White ethnocentrism (Corvin & Wiggins, 1989), and that that ethnocentrism is a pervasive and problematic attitude for us all.

Despite the wide range of differences among people, diversity is not yet valued and celebrated. We do not yet fully respect those who differ from the majority. Indeed, racism is often an attempt to control diversity, for differences still make us feel uncomfortable, less secure, and, above all, threatened. Ironically, those therapists most prone to ethnocentrism seldom allow themselves to recognize that imposition of monoculturalism is identified, by some theorists, as a characteristic of the adolescent developmental stage, or that such a "herd instinct" cannot be easily reconciled with a quest for autonomy. The inability to accommodate ambiguity, the tendency to polarize, and the simplistic reasoning of duality are all characteristics of less than mature emotional and cognitive development. They are also central to the mindset of racism.

Psychotherapists must be aware of the possibility of the insidious, pervasive and inadvertent internalization of intolerance, which may take the form of disdain for deviations from their preferred standard, and must be particularly sensitive to their role in working with members of oppressed groups. Hare-Mustin, Marecek, Kaplan, and Liss-Levinson (1979) describe how members of these groups often enter therapy in a help-seeking posture, not a self-protective one; that the therapy situation is a novel one for most clients; and that some clients, who have been denied power historically, may not be prepared to assert their rights, especially if their complaints are typically unheeded. Therapists who must obtain informed consent for a particular technique or disclosure, for example, must be especially careful to insure that genuine informed consent is in fact obtained.

Finally, therapists must be aware of how training and learning about human behavior takes place in a sociocultural context. Our typical training does not emphasize the unique frame of reference and psychosocial history of culturally different clients. Moreover, our learning process entails development of a "cognitive map of the counseling process and a related 'psychology' of humanity" (Holiman & Lauver, 1987). The counselor's own cultural background and experiences serve as powerful filters to the acquisition of that cognitive map and view of humanity. This filtering process not only inhibits learning about cultural diversity, but also results in the tendency and desire to work with clients most culturally similar to oneself. It also discourages our appreciation of the importance of understanding behavior, attitudes, and feelings from the perspective of the culturally different individual. As a result, either we do not bond with our culturally different clients, or we risk errors in assessment, diagnosis, and treatment of those clients—sometimes both. Before we try to understand our clients, we must first be aware of our tendencies toward inappropriate inferences when we assess others' behaviors different from our own worldviews.

KNOWLEDGE OF THE CLIENT

Gender, ethnicity, and socioeconomic class are core components of an individual's identity. The Latina woman's culture, history, and experience with oppression causes variations in human behavior and development. Visible behavior may not mean the same to the client as it seems to the clinician, so that understanding these aspects of Latinas' cultural context is crucial for the psychotherapist. At the same time, we must remember that the descriptions that follow in this section are applicable to some Latinas, some of the time, for a period of time. Many differences exist within groups, and the groups that make up Latina women in the United States are dynamic and constantly in flux, as are values, behaviors, and attitudes. Conceptions of gender roles are changing for men and women as we enter the 21st century, both for White cultures and for the cultures of Latinos.

The following scenarios are created from years of clinical observation and experience, as well as from research conducted about Latina women. Some are fictional, others are composites of cases and have been modified to protect confidentiality. No case identifies any one person. There are no clear ways to conceptualize or intervene, but the cases are presented to stimulate discussion, and to encourage the reader to draw conclusions based on the information presented in this chapter. I also refer to these cases later in the chapter.

Scenario 1. A 35-year-old Chicana woman enters therapy, reporting depressive symptoms. She reports that she has been distraught about and feels "stuck" in her grief for an aged aunt who died several months previously. As you explore, you discover that the aunt had served as the primary nurturer in this woman's life. Furthermore, you discover that this woman, who is a professional with advanced degrees, is suffering from incredible guilt because she "failed" to be at her aunt's deathbed, even though the aunt had asked for her. Your client had chosen to attend a professional meeting to do "networking," basing her decision on the fact that her aunt had been sick on and off for several months. How do you proceed?

Scenario 2. You co-lead a Latina Women's Support Group that consists of Chicana, Puerto Rican, and Mexican group members. You discover that all but one of the ten members of your group has either been sexually molested as a child, or has experienced rape or other sexual assault. The question arises in your mind, Is there a higher incidence of sexual abuse among Latino groups?

Scenario 3. A 32-year-old Chicana whose gentle, polite style has resulted in being "run over" and mistreated both at work and at home, enters therapy as a result of a white woman's suggestion. She cannot afford your fee. After negotiating a sliding scale fee, she reports that she can only come once a month. Furthermore, she reports doubt about the "assertive style" that her friend uses and is fearful that the therapist will also insist that the Chicana client use that style, as her friend has been insisting. How should you proceed?

Scenario 4. A 23-year-old university female student enters therapy in crisis over a racist statement that a roommate made about Latinos. The client, half European American (father) and half Latina (mother), has never "claimed" her identity to herself, much less to peers such as roommates. She had been told by both parents to "pass" as White if she could. She has become very concerned about gender, race, and class issues, recently gave a talk about feminism, and is now confused about the ethnic aspect of her identity. She is beginning to be aware of the hurt and anger that is emerging toward her roommates and her parents. What direction should therapy take?

Demographics

The term "Latina" comprises a very diverse group of people. A publication from the U.S. Census Bureau (1991) reports that Latinos increased by 53%

to 22.4 million since 1980, 9% of the U.S. population, compared to a 9% increase for the total population. Approximately half of this growth was due to foreign immigration and half was due to births to Latinos in the United States (Chapa & Valencia, 1993). Unfortunately, research surveys, census information, and other statistics rarely provide breakdowns of information within Latino groups. This is a problem since Latinos comprise an aggregation of several distinct national origin subgroups (Chapa & Valencia, 1993), and research has found differences among Puerto Rican, Mexican, and Cuban, Central, and South Americans (Amaro, Russo, & Johnson, 1987). Latinos living on the U.S. mainland have the following backgrounds: the Mexican-origin population constitutes 60%; South Americans, Central Americans, and other Latinos 22%; Puerto Ricans 12%; and Cubans 5% of the total Latino population.

The various Latino groups are concentrated in different regions of the country: Mexicans in the Southwest and Midwest, Puerto Ricans in the Northeast, Cubans in the Southeast. The other Latino populations are found in areas with concentrations of Mexican, Puerto Rican, or Cuban populations (Chapa & Valencia, 1993). Chapa and Valencia (1993) point out that Latinos are highly urbanized, and that 67% of all U.S. Latinos reside in 16 metropolitan areas.

Various sociodemographic characteristics of Latinos are relevant to mental health, including education attainment, employment, generation and immigration status, family income, family size, and language status. Chapa and Valencia (1993) provide a thorough overview of those data for Latinos. It is important to note that a large percentage of Latinos are of the lower class, regardless of generational status in the United States (Padilla, Salgado de Snyder, Cervantes, & Baezconde-Garbanati, 1987). Any study involving Latinos should therefore control for social class, either experimentally or statistically. Unfortunately, many studies have been conducted comparing lower-class Latinos to middle-class Anglo Americans in which differences were attributed to culture rather than social class (Padilla et al., 1987). More research is needed to determine the effects of poverty on Latinos, especially since Chapa and Valencia (1993) point out that many educational and economic measures show no indication that Latinos are achieving parity, and some measures indicate relative and absolute declines even among Latino families who have been in the United States for a number of generations. There is no doubt that poverty is clearly stressful, damaging to a sense of well-being, and results in numerous and complex disadvantages. Yet we must not automatically assume knowledge about the effects of poverty on each geographical cultural group. A report by Winkler (1990) in the *Chronicle of Higher Education* cited evidence of "cultural vitality," coined by Dr. David E. Hayes-Bautista, a professor of Medicine at UCLA. Researchers examined some of California's poor Latina population, and their findings promoted debate over the traditional definitions of the "underclass." Some of Dr. Hayes-Bautista's research findings clearly invalidated characteristics typically associated with the "underclass" portrayed in other reports.

For example, poor Latinos were twice as likely to live in traditional family structures compared to either poor Blacks or Whites; Latinos had the highest rates of working males, higher life expectancy, with a 50% lower rate of violent deaths compared to Blacks, and 20% lower compared to Whites. Furthermore, immigrant Latinos exhibited healthier behavior than Latinos born in this country. These unexpected findings point to the importance of using well-conducted research, as foundation for our understanding of Latinos, rather than speculative assumptions.

As the United States shifts to an economy based on technology and information, the American worker must become increasingly skilled, trained, and educated. Unfortunately, the educational rates of attainment for Latinos remain low. Educational demographics are important, since attainment of education is highly correlated to success and power in the United States society, which in turn are related to well-being and mental health. In a study of 18- and 19-year-old Latinos, the National Council of La Raza found that in 1988, 31% had dropped out of high school, compared to 18% of African Americans, and 14% of European Americans at the same age. According to other figures 40 to 50% of all Latino students leave school before the tenth grade. A report (1990) by the United States Census Bureau found that three out of ten Latino high-school graduates aged 18 to 24 were enrolled in college in 1988, about the same percentage as in 1978; thus, over the past decade there appears to have been little or no improvement in the Latinos overall college attendance rates. A recent (1991) report from the American College Testing service indicated that Latinos had the lowest educational attainment rates compared to other groups.

There is some evidence that Latina women, particularly Mexican Americans, fare even worse. Mexican American women are reported in some studies to have the lowest educational attainment rates, the highest levels of unemployment, and the highest poverty levels of any group in the United States, including Mexican American men, African Americans of both sexes, and women of all groups (Chacon, Cohen, Camerena, Gonzalez, & Strover, 1985). The problem of educational attainment for Latinos is a complex one, and cannot be adequately addressed here. Suffice it to say that the relatively low levels of educational attainment, low income, and lack of access to key resources in society contribute to many of the problems for Latina women.

Ethnic and Gender Identity

Identity is a very important factor affecting mental health. It involves the way one views oneself in regard to qualities, characteristics, and values. Social psychologists describe the development of one's identity as partly based on the messages one receives from significant others about oneself.

In addition, identity is formed as a result of messages in society about one's primary reference group.

What are the messages in society about Latinas? The lack of positive images in the media, the lack of positive role models in positions of power, and the promotion of negative stereotypes and expectations of Latinas contribute to their second-class status. Some exceptions are emerging, such as the national newspaper *Vista*, which highlights positive contributions and achievements of Hispanic men and women. Nevertheless, Latinas are still generally affected by the triply oppressive experiences associated with being female, ethnic, and, often, poor. Latinas frequently come from families who themselves have had few opportunities and options in life, and do not have options in their repertoire to offer to their daughters.

Ramirez (1991) describes how minorities often experience "feeling different," including feelings of alienation and loneliness. He describes how the majority society imposes pressures on minority cultures to conform, to abandon their individuality, and to force themselves into the fictional ideal molds and patterns created by those who have power and influence. The members of these cultures are made to feel different and inferior, as if there were something wrong with them. The end result is often the rejection of oneself in order to "fit in" and to appear less different.

Dr. Teresa Bernardez, a professor of psychiatry in the College of Human Medicine at Michigan State University, in describing the various sources of depression for women at a Women and Self-Esteem conference (1990), noted that when a woman is not provided with people around her who are able to communicate appreciation for that woman's uniqueness and difference, damage to the self occurs. When caretakers, significant others, and society do not convey a caring attitude, with expectations that women will succeed, these women then fail to discover the abilities in themselves. Confidence does not develop and/or is eroded. When a Latina does not experience individuals who register with sensitivity and admiration the possibilities and visions for that woman, she then runs the risk of resigned despair, of finding herself on a "dead-end street."

Unfortunately, the restrictive gender and sex-role stereotyping that characterizes early socialization fails to equip girls with skills and competence, undermines self-confidence, and lays a foundation for the development of mental health problems in adulthood (Gilligan, Rogers, & Tolman, 1991) Indeed, one of the most pervasive issues for women, including Latinas, is lack of confidence, tendency to blame self or lack of ability for failures, and failure to take credit for successes.

Encounters with racism, regardless of age, are traumatic. Early in life, those experiences result in a feeling of lack of safety, and create dissonance and confusion. These experiences may result in a variety of responses and coping strategies. If one has been "inoculated" with a sense of self-pride, and given strong messages of entitlement and appreciation of one's group, then an individual may not internalize the negative messages so much.

However, most people have to develop a cognitive, emotional, and behavioral map of how to deal with the hurt, including denial, anger, and rage, achievement, perfectionism, defensiveness, and strategizing.

Recurring racist events may lead to depression, anxiety, and posttraumatic stress disorder. Increased anxiety, nightmares, feelings of lack of safety, and irritability are some symptoms which Latinas may exhibit in response to such traumas. Each individual who experiences discriminatory behavior has to struggle to incorporate and deal with the painful experience. It takes extra effort not to feel badly about oneself; it takes extra effort to know what do with hurt and anger. It is important in psychotherapy to talk openly about these aspects of a Latina woman's life, and to discuss these issues as due more to institutional and systemic discrimination than to personal inadequacy. At the same time, skills (assertiveness, conflict management) and strategies (positive self-talk, seeking support strategies) in dealing with discrimination are part of the process of empowerment for a Latina. The negative expectations a college professor has of a Latina advisee, and the "glass ceiling" she experiences at work because her boss assumes that her style would not be effective in advanced positions, are examples of subtle but painful oppression. Helping a Latina client face these issues can contribute to a more positive sense of identity, which is a major aspect of mental health and well-being.

Cultural Characteristics

The importance and value of the family is perhaps one of the most salient and empirically supported characteristics of the Latino culture. Ramirez and Arce (1981) reviewed relevant empirical literature on the Chicano family, for example, in an attempt to explore the validity of various family issues that have been conceptually confusing and distorted in the social science literature. They present the following characteristics of Chicano families:

> a strong, persistent familistic orientation; a widespread existence of highly integrated extended kinship systems, even for Chicanos who are three or more generations removed from Mexico; and the consistent preference of Chicanos for relying on the extended family for support, as the primary means for coping with emotional stress. (p. 15)

In an investigation of Latino familism and acculturation, Sabogal, Marin, Otero-Sabogal, Marin, and Perez-Stable (1987) identified three separate dimensions of familism: family obligations (perceived obligation to provide material and emotional support to extended family members), perceived support from family (perception of family members as reliable providers of help), and family as referents (relatives as behavioral and attitudinal models of identity). They found that acculturation was a salient variable in predicting both the familial obligations and family as referents aspects of familism. Perceived support from the family seemed to be the most stable dimension of familism, as it did not decrease significantly with acculturation. Although two of the dimensions decreased with acculturation, even highly acculturated Latinos were more familistic than White non-Hispanics on all dimensions that were examined. Furthermore, the dimensions of family obligations, support from family, and family as referents were found to be core characteristics of Latino culture that did not vary among the subgroups who participated in the study—Mexican Americans, Cuban Americans, and Central Americans—despite levels of acculturation.

The implication of this research is that the individuation process, a salient therapeutic issue in most Western psychotherapies may proceed differently for those from Latino cultures. Additionally, the importance of such values as independence, individuality, and competition may be different for Latinas than the traditional psychotherapist may expect.

Indeed, the client in Scenario 1, despite the fact that she was a third-generation, relatively acculturated Latina, still experienced the dilemma of pulls in the professional world to make professional responsibilities high priority, despite her family norm of honoring older members of the family by one's presence, particularly at times of illness and death. Helping her struggle through the guilt meant not diminishing the importance of either of her competing values and regrets about choices, but rather encouraging her to let go of the perfectionistic harshness with which she judged herself. She could do so when the therapist allowed her to have her regrets, grief, and wishes about different choices.

Gender Roles

Much has been written about the rigidity of gender roles in the traditional Latino culture. Many mental health workers automatically assume that derogatory portrayals of the socialization processes regarding gender roles in the Latino family are true. The most common stereotype is that of an authoritarian husband and submissive wife. In fact, very few studies have actually assessed the socialization processes of Latino families. A study by Zapata and Jaramillo (1981) used Adlerian-style interviews to examine the socialization of sex-role stereotypes. They concluded that gender-related interactions within the Mexican American family were more complex than previously assumed. Parents did not perceive themselves as prescribing rigid sex roles to their children, but siblings reported perceptions that females acted in a more socially cooperative manner. Zapata and Jaramillo suggested that the socializing processes of Mexican American families may not be as different from majority culture as was earlier believed. They further concluded that a dynamic view of the Latino family may be more accurate than the static, rigid view that has been taken in past research. Indeed, the myth of male dominance in the Latino family, especially in regard to decision-making, has been reviewed by others (Bernal, 1982; Comas-Díaz, 1989; Cromwell & Ruiz, 1979). Cromwell and Ruiz (1979), for example, concluded that the notion of male dominance in marital decision-making was a myth. Their conclusion was based on an intensive analysis of four major studies on marital decision-making within Mexican and Chicano families. While they did acknowledge that Latino males may behave differently from non-Latino males in their family and marital lives, they concluded that such behavior did not necessarily take the inappropriate forms suggested by the myth of the *macho*, with its strong connotations of social deviance.

In my experience, families that are relatively healthy and functional, where roles are traditionally assigned, exhibit a mutuality and respect for the ascribed roles. In those healthy families, the traditional roles (e.g., working father, homemaker mother) do not exclude equity in decision making and conflict resolution. However, in dysfunctional families, traditional roles are carried out in a more oppressive and pathological manner, with power battles, abusive behavior, poor conflict resolution, and low marital satisfaction. There is some evidence that Latinas internalize the expectation to nurture, care for, and maintain the family unity and connections. The Latina may therefore deny or ignore her needs in order to keep the family intact, even in the face of abuse, lack of happiness, or unsuccessful marriage. In addition, there is evidence that family support is positively associated with success in college for Chicanas (Gandará, 1982; Vasquez, 1982), and that Chicanas' strong emphasis on domestic responsibilities is related to poor progress in academic programs (Chacon, Cohen, & Strover, 1986).

The actual dynamic variation that exists among Latino families must be considered, and the tendency to pathologize Latino families simply because of traditional values must be avoided. Yet, some elements of the assignment of traditional roles to men and women in any culture, while adaptive in agricultural and other societies, may become problematic in a dynamic, technological society (Vasquez, 1984). Especially for those women who are in traditional and dysfunctional relationships, symptoms of mental and physical illnesses, such as depression, anxiety, and psychosomatic symptoms may be evident.

Mental Health Issues

Latina women are at high risk of experiencing mental health problems. However, the extent of this risk for Latinos in general, and to some degree for Latina women, is only beginning to be understood. Epidemiological studies on topics such as alcoholism among Latinos are relatively recent, and often do not break down gender differences.

Depressive disorders and depressive symptomatology have been examined, as well as risk factors associated with depression. Most studies

(Canino et al., 1987; Salgado de Snyder, 1987) are consistent with previous research on other groups, which shows that depression is significantly more prevalent in Latino (in these studies Puerto Rican and Mexican) women than in men. Gender differences are typically hypothesized to be due to social causation. That is, many of women's traditional roles are given low societal value; roles may be unrewarding; women's work outside the home may be associated with gender, ethnic, and class discrimination; in women, overt manifestation of anger is discouraged; and women feel (and often have) less control in their lives.

Some research is beginning to shed light on the specific manifestations of depression for Latinas. For example, Salgado de Snyder (1987) found that women immigrants who in the last three months experienced discrimination, sex-role conflicts, and concern about starting a family in this country had significantly higher depression scores than did women who did not report experiencing those situations. Thus Mexican women immigrants with those experiences may be at a higher risk for the development of psychological problems.

In a study examining family and work predictors of psychological well-being among Latina women professionals, Amaro et al. (1987) found that income was the most consistently related demographic factor across all measures of psychological well-being.

This study of a very select population of highly educated, high-income Latina women in professional and managerial positions also showed that Latina women's psychological well-being is related to the experience of discrimination, reported by more than 82% of the sample. Furthermore, women in some Latino groups enjoyed better mental health than others. For example, Puerto Rican women were more likely than Mexican American women to report psychological distress symptoms, whereas Cubans reported less stress in balancing partner and professional roles than did Mexican Americans. These findings point to the critical need for research involving separate analyses for women of diverse Latino backgrounds; clinically, they imply that we must remain abreast of such research developments and carefully assess the situations of our individual clients. Never assume that a general finding for a particular Latino group applies to all Latino groups, or to all individuals within the particular group.

A report by the American Psychological Association's National Task Force on Women and Depression (McGrath, Keita, Strickland, & Russo, 1990) more fully described the risk factors, research, and treatment issues in regard to women and depression, including Latinas. While no one theory or set of theories fully explains gender differences in depression, many helpful considerations for therapists are provided. For example, the rate of sexual and physical abuse of females is a major factor in women's depression. One third to one half of all women have had a significant experience of physical or sexual abuse before the age of 21. This points to the probability that depressive symptoms may be long-standing effects of posttraumatic stress syndrome for many women. Additionally, women in unhappy marriages are three times as likely to be depressed as married men and single women. Mothers of young children, especially several young children, are highly vulnerable to depression. Finally, the report summarizes that poverty is a "pathway to depression" (p. xii).

Violence against Latinas is an issue of concern to clinicians. Wife abuse is found in all social, economic, religious, ethnic, and educational levels. Mixed data are found in regard to variations of incidence among those groups. Studies report a range of 26% to 60% incidence for all couples (Torres, 1986). While no studies have indicated a higher or lower incidence of spousal abuse among Latino groups, some research does indicate a higher incidence of wife abuse in lower socioeconomic classes. Other factors contributing to spousal abuse include violent behavior in pervious generations, high levels of stress, social isolation, pregnancy, sex-role stereotyping, and prevalence of alcohol and drugs (Walker, 1989).

As with wife abuse, rape is suspected to be underreported by Latina women, as it is in the general population. Nevertheless, perhaps because of the distrust of public agencies, women of color are less likely to report rape than nonminority women (Feldman-Summers & Ashworth, 1981). Violence against women is a major problem in society; for the Latina, it is an additional oppressive experience that can result in depression, poor self-esteem, and other physical and mental disorders.

Very little information is available in regard to sexual abuse among Latino families. In one study, however, the prevalence rates of child sexual victimization were reported to be lower for Latinos (3.0%) when compared to non-Latino Whites (8.7%) (Siegel, Sorenson, Golding, Burnam, & Stein, 1987). Thus, as clinicians, we must be aware that individual and group clients are a self-selected group of individuals, and a large proportion of sexually abused or assaulted clients means that these clients are suffering from long-term adjustment difficulties. Therapists must not generalize from situations such as that in Scenario 2, where 9 out of 10 group members had experienced some form of sexual violence. Clinicians must remember that clients often self-select for treatment in appropriate ways—for example, to work through wounds from earlier emotional damage—but characteristics such as a high incidence of rape experiences among clients should not alone be considered evidence of high incidence in the Latina population quite generally. Wyatt (1990) maintains that there may be some aspects of ethnic minority children's lives that affect long-term adjustment to these traumatic experiences. Other forms of victimization (discrimination, poverty), may evoke posttraumatic stress disorder, for example.

Adolescent pregnancy has become a major social problem with the increase in pregnancy rates in the last decade. In 1978, over 19% of all teenage women in the United States had had unplanned pregnancies. Recent figures indicate that teen birthrates among Latinos are higher than those of non-Latino White women (Padilla et al., 1987). Interestingly enough, Becerra and De Ana (1984, as cited in Padilla et al., 1987), who conducted one of the few studies on Mexican American adolescent pregnancies, found that high level of acculturation was related to high levels of sexual activity and to low usage of contraceptive devices. That is, the more acculturated Mexican American adolescents are at higher risk for unwanted pregnancies than are those less acculturated. Padilla et al. (1987) point out that many factors other than acculturation have not been adequately studied in Latino adolescents, such as educational level of mothers, social support received from the mother, adolescents' self-esteem, use and non-use of contraception, information about human reproduction, etc.

Suicide risk among Latinos has also been ignored among researchers. Padilla et al. (1987) summarized two studies, which reported lower rates of suicide among Latinos when compared to Whites. Important differences with respect to gender and age were found. The ratio of male to female suicides among Latinos was almost twice that of the male–female suicide ratio evidenced for non-Latinos. Additionally, 25% of Latina females and 33% of Latino males who committed suicide were found to be under 25 years of age. Unfortunately, the incidence of Latino homicide rates appears to be quite high: 2½ times the homicide rates found for Whites. Socioeconomic conditions and stressful urban living conditions are offered as possible reasons for the higher rates. These distressful realities either directly or indirectly affect the lives and well-being of the Latina women with whom we work.

AIDS as an issue for Hispanics and women was reported in the February 1991 issue of the *Monitor* (American Psychological Association). A study by Hortensia Amaro found misconceptions about AIDS and transmission of HIV that causes AIDS in large portions of four Latino subgroups studied, including women of childbearing age. The other groups included were drug users, adolescents and gay men. At the time of the study, Latinos accounted for more than 15% of the total AIDS cases diagnosed in the United States, but made up only 7.8% of the U.S. population. The study reported that many programs have attempted to educate women about the need for condom use with their partners, but have sometimes overlooked the critical role of educating men. This health crisis has numerous implications for mental health.

Employment issues are also of concern for Latina women. A person's employment and her attitude toward work are important characteristics affecting mental health. For most persons, work is a major life activity. A good job may represent a goal allowing escape from poverty for immigrants, or it can be an occupation that contributes to a positive sense of identity or well-being. It can also constitute a tedious unavoidable task. We know that stress in the workplace is pervasive and has extensive costly consequences in dollars and physical health and psychological well-being. We also know that while high-stress jobs can have negative consequences, worker control (the fact and/or the perception that one has some degree of choice in work tasks, etc.) or lack thereof, is the more meaningful predictor of physical problems such as cardiovascular response.

As of 1990, 75% of those entering the American workforce are minorities and women. Thus, women and ethnic minorities are predicted to dominate our labor pool in the near future. Patterns of prejudice, bias, and in-group preference will consequently have to be modified (Jones, 1990). Women and minorities face a "glass ceiling" that limits their advancement toward top management in organizations throughout U.S. society. The glass ceiling is a popular concept of the 1980s, describing a barrier so subtle that it is transparent, yet so strong that it prevents women and persons of color from moving up in the management hierarchy (Morrison & Von Glinow, 1990). Morrison and Von Glinow cite data that dispute that sex and race deficiencies account for the lack of representation in management ranks. Discrimination and other systemic barriers, including sexual harassment, are proposed as explanations. Discrimination was one of the factors described by Amaro et al. (1987) as associated with Latina professional women's mental health distress symptoms and with their lower satisfaction in their personal lives.

The unique experience of the Latina must be assessed as an "overlay" to other more traditional sociohistorical life factors that differentiate all individuals (i.e., family size, birth order, childhood illnesses, family mobility, family deaths and divorces, type of parenting received, etc.). Each Latina's experiences must be assessed to determine more accurately her particular reality and mental health needs. This section has articulated issues that, recognized and addressed, can contribute to the therapist's better understanding of Latinas.

THERAPEUTIC INTERVENTION

Individual Psychotherapy

Regardless of theoretical approach to treatment, effective therapy with Latina women incorporates elements of both feminist therapy and multicultural treatment. Both feminist and cross-cultural therapies are based on philosophies that hold as a basic tenet that external factors are examined as causative in the client's problems. Approaches are endorsed that result in empowerment of the client to engage in change if she so chooses, rather than those that pathologize or blame her. Her strengths rather than her weaknesses are emphasized and validated. Care, respect, and conditions conducive to trust are promoted. Perhaps one of the most important functions of the therapist of a Latina is to communicate a caring attitude that discovers the abilities in the client, registers with sensitivity, respect, and admiration the possibilities and visions for the client, and is able to delight in what is unique, special, and novel in that client. Believing in a Latina client can do much to promote the confidence that has probably been eroded by the experience of life in this society.

For example, consider the group members in Scenario 2. Nine out of ten experienced sexual abuse and felt some degree of guilt and responsibility for that abuse. In addition to facilitating expressions of care, anger, and concern for each other about the experiences, the effective therapist would help group members understand how society condones such behavior toward women. The group would explore the differences between the socialization of the genders: that men are seen as entitled to having their needs met, without regard to women's feelings; that women are socialized to feel responsible for the well-being of others. This is an important intervention in decreasing the toxic guilt that women carry when they've been abused. Women in general tend to assume blame and responsibility for failure, or for negative, painful experiences. The role of the therapist is to help the client have compassion and care for herself, and to learn to expect it from significant others.

As therapists, we must guard against our tendency to apply psychotherapy in a manner that encourages our clients to adapt to unhealthy environments, rather than empowering them to change those environments or leave them. Amaro and Russo (1987) call for the cultural sensitivity of services for Latina women, and they cite feminist criticism of psychotherapy as a form of social control. We cannot afford to ignore the truth that exists in that generalization. For example, "helping" a woman modulate her anger, or express it in a "sensitive, tactful" manner to an abusive, sadistic husband or to an oppressive boss, rather than exploring other options such as to leave those environments, may collude with the oppression she is experiencing. Offering choices while examining potential consequences of those options is more freeing, empowering, and effective.

Often, well-meaning therapists discourage women's drive to maintain and need relationships by labeling women as dependent or codependent in the pathological sense, for wanting to care for others. The effective therapist validates the qualities and characteristics of care and nurturing of the Latina; in addition, the effective therapist teaches the Latina client to apply the same principles of care and nurturing to herself. Discouraging a Latina mother from caring "too much" for her children can be confusing. A more effective approach would be to validate her care, and to also help her learn to listen to her inner voice in regard to the point at which "giving too much" violates her own needs and identity as a person. One client, for example, found herself constantly depressed in response to the life struggles of her three adult children. In therapy, we discussed the value of caring for her children, but also the notion of balancing her own care for herself. For a period of time, we "practiced" figuring out the ways in which she could indeed care, listen, and help within certain bounds, but not feel she had to come up with the resolution of every problem, and especially not "take on" the pain, depression, and angst of her children, which was conceptualized as a natural part of life's struggle.

Comas-Díaz (1987) challenges therapists to apply carefully the integration of feminist principles into practice with Latina women. She urges feminist therapists to appreciate the unique experiences of power and oppression, transculturation (process whereby a conflict in opposing cultural values results in emergence of a new culture, a very different process from acculturation), and other cultural experiences of Latinas. She also describes how assertiveness training can be effectively used with Puerto Rican women, when a cultural component incorporated into the training "translates" the concept to Puerto Rican women in an acceptable manner.

The Chicana in Scenario 3, who was fearful of having to be assertive like her white female friend, was much more willing to consider developing communication skills which articulated how she felt, what she preferred, and what was experienced as disrespectful to her. These assertive skills were incorporated into her style, and conveyed in a manner with which she felt comfortable. She did leave her job for one with more responsibility (which she had been told by her previous boss that she could not handle), and has since received two promotions.

Traditional definitions or models of "power over" or "power for oneself" often leave Hispanic women feeling unable to act, since they perceive such behavior as incompatible with consideration of others, or they anticipate it may lead away from connection and bonding. Jean Baker Miller's (1988) proposed definition of "power" as the "capacity to move or to produce change" rather than "power over" is a preferred construct. Additionally, Surrey (1987) defines empowerment as the motivation, freedom and capacity to act purposefully, with mobilization of the energy, resources, strengths or power of each person through a mutual relational process. The therapist can better help many Latinas by exploring direct and healthy ways to be powerful and by empowering through awareness and expression of feelings, reactions, and needs in more effective ways.

Vasquez-Nuttal, Romero-Garcia, and De Leon (1987) describe how cultural sensitivity should incorporate recognition of the changes in Latina women's roles and circumstances, rather than reinforcing disadvantaged social and economic status for such women. In particular, Vasquez-Nuttal et al. review more recent psychosocial studies that question the traditional portrayal of male–female roles and allocation of power in Latino families. More research is needed to determine how Latinas are guiding their lives in ways that are compatible with cultural expectations, societal demands, and dynamic changes in gender roles.

Group Psychotherapy

Group psychotherapy has long been regarded as treatment of choice for subgroup populations. Latina women's groups may be geared to those likely to benefit from validation of gender and ethnic identity. Group members help one another realize that they can nurture themselves as well as others, that they can give and receive support and nurturance from other women. Latinas often better learn to value themselves and other women as a result of group membership; consequently, group leader(s) should promote interaction that builds connection and enhances everyone's personal power.

Empowering group interactions increase zest, knowledge, self-worth, salience, and desire for more connection. The capacity for connection depends on the maintenance of fluid ego boundaries and responsiveness to the thoughts, perceptions, and feeling states of others (Surrey, 1987). In the tradition of feminist therapy, an effective group leader would model such behaviors, being careful to promote self-nurturance as well as nurturance of others. She would recognize and reinforce the positive aspects of Latinas' tendency to care for others, and raise the possibility that some group members may not be applying the same concept of care to themselves.

The leader of a Latina women's group may need to rethink frequently asked questions. As these women deviate from the traditional models of power and action they will encounter the widely recognized "fear of owning one's power," "identification with the victim," and "fear of success." Instead of asking, "Is she being too passive?" or, "Can she learn to be more active on her own behalf?" it may prove more growth-enhancing and validating to ask, "Is she being responsibly interactive?" or, "Has she established a relational context where mutual power is encouraged and facilitated?" (Surrey, 1987). And, as with individual therapy, it is important for group therapy leaders to individualize the members, knowing that they may be of different socioeconomic class, different acculturation levels, and/ or from different subgroup populations.

Groups provide members an opportunity to focus on issues that are uniquely or primarily the concerns of Latina women and explore them from the Latina's perspective. I (with Ay Ling Han) have developed a "theme-oriented" group for Latina women. The themes, around which various activities have been designed, include: family relationships (mother, father, siblings); relationships with significant others (spouses, partners, friends); cultural conflicts, strengths, and identification; barriers to achievement; confidence enhancement; dealing with anger and other feelings; empowerment; skill building (communication, assertiveness, and risk-taking); and sexuality. Typically, each of these themes take one to three $1\frac{1}{2}$-hour weekly sessions, during which structured activities may be used to stimulate issues to be worked upon.

For example, the very first session is begun with an activity designed to elicit the Latina's identity issues, which are often related to relationship with mother. Members are asked to introduce themselves to group members the way their mothers would introduce themselves. After each member has done so, members express reactions, feelings, and concerns to one another, based on the nature of the introductions. While the group is structured with activities such as this one, lots of room is provided for in-depth exploration of feelings and issues.

Advocacy

Often, improving a Latina client's mental health may require direct advocacy activities, such as writing a letter (with appropriate releases) for a student to reenter school. Advocacy may also include engaging in efforts to effect policies, laws, and judicial decisions. Using one's expertise and knowledge of how the various forces effect the mental health of Latinas to educate others and effect situational change is a shared responsibility of all therapists of Latinas.

A CLINICAL CASE

The following is a summary of an illustrative case. Identifying data have been changed in order to protect confidentiality.

Angela was a 22-year-old Latina who was a junior when she came to the University Counseling Center. Her presenting concern was depression, which she reported experiencing for most of high school. She also reported high degrees of isolation and loneliness, and the feeling that she belonged to no part of any group (social, cultural, professional, or otherwise). She came from a poor, working-class background, and was the daughter of a single parent. She had two younger siblings. She and her mother and siblings had lived with several relatives over the years. Her father had been briefly married to her mother, but lived with them only infrequently despite 10 years of marriage. Angela rarely saw her father, and he had provided virtually no child support on a regular basis. Angela still lived at home, and complained of her mother being overly involved, protective, and demanding. Yet, she had few resources with which to consider moving either into a dorm or an apartment. She occasionally worked, but found it difficult and time-consuming to keep up with her studies. Her grade-point average was approximately 2.8 (on a 4.0 scale), and her mother wanted her to be an engineer.

  The initial treatment plan consisted of developing a warm and trusting relationship, assessing sources of depression, and having a psychiatric evaluation, given the chronic and severe nature of the depression. While women tend to be overmedicated for treatment of depression, and while I am conservative in regard to referral for psychotropic intervention, this case clearly presented the possibility of chemical, biological depression.

  In establishing the relationship, Angela's insecurities and ambivalence about her need for me in her life became clear. She quickly bonded, but often apologized for existing, called me "Dr. Vasquez," long after I offered the option of calling me by my first name, and often called me or telephone counseling with her fears and anxieties about a negative assumption she'd made in "second guessing" some aspect of our last session. I began to recognize in her behavior a terror of being abandoned, and an incredible lack of confidence in general, but especially in her right to be a client. Given the time-limited nature of our agency's policies, I quickly decided that I would advocate for a lengthy extension for this client. It was important that I use my "chip" to see a long-term client in my organization with someone who did not have resources to get outside community help, and who I judged could benefit especially from a Latina therapist. Given her identity confusion and loneliness, I felt that a Latina therapist would help her introject some positive elements of her cultural identity. As in many modern day Latino families, some cultural traditions were maintained, others were not. For example, her family had an important extended family network, with many advantages and disadvantages. My client often felt supported by extended family relatives; on the other hand, the grandmother in particular frowned upon her living alone without being married. Other cultural characteristics were not present; my client did not speak Spanish, for example.

In addition to accessing extended therapy for Angela as an advocacy activity, the psychiatrist and I also provided key referral sources for Angela and her mother to seek methods to acquire regular child support from the father for the younger children. The state had new laws that allowed for garnishing of wages, and when the family had no money to pay for Angela's antidepressants, this intervention came to mind. This type of advocacy is one seldom used by most mental health professionals, with the exception of social workers. Yet, it was a powerful way to enlist the support of the mother for Angela's continuance in therapy (which had been threatening to the mother). Naturally, appropriate and limited releases were acquired from Angela to engage in this process.

Angela's initial behavior during the first few weeks of therapy was typical of those clients often labeled "dependent." My approach consisted of validating her need to feel connected, and assuring her that as long as it was within my power, she was not to be abandoned, due to her "mess-ups" in therapy. In addition, it was important that I be clear about my personal and professional limitations as well as those of the agency, in meeting her needs, in order for her not to interpret them as rejection of her. In other words, it was important during the first few weeks of therapy to be clear about our termination time (thus clearly identifying our time together), the times in which she could try to reach me, and about what issues (crisis, suicidal ideation, need for reassurance, etc.). This "boundary setting" was done in as humanistic and interactive a manner possible, with some flexibility for negotiation, so that she could feel power in the relationship. In other words, I did not lay the rules out for her, but the boundaries emerged from two or three sessions (and occasionally later as needed) of negotiation of what her needs were, and what would work for her, as well as for me and for the agency. At all times, I validated her needs as normal to her situation, and did not convey that she was wrong or bad for wanting what she wanted.

In examining possible external sources of depression, we found several. While she had a generally positive nurturing experience from her mother,

Angela and her family often lived with extended family members, some of whom were kind, but some of whom were physically, emotionally, and sexually abusive to Angela. Therapy consisted of helping Angela realize and work through the notion that some members of her extended family were dysfunctional, and that despite the wonderful network and kinship of her Latino culture, it was tragic that some members of that family were abusive. It was also a tragedy that her mother had to work long hours, often evening hours. This resulted in Angela's inconsistent nurturing and experience of abandonment. She also came to understand the abandonment she experienced from her father, who was mostly a shadowy, distant figure to her, even during the brief times he was around. She also felt overly responsible and sad about the caretaking of her siblings. She was very devoted to them, but often made them a priority over her own needs, frequently canceling her own social plans if one of them wanted her attention.

The treatment itself involved several aspects: she did take antidepressants, which helped. Additionally, we explored the various forms of abuse, which were painful, and which resulted in the lack of confidence, low self-esteem, and lack of efficacy she felt. Not only did I insist over and over that she was not to blame for the abuse, but that she was a wondrous survivor, who had accomplished much, given the lack of support. The exploration of memories often evoked posttraumatic stress disorder symptoms, such as anxiety, nightmares, irritability, increased feelings of vulnerability, and suicidal ideation, which we had to attend to. We also explored her mixed feelings about the role of her mother. Facilitating anger for her mother's lack of protection is a traditional therapeutic intervention, but for many Latina women, especially in this case, where her mother was one of the few sources of support, that anger had to be balanced with an understanding that despite her historical (and current) parenting errors, her mother did the best she knew how to do, and was herself a survivor of much abuse and distressful living. We worked on skills in communication and conflict management that would allow her to deal more effectively with her mother (in getting some degree of separation), and with other family members, professors, and peers. Her challenge of a professor who made a racist implication in class was a very powerful and important experience for her. Although she ended up dropping the class because of his hostile rebuke, she felt empowered, supported by a couple of students, and more assertive. She felt that she had spoken up for her integrity and identity.

Perhaps one of the most important elements of the therapeutic intervention was my attempt to be someone in her life who conveyed a consistent caring attitude that allowed her to discover her abilities. She was able to explore options other than engineering, and discover that her grade-point average went up both when the antidepressants worked, and when she chose a major more to her liking and "fit." I was able to convey in all kinds of ways that her uniqueness, despite her lack of a beauty similar to that of White women, or her lack of ability to speak Spanish, like that of other Latinos, was indeed special. She was beautiful; she was a "legitimate" full-blown Latina. Referring her to the Hispanic woman's group, and encouraging her to join the professional Hispanic organization in her major were helpful strategies in that regard. My ability to convey genuine respect for her as a person, and to listen without defensiveness when she was finally able to express anger and disappointment in me, were key elements in her empowerment in her relationship with me.

Therapy consisted of almost 2 years of regular weekly therapy. At termination, she declared that the most important thing I did for her was demonstrate that I "believed in her." My consistency, and my ability to be honest and genuine about my care as well as negotiate my limits in a respectful way were important. Indeed, I was able to convey and mirror the admiration that she evoked, and that she was then able to see in the eyes of others. The seeds of confidence, which were fortunately planted by her mother's positive aspects of parenting, grew and allowed her to take more risks in her life, and to envision more options than a Latina woman in her experience had been allowed. This former client, who at one point was told by an engineering professor that she'd "never make it" in graduate school, (and which she heard as "you're not graduate school material at all," and which her grade-point average at the time confirmed) has successfully completed a graduate program in another, better suited field.

SUMMARY

Effective psychotherapy with Latinas requires knowledge of the clinician's personal and professional attitudes, beliefs, and knowledge. Despite the challenges, we as clinicians must avoid negative and inappropriate stereotypes, and prevent the replication of the experience of discrimination in the therapeutic experience. Knowledge and understanding of the individual and her sociocultural and environmental experiences as a Latina are important as tools to assess appropriate applications of the client's reality. We must also be aware of the aspects of our training that are irrelevant or even harmful to our clients. Labeling Latinas' need to nurture, care and connect as "dependent" in a pathological manner can be inappropriate, as can be the failure to help a Latina learn to apply the same standard of care to herself.

Since Latinos make up almost 10% of the United States population, and will by the year 2020 be the largest minority group, it behooves the therapist to learn to appreciate, value and work effectively with differences. By then, one of every three Americans will be a person of color.

Feminist and multicultural approaches to both individual and group psychotherapy contribute a philosophy, more than technique, that encourages the examination of external factors as causative in the client's problems. The client's strengths rather than weaknesses are emphasized and validated, and approaches are endorsed that result in empowerment of the client to engage in change if she chooses. The Latina often enters therapy with a significant lack of confidence, resulting from the lack of societal validation of her worth, and a clear message that she is responsible for her problems. The role of the therapist is thus not only to impart skills and understanding, but to convey a caring attitude that discovers the abilities of the client, that registers with sensitivity and admiration the possibilities and visions for that client, and that delights in what is unique, different, and special about her (Bernardez, 1990).

Advocacy, undertaking activities that enhance the ultimate well-being of Latinas, is an unavoidable responsibility. Resources have much to do with one's sense of well-being, and often those with the least access to those resources (economic power, political power, decision-making in organizational structures) are Latina women. Using our resources to provide access to resources directly for a client, or to change policies, laws, and other institutions that affect Latinas is a social, moral, and professional responsibility.

Through ongoing training, supervision, consultation, and other mechanisms, therapists can greatly enhance their potential to provide competent and ethical psychotherapy to Latinas.

REFERENCES

Amaro, H., & Russo, N. F. (1987). Hispanic women and mental health: An overview of contemporary issues in research and practice. *Psychology of Women Quarterly. 11*, 393–408.

Amaro, H., Russo, N. F., & Johnson, J. (1987). Family and work predictors of psychological well-being among Hispanic women professionals. *Psychology of Women Quarterly. 11*, 505–522.

American College Testing (1991). *Reference norms for spring, 1990 ACT-tested high school graduates.* Iowa City, IA: Research Services Department, American College Testing Service.

American Psychological Association. (1991, February). Hispanics lack knowledge about AIDS. *American Psychological Association Monitor*, p. 31.

Bernardez, T. (1990) *Older women: Inventing our lives* [Audiotape]. Topeka, KS: Menninger Foundation.

Bernal, G. (1982). Cuban families. In M. McGoldrick, J. K. Pearce, & J. Giordano (Eds.), *Ethnicity and family therapy* (pp. 187–297). New York: Guilford Press.

Canino, G. J., Rubio-Stipec, M., Shrout, P., Bravo, M., Stolberg, R., & Bird, H. R. (1987). Sex differences and depression in Puerto Rico. *Psychology of Women Quarterly, 11*, 443–460.

Casas, J. M., & Vasquez, M. J. T. (1989). Counseling the Hispanic client: A theoretical and applied perspective. In P. B. Pedersen, J. G. Draguns, W. J. Lonner, & J. E. Trimble (Eds.), *Counseling across cultures* (3rd ed., pp. 153–176). Honolulu: University of Hawaii Press.

Chacon, M., Cohen, E., Camerena, M., Gonzalez, J., & Strover, S. (1985). *Chicanas in California post-secondary education: A comparative study of barriers to program progress.* Stanford, CA: Center for Chicano Research.

Chacon, M., Cohen, E., & Strover, S. (1986) Chicanas and Chicanos: Barriers to progress in higher education. In M. A. Olivas (Ed.), *Latino college students* (pp. 296–324). New York: Teachers College, Columbia University Press.

Chapa, J., & Valencia, R. R. (1993). Latino population growth, demographic characteristics, and educational stagnation: An examination of recent trends. *Hispanic Journal of Behavioral Sciences, 15*, 165–187.

Comas-Díaz, L. (1987). Feminist therapy with mainland Puerto Rican women. *Psychology of Women Quarterly, 11*, 461–474.

Comas-Díaz, L. (1989). Culturally relevant issues and treatment implications for Hispanics. In D. R. Koslow & E. P. Salett (Eds.), *Crossing cultures in mental health* (pp. 31–48). Washington, DC: SIETAR International.

Corvin, S. A., & Wiggins, F. (1989). An antiracism training model for White professionals. *Journal of Multicultural Counseling and Development, 17*, 107–114.

Cromwell, R. E., & Ruiz, R. A. (1979). The myth of macho dominance in decision making within Mexican and Chicano families. *Hispanic Journal of Behavioral Sciences, 1*, 355–373.

Feldman-Summers, S., & Ashworth, C. D. (1981). Factors related to intentions to report rape. *Journal of Social Issues, 4*, 53–70.

Gandara, P. (1982). Passing through the eye of a needle: High-achieving Chicanas. *Hispanic Journal of Behavioral Sciences, 4*, 167–179.

Gilligan, C., Rogers, A. G., & Tolman, D. L. (Eds.). (1991). *Women, girls and psychotherapy: Reframing resistance.* Binghamton, NY: Harrington Park Press.

Goodyear, R. K., & Sinnett, E. R. (1984). Current and emerging ethical issues for counseling psychology. *Counseling Psychologist, 12*, 87–98.

Hare-Mustin, R. T., Maracek, J., Kaplan, A. G., & Liss-Levinson, N. (1979). Rights of clients, responsibilities of therapists. *American Psychologist, 34*, 3–16.

Holiman, M., & Lauver, P. J. (1987). The counselor culture and client-centered practice. *Counselor Education and Supervision, 26*, 184–191.

Jones, J. M. (1990, July). Psychology goes to work. *Advancing the Public Interest, 11*, p. 3.

Katz, J. H., & Ivey, A. G. (1977). White awareness: The frontier of racism awareness training. *Personnel and Guidance Journal, 55*, 485–489.

McGrath, E., Keita, G. P., Strickland, B. R., & Russo, N. F. (1990). *Women and depression: Risk factors and treatment issues* (Final Report of the American Psychological Association's National Task Force on Women and Depression). Washington, DC: American Psychological Association.

Miller, J. B. (1988). *Connections, disconnections and violations* (Work in Progress No. 33). Wellesley, MA: Stone Center Working Papers Series.

Morrison, A. M., & Von Glinow, M. A. (1990). Women and minorities in management. *American Psychologist, 45*, 200–208.

National Council of La Raza. (1990). *Hispanic education: A statistical portrait.* Washington, DC: Author.

Padilla, A. M., Salgado de Snyder, N., Cervantes, R. C., & Baezconde-Garbanati, L. (1987, Summer). Self-regulation and risk-taking behavior: A Hispanic perspective. In *Research Bulletin* (pp. 1–5). Los Angeles: Spanish Speaking Mental Health Research Center.

Pinderhuges, E. (1989). *Understanding race, ethnicity and power: The key to efficacy in clinical practice.* New York: Free Press.

Pope, K. S., & Vasquez, M. J. T. (1991). *Ethics in psychotherapy and counseling: A practical guide for psychologists.* San Francisco: Jossey-Bass.

Ramirez, M. III (1991). *Psychotherapy and counseling with minorities: A cognitive approach to individual and cultural differences.* New York: Pergamon Press.

Ramirez, O., & Arce, C. (1981). The contemporary Chicano family: An empirically-based review. In A. Baron (Ed.), *Explorations in Chicano psychology* (pp. 3–28). New York: Praeger Press.

Sabogal, F., Marin, G., Otero-Sabogal, R., Marin, B. V., & Perez-Stable, E. J. (1987). Hispanic familism and acculturation: What changes and what doesn't? *Hispanic Journal of Behavioral Sciences, 9,* 397–412.

Salgado de Snyder, V. N. (1987). Factors associated with acculturative stress and depressive symptomatology among married Mexican immigrant women. *Psychology of Women Quarterly, 11,* 475–488.

Siegel, J. M., Sorenson, S. B., Golding, J. M., Burnam, M. A., & Stein, J. A. (1987). The prevalence of childhood sexual assault: The Los Angeles Epidemiology Catchment Area Project. *Journal of Epidemiology, 126,* 1141–1153.

Surrey, J. L. (1987). *Relationship and empowerment* (Work in Progress No. 30). Wellesley, MA: Stone Center Working Papers Series.

Torres, S. (1986). *A comparative analysis of wife abuse among Anglo-American and Mexican-American battered women: Attitudes, nature, severity, frequency, and response to the abuse.* Unpublished doctoral dissertation, University of Texas at Austin.

U.S. Bureau of the Census. (1990). School enrollment—Social and economic characteristics of students: October 1987 and 1988. *Current population reports* (Ser. P-20, no. 443). Washington, DC: U.S. Government Printing Office.

U.S. Bureau of the Census (1991). *Resident population distribution for the United States, region, and states by race and Hispanic origin: 1990* (Census Bureau Press Release No. CB91-100). Washington, DC: U.S. Government Printing Office.

Vasquez-Nuttal, E., Romero-Garcia, I., & De Leon, B. (1987). Sex roles and perceptions of femininity and masculinity of Hispanic women: A review of the literature. *Psychology of Women Quarterly, 11,* 409–426.

Vasquez, M. J. T. (1982). Confronting barriers to participation of Mexican American women in higher education. *Hispanic Journal of Behavioral Sciences, 4,* 147–165.

Vasquez, M. J. T. (1984). Power and status of the Chicana: A social-psychological perspective. In J. L. Martinez & R. H. Mendoza (Eds.), *Chicano psychology* (2nd ed., pp. 269–287). New York: Academic Press.

Walker, L. E. A. (1989). *Terrifying love: Why battered women kill and how society responds.* New York: Harper & Row.

Wampold, B. E., Casas, J. M., & Atkinson, D. R. (1981). Ethnic bias in counseling: An information processing approach. *Journal of Counseling Psychology, 28,* 498–503.

Wilkinson, D. Y. (1980). Minority women: Sociocultural issues. In A. Brodsky & R. Hare-Mustin (Eds.), *Women and psychotherapy* (pp. 285–304). New York: Guilford Press.

Winkler, K. J. (1990, October 10). Evidence of "cultural vitality." *Chronicle of Higher Education,* pp. A5, A8.

Wyatt, G. E. (1990). Sexual abuse of ethnic minority children: Identifying dimensions of victimization. *Professional Psychology: Research and Practice, 21,* 338–343.

Zapata , J. T., & Jaramillo, P. T. (1981) The Mexican American family: An Adlerian perspective. *Hispanic Journal of Behavioral Sciences, 3,* 275–290.

5

West Indian Women of Color: The Jamaican Woman

Janet R. Brice-Baker

Where does the West Indian woman of color fit into the tapestry of women from around the world? She is certainly one of the multicolored threads of the weave, but which one? To answer these questions we must identify and endeavor to understand the people of whom we speak.

The appellation "West Indies" is a misnomer. These islands were inadvertently discovered by Christopher Columbus in the late 1400s as he attempted to find a shorter trade route to India. When he arrived in what is now known as the Caribbean Sea he believed himself to be approaching India's western shore.

Geographically, the terms Caribbean and West Indian are used interchangeably. The West Indies are in fact subsumed under the label Caribbean, which includes Central America and the West Indies. The islands of the West Indies are divided into three areas—the Greater Antilles, the Lesser Antilles, and the Bahamas—which constitute approximately 300,000 square miles of land. Roughly 208,000 square miles of that land is in Central America, with the remaining 92,000 accounted for by the islands of the West Indies (Augelli, 1973).

The people of the Caribbean have a rich blend of languages, religions, and ethnic diversities. Some are descendants of the European settlers from England, France, Spain, and the Netherlands. Others are descended from the African people, brought to the islands as slaves, and from the Indians who lived on the islands originally. The Mayan Indians were natives of Central America, the Arawak Indians were native to the Bahamas and the Greater Antilles, while the Carib Indians first populated the Lesser Antilles. There are in addition, Asian descendants of the Chinese, East Indians, and Syrians, who were brought to the islands to work the plantations. Finally, the population includes two groups of mixed people: the Mestizos, a blend of Indian and French lineages, and the Mulattoes, a blend of White and Black (Augelli, 1973).

The languages spoken in the Caribbean reflect the diversity of the people. Dutch is the official language of the Netherlands Antilles. English is spoken in the Bahamas, Barbados, Jamaica, Trinidad, and Tobago. French is the language of Haiti, Guadeloupe, and Martinique, while Spanish is heard in Cuba, Puerto Rico, and the Dominican Republic. In addition to these languages there are several patois, or "the blend of a provincial dialect with a standard form of a language" (Augelli, 1973). Two very prominent ones are Creole—a mixture of French, English, Spanish, and African languages—and Papiamento—a mixture of Spanish, Dutch, and English (Augelli, 1973).

Familiarity with the people of this culture requires in particular an understanding of their religious practices. Generally, religion provides us with insight into the many values of a people and teaches us how they organize their world and explain the events occurring in it. Within the traditional realm, it is not surprising that the two major religions of the Caribbean are Catholicism and Protestantism, since three quarters of the people there live in countries colonized by Spain or France (Augelli, 1973).

Asians practice either Hinduism or Islamism. Non-Western beliefs include *obeah, espiritismo, santeria,* and *vodun,* which are frequently practiced by mediums, to whom West Indians communicate their problems. The relevance to psychotherapy of these belief systems will be discussed in a later part of this chapter, but first their major tenets will be defined.

Obeah, also known as witchcraft, is not considered a religion. It is, however, an amalgam of Protestantism and some of the African Ashanti religious beliefs and is widespread throughout the Bahamas, the Virgin Islands, and the British West Indies (Lefley, 1981). It is practiced by people who are believed to have special powers, which are used to contend with things that are threatening and therefore deemed evil (Neki et al., 1986). It is a "means of structuring and expressing intense feelings, . . . a mechanism for organizing uncontrollable and unpredictable forces impinging on the individual" (Lefley, 1981, p. 7).

Miss R., a single mother in her mid-40s, had been in therapy for the past 5 months. During that time she disclosed to the therapist that she had been romantically involved with the minister of her church. According to Miss R., the relationship was severed by him quite some time ago. She was unclear about the reasons. At times she stated that it was because he didn't want the responsibility of a retarded stepdaughter and other times because he was living with another woman. These things were always reported by Miss R. with a blunted affect. The therapist noticed that Miss R. was never able to express any anger toward this man for rejecting her. In fact, her predominant mood was depression.

One day she reported coming home to an empty house and having the distinct feeling that someone had been there in her absence. She stated that she ran up to her bedroom in search of a red scarf, only to find that it was missing. At that point she knew that he had taken possession of her scarf to work *obeah* on her. She became sick to her stomach and vomited. She said, "I knew that I had to find someone to counter his magic."

This was the closest she had gotten to identifying any conflict in the relationship. Apparently, the feeling of anger was too intense for her to discuss directly with the therapist.

Another belief system of Black people in the Caribbean is African Cuban *santeria*. Once practiced only by Black people of the lower classes, it has more recently gained popularity among other socioeconomic classes and races. The deities are referred to as *orichas*, and people seek them out to cope with problems. A typical West Indian woman believing in *santeria* would strive, throughout her life, to form a positive relationship with the *orichas* so that they would work on her behalf (Lefley, 1981).

Espiritismo deals with the seen and unseen worlds (Lefley, 1981), and is practiced primarily by Puerto Ricans (Sandoval, 1979). While the vast majority of Puerto Ricans are devout practicing Roman Catholics, their devotion is not mutually exclusive of a belief in the spirit world. A very basic tenet of this belief system is that

> the visible world is surrounded and inhabited by good and evil spirits who influence human behavior. According to this belief, spirits can either protect or harm, as well as prevent or cause illness. Every person is seen as having spirits of protection; the protection can be increased by good deeds or decreased by evil deeds. (García-Preto, 1982, p. 169)

Last, but certainly not least, is the practice of *voodoo* or *vodun*. Leyburn (1966) defines *vodun* as "a set of beliefs and practices which claim to deal with the spiritual forces of the universe and attempts to keep the individual in harmonious relationship with them as they affect her life" (p. 134). The men who possess these powers are called *houngans* and the females *mambos*. Their rituals involve animal sacrifices, possession, and trance. Like *espiritisimo*, *vodun* divides the world into the visible sphere, which includes people and all material things, and the invisible sphere, which includes the dead and spirits (Lefley, 1981). All of these belief systems exist in conjunction with the beliefs of the mainstream European faiths.

West Indian women from the island of Jamaica constitute the focus of this chapter. Since there is no uniform composite of the Caribbean woman, any attempt to explore all of the different groups they represent in a truly meaningful way is well beyond the scope of this chapter. I thus present relevant historical, sociological, and psychological information about the Jamaican female, interspersing appropriate clinical case material to illustrate certain points, with names and other identifying data changed to protect confidentiality.

IMMIGRATION: REASONS AND OBJECTIVES

Unlike some immigrants, Jamaican women do not come to the United States to escape persecution, nor were they brought here forcefully as slaves. Their reasons for immigrating are as varied as the number of women who make the trip. Because a Jamaican female client may very well be a first- or second-generation "American"—in contrast to an American client of European ancestry, whose family is likely to have been here for generations—her reasons for immigration will have more of an impact on her functioning, and therefore on her mental health, than they would for someone whose family immigrated many generations ago.

A major portion of Jamaicans immigrate for financial reasons, seeking work when they were unable to find any at home, or seeking better paying jobs than the ones they already had. Others immigrate for educational reasons, assuming that they will get a better education in the United States, and thus a better job.

Education is greatly valued in Jamaican culture. Sowell (1981) points out that West Indians are overrepresented among Blacks in professional occupations in the United States. It should be noted, however, that this value for education is tempered by pragmatism. Although education is emphasized, all adults are encouraged to educate themselves in fields of study that will lead to lucrative and steady work, and they are also admonished not to stay in school too long, so as to avoid accruing debts and delaying their entry into the workforce.

Miss B. graduated with honors from her local high school and went on to attend an Eastern Ivy League college. She entered as a pre-med major, much to her family's delight. It was assumed that her income as a physician would be lucrative and that she would be an important resource to her family. Throughout the first year of her studies she had the unfailing support of her family, who looked forward to her becoming a physician. Midway through her junior year Miss B. enrolled in some liberal arts courses in addition to her science and math curriculum. She developed an interest in sociology and decided to change her major and pursue a doctorate degree in that discipline. Trips home to visit her parents became tension filled as she tried to conceal the fact that she had changed her major. It was difficult for her to respond to her family's questions about her science courses, since she was not taking any. Miss B. eventually stopped making trips home during school breaks because she could not stand to hear her parents boast about the "doctor in the family." Miss B. developed headaches that became increasingly debilitating. She had trouble getting up in the morning and her appetite increased. She was unable to concentrate on school work and her grades dropped significantly.

A roommate of Miss B.'s encouraged her to go to therapy. In the course of treatment it became evident that Miss B.'s depression was precipitated by her decision not to become a physician and her anticipation of her parent's response. She doubted her parents' ability or willingness to understand her career choice, since they would be hard pressed to see steady work coming from a Ph.D. in sociology.

The decision regarding who immigrates is dictated by the immigration laws and by the avilability of jobs at any given time. Jamaican women are frequently the family members chosen to immigrate because employment opportunities for them are ample, particularly in the area of domestic work or live-in babysitting. After sufficient money is accumulated and a home is established, husbands are sent for, followed by the children. Being chosen as the one to immigrate to the United States carries major responsibilities; sending money home, sponsoring other family members' immigration, securing items not available or too expensive in Jamaica, and purchasing property.

This last responsibility is first on the Jamaican woman's agenda. Owning a home serves two important purposes: It provides a place for relatives to stay when they come to the United States, and it often enables her to rent one bedroom out, thereby acquiring additional income. It is common for Jamaicans, to move, over the years, into increasingly larger apartments or houses. This is not simply to expand their living space but also to increase their rental income (Brice, 1982).

Miss C. had worked three jobs in order to save enough money to buy a house. Her mortgage application was rejected because she couldn't show sufficient income, since only one of her jobs was "on the books." The salary from that job alone did not qualify her for the mortgage amount she had requested. She expressed embarrassment and a sense of failure because this purchase would have enabled her to help bring other relatives to this country. She was left with a feeling of having let her family down with her failure to meet this obligation.

The financial objectives of the Jamaican immigrant are so central that she often works several jobs to meet her obligations. Then as soon as enough money is saved, she will purchase real estate. It should also be understood that many Jamaicans are distrustful of banks and the stockmarket. Quite a few older Jamaicans experienced the stock market crash of 1929 and the resulting economic depression, and it is not uncommon to find older Jamaican women keeping large sums of cash in their homes. Another way they have developed to save money without having to use banks is the "rotating credit association" (Regis, 1988): A group of women will contribute some previously determined amount of money weekly into a pot. At the end of the week one woman gets the contents of the pot, with a different women receiving the sum each week. This has helped many women save considerable amounts, even in lean times.

Ownership of property has one final significance to Jamaicans. Historically, slaves (in the islands as elsewhere) were not allowed to own property. After emancipation, when the right to vote became an issue, only those Jamaicans who had acquired land were then allowed to vote. Property, therefore, has in many ways been equated with status. This, in conjunction with their distrust of banks and the stockmarket, predispose Jamaican women to view real estate as an important factor in securing their family's future.

Stress of Immigration

For many Jamaican women, the stresses inherent in immigration are likely to precipitate symptoms for which she will seek help. Primary among these stressors is the differences in language. As previously mentioned, a variety of languages are spoken in the West Indies. If a West Indian woman's native language is Spanish, French, Dutch, or one of the patois, she must learn English. Even among English-speaking West Indian women there are many different patois as well, each with their own structure, grammar, and syntax. No matter what her language background, the Jamaican woman will speak English with an accent and will sound foreign to Americans. An issue for a Black person of any origin, who desires assimilation in the United States is that skin color immediately sets her or him apart. Although melodic and lilting, the accent of the Jamacian becomes one more thing that immediately distinguishes her or him from Whites and from other Blacks. Whether or not Jamaicans find it advantageous or disadvantageous to be viewed as distinct and different from African American Blacks is the subject of much debate and is explored later in this chapter.

The immigrant West Indian woman must accommodate a variety of concrete changes in her living conditions such as climate, dress, and diet. Coming from very tropical locations, many West Indian immigrants find the winters in the United States rather brutal. I am familiar with older Jamaicans who were forced to return to their homeland because they could not withstand even the mildest winters in the cities of the Northeast and the physical confinement that accompanies them. Many older people have arthritic conditions that are exacerbated by the cold, while others may risk severe illness as a result of not knowing how to properly dress for the cold. In any locale warm weather makes it easier for people to get around and to spend more time outdoors. Most are less likely to walk somewhere if they are not dressed for the cold, and less likely to drive if they have had little or no experience driving on snow and ice covered roads. Thus weather conditions often interfere with mobility and contact with support networks.

Depending on where she settles in the United States, the Jamaican woman may also have trouble obtaining the foods she is accustomed to.

Some of the foods indigenous to the islands are not widely available in United States supermarkets, and when available are often overpriced and unfamiliar to store clerks.

The type of work that a West Indian woman undertakes when she arrives in the United States depends on a number of factors: her age, the amount of money she needs to earn, her immigration status, and her job qualifications. I mention qualifications last because West Indian immigrants have a history of having to take menial jobs regardless of their level of education or previous work experience. Not only do they come up against racist hiring practices, but often they are passed over because an employer will assume that their Carribean education was inferior to what they would have received here. Such underemployment not only has the effect of decreasing their self-esteem and sense of worth, but often makes them disdainful of African Americans, who they perceive as being lazy and wasteful of opportunity in their unwillingness to take menial and possibly degrading jobs.

In traveling to and from multiple jobs the West Indian woman is confronted with the need to orient herself to the surrounding city, which is often equivalent in size to the entire island that she left behind. Transportation systems in urban cities are complex and confusing. Housing arrangements do not reflect longstanding kinship and neighbor patterns as in the West Indies. Instead, people live in close proximity to one another but do not necessarily know one another so that strangers are in abundance. Because the cities are so large, even if she has a relative or family friend from home living in the same city, the Jamaican woman may find maintaining contact difficult.

Additional stressors exist for the Jamaican woman who is here illegally. Caution must be taken at all times to avoid discovery, which makes her unable to take legitimate jobs that require social security numbers and tax disclosures. Instead she must work "under-the-table" jobs, for low wages and under often intolerable conditions in exchange for secrecy about her illegal alien status. Such women cannot register to vote, they cannot get driver's licenses, they cannot buy property, and they cannot open bank accounts. They are totally at the mercy of their employer, about whom they may have ambivalent feelings: On the one hand, the employer has given them an opportunity to earn some money in this country, on the other hand, that same employer is free to treat the illegal alien in any way he or she pleases, knowing that the threat of deportation hangs constantly over the immigrant's head.

Any health provider working with this population should tread carefully. Refusals to provide information such as an address, place of employment, and the like may arise from the fact that the woman is an illegal resident and is afraid that such information given to "authority" figures will result in deportation. One should also be aware that these same fears can pose barriers to seeking assistance in other areas as well: crime victims, for example, may be unwilling to make a police complaint or contact a lawyer, or the physically ill may refuse to go to a clinic or hospital. One wonders why someone who has been a victim or who is truly suffering would fail to take such steps, but it is more understandable when one takes into account the potential consequences for an illegal alien of pursuing these options.

The separation from spouses, children, and extended family constitutes another major stressor. Wray and McLaren (1976) in their study of Jamaican children found that 71.2% of their sample experienced parent–child separation symptoms as a consequence of immigration. they also found that "migration as a disruptive factor of family life affected more boys than girls" (p. 253), a gender difference worth exploring further, as are its effects on adults. Reuniting the family, however, is not always stress-free. A woman may experience marital strain once she is reunited with a husband she has not seen for months. Children may not follow limits set by a mother who has not been around to discipline them on a routine basis. They may even resent her for her initial abandonment and for their own separation from home and friends, to a country where it is hard to fit into either the Black or White community.

Allen (1988) discusses the issue of "double discrimination," using this phrase to refer to the difficulties Jamaicans have had developing relationships with White and Black Americans. While they often expect racist attitudes from individual Whites, they are usually unprepared for the level of personal and institutional racism they face in the United States. In the West Indies skin color preferences exist and are used to make social distinctions, but status is most strongly associated with education and income. The majority of Black people in the United States are viewed by the dominant culture as if they are all the same regardless of class and educational distinctions. Therefore, while the West Indian woman may be one of a few doctors or lawyers in her entire parish, which would place her high up in the social hierarchy, on entering the United States she may find that her status as a professional does not protect her from racial discrimination.

WEST INDIAN AND AFRICAN AMERICAN WOMEN

The exploration of differences between West Indians and African Americans is often controversial. It has been suggested that highlighting differences between groups of Black people is divisive and therefore damaging to attempts at political unity between the two groups in the United States. This argument implies that when one talks about the differences between two ethnic groups in the United States, one encourages the idealization of one group and the devaluation of the other.

Diversity does exist nevertheless among Black persons as a group, which is particularly important for us as therapists, to be aware of and recognize. Clinical experience informs us that individuals can experience the same situation differently or express their experience in a variety of ways. Furthermore, there is no reason to expect the Black community to be any more homogenous than the White community.

Slavery and racial discrimination are examples of common historical experience within groups of Black persons. In the Caribbean, unlike in the United States, Black people were in the racial majority, and the emancipation of slaves was achieved with far less bloodshed and violence. I contend that there was also a difference in the attitudes of landowners in the South than those in the Caribbean. Landowners in the South considered the South their home, while landowners in the Caribbean were often colonizers who saw the plantations as an investment. Hence Southern landowners' fear of Blacks owning land, voting, and participating equally in American society betrayed their feelings of territoriality, which were consequently deeper than Caribbean landowners, who were often absent from their property altogether. The danger in White Southener's eyes lay in the Black slaves being moved from the status of livestock to that of equals, upsetting the prevailing social structure and privileges that White Americans accrued as a function of that structure. Hence, the Jamaican woman who comes to this country has a very different view of race relations from those who were born and raised here. Her immigration to the United States is usually voluntary and designed to enhance her lifestyle and economic well-being, while for many African American women their presence in the United States is part of a degrading legacy. West Indian women come from a country in which they are accustomed to being part of the majority, unlike African American women, who have a more disparaged ethnic identity (Best, 1975). People from the West Indies identify themselves in two ways: by the island they grew up on or by the country that colonized that island. African Americans do not have the same sense of nationality. Maintaining the slavery system depended upon creating a distorted image of Africans, concealing their true history, and presenting the distorted version to both Black and White Americans. African Americans can rarely name a country within the continent of Africa and call it the home of their ancestors. The fear of slave uprisings was so great that members of the same African tribes were deliberately separated and forbidden to read or write or speak to one another. They were in addition forbidden to engage in any familiar cultural or religious practices. While many of these same attempts to separate Caribbean slaves may have been made, their effectiveness on islands that were smaller than many urban cities were most likely limited.

Another difference between the two groups is reflected in both their experiences and views about their ability to make social and economic progress in this country. It has been suggested that the Jamaican woman feels more optimistic about her chances at a good life in the United States than the African American woman. She comes here in search of the work that will enable her to have the money she needs to make a better life. In this light, the United States is seen as the land of opportunity, where the only obstacle to success is one's own "laziness." The reader must keep in mind the pervasive influence of the English and Protestantism on the Jamaican's high value of the work ethic. Most West Indian women have multiple jobs and work not only to make ends meet but also to make life better for themselves and successive generations. Attribution for failure to obtain material wealth is internalized, leading to guilt and self-blame.

Whether or not Jamaican women have reason to feel optimistic about the life situations immigration to the United States affords is debatable. It all depends on what yardstick is used to measure the benefits of immigrating. If material possessions and monetary wealth are the goals sought, there is reason to be optimistic. The Jamaican immigrant is able to raise her family's standard of living in Jamaica when she sends money and needed items home. If, on the other hand, the treatment of people of color in the United States by Whites is the measure, there is no reason for optimism. West Indians can be naive about the existence and power of institutional racism in America. When they fail to realize certain ambitions they may be oblivious to the ways that systems presumed to protect them can act to harm them. The Jamaican woman's awareness of discrimination will be tempered by whether or not she is an immigrant or a second-, third-, or fourth-generation resident in this country, whether or not she intends to make the United States her home or return to Jamaica, whether or not her support network in this country is other Jamaicans or African Americans, how much of an affinity she has for things European, what type of work she does, and where she chooses to live.

FAMILY STRUCTURE

The psychotherapist who works with the Jamaican female patient must familiarize him or herself with the family environment of which the patient is a part. Henriques (1968) identifies four types of family constellations: the Christian family, faithful concubinage, maternal or grandmother family, and the keeper family. It must be kept in mind that the prevalence of any one type of family is to a large degree dictated by socioeconomic class.

The decision to marry is one that is given a great deal of thought in Jamaican culture. When one marries is not dictated by the age of the participants or their mutual affection but rather by their financial preparedness.

The Christian family consists of a legally married couple and their progeny. Sex roles in the Christian family are very clearly prescribed. Formally, the man's role in the family is predominantly financial. He is not even considered eligible for marriage until he has saved sufficient money to support his wife and purchase a house. Additionally, he is expected to contribute to the support of his family of origin and extended family. This savings plan can take quite some time, and as a result the average age of a Jamaican male at marriage is roughly 10 years older than the average age of a male marrying in the United States (Schlesinger, 1968). While the man is the major wage earner he is not always the sole wage earner; the woman may be employed as well.

Aside from economic responsibilities, the male makes all the major decisions in the family. The influence of the female is restricted to the household and children. She is formally in charge of the children and their schedules. She is also responsible for preparation of meals, cleaning, laundry, and grocery shopping. If the couple is fortunate enough to have a servant, the wife may not actually perform the tasks mentioned above, but she is still responsible for directing that servant's work and seeing to its completion. It should be noted that a woman's "say" in the marriage is directly proportional to her earning power: As that earning power increases so does her power in the family.

Concubinage involves "cohabitation of a man and woman without legal and religious sanction" (Clarke, 1957, p. 30). It tends to be more prevalent among the underclass and is an arrangement that suits the lifestyle of a man who must go from place to place to secure work. From the woman's perspective, this cohabitation arrangement can be beneficial financially if she is not able to support herself and her children on what she earns alone. These relationships are further characterized by their temporary nature and the inferior status they give women. What is meant by the latter is that men and women enter into these arrangements with the understanding that the woman is not his "lady" but that her role is to look after the man's needs (cooking, cleaning, etc.), even though she also is likely to be employed outside the house.

Faithful concubinage is a form of concubinage that carries the promise of stability. The woman *is* considered the man's "lady" and he promises her and her family that he will look after them (Clarke, 1957). In many instances this type of arrangement is viewed as a testing ground for marriage.

There are two kinds of maternal families. In one type a couple exits but the grandmother makes the major decisions in the family, while the man is just a "figurehead." In the second type, the male is totally absent and the grandmother fills the parental void left by the absence of the father. In both cases the marriages are legal; what distinguishes the maternal family from the others is the presence of three generations in the household. Moreover, the female's power is overt and extends to areas beyond household concerns.

In the keeper family, a woman and man decide to live together, with no legal ties in a temporary arrangement. This type differs from the Christian family and faithful concubinage in that the woman never works outside the home and the man always provides for the family.

Families in the lower classes are generally among the latter three of Henriques's family constellations, whereas those in the middle classes tend to fall into the Christian family category.

Middle-class family structure can best be understood by examining the criteria for determining one's membership in this group. Occupation, family backround, and skin color are the most prominent requirements. There was a period directly after the end of slavery when Jamaicans were interested in their family roots. At that time, being descended from a White male was viewed as advantageous. Having those particular roots no longer carries the same prestige, but Jamaican women still refer to different families as "good" families and "bad" families. Being from a "good family" was closely related to the family's skin color. Light-skinned people often comprised the ranks of the middle and upper classes because more opportunities were made available to them and their earning power increased. Today, even though people no longer formally admit to making judgments on the basis of skin shades, and although there are dark-skinned people with education and money, many Jamaican women (of all classes) still attach significance to skin color and will consider it when choosing a spouse. It is not unheard of for Jamaican women to marry White or Asian men. In some instances such a union would be openly encouraged if it was thought that there were no suitable Black Jamaican men for that woman.

Mary was the oldest child in the Blake family, a middle-class Jamaican family from Kingston. Her complexion was the color of cocoa, while her husband's complexion was ebony. This match was seen as imminently suitable, since the husband was an ambassador and therefore his position in society canceled out the "negative" element of his dark skin color.

Mary's sister Rose, on the other hand, dated a German man for several years. She eventually settled in the United Kingdom and married a White British man. One of their male cousins, a dark-skinned divinity student, married a Chinese woman from the island. These latter two marriages were looked upon as favorably as was Mary's marriage. The White husband and the Chinese wife insured that the skin color of the offspring would be appropriately "light."

Readiness for marriage is primarily determined by economic success. Therefore, the existence of such success in the upper classes makes the "Christian family" the dominant family form. Among this group of people we can also see the pervasive influence of English culture. Despite the overt support of monogamy the Jamaican man usually keeps a mistress and maintains her and his children by her (referred to as "outside children") in a separate household. The fact that the practice is given a name—"twin households"—suggests the extent of its prevalence. The reasons given for this practice are varied. One argument suggests that as one moves from the lower to the upper classes, how a mate is chosen has increasingly less to do with personal attraction. It is thus presumed that the husband from an upper-class family must go outside of the marriage to obtain sexual fulfillment, which is continued as long as he is able to support both households financially. There is a clear double standard in this practice, since wives are not expected or encouraged to do the same. A woman's involvement in an extramarital relationship would be censured by both men and women, whereas, although wives are not necessarily happy about their husband's infidelity, they tend not to do anything about it. Divorce is unlikely. If the husband is discreet and takes care of his family, the infidelity may not be discussed openly at all, but if he is not discreet, then some action would have to be taken. Some women may take the children and leave, while others may consult an *obeah* woman. Any course of action would have to include saving face and keeping up appearances. In some cases, a woman's greatest ally in marriage is her mother-in-law. Although there is a strong mother–son bond, a mother will look to her daughter-in-law to help support the son accomplish great things. In situations where the son may be in danger of jeopardizing or disgracing the family, a wife could count on her mother-in-law for help.

CHILD-REARING PRACTICES

Children in the lower classes are expected to be obedient, respectful of their elders and authority figures, and responsible for the completion of household chores. They are not considered the equals of adults and therefore their opinions on family matters are not solicited. A child does not talk back to his or her elders. Adult friends of the family are called "aunt" or "uncle"; to call them by their first names alone would be disrespectful. Discipline can take a number of forms. Spankings are the primary form of discipline and are often accompanied by a verbal reprimand or "tongue lashing." Limits are imposed on younger children with stories about ghosts or "duppies" who are "stone throwing spirits" (Henriques, 1968, p. 33).

Payne's (1989) study demonstrates just how widespread the belief in spanking is. She found that 70% of her sample approved of corporal punishment for minor children. Decisions about when its use was appropriate was not random. In fact, the author found quite a bit of "consensus about when it is unsuitable and/or abusive," continuing, "the majority considered serious disadvantages to arise only if parents resorted to punishment in an unsystematic, excessive or self-serving manner" (p. 389). Such findings strongly indicate that Jamaican mothers will have some difficulty understanding the child protective system of this country. However, assuming that a mother is charged with child abuse, it is imperative that professionals involved extend their inquiry beyond the simple verification of whether or not a child was hit. A careful exploration must be made about motives and intentions.

In middle-class families the discipline of young children is accomplished through "reasoning" as opposed to spankings. Children are not expected to "tow the line" until they reach adolescence. This is in contrast to the upper-class family, in which indulgence tends to be practiced throughout the child's life as a minor.

Women have primary responsibility for child rearing in the middle and lower classes. In the upper classes nannies are hired to deal with the everyday care of the children, although mothers are expected to supervise the nanny. A nanny is viewed as a status symbol, and women are freed and expected to involve themselves in charity and social events. Children, regardless of class, are appointed godparents. The godparents assume responsibility for the child's religious upbringing. In the event that something happens to the parents, the godparents are duty bound to assume the responsibility of raising the children.

In some instances children are separated from their parents. It is not unusual for school-aged children to be sent to live with extended family because no one is home to supervise them while the parents work. A relative living close to a more desirable school may also precipitate this temporary change in the child's residence so that the child may benefit from attending a better school. Sometimes the arrangement is made for the benefit of a relative. For example, a child may be sent to be a companion for a childless woman or a woman whose children are adults living elsewhere (Sanford, 1974).

GENDER ISSUES

In Jamaican culture sex roles are fairly stereotyped and rigid. Girls are expected to be obedient, feminine, and attractive, to be refined and cultured, to be bright and educated—but not to outstrip a man. A girl is taught to bear and raise children, to encourage her mate and generally to be the mainstay of her family.

This is quite a tall order, and it can create many double binds for the Jamaican girl. For example, her education is strongly encouraged because it is seen as the means to secure and steady employment. However, if she stays in school "too long" (a period for which there is no precise definition) and remains unmarried, another message is given, one communicated by the maxim, "Don't stay in school too long and educate yourself out of a husband."

Exposure to the arts is considered just as important as formal education; it is viewed as enhancing a girl's femininity while also increasing her chances of social mobility. To this end, time and money are set aside for music lessons, dance lessons, trips to museums, and so on. If there is an older female in the family who is particularly talented in one area, she may be asked to start a young (i.e., latency-age) girl off with lessons. Once again, a dilemma presents itself if the girl develops a talent for or becomes too interested in these lessons. When she gets older she is by no means to consider a career in the arts, for jobs in these fields are viewed by Jamaicans as too unstable.

One issue confronting the therapist working with the Jamaican woman may be her fear of success. Being successful is quite a paradox. On the one hand, achievement is encouraged to ensure security through steady work and the acquisition of a husband, but, on the other hand, the achievements of a talented girl able to achieve great things is stifled at a certain point. This has an effect on a woman's self-esteem, because the message is that a woman's status is acquired through her husband and who he is. Where does this leave the woman who ignores the admonitions to slow down? It leaves her in what the culture considers a socially awkward position: a woman who is financially secure and professionally successful but has no husband. If the woman happens to be dark-skinned and successful, her chances of marrying are drastically reduced. A man is more likely to marry a light-skinned woman who could improve his social status.

Skin color is one area over which people have no control in their lives. Although publicly people in the islands and the United States deny the existence of preferential treatment based on skin color, privately many decisions are made with this in mind. Lighter skinned Blacks are considered more attractive than darker skinned Blacks (Garvey, 1973). Nevertheless, skin color is only one of the factors in the larger issue of physical attractiveness and self-esteem. Miller (1969), in his study of Chinese, Black, and White adolescents in Kingston, Jamaica found the following: (1) the darker skinned Black subjects were more dissatisfied with their hair than the White, Chinese, or lighter skinned Black subjects; (2) only the Black subjects raised the issue of lips and skin color, and it was the darker skinned Black subjects who expressed dissatisfaction with those features; (3) their conceptualizations of a "beautiful girl" and a "handsome boy" were identical in terms of facial features and skin color, with an emphasis on fair skin and Caucasian features; and (4) their descriptions of the average Jamaican differed sharply from those considered beautiful. "The average Jamaican described by these adolescents was basically Negroid in character. What is interesting is that the concept of the average Jamaican is very far removed from the concept of the handsome boy or beautiful girl" (Miller, 1969, p. 87).

Double standards in male and female socialization patterns abound. Males are expected to "raise a little hell" and "sow some wild oats" in their youth. They are supposed to father children, get steady work, and, when able, to marry. Affairs or "outside" relationships are allowed if not expected. Masculinity is verified by the man's ability to make babies and money.

A problem for boys is that often, due to the absence of fathers, their mothers are responsible for socialization. This means that the predominant role models at home are female. Allen (1988) suggests that this lack of a source of knowledge about being a husband and father cuts across class lines. The resulting gender identity confusion can lead to low self-esteem. That sense of inadequacy can lead to symptom formation.

SEXUALITY

Sexuality in Jamaican culture represents a cultural paradox. Despite the formal emphasis on propriety, premarital sex and children born out of wedlock are not uncommon occurrences. Sex education is rarely done overtly or purposefully. Much of what a young woman learns as a child or adolescent she infers indirectly from nonverbal information. Unwed pregnancies of the young are not categorically frowned upon. A family's attitude about such a situation is largely determined by the attributes of the unwed father. If he is perceived as lazy, has no ambition, and lacks a source of income, he will be scorned. On the other hand, if he should prove industrious and hard working the family will welcome him and support the relationship. A precipitous marriage is not likely to be encouraged if the man is not a good financial prospect.

Unwed pregnancies of older women who are mistresses to married men are viewed differently. If the man is financially secure he will maintain two separate households. The "outside" children may even carry his name and receive the same benefits as his legitimate children. Reactions to the mistress are mixed. Some may find her morally lacking, while others may admire her ability to gain entry into the upper class. Although no statistics were available, there is reason to believe that the abortion rate among Jamaicans is quite low. First, the number of Catholic and Protestant believers constitutes a relatively high percentage of the population. In the West Indies being born out of wedlock does not carry the same level of stigma as it does in the United States, since there are enough people willing to take unwanted children.

I have confined my comments mainly to heterosexual behavior because there is very little other data available; the theoretical or research literature about homosexuality in the Jamaican culture is almost nonexistent. This absence itself may be quite telling, indicative of certain attitudes on the subject rather than an absence of lesbians in the population. One study was done by Brown and Amoroso (1975) in Trinidad. They sought to compare data collected on the attitudes of West Indians toward homosexuality with data previously collected on Canadians and Brazilians. Results indicated that West Indian males were less homophobic than Brazilians but more homophobic than Canadian males. The West Indian females overall were less homophobic than their male counterparts.

In a culture where sex roles are fairly rigid and propriety is of the utmost importance one would not expect homosexuality to be condoned. When I have spoken informally with my West Indian colleagues, they have suggested that not only is homosexuality not condoned, it is not even recognized—hence its absence in the literature. If a woman wants to make public her sexual orientation, she risks being ostracized from the family. The issues of Black lesbians are addressed further in Chapter 14 of this book. The reader may also consult the autobiographical literature available on Black Caribbean lesbians (Lorde, 1982).

PSYCHOTHERAPY

The aspects of life that could be considered problematic by the Jamaican female encompass a wide range of issues. That range may be conceptualized in terms of three broad areas: concrete issues, interpersonal issues, and individual or intrapsychic issues. The first area includes money, citizenship status, ability to support family, and financing education and health. Getting along with a spouse, discipline issues with children, and problems with extended family or in-laws comprise the interpersonal realm. The final area may reflect poor self-esteem (including questions regarding physical attractiveness) and concerns about propriety, which will manifest itself as shame or embarrassment. It should be noted that what separates this cultural group from others is not necessarily the type of problems but how they are experienced, what is seen as their etiology, at what point Jamaican women seek help, and where they go for that help.

In general Jamaicans do not talk about problems. Feelings are seldom, if ever, revealed verbally. Mental health problems are not labeled as such and would not be discussed. Men handle psychological distress by going out with other men, while women deal with pain in church and by investing themselves in their children. If a child expresses any feelings that the family is not willing to recognize or if he or she is acting out, that behavior will be seen as a sign of ungratefulness.

One clear expression of a cry for help is suicide. Burke's (1985) study found a very low suicide rate in Jamaica when compared to the other islands. The rate was 1.4 in 100,000 with a gender ratio of 12 males to 1 female. Burke found no clear explanation for the low suicide rate among Jamaican women, and could only hypothesize that it was somehow related to their role in society. Mahy (1987) reported rather disturbing findings that indicate a rise in the number of attempted and completed suicides among women in Barbados. The female teenagers in the Mahy study attempted suicide after conflict with a parent, and the females in the 25- to 29-year-old group attempted suicide after a conflict with a lover. Both studies raise questions that still need to be examined, particularly as to why the suicide rate in Jamaica is so much lower than the rest of the Caribbean, and how one can explain the sex difference.

When a problem is recognized an individual will try to solve it on her own. If she is not successful the next step would be to consult an older family member. Senior family members are held in high regard, which is consistent with African cultural derivatives that value the wisdom of elders. Although there is an appreciation for education or "book learning," older people are seen as having "life experience," whence wisdom is said to come. One can understand why a Jamaican woman would not go to a mental health facility, considering the history of psychiatry in Jamaica. The fist psychiatric hospital in Jamaica was Bellevue Hospital, established in Kingston in 1873. It has grown into a "monolithic custodial institution of over 3,000 beds, accepting patients from the remotest areas of the island, with the police as the major referral source" (Hickling, 1976, p. 101).

Where a Jamaican woman does go for help depends on the level of her distress and her perception of the etiology of her problem. Some women believe their problem is within themselves (e.g., "I'm not working hard enough"). Others may externalize problems, viewing them as a run of bad luck or the result of witchcraft. A therapist should not make the assumption that a belief in *obeah* is strictly reserved for the lower classes, or is in itself a sign of pathology. There are many middle- and upper-class West Indian women who believe in *obeah* but fear that acknowledging such beliefs would bring them into disfavor among their upper-class peers.

A therapist cannot treat a Jamaican woman without familiarizing him- or herself with the many ways that *obeah* can come up as an issue in therapy (Neki et al., 1986, does an excellent job of outlining this). Frequently it is used by the patient to explain situations in her life that are not going well. "The spiritualistic interpretations of the mentally ill are simple, credible, and given in a setting free of the stigma associated with psychiatric treatment" (Roger & Hollingshead, 1965, pp. 259–260). It can be used to control overwhelming or intense emotions like anger by projecting those unacceptable feelings onto the witchdoctor. Women consult the witchdoctor to allay their fears, to validate their perceptions, and to get a plan of action—not unlike the reasons people go to psychotherapists. We know from outcome studies in psychotherapy that the instillation of hope and feelings of self-efficacy are important factors in getting well. There are, however, other ways that *obeah* may come up in therapy in a more negative way. The fact that this is a cultural syntonic belief does not mean that it cannot be used in pathological and maladaptive ways. It may be the symptom of a psychotic process or it may be a way for the woman to deny problems.

Michelle, a 19-year-old Jamaican woman, came to our clinic for treatment of anxiety symptoms. After interviewing Michelle it became apparent to the therapist that a great deal of her anxiety had to do with her relationship with her boyfriend. She told the therapist that she had stolen another woman's boyfriend. She believed that her distress was the result of being *obeahed* by someone the other woman had consulted. One area of concern for the therapist was a recurring stomach pain that Michelle complained about. The therapist advised her to go see a physician. Michelle refused, stating that the doctor's magic would not be powerful enough to counter that of the *obeah* woman. Weeks later Michelle failed an appointment and did not call. The therapist phoned the home to find that Michelle had been hospitalized due to a perforated ulcer. In this instance the patient's strong belief in *obeah* prevented her from seeking the appropriate medical treatment.

Neki et al. further explain that the person who believes in *obeah* will have mixed feelings about the therapist, because a person capable of grappling with the powers of a witch has to be pretty powerful him- or herself and thus is someone to be feared. The woman who is not a believer of witchcraft will view the therapist as an authority figure. The older the therapist is and the more credentials she or he possesses, the more respect is granted.

The race of the therapist is a crucial issue. There has been no research to date that looks at the effects of the specific therapy dyads of Black therapist–Jamaican patient or White therapist–Jamaican patient. However, I caution therapists of both races. For the White therapist the absence of knowledge about Blacks in this country and in Jamaica can result in the therapist completely missing issues important to the patient, or misunderstanding them. There may be a tendency to idealize the patient as the "good" Black and ignore racial issues that might make the therapist uncomfortable. Another problem that may arise in an attempt by the White therapist to overcompensate for discriminatory feelings is the attribution of too much weight to racial issues, to the exclusion of intrapsychic ones.

The Black American therapist–Jamaican patient dyad is not without its problems.

Coral was a 34-year-old Jamaican attorney in a prestigious Wall Street firm. She had attended the top schools in the country and clerked at one of the best law firms. Her credentials and experience were the best. For this reason it was very puzzling to her when she did not make partner and a less qualified White associate did. After hearing the news she analyzed herself and her training, looking for where she had made a mistake. Weeks of doing this "post mortem" left her feeling depressed. She slept little and her appetite diminished. She lost interest in recreational activities and stopped seeing friends.

Coral's therapist was Dr. B., an African American psychologist. Like Coral, Dr. B. had attended the finest schools to attain her doctorate degree. However, in addition to devoting herself to her studies, she was also very involved with the Black Civil Rights movement. Within moments of hearing Coral's situation, Dr. B. jumped to the conclusion that Coral had been the victim of racism. While that may have been the case, it turned out to be the sole focus of Dr. B.'s work with Coral. She lost all objectivity and insisted that Coral accept her view. Coral got the message that she wasn't "really Black" if she didn't see the racism in this situation, and she left treatment shortly thereafter.

Because of the pervasiveness of discrimination in this country there is a desire for minority people to want to bond. Identifying with the patient and glossing over differences can lead to misunderstandings, as can a Black therapist's need to distance her- or himself from the patient. The therapist may reject the Jamaican patient, viewing her as "elitist" and desiring to be White.

Overall, it can be said that psychotherapy is not the first or even the second resource Jamaican women are likely to tap whenever a problem arises. If she arrives in a therapist's office it is likely that she is very acculturated to American ways or that she has been referred by an agency (school, medical center, church, etc.). In the latter instance the Jamaican woman will present herself for therapy but will not immediately be convinced of its efficacy. The therapist should not assume that ignorance of the psychotherapeutic process is something endemic to the lower classes. Some very sophisticated and educated Jamaican women may be unfamiliar with therapy because of its cultural incompatibility.

Measures can be taken by the therapist to join with this patient. As stated above, formality and propriety are important, as is giving consideration to her work schedule when making appointments. Her work hours may be erratic or she may go from one job to another, leaving little free time. This should not immediately be seen as resistance avoidance. If she is not working in a professional capacity it may be difficult for her to take time off without losing pay.

Jamaican women are quite stoic and may not admit to having symptoms or difficulty coping for some time, a reluctance that should not always be used as a barometer of trust. Continued attendance and asking the therapist's opinion are good indications of trust in the therapeutic relationship.

SUMMARY

Treating the Jamaican female can be very challenging and rewarding. Jamaican families have multiple strengths. Individuals are strong and hard working, and the nuclear and extended families have tremendous loyalty ties to one another. A sense of duty works in both directions: elders to children and children to elders. Family boundaries are quite fluid, allowing for a variety of family constellations and insurance that vulnerable members (i.e., young children, the elderly, the infirm, etc.) are always taken care of. These strengths should be emphasized and capitalized on in any therapy.

IMPLICATIONS FOR FURTHER RESEARCH

1. It would be helpful to examine the perceptions that Jamaican women have about psychotherapeutic services. This could be approached from two sides: the expectations of those who have never been in therapy versus the impressions of those who have experienced treatment.

2. There have been very good studies done in the area of Black children's perceptions of what is "good" and what is "pretty" when they are shown pictures of children of varying skin shades. Useful information would be obtained from a study that addresses Jamaican women's perceptions of "goodness, prettiness, successfulness, and happiness" as they relate to pictures of Black women of various skin colors.

3. There is a paucity of literature—research or theoretical—on the lesbian Jamaican woman and her relationships.

4. An investigation of what accounts for the gender differences in response to parent–child separation could provide useful data for therapy.

5. Assessing the clinical implications for adult women of separation from their children would be helpful.

6. Important insight could be gained from examining whether Jamaican women, who have grown up in a country where the majority of the people look like them, have higher self-esteem than African American women, who have grown up as part of a numercial minority.

7. It would be useful to know what some of the mental health issues are for women who are mistresses, as well as what the issues are for women whose husbands keep mistresses.

8. Ascertaining what the Jamaican woman's perception of the traits that make for a mentally healthy adult woman would increase therapeutic effectiveness.

9. A very interesting study could result from contrasting Jamaican women's perceived ability to obtain success in the United States with their actual attainment.

10. There is much to learn about *obeah*. If it is a vehicle for dealing with overwhelming feelings then it would be worthwhile to examine its efficacy as a deterrent to the self-injurious behavior that comes from intense anger.

REFERENCES

Allen, E. (1988). West Indians. In L. Comas-Díaz & E. Griffith (Eds.), *Clinical guidelines in cross-cultural mental health* (pp. 305–333). New York: Wiley.
Augelli, J. P. (Ed.). (1973). *Caribbean lands*. Grand Rapids, MI: Fidler.
Best, T. (1975). West Indians and Afro-Americans: A partnership. *Crisis, 82*, 389.
Brice, J. (1982). West Indians. In M. McGoldrick, J. K. Pearce, & J. Giordano (Eds.), *Ethnicity and family therapy* (pp. 123–133). New York: Guilford Press.

Brown, M., & Amoroso, D. (1975, December). Attitudes toward homosexuality among West Indian male and female college students. *Journal of Social Psychology 97*(2), 163–168.

Burke, A. (1985). Suicide in Jamaica. *West Indian Medical Journal, 34,* 48–53.

Clarke, E. (1957). *My mother who fathered me: A study of the family in three selected communities in Jamaica.* London: Allen & Unwin.

Garcia-Preto, N. (1982). Puerto Rican families. In M. McGoldrick, J. K. Pearce, & J. Giordano (Eds.), *Ethnicity and family therapy* (pp. 164–186). New York: Guilford Press.

Garvey, M. (1973). The race question in Jamaica. In D. Lowenthal & L. Comitas (Eds.), *The consequences of class and color* (pp. 4–11). New York: Anchor Books.

Henriques, F. (1968). *Family and colour in Jamaica.* London: MacGibbon & Kee.

Hickling, F. (1976). The effects of a community psychiatric service on the mental hospital population in Jamaica. *West Indian Medical Journal, 25,* 101–106.

Lefley, H. (1981). Psychotherapy and cultural adaptation in the Caribbean. *International Journal of Group Tensions, 11*(4), 3–16.

Leyburn, J. G. (1966). *The Haitian people.* New Haven, CT: Yale University Press.

Lorde, A. (1982). *Zami: A new spelling of my name.* Freedom, CA: Crossing Press.

Mahy, G. (1987). Attempted suicide in Barbados. *West Indian Medical Journal, 36,* 31–34.

Miller, E. (1969). Body image, physical beauty and color among Jamaican adolescents. *Social and Economic Studies, 18*(1), 72–89.

Neki, J., Jornet, B., Ndase, N., Kilonzo, G., Haule, J., & Duninage, G. (1986). Witchcraft and psychotherapy. *British Journal of Psychiatry, 149,* 145–155.

Payne, M. (1989). Use and abuse of corporal punishment: A Caribbean view. *Child Abuse and Neglect, 13,* 389–401.

Regis, H. (1988). A theoretical framework for the study of the psychological sense of community of English speaking Caribbean immigrants. *Journal of Black Psychology, 15*(1), 57–76.

Rogler, L., & Hollingshead, A. (1965). *Trapped: Families and schizophrenia,* New York: Krieger.

Sandoval, M. (1979). Santeria as mental health care system: A historical overview. *Social Science and Medicine, 13,* 137–151.

Sanford, M. (1974). A socialization in ambiguity: Child lending in a British West Indian society. *Ethnology, 13*(4), 393–400.

Schlesinger, B. (1968). Family patterns in the English speaking Caribbean. *Journal of Marriage and the Family, 30,* 149–154.

Sowell, T. (1981). *Ethnic America.* New York: Basic Books.

Wray, S., & McLaren, E. (1976). Parent–child separation as a determinant of psychotherapy in children: A Jamaican study. *West Indian Medical Journal, 25,* 251–257.

Women of the Indian Subcontinent

Kushalata Jayakar

Women of Indian descent constitute a large and distinct cultural group. They are, however, rarely the formal focus of attention in psychology texts about women or in the training of psychotherapists who treat women. The psychosocial development of Indian women occurs in the context of a complicated and often paradoxical culture, about which little is known by Westerners.

When I first undertook the task of writing this chapter, I initiated a series of discussions with other Indian women to elicit different perspectives on this issue. Questions arose, with surprising regularity, as to why a chapter on Indian women would appear in a book on "women of color." A surprising number of my Indian colleagues vehemently expressed their contention that Indians were not persons of color, but rather White. The vehemence with which these contentions were presented gave rise to what was for me a new realization. Having been born and raised in India as an Indian woman, I was always and clearly not White, and therefore a person of color. This was true during the "colonial time" or "Raj" as Westerners know it, and is currently true in most parts of the world, particularly in South Africa. In further discussions, it was revealed that most Indians who viewed themselves as Whites were of the Brahmin caste. This perspective seems to be another remnant of the old caste system deeply embedded in the Indian psyche. The system contributes heavily to a frame of mind that leads Indians to divide themselves into Whites, who are considered superior, and persons of color, who are considered inferior. Social status is a function of caste and/or physical appearance.

This issue of caste clearly articulates one of the dilemmas in treating Indians. How Indians are viewed by Westerners, both White and non-White, and how Indians view themselves, may be quite different; the tendency to perceive all Indians as if they were culturally the same as one another or as if they were the same as other persons of color is problematic in clinical practice.

In this chapter I will explore the issue of color and other pertinent aspects of Indian history and culture, including their effects on the development and maturation of Indian women. Indian women come from many major religious groups: they are Muslim, Sikh, Parsi, and others. While a detailed discussion of them is beyond the scope of this chapter, the role of the specific group a client belongs to as well as her religious practices and beliefs is clearly relevant to any clinical assessment. My comments here regarding women's roles pertain primarily to Hindu women, who are the majority, and Muslim women, the largest minority. I will also address gender roles in Indian families and the relevance of all of these issues in the mental health and psychotherapeutic treatment of Indian women.

INDIA'S BORDERS

India is a vast country of 1,269,346 square miles, spread between the mighty Himalayas and the Arabian Sea. It is a country that has been repeatedly invaded by outsiders, from Alexander the Great to Genghis Khan to the Great Mughals. The last invaders were the British in the 17th century (Brata, 1985). India assumed a new identity within the country itself after each invasion. Originally, curiosity and greed drove explorers toward India, which some 600 years ago was among the richest countries in the world. Explorers came and brought with them their cultures, religions, and their languages. India absorbed parts of each new culture and altered itself while maintaining its own ancient cultural base. This capacity to tolerate outside influence without changing major aspects of the original structure of society contributes to the paradoxical nature of India's culture. With each new invader India changed, perhaps for the better *and* for the worse. Islamic rulers enriched India with the development of art and architecture such as the inimitable Taj Mahal, but the introduction of their new and completely different religion, Islam, eventually led to the partition of the country into what is now known as original India, Pakistan, and Bangladesh.

Prior to the British invasion, in the 16th century, India was a country composed of small independent states, each governed by individual rulers. The British conquered each state and eventually gained control of the entire country, maintaining control until India's independence in 1947. For the British, India was never a home, but merely an occupied colony to which they were always the conquerors and outsiders. The non-Whiteness of Indians became a major issue at the time of the British invasion. Indians were clearly perceived by the British as people of color or as "black" people. Inferior status was linked to skin color in a profound way, darker skin being explicitly associated with inferiority. British influence contributed heavily to the paradoxes we continue to see in India at the present time.

In actuality, a large part of northern India's population consists of a fair-skinned Aryan people. As one moves to different parts of India, the climate and population change dramatically. The people of the Southern, warmer regions appear shorter and darker, indicating Dravidian ancestry. In the east and northeast there is evidence of Mongol ancestry.

Skin color, although varying tremendously throughout the country, was not as important in pre–British India as a person's caste in determining social status and drawing segregation lines. Here the impact of British influence is undeniable in its subjugation and view of the entire country as non-White. Brata (1985) writes that it was paradoxically the shared experience of foreign domination that brought Indians together in many ways. As the foreign rule became more powerful and oppressive, many Indians allied themselves against the outside invader, overlooking class distinctions.

The majority of Indians today read, write, and speak the English language. This may be attributed in part to immigration qualifications. In India a significant amount of elementary education is in English, as is almost all secondary, university, and scientific education. The Indian immigrant's level of fluency in English contrasts with that of Latin and other Asian immigrants, many of whom were not colonized by English-speaking nations. English fluency has helped to hasten the absorption of Indian immigrants into the mainstream labor force more readily than other immigrants.

The need to accommodate the influence of the West in the development of the education system grew, increasing the dichotomy between the old and new Indias. The country's present paradoxes represent the continuation of attitudes adopted during years of foreign rule. These changes occurred quite rapidly and were most evident in urban India. The city of Bombay is as cosmopolitan as the city of New York and contrasts sharply with the stagnant ways of a rural India, which lags hundreds of years behind.

INDIA'S PEOPLE

Currently, all immigrants coming from beyond Europe and the Middle Eastern countries or the countries on the other side of the Pacific Ocean are lumped together as "Asian American." Saran (1985) notes that there are no real ties or similarities, ethnic or phenotypic, between Indians and other Asians or the people from the Orient. Indians are distinct in their cultural properties from other Asians, a factor that becomes obvious when one grows familiar with the Indian psyche.

India is a country filled with paradoxes and contradictions. It is a society that is described as simultaneously advanced and ancient, one of grinding poverty and extravagant wealth, politically democratic yet authoritarian and corrupt in just as many ways (Brata, 1985). It is in these respects similar to the United States as well as many other developing or "third world" countries.

Some 25 years ago, as a medical student in India, it was my common observation that 45–50% of the medical school enrollment was female. India is one of the few countries where a capable woman remained at the helm of the government for over two decades, long before England ever elected a woman to head the government. Women lawyers argue in both civil and criminal courts, and the number of women in the medical field in India is virtually equal to the number of men in all medical specialties. This occurred long before the system of limited quotas of females was lifted in the U.S. medical schools. Additionally, DurgaKali, India's most powerful diety worshipped by Hindus, is a goddess. Yet, India is also a country where 12- to 15-year-old daughters are sold to wealthy Arabs for a minimal price, and brides are burned to death by their husbands in order to obtain multiple dowries (Bumiller, 1990; "Child Bride," 1991; "Discarding Daughters," 1990; "India," 1990; Luthra, 1989; Paul, 1986; Ramu, 1988; Singh, 1990). Since the advent of modern medical techniques that reveal the gender of the fetus, 99% of aborted fetuses were female, resulting in a significant decline in the number of females in the population (Bumiller, 1990; "Discarding Daughters," 1990; "India," 1990; Freed & Freed, 1989; Kristof, 1991; Singh, 1990).

Although this state of affairs has remained consistent over many years, even as an Indian woman I was only vaguely aware of it until I left home 25 years ago, fresh out of medical school and eager to explore the mighty West. I became particularly conscious of the contrast between the cultures of the United States and India when I first revisited India after living for some time in the United States. Many women currently living in India are oblivious to the great contrast between India and the United States, and to the adjustments they would face on immigration. The extent of contrast between the two countries may not even be apparent until one returns to India after having been away for some time.

Indian Immigrants in the United States

Indian immigration in the United States was minuscule prior to the mid-1960s. According to data from the U.S. Bureau of Census (Bachu, 1985), the earliest record of Indians in the United States was found in 1790. Later, immigration in small numbers was noted between 1897 and 1920, Indians serving for the most part as a labor force from British Columbia and Canada. Further immigration of Indians was officially prohibited in 1946 (Bachu, 1985). Those Indians who were in the United States at that time were not granted citizenship until 1970, because of the laws in place until that time (Saran, 1985).

The major wave of immigration of Indians came after the 1965 amendment to the Immigration and Naturalization Act. The majority of this group consisted of young adults from middle- to upper-middle-class backgrounds. Most of this group had at least four years of college; a majority of them had postgraduate or professional degrees, usually in engineering or medicine. This was in part a reflection of highly selective or discriminatory immigration criteria that required immigrants to be self-sufficient or supported by their sponsors.

Of the immigrants from India, 80% were single or married young adults (Saran, 1985). Most of the women who immigrated to the United States came primarily as wives or daughters of the male immigrants who came to the United States after the mid-1960s. An extremely small number of educated women immigrated independently (Asian Women United of California, 1989; Mitter, 1991; Ramu, 1989). Single men returned "home" to "fetch" the brides selected for them by their families—a practice as common now as it was 30 years ago (Gupta, 1991; Paul, 1986; Saran, 1985). In arranged marriages, a bride's higher level of education is viewed as an asset, and thus many women who enter this country as homemakers often enter the workforce eventually (Rao & Nandini, 1985). Formal levels of education allow Indian women to be able to function at various levels. They are employed as teachers, from kindergarten and special education to the college level. They are represented in the ranks of accountants, practicing physicians, social workers, administrators, and entrepreneurs running their own businesses, as well as on Wall Street in the corporate world alongside men (Dasgupta, 1986; Ramu, 1989; Sethi & Allen, 1984).

There does not appear to be any one reason for the immigration of the majority of Indians to the United States. Significant numbers came for research, the cultural experience of Western society and glamour, the promise of "freedom" and an open society (I. Puri, personal communication, December 1, 1990). The sheer numbers of immigrants are no doubt largely the result of the favorable changes in immigration laws since 1965, but other possible reasons for immigration emerge. The first and foremost appears to be financial, the U.S. economy being stronger than India's, and secondly there has always been a fascination with the West among many Indians. Indians who travel to the West—considered by many to be the land of the superior, "ruler" White race—and return seem to carry some magical attraction. It is as if their association with the superior, ruler race makes them superior to other Indians. This is perhaps a residual effect of British rule. A smaller number of individuals come to the United States specifically for higher education, through government-sponsored financial aid or scholarships, or spending on their own.

As the size of the Indian community in America increased in the 1960s and 1970s, business and career opportunities opened up; for example, there are many businesses in the New York City area serving the needs of Indians exclusively. These flourishing establishments include garment or sari stores, jewelry, electronic, grocery, and condiment stores, and a multitude of Indian restaurants. I can remember coming to America in the late 1960s and finding only two Indian groceries and one sari store in all of Manhattan; now there are hundreds.

INDIAN LANGUAGE AND CULTURE

Most Indian immigrants do not speak with each other in their native tongues to the extent that other nonnative English-speaking immigrants do, generally tending to communicate with one another in English. A major reason for this is the existence of many different languages among Indians themselves. India has a minimum of 18 languages and many more dialects. Although Hindi is the official language of the country, very few use it to communicate socially or officially, even in India. They generally speak with each other in English. The pervasive use of English was another unifying legacy left behind by the British. One important feature must be noted in understanding the Indian's spoken English, however. Often, Indian sentence constructions sound literal and awkward to American ears, which can be a source of confusion and misunderstanding in communications between Indians and Americans. This happens primarily because the grammatical construction of Indian languages is quite different from that of the English language. This issue is a particularly salient one in verbal psychotherapies where language, subtleties in word meanings and usage, and expressions are presumed to have deeper meaning and are used to reflect the capacity for abstract reasoning. For example, an Indian woman who calls herself "homely" means that she is home loving, not that she is unattractive.

Even though most Indians speak English and have been readily absorbed into the mainstream American workforce, the majority have remained unchanged in their basic spiritual beliefs. These beliefs heavily influence the Indian woman's view of the world and her place in it. There is a strong fatalistic view of life based on an understanding of one's *dharma* and *karma* (Dhruvarajan, 1990; Mitter, 1991). Dharma, basically a Hindu concept, is defined as the traditional established order, including all individual, moral, social, and religious duties (Roland, 1989). Every person has his or her own individual dharma (*swadharma*), which is determined less by abstract moral principles than by contextual factors such as stage in the life cycle, particular hierarchical relationships, caste, and individual temperament (Dhruvarajan, 1990). The Western doctrine of individual human rights is profoundly alien to the Indian, who pursues "adjustments" rather than "rights." For the Indian woman, therefore, identity is always based on relationships such as mother, daughter, niece, sister, pupil, and so on. Identities outside of these relationships may seem inconceivable to her (Altekar, 1983; Dasgupta, 1986; Everett, 1981; Mitter, 1991).

Western concepts of human development stress autonomy and initiative in young children, and moratoria and synthesis in adolescence and young adulthood, as central universalized schema (Erikson, 1946; Vaidyanathan, 1989). This schema may not however apply to Indian development. The Indian child must respond to the culture's active encouragement of dependency and active discouragement of independence in the earlier stages of childhood. Western developmental schemes also fail to take into account or explore meaningfully the Indian child's negotiation of the severe crackdown and restriction of behavior in familial hierarchical relationships from ages 4 or 5 through adolescence (Roland, 1989). These factors are all culturally relevant, with implications for the psychotherapeutic alliance and relationship.

Karma can be defined literally as deeds or actions, but, in its broader meaning life is viewed as a continuous cycle of birth, death, rebirth, and death (Dhruvarajan, 1990; Mitter, 1991). It is believed that one's destiny is to repeat this cycle indefinitely unless one performs deeds that allow one to be reborn in a higher form. For example, one may progress from an insect to a mammal and finally to a human form endowed with the capacity to think. The performance of evil deeds in one's present life will result in condemnation to rebirth in a lower form. Conversely, if one gives up all material or worldly attachments that are a function of five human emotions, lust, anger, greed, want, and envy, the cycle of karma is broken and one enters the stage of *Nirvana* or *Moksha* (Dhruvarajan, 1990; Mitter, 1991; Sethi & Allen, 1984).

INDIAN WOMEN AND DOMESTIC RELATIONSHIPS

The strong belief in dharma and karma and the fatalistic view of life is reflected in the Indian tradition of arranged marriages. Although this is changing somewhat in larger cities and may not be followed in all individual families, the arranged marriage remains the primary route to marriage both in India and in the United States among Indians (Bumiller, 1990; Kanekar & Kolsawalia, 1983; Liddle & Joshi, 1986; Luthra, 1989; Mandelbaum, 1986). This is true for almost all of rural India and remains true for a high percentage of the urban educated population as well. The usual procedure begins with the assumption that a marriage does not occur between two individuals but between two families. Therefore, the compatibility of the two families is of paramount importance. Secondly, it is an accepted fact that parents always know what is best for their children, even if the "children" are professional, well-established adults. To question the judgment or motives of one's parents is considered blasphemous. It is believed that the young, by virtue of their youth and inexperience, are bound to use immature judgment and give in to youthful infatuation. Most well-educated Indians, both women and men alike, accept this as their dharma or prescribed duty (Ramu, 1988; Rao & Nandini, 1985; Saran, 1985). Many therefore accept the belief that love will simply "happen" once they are married.

A bride is chosen in a fairly established manner. A matchmaker presents information about suitable individuals to the two families. Descriptions of the individuals are exchanged, along with photographs. On a fixed date, chosen as auspicious according to astrological signs, the family members of the male visit the home of the chosen "girl." The girl is observed by members of the prospective groom's family while she is engaged in the duties of supposedly entertaining them by bringing them snacks or drinks. She may be asked to sit down so that the elders may ask her questions. This is done in order to take note of her speech, physical appearance, and the color of her skin. Fair skin is greatly valued and presumed to rule out other "defects" or weaknesses. The manner and extent to which women and women of color are objectified in this process is obvious.

While the aforementioned description captures the essence of the process, it may also present extremes. In contemporary situations the process may be modified such that a prospective couple may be brought to a restaurant with chaperones, and allowed to chat briefly. On the other hand, many families arrange the entire process themselves. The bride and groom in this case may not see each other face to face until the wedding. The ceremony in which a bride's face is unveiled has been a romanticized ritual in both Hindu and Muslim weddings.

It should be noted that the groom and his family have the greater option of refusing to marry a chosen female. Women who refuse marriage with a chosen male face more severe repercussions than men, who are "allowed" to refuse several brides. Another aspect of arranged marriages is that of the dowry (Paul, 1986; Sethi & Allen, 1984). According to ancient Hindu custom, the bride's family is obligated to give a dowry consisting of cash and gifts to the groom. How much the groom may require is usually a function of his social standing and occupation. The higher his status, the higher the price he can demand of his bride's family. There is a stigma attached to remaining unmarried and to avoid it a family will do their utmost to pay the required amounts, rather than risk the humiliation of not being able to find a husband for their daughter (Ramu, 1988; Rao & Nandini, 1985; Luthra, 1989).

It is clinically important to raise a number of questions at this point about the socialization of women in this culture and its effect on the state of mind of many of the women who find themselves in these situations. The names of the women discussed in the case examples have been omitted and their identifying characteristics altered to protect their confidentiality.

The effects of the low status of women and the realities of arranged marriages can be seen in the following case examples.

Both women have been married for at least 15 to 20 years and, from all outside appearances, would be considered "happy" in their marriages. Both women come from upper-middle-class families and were college educated. Both reside in the United States as do other members of their immediate families. By all external accounts they would be considered modern professional women. When asked about their marriages and their level of satisfaction in the marriage, both began by discussing their respective wedding nights.

M. reported that she had never seen or spoken to her husband before they were married. She noted that she would not look at the photograph of him out of fear that she might not like him but would be unable to refuse a marriage which had already been arranged by elders. M. is a quite beautiful woman and reports that her groom was extremely pleased with her appearance. She also reports, however, that she was terrified of having sexual intercourse with a stranger and in a most unexpected fashion found that she was menstruating on her wedding night. Despite this most unwelcome situation, the marriage was consummated later and eventually they had children. Apparently, the marriage is regarded by the parents as successful and they pat themselves on the back for what they consider having done well for their daughter. M., however, laments that she has never had a successful sexual experience nor has she ever achieved orgasm. Indeed, she states that she does not know what she is supposed to feel, rather, she experiences sex as an "agonizing" activity, akin to molestation, which she endures with "clenched fists." M. says that she waits for the day when her husband "tires of this punishing activity."

The second woman was more fortunate than the first. She reported that her husband was gentle and sensitive to her fears of being intimate with someone whom she regarded as a stranger, and quite rightly so. He agreed to not approach her sexually for quite some time after their marriage. Both felt this afforded them the opportunity to "get to know each other better." Only after she felt comfortable with him did he approach her sexually.

Another individual, now divorced, described her wedding night as an "agony." She too had refused to look at her prospective husband's photograph for the reason described before. The prospective bridegroom had refused the offer to meet in person, thinking that he might be rejected because of his dark skin, since dark skin in India is considered a major negative factor in the marriage market. The families in this case agreed that the marriage would proceed and the reluctant pair found themselves betrothed. On the wedding night the woman was anxious and unwilling to have sexual intercourse with her new husband, who ultimately forced her to do so. Later he explained that it would have been scandalous if anyone had found out that he had not done what he was expected to. They would, in his view, naturally question his "manliness." It was not clear how or who would report on him, especially since no one would ever ask his wife about such matters. Their relationship worsened. Following persistent emotional and physical violence, the marriage ended in divorce. This woman, initially quite attractive by conventional standards, became severely obese. In discussing her understanding of her obesity she revealed, "I am shielding my body and sexuality under layers of fat . . . no man will ever come near me again."

While these case histories focus on the rituals of arranged marriages, they may be used to illustrate the broader issues of family structure, relationships, expectations between parents and children, and the cultural attitudes toward females. Generally, children, even as adults, are expected to do whatever their families want them to do (Liddle & Joshi, 1986; Mitter, 1991). The needs of the family and what may be obtained for the family via marital alliance is considered primary. The feelings of spontaneous attractions and affections of the individuals involved seem to have little importance.

With respect to developmental issues, Indian women arguably go through the phases of the life cycle with far less turmoil than Western women. There does not appear to be the fear or fright of seniority or age in Indian women, for it is with age that they may finally savor the power and reverence accorded an elder (Mitter, 1991). Motherhood is welcomed and considered the epitome of womanhood. Childlessness or barrenness is absolutely frowned upon and may be considered the ultimate shame. Many cases of divorce have ensued simply for infertility, which is always presumed to be the woman's problem or responsibility (Altekar, 1983; Mitter, 1991; Rao & Nandini, 1985).

Singh (1990) writes that the female child born in India, if she is fortunate enough not to be aborted, faces prejudice and discrimination at every stage of her life, right from birth. It is not uncommon for female children to be breast-fed for shorter periods of time than their male counterparts. Later, the distribution of nutritious foods within the family favors the male children (Kristof, 1991). Singh (1990) and Luthra (1989) attribute these practices to the notion that females are viewed from birth as moral and economic liabilities; their families are eager to see them become the responsibility of some other family. This view contributes to the prevalence of child marriages (women married below the age of 16 years) and results in higher rates of premature domestic responsibilities, the trauma of pregnancy, and premature child care responsibilities ("Child Bride," 1991; Sethi & Allen, 1984; Singh, 1990). While many of these practices are formally against the law, the laws, created during British rule, did and still do little to challenge this behavior even when it is overt.

Females are in many ways treated like property, to be displayed, judged, and valued according to their physical attributes (Bumiller, 1990; Mandelbaum, 1986; Paul, 1986). Additionally, stories of the wedding night experience highlight the blatant lack of attention given to the importance of sexual satisfaction for women, and sexual education in modern Indian culture for both men and women (Kanekar & Kolsawalia, 1983; Luthra, 1989).

It might be tempting to conclude that Indian parents are inherently cruel and insensitive. What other explanation is there for this inhumane treatment, generation after generation? To understand this conclusion we must go back to the concept of dharma and expected social roles. Dharma is the duty bestowed on an individual by virtue of his or her being in a given place or space at a given time. A person is essentially a fluid self, changing and interchanging with others or easily accommodating and adjusting. This concept is completely at odds with Western culture's emphasis on individualism (Vaidyanathan, 1989). In Indian culture, the individual's role is to follow the expected path. Self-awareness and actualizing one's own personal needs, wishes, or desires, are considered selfish, Western, and essentially unacceptable. One of the major hurdles with an Indian patient, particularly in dynamic psychotherapy, involves making the patient's concerns about her own emotional needs more ego-syntonic (Altekar, 1983; Saran, 1985).

GENDER ROLES

Gender roles within the extended family structure are quite well defined, as is everything else. Each individual is assigned a role within the family hierarchy, with males at the top of that hierarchy. As previously mentioned, the raising of sons is very different from the raising of daughters (Bumiller, 1990; Mitter, 1991). Sons are prepared to be the breadwinners of their families, as well as the caretakers of parents and any other elders within the extended family structure. Daughters are prepared to be daughters-in-law in a family, wherever they go (Mandelbaum, 1986; Mitter, 1991; Ramu, 1988). Right from birth, a female child is literally considered "*kisi aurki amanat,*" which means someone else's property.

This phenomenon highlights similarities with other Eastern cultures. To promise a girl in marriage from the time she is an infant is as common in India as it is in China, as is the idea that she is someone's property. The second story in *The Joy Luck Club* (Tan, 1989) illustrates this point. Being obedient and agreeable are the virtues most valued in women and are consistent with the function of a piece of property, that is, to serve the wishes of its owner (Mandelbaum, 1986; Mitter, 1991). This status does not change for a female for most of her life, as a child, student, wife, or even a working professional, who may be considered a subordinate (Ramu, 1988; Rao & Nandini, 1985).

This also highlights the similarities in the Western culture. It has been observed that Indian women seem to be rapidly Americanized or easily adaptable to American ways (Saran, 1985; Sethi & Allen, 1984). This pattern is perceived to be the case both socially and in the workplace. While this adaptability is often viewed as a virtue, it is also a clear function of the Indian woman's socialization as a woman (Liddle & Joshi, 1986; Saran, 1985; Sethi & Allen, 1984). This socialization emphasizes the development of a capacity to adapt to a changed environment without much resistance, and to do what the external environment or authority figure expects her to do. Hence, one may observe an Indian woman wearing American attire and appearing to relate and function like any other American professional woman (Saran, 1985). It would be a great surprise to see this same woman become a docile daughter-in-law, wearing a traditional Indian costume and serving the elders and in-laws with whom she shares her home, yet this is what she must do. She is required to sense quickly what is expected of her under different situations, change her attitude and behave accordingly (Sethi & Allen, 1984). Roland (1989) writes that this capacity for adaptive behavior is the reflection of a profoundly internalized ego ideal that is strongly oriented toward obtaining approval from others. Approval from others enhances feelings of inner esteem, rather than one's individual achievements.

The concept of fixed gender roles has made it nearly impossible for many Indian women even to consider the freedom of thinking about let alone practicing a more egalitarian attitude. Clinicians working with Indian women will need to monitor their own responses to the client who assumes this posture. One must be careful not to lose patience and move the client too quickly past this view. The therapist who feels that women should be more active and assertive may impose this value on the client before she is ready to entertain the possibility. For many Indian women, even the idea may be new, and her family is not apt to be supportive of such a change. The therapist must follow the client, helping her to move at her own pace in exploring new perspectives and styles.

A constant alternating of behaviors to accommodate others is a major source of psychological strain among many professional Indian women, and in relationships between Indian women and men. After doing this accommodating dance in a bicultural environment for many years, the switching between two different and contradictory worlds may compel some Indian women to make a choice between the two (Mandelbaum, 1986; Ramu, 1988; Sethi & Allen, 1984). Psychotherapy can be helpful in assisting these women in integrating two apparently disparate worlds. For the healthy individual, this can be a step toward the process of self-actualization and, though delayed, perhaps true individuation. It can, however, precipitate marital discord, for which these women pay a great price. Divorces initiated by professional Indian women are becoming more common and many undergo major emotional problems after initiating such actions. In part this may be attributed to deep feelings of ambivalence about giving up their habitual attitudes. These women frequently harbor deeply embedded conflicts between meeting their own needs and focusing on the desires of others. The partners of women in these evolving states experience emotional upheaval as well.

As previously stated, many Indian men in America prefer Indian-born and raised women for brides (Brata, 1985; Kanekar & Kolsawalia, 1983; Luthra, 1989). The perception is that such a woman is less likely to reject traditional ways. Aside from providing purity and chastity, the traditional bride provides the security of someone who will adapt and make compromises in the family and will act in accordance with her husband's needs.

When an Indian woman is rapidly "Westernized," and thus expects some recognition for her own achievements, it can be both challenging and unacceptable to her husband. Because of their traditional expectations, the husbands of these women feel angry and threatened, giving rise to both emotional and sexual strain in both partners. The conflict and emotional strain within these marriages are often reflected in serious mental breakdowns of partners and, in some extreme cases, wife battering. (This occurs regardless of the socioeconomic levels of the families.) The husbands in these relationships may respond to changes in their wives by becoming much more controlling in the relationship, which may be explained as a reaction to their own feelings of insecurity and fears of loss of control as well as the imminent possibility of divorce and abandonment. Some men may respond by becoming emotionally withdrawn and distant. It is important for the therapist to remember that Indian women and men were often raised with very different assumptions about their roles than those reflected in Western cultures. Even among those persons who desire to change their attitudes and behaviors, they do so with great ambivalence and with the psychic pain that accompanies it.

The Americanization of Indian women may also involve their increased expectation of open demonstrations of physical love from their husbands, consistent with romanticized notions of relationships depicted in American films and popular television programs. Women who adopt these expectations are often frustrated and disappointed if their husbands are unwilling to give up deep-rooted traditional beliefs about husbands' and wives' behavior toward each other (Roland, 1989).

Many sophisticated and insightful Indian women have related to me that their husbands simply cannot tolerate much assertiveness on their part. I suspect that this must have multiple determinants. Among these is that of the husband's threatened superior position in the social hierarchy (Kanekar & Kolsawalia, 1983; Mandelbaum, 1986; Roland, 1989). Another is the husband's unconscious perception of his wife's assertiveness as a kind of covert power, like his mother's power. Put simply, the husband would begin to experience his wife as the powerful mother. It must be understood that many Indian women correctly presume that asserting themselves will profoundly disturb the equilibrium in the marital relationship, and they can expect no support from their families in these matters. Therefore, they often give in to many of their husband's demands, even when these involve making major career concessions. If such relationships are to survive these crises, therapists must be willing to work with both partners or to facilitate such work whenever possible.

The Indian woman in America must walk the tightrope of being neither too powerful to avoid being perceived as a threat to her husband, nor too weak to maintain her identity as a modern woman in a society where individualism is stressed.

SEXUALITY AND ATTITUDES TOWARD SEX

A formal review of the psychological literature in the area of sexual practices and attitudes of Indians or Indian Americans yields relatively little, and such an absence betrays the level at which this is a taboo topic. Despite the absence of formal discussion and investigation on the subject, it is clearly an area of concern to Indian men and women and shapes their relationships with one another.

Many Indian men, after immigrating to the United States, date and have sexual intimacies with American women but return to India to find a bride, whom they insist be a virgin. The hypocrisy is blatant. Moreover, despite the value of a traditional Indian bride, the Indian woman who can speak fluent English, dance in a Western style, and move about comfortably within Western social schemes will be more marketable as a prospective wife (Bumiller, 1990; Dasgupta, 1986). Many Indian husbands nevertheless complain bitterly about their "Westernized" wives and particularly about any friendships their wives may have with other males, even in the context of work.

One of the major areas of concern for Indian Americans raising children in the United States revolves around the subject of dating (Saran, 1985). In the 1990 meetings of the American Psychiatric Association, the subject of child rearing among Indian immigrants was debated. While most of the speakers were educated Indian professionals, they all expressed concern over the issue of dating among adolescents of Indian origin, with the assumption that dating certainly meant having premarital sex. Some parents send their teenage children back to India to continue their studies under the watchful eye of their grandparents, in order to avoid the "catastrophe" of premarital sex. Others are so anxious at the possible "spoiling" of their daughters before they can be safely married that they actually arrange for them to be married prior to their 15th birthdays ("Child Bride," 1991; Saran, 1985; Singh, 1990).

The lack of change in attitudes of immigrant Indian parents and their traditional expectations and values is a major source of strain among the Indian families residing in the United States. Parent–child relationships are a significant issue in Indian communities. As second and third generation children become more acculturated than their parents and grandparents, these issues will warrant serious attention from mental health professionals.

India is a country that maintains conservative attitudes about sex and dating, and one in which discussion of sexuality is virtually nonexistent (Liddle & Joshi, 1986; Mitter, 1991). Ironically, it is also the same country where the *Kama Sutra*, the encyclopedia of human sexuality, originated. The masses in India, in part due to illiteracy, are totally ignorant of their erotic tradition, while American culture is considered immoral by many Indians because of what is perceived to be its uninhibited and public expression of sexuality. I have encountered many women in treatment who had no idea how they were "supposed" to feel in a relationship or during sexual relations. They based their assumptions and in large measure their behavior around American movies, as if these films were an accurate and literal reflection of American life and relationships, rather than fictionalized and dramatized accounts.

As there is little information about sexuality in general among the immigrant population, there is even less information or discussion about unconventional or unacceptable aspects of sexuality or sexual behavior. There is some evidence, however, that incest was and is regarded a sin. Gregerson and Watts (1983, p. 219) quote ancient law in the matter of incest: "He who has sexual intercourse with sisters by the same mother, wife of a friend or of a son, with unmarried girl and with female of lower caste shall perform penance."

Homosexuality among men is considered "defiling," although there are known male transvestite prostitutes in the city of Bombay, some of whom are considered to be eunuchs. Pedophilia is against the law, but several cases have been cited in the newspapers. Female homosexuality is never mentioned in the literature I have reviewed except in Gregerson and Watts (1983). It is not generally discussed or overtly acknowledged within the culture. If one asked the average Indian about it, they would no doubt say that lesbianism does not exist among Indian women. Among those Indian women whom I and my Indian colleagues in psychiatry have treated, none have disclosed or suggested that they might be lesbian. This raises a number of questions concerning the failure to observe the phenomenon, since certainly as many forms of sexual behavior exist among Indians as exist among other human beings. The fact that Indian lesbians are rarely observed or openly acknowledged does not mean that they do not exist; rather, there may be a range of factors that mitigates against their disclosure among Indians.

One speculation is related to cultural transference between an Indian patient and Indian therapist. The culture's overt rejection of lesbian relationships might lead the client to assume that most other Indians will reject her, regardless of their level of education or profession. In this case, the Indian lesbian might be less likely to disclose herself to another Indian, even if she is her psychiatrist. The denial of such relationships also suggests the level at which they are deemed unacceptable among Indians. Another possibility is that lesbianism is not noticed as "different" or distinguishable in a culture where emotionally intimate relationships between women, married or unmarried, are common. Such closeness is acceptable and encouraged among Indian women. In fact, nonsexual physical contact between Indian men is encouraged as well, to a degree that is at variance with their American male counterparts. In contrast, Indian society discourages close heterosexual relationships and friendships between men and women. A detailed exploration of issues relevant to Indian lesbians is beyond the scope of this chapter, but a more detailed discussion concerning lesbians of color can be found in Chapter 14 of this volume.

In clinical practice, a major problem encountered in therapy with Indian women is the difficulty of raising, acknowledging, and discussing issues of sexuality of any sort. This is clearly connected to the tradition of treating such issues as subjects that are forbidden and that "good," "virtuous" women know nothing about (Moghaddam, Ditto, & Taylor, 1990). Addressing unconventional aspects of sexuality is an even more sensitive issue. The therapist must be tactful and patient in approaching such issues, to a greater degree than in therapy with women from the Western cultural mainstream. For many Indian women, to acknowledge an awareness of sexual matters is to be immoral or bad.

EDUCATION

In Western culture, education is valued as a tool in the achievement of enlightenment and career advancement. While Indians recognize the self-enhancing properties of education, their reasons for seeking it out are more pragmatic and traditional, and somewhat different for males and females. Education is seen only as the vehicle for earning better wages. The choice of educational path is determined by the family, with earning money as the particular goal in mind. Among college-educated, middle-class Indians, the standard is almost routinely to enter medicine, engineering, law, teaching, or, more recently, business (Saran, 1985).

Among women, teaching and medicine are routinely encouraged, regardless of the wishes, aptitude, or inclinations of the student. In medicine, certain specializations are viewed as more appropriate for women because they require minimum physical contact with the opposite sex (e.g., pediatrics, obstetrics, and gynecology). Entering psychiatry as a specialty was presumed to be inappropriate for a woman and even dangerous, although in major metropolitan cities this is changing to some extent (Ramu, 1989; Sethi & Allen, 1984).

It is common for Indian women to open their own businesses, most often beauty parlors, travel agencies, real estate agencies, clothing shops, factories, and interior design companies. Indian women in the United States are making various professional choices of their own, but in India the old ways of thinking still persist. The more commonly understood purpose of college education for an Indian woman was to increase her value on the marriage market. It is routinely accepted that the higher the Indian woman's level of education, the higher her ornamental value as a daughter-in-law in a family (Mitter, 1991; Ramu, 1988, 1989; Rao & Nandini, 1985). It must be noted that the operative relationship here is as a daughter-in-law, not a wife. An extremely high education in an average-looking girl can at times become a liability rather than an asset, because she then may be more advanced educationally than her would-be husband. A girl who is uneducated, reasonably attractive but wealthy is considered a more acceptable bride. In Indian families, funds are set aside for a son's education and a daughter's dowry regardless of the desires or intellectual capacity of individual children (Paul, 1986). Despite this practice it is not uncommon for modern Indian women to have college degrees. As more of these women are attaining such status and interacting with more people outside of Indian culture, they suffer from various emotional conflicts.

One of the effects of interacting in Western educational institutions for Indian women is that they develop a sense of their own capabilities and power. They also learn more about freedom of thought. Since most of these institutions are coeducational, particularly at the graduate and postgraduate levels, sexual attractions are likely to be aroused through increased daily contact with the opposite sex. Despite this, major cultural limits are set by the family on intimacy and relationships. For an Indian woman, merely being seen with a male in public may be perceived by other Indians as immoral behavior.

A newly married young woman was reprimanded severely by her father-in-law. The young woman in question returned home after 11 p.m., riding behind her brother on a motorcycle. According to her father-in-law, she was seen in public with a man whom no one would know was her brother. As such, he assumed that the young woman would be seen as morally loose and perhaps promiscuous.

Education is not always the path to liberation for Indian women, as can be seen in another case.

An older sister was expected to continue her education and work chiefly to support her younger siblings. This was particularly for the purpose of helping younger brothers obtain the funds needed to be educated. It was the family's expectation that she make the ultimate sacrifice of remaining single and a virgin. While her education enabled, freed, and caused her to think more independently, she was still not free to live independently. In this case her education only increased the burden of her family's dependence on her. Her education was permissible in that it assisted the family in reaching traditional goals, those of educating and preparing the sons of the family.

COPING STRATEGIES AND ATTITUDES TOWARD MENTAL HEALTH

Indian women are reluctant to seek professional help for stress or psychological problems. In their view, time will solve their problems and psychotherapy is thus unnecessary or unsuitable. Because help is not sought until the problem is viewed as impossible to control, major depressions and suicide attempts are not uncommon consequences. Another factor that mitigates against seeking help is the distrust of American therapists. The basis for many therapies in which an individual is treated as an individual does not fit the Indian view of themselves in relation to family and loved ones. When help is sought, there may be the expectation that the therapist will serve as benefactor and guru and give specific advice, rather than helping the individual understand her role in the present problem.

Seeking out an Indian therapist creates other problems. The Indian community is small in size and contains a large number of people in a well-defined geographical area. The families of clients may worry about maintaining their anonymity and privacy, especially since a strong stigma is still attached to the presence of mental illness in a family. This is reflected in the common inquiry made during the process of arranging marriages about the presence or absence of mental illness in the immediate and extended families of the prospective bride and bridegroom. This also reflects the view that mental illness is familial or inherited by definition.

Given the range of cultural paradoxes confronting Indian women, we must now ask how she copes with these conflicts and continues to function. Denial is a common defensive operation. Clinically, one observes a woman who behaves as if her own needs do not matter, as if she is as fluid and colorless as water, flowing into and remaining in the container into which she is placed. If she has some level of self-awareness, her conflict may be conscious and observable to the therapist. She may even rebel. When married women successfully rebel against the wishes of their spouses, the spouse may be perceived as weak by other Indians, even though he may in fact be enlightened. In either case, the woman may be seen as a capable, successful woman by her professional peers, while simultaneously deemed a "shrew" by her husband and perhaps both their families.

When denial is no longer successful, these women may initially experience physical and psychosomatic illnesses, for which they may present to a medical doctor rather than a psychotherapist. These complaints may range from skin allergies, rashes, headaches, and ulcers to hysterical seizures. Hysterical conversions are not uncommon but appear to occur in Indian women with less frequency in the United States than in India, where they are prevalent. This may be partially explained by the fact that physical symptoms are more readily acceptable than emotional or mental symptoms in India. In the United States it is more permissible to discuss one's feelings. In India, the treatment for these complaints are invariably modern psychotropic drugs, electroshock therapy or spiritual rituals, depending on the beliefs of the family. It is not uncommon to use a combination of these modalities. Indian women also frequently express a general lack of awareness or insight into these maladies. It is quite natural for Indian women and their families to blame some external factor, including supernatural forces, for these illnesses, rather than delving into possible emotional factors.

Western concepts of psychotherapy, which stress looking within or taking personal responsibility for one's own life experiences, are alien concepts that may appear to contradict the principles of karma and dharma. It is likely that many Indian women would accept medicines, prayers, or rituals, or even severe punishments under the guise of treatment before seeking any insight-oriented psychotherapy. In some cases behavior modification is more acceptable than psychodynamic forms of psychotherapy.

The majority of these difficulties are naturally extended among the Indian American immigrant woman at many levels. It is not at all unusual for a bright, articulate, and "Westernized" woman to request advice and/ or medicine from a therapist for the purpose of making her "feel better" or to make her husband and in-laws "like" her. The woman would feel more comfortable taking advice or medicine than she would considering what may be causing her symptoms—perhaps certain actions or feelings toward the family members and the conflicts between them. It is also not uncommon to seek some symbols or religious objects in order to keep the "evil eye" or the presumed external source of the problem away. Just as conflicts over expressions of power and anger are denied, so is an awareness and expression of sexuality. Thus, Indian women often display behavior noted by Westerners as histrionic, hysterical, or naive. It must be noted that Indian movies are filled with grotesque and blatant sexuality and are a regular staple of the entertainment diet for a growing Indian girl. Yet such overt behavior in real life is considered unacceptable and immoral. This leaves the Indian woman with few options for directly expressing certain feelings. Hence what is perceived as coquettish flirting or even teasing may represent an indirect way of expressing sexuality. If asked about it or confronted, the Indian woman must not only deny it to the observer but to herself as well. She may protest vehemently and feel insulted. Indian culture mandates that women appear sexually naive, to the point of seeming childlike. Such behavior might be better understood as normative within the culture. We must explore the cases of individual patients to see how much of this behavior, on the one hand, is consciously designed to satisfy external expectations without a concomitant internalization of the cultural mandate. On the other hand, the situation may truly be a hysterical phenomenon caused by an unconscious denial of the sexual knowledge so prescribed for Indian women. A woman having such knowledge is very often considered "Westernized," which is equated with being "morally loose." The answer lies in the careful evaluation of each client and her own individual dilemma within her cultural framework.

It is important for psychotherapists who work with Indian women to make careful distinctions between the appearance of being integrated into American culture versus the reality of it. What many Indian women internalize as "American" is a popularized "Hollywood" portrayal of American life and not a realistic one. Whether we observe her moving through American life as a "hip" teenager, or as a well-educated professional woman, we cannot presume that this gives us a true picture of how she views herself or how she is viewed and functions within her family relationships.

Another factor we must appreciate in communicating with Indian women is that despite the high level of English fluency in many individuals, English is usually not their first language. There may be a subjective process of translation occurring that is invisible to the Western eye. Clinically, it is worthwhile to determine if the client dreams in her native language or in English. There is clinical evidence that suggests that translation may be less of an issue when the client's dreams are in English. This language difference may explain difficulties in communicating subtleties, particularly jokes, riddles, or colloquialisms that are heavily language and culture based.

SUMMARY

Indian American women face the task of adjusting from a slowly changing, passive Indian culture to a rapidly changing, assertive American culture. The latter is at a different and more active stage of transition regarding women's roles and rights and sexual matters. An entry into this new culture requires that these women leap very rapidly into a new position, skipping the steps in between, which American women have had the opportunity to go through and process.

Conflicts arise and are unavoidable in any group in transition. The mother society in India, however, is proud of its accomplishments and is eager to display a successful picture. As such, it tends to deny signs of distress and malfunction within the group. Indian women's psychological problems are therefore often unrecognized or denied or may remain untreated even if they are acknowledged. In situations where individual support systems, families and husbands, are sensitive to the stresses of assimilation in themselves, the Indian woman may be more easily encouraged to move toward a more satisfying adjustment. While there are many instances of such enlightened individuals, there are just as many for whom these issues remain denied, forbidden and a matter of shame. This chapter has focused on the plight of these latter women and their families.

REFERENCES

Altekar, A. S. (1983). *The position of women in Hindu civilization: From prehistoric times to the present day.* Delhi: Motilal Banarsidass.

Asian Women United of California (Eds.). (1989). *Making waves: An anthology of writings by and about Asian American women.* Boston: Beacon Press.

Bachu, A. (1985). *Socioeconomic, demographic, and linguistic characteristics of Asian Indian migrants in the United States.* Washington, DC: U.S. Bureau of Census.

Brata, S. (1985). *India labyrinths in the lotus land.* New York: William Morrow.

Bumiller, E. (1990). *May you be the mother of a hundred sons: A journey among the women of India.* New York: Fawcett Columbine.

Child bride for sale. (1991, October 27). *New York Times,* p. E7.

Dasgupta, S. D. (1986). Marching to a different drummer? Sex roles of Asian Indian women in the United States. *Women and Therapy,* 5(2–3), 297–311.

Dhruvarajan, V. (1990). Religious ideology, Hindu women, and development in India. *Journal of Social Issues, 46,* 57–69.

Discarding daughters. (1990, Fall). *Time, 36*(19).

Erikson, E. (1946). *Ego development and historical change in identity and the life cycle.* New York: International Universities Press.

Everett, J. (1981). Approaches to the "woman question" in India: From maternalism to mobilization. *Women's Studies International Quarterly, 4,* 169–178.

Freed, R.S., & Freed, S.A. (1989). Beliefs and practices resulting in female deaths and fewer females than males in India. *Population and Environment: A Journal of Interdisciplinary Studies, 10*(3), 144–161.

Gregerson, E., & Watts, F. (Eds.). (1983). *Sexual practices: The story of human sexuality.* New York: Franklin Watts.

Gupta, U. (1991, June–July). Out of India. *New York Woman,* pp. 46–47.

India: Till death do us part. (1990, Fall). *Time, 36*(19), p. 39.

Kakar, S. (1978). *The innerworld: A psychoanalytic study of childhood and society in India.* Delhi: Oxford University Press.

Kanekar, S., & Kolsawalia, M.B. (1983). Sex and respectability: The double standard, Indian style. *Personality Study and Group Behavior, 3*(1), 12–15.

Kristof, N. D. (1991, November 5). Stark data on women: 100 million are missing. *New York Times,* pp. C1, C12.

Liddle, J., & Joshi, R. (1986). *Daughters of independence: Gender, caste and class in India.* London: Zed.

Luthra, R. (1989). Matchmaking in the classifieds of the immigrant Indian Press. In Asian Women United of California (Eds.), *Making waves: An anthology of writings by and about Asian American women* (p. 344). Boston: Beacon Press.

Mandelbaum, D. G. (1986). *Women's seclusion and men's honor: Sex roles in North India, Bangladesh and Pakistan.* Tucson: University of Arizona Press.

Mitter, S. S. (1991). *Dharma's daughters.* New Brunswick, NJ: Rutgers University Press.

Moghaddam, F. M., Ditto, B., & Taylor, D. M. (1990). Attitudes and attributions related to psychological symptomatology in Indian immigrant women. *Journal of Cross Cultural Psychology, 21*(3), 335–350.

Paul, M. C. (1986). *Dowry and position of women in India.* New Delhi: Inter-India Publications.

Ramu, G. N. (1988). Marital roles and power: Perceptions and reality in the urban setting. *Journal of Comparative Family Studies, 19*(2), 207–227.

Ramu, G. N. (1989). *Women, work and marriage in urban India.* New Delhi: Sage.

Rao, V. V. P, & Nandini, V. (1985). *Marriage, the family and women in India.* New Delhi: Heritage Publishers.

Roland, A. (1989). *In search of self in India and Japan.* Princeton, NJ: Princeton University Press.

Saran, P. (1985). *The Asian Indian experience in the United States.* Cambridge, MA: Schenkman.

Sethi, R. R., & Allen, M. J. (1984). Sex-role stereotypes in northern India and the United States. *Sex Roles, 11*(7–8), 615–626.

Singh, A. (1990, November). The plight of the girl child in India. *India Today,* pp. 2–3.

Tan, A. (1989). *The joy luck club.* New York: Ballantine Books.

Vaidyanathan, T. G. (1989, Fall). Authority and identity in India. *Daedalus: Journal of the American Academy of Arts and Sciences, 118*(4).

II

THEORETICAL AND APPLIED FRAMEWORKS

Overview: Gender and Ethnicity in the Healing Process

Lillian Comas-Díaz
Beverly Greene

WOMEN OF COLOR AND MENTAL HEALTH SERVICES

The history of the delivery of mental health services to women of color has been closely tied to the history of mental health services to people of color in general. The sociopolitical context of the Civil Rights movement provided the impetus for an examination of how appropriately mental health services meet the needs of people of color. The women's liberation movement and the advent of feminism offered a niche where issues of gender, race, and ethnicity could be examined within the clinical arena (Comas-Díaz, 1991).

The effectiveness of traditional mental health services with women and men of color has been questioned (Sue, 1988). This inquiry was based on the predominance of cultural, racial, and gender bias in mental health treatment (Brown, 1990; Katz & Taylor, 1988; Trimble, 1990). As an illustration, it has been argued that North American mental health treatment reflects a White male European orientation (Katz & Taylor, 1988) as well as a middle-class orientation (Pinderhughes, 1989). The emphasis on individualism, rational and scientific thinking, free expression of thought, tolerance of dissent (Kinzie, 1978), and internal locus of control have socially constructed the dominant paradigms of psychotherapeutic theory and practice. Some people of color with a non–middle-class orientation may prefer psychotherapeutic approaches that are directive, offer advice, work with systems and significant others toward increasing interdependence (Pinderhughes, 1989), and which are contextual, holistic, and acknowledge modes of behaving according to an external locus of control (Comas-Díaz, 1992).

The initial stage of development in the assessment of mental health services for people of color involved attempts to strengthen the weaknesses of traditional services in treating women and men of color (President's Commission on Mental Health, 1978). The culturalism movement in mental health was an example of this type of solution. Culturalism involves the emphasis of culture-specific themes and techniques in mental health treatment (De La Cancela & Zavala, 1983). For instance, it includes the use of folk healing for culture-bound syndromes such as *susto* or *espanto* (sudden fright), evil eye, *ataque*, *koro*, and *amok* (Kiev, 1972; Simons & Hughes, 1993). The historical exclusion of many people of color from the health care system resulted in their dependence on indigenous healers (Baker, 1988). Therefore, culturalism involves the utilization of community and indigenous resources such as paraprofessionals, clergy, teachers, and the network of individuals (known as the *servidor* system) residing in and/or delivering services to ethnic minority communities (Escobar & Randolph, 1982). A significant number of these people are women of color, and this indicates their central positions within their communities.

According to Comas-Díaz (1992), the delivery of psychotherapeutic services to women and men of color has evolved historically through different developmental stages. The current stage is a revisionist, moving from the question of effectiveness of treatment to examining the process variables of race, culture, and ethnicity. Although the influence of culture, ethnicity, and race on the psychotherapeutic process with people of color has been historically acknowledged (Devereux, 1953; Ticho, 1971), these variables are receiving more attention and are emerging as key factors in mental health treatment (Comas-Díaz & Griffith, 1988; DeAngelis, 1990; Dudley & Rawlins, 1985; Harris, 1990; McGoldrick, Pearce, & Giordano, 1982). Similarly, gender issues have been identified as crucial factors in mental health treatment (Brody & Hare-Mustin, 1980; Jordan, Kaplan, Miller, Stiver, & Surrey, 1991; Walters, Carter, Papp, & Silverstein, 1988).

WOMEN OF COLOR: GENDER AND ETHNICITY

The relevance of the interaction of ethnicity and gender as a variable in mental health treatment with women of color has also been acknowledged (Brown & Root, 1990; McGoldrick, García-Preto, Hines, & Lee, 1989). The significance of gender is culturally determined and its articulation is ongoing (Lott, 1991). Therefore, the gender–race interaction in women of color needs to be examined through its dynamic and evolving cultural lens. Similarly, the lives of women of color need to be examined from a racial minority and feminist perspective, one that recognizes that both racism and sexism exist and are extremely oppressive of women of color. For example, Gould (1985) argues that racism and sexism interact to produce gender-specific race effects and race-specific gender effects, which need to be stressed apart from the separate effects of racism and sexism in the lives of women of color.

The relevance of gender often tends to subordinate the importance of race for women of color. As an illustration, Brody (1987) has indicated that racial homogeneity for client and therapist is less important than the bonding thread of interpersonal trust in the same-gender dyad, where a climate of equality is cultivated. Consequently, this assertion seems to reinforce the subordination of race for gender in the mental health literature, neglecting the combined effect of the gender and race/ethnicity in the lives of women of color (Greene, 1994). This assertion may also be indicative of the covert ethnocentrism found among some White feminist therapists who discount the centrality that race and ethnicity have in the lives of women of color. Moreover, research has suggested that race and gender of both client and therapist significantly influence diagnosis (Loring & Powell, 1988).

The realities of women of color reflect the confluence of gender, race, ethnicity, class, biology, sexual orientation, physical ability, religion/spirituality, as well as contextual variables such as historical and sociopolitical factors. Once clinicians understand that these variables are simultaneous and intersecting systems of relationship and meaning, they can also understand the different ways that other categories of experience intersect in women's lives (Andersen & Collins, 1991). Clinical realities are negotiated by clinicians and clients not merely in terms of theoretical models but also in subjective contexts (Comas-Díaz & Jacobsen, 1991). Multilayered gender-, race-, and ethnoculture-based perceptions tend to influence both the process and outcome of clinical work. More specifically, a failure to recognize the combined influence and impact of racial and gender parameters can seriously compromise the effectiveness of mental health treatment.

The future of mental health treatment with women and men of color will involve an integrative and comprehensive framework addressing the multiple contextual parameters inherent in the reality of being a minority individual (Comas-Díaz, 1992; Greene, 1994).

TRADITIONAL MENTAL HEALTH SERVICES: REVISION AND REFORMULATION

Women of color present a challenge to traditionally trained mental health professionals. Due to the combined effects of gender and ethnicity, they often are in double jeopardy with respect to their mental health status (Olmedo & Parron, 1981). Moreover, not only has ethnicity and gender interaction frequently been neglected in the mental health assessment and treatment, but there has also been a dearth of information about the epidemiology of mental disorders in women of color. Part of this problem is due to a lack of data collected about the combined effects of ethnicity and gender, as women of color are included either under their ethnic minority group or under the general category of women (Olmedo & Parron, 1981). Notwithstanding their marginality, women of color often seek and receive mental health services more than their male counterparts, although it is unclear how effective these services are. The interaction of race, gender, class, ethnicity, culture, and sexual orientation provides a blueprint for effective mental health treatment of women of color. However, the challenge to clinicians who follow traditional treatment is to intervene in ways that respect race, gender, ethnicity, and sexuality, and at the same time to challenge inequities in the realities of women of color.

The authors in this section of the book, "Theoretical and Applied Frameworks," accept this challenge and explore the integration of an orientation informed by ethnoculture, race, and gender into different therapeutic approaches. It presents diverse therapeutic perspectives and critically examines their relevance to the experiences of women of color. These perspectives include psychodynamic, cognitive–behavioral, feminist, family systems, and integrative approaches.

The chapters in this section postulate that traditional psychotherapeutic orientations need to be expanded and integrated into the realities of women of color in order to be effective. Jean Lau Chin's chapter advocates a psychodynamic understanding of what women of color experience during the healing process (Chapter 7), while Sandra Lewis' chapter asserts the efficacy of cognitive–behavioral approaches when they are tailored to women's special needs (Chapter 8). The relevance of the family and collective context is acknowledged by Nancy Boyd-Franklin and Nydia García-Preto in their chapter on family therapy orientations (Chapter 9); while in Chapter 10 Oliva M. Espín discusses the applicability of feminist approaches to empowering women of color. Comas-Díaz presents an integrative approach specifically developed for women of color in Chapter 11. And finally, given the potential for misdiagnosis and mistreatment using psychotropic medications, we have included a chapter on psychopharmacological treatment with women of color authored by Frederick M. Jacobsen (Chapter 12).

There are other therapeutic approaches that are not presented in this volume because of an unavailability of authors and other realistic limitations. Unfortunately, we have not been able to include a chapter on substance abuse treatment and rehabilitation. Substance abuse is an alarming problem in many communities of people of color and may be considered a coping strategy for escaping an oppressive situation (Spiegel, Tate, Aiken, & Christian, 1985). We believe that in order to be effective the practitioner working with women of color needs to be familiar with alcohol and substance abuse prevention and treatment. Given this context, here is a brief overview of these issues.

SUBSTANCE ABUSE TREATMENT

People of color do not abuse substances more than other groups (National Institute on Drug Abuse, 1992), but substance abuse is often associated with violence, AIDS, physical illness, and many other epidemiological and health problems that affect their lives. Substance abuse can affect women of color regardless of their socioeconomic class. For women with low incomes, street drugs, through their availability, become the drugs of choice, while addiction for middle-class women of color often involves prescription medication. Frederick M. Jacobsen discusses the problem of drug prescription for women of color (Chapter 12).

Because alcohol is legal, alcohol abuse is a serious problem for women of color as it is for the vast of the population. It is important, though, to recognize the differences in alcohol abuse not only between men and women but also among women of different racial and ethnic groups (National Institute on Alcohol Abuse and Alcoholism, 1990). African American women are more likely to abstain entirely from alcohol (46%) than White women (34%) (Herd, 1988). However, an equal proportion of African American and White women drink heavily (Wilsnack, Wilsnack, & Klassen, 1984). But while African American women report fewer alcohol-related personal and social problems than do White women, a greater proportion of African American women experience alcohol-related health problems (Herd, 1989).

Self-reports by Latinas indicate that they are infrequent drinkers or abstainers (Caetano, 1989). However, this may change as Latinas enter new social and work arenas. For example, Gilbert (1987) found that reports of abstention are greater among immigrant Hispanic women, while reports of moderate or heavy drinking are greater among younger, American-born Hispanic women. Among American Indian women, alcoholism may be considered an epidemic health problem (LaFromboise and colleagues, Chapter 2, this volume).

Some women of color have been revealed to be at high risk, given the current awareness of fetal alcohol syndrome (FAS). According to a Centers for Disease Control catchment area study, the incidence of FAS per 10,000 total births was Asians 0.3, Hispanics/Latinos 0.8, Whites 0.9, Blacks 6.0, and American Indians 20.9 (Chavez, Cordero, & Becerra, 1989). Although the incidence of FAS varies among the different groups of American Indians (May, Hymbaugh, Aase, & Samet, 1983), recent estimates suggest that 40% of American Indian women meet the criteria for alcohol dependency (LaDue & O'Hara, 1992). Among African Americans the risk of FAS remains significantly higher in comparison with Whites, even after the frequency of maternal alcohol intake, occurrence of chronic alcohol problems, and number of children borne have been adjusted (Sokol et al., 1986). The question of some kind of genetic susceptibility among some people of color has been raised (National Institute on Alcohol Abuse and Alcoholism, 1991), and the incidence of FAS does appear to have profound implications for American Indian and African American women. Unfortunately, it is beyond the scope of this overview to discuss so complex an issue in detail.

It is crucial to have a culturally relevant and gender-informed treatment for women of color who are substance abusers. An example of such an approach is the "future past" technique developed by Comas-Díaz (1986) for the group treatment of alcoholic Latinas. In this technique, older women demonstrate to younger women the effects of alcoholism and substance abuse by clarifying through their own history, the potential future of the younger women if they continue drinking—thus, the *future past*. Whether women of color are substance abusers or not, the likelihood that a significant other has this problem may be relatively high. Consequently, the clinician's knowledge of substance use and abuse could be very helpful in working with women who interact with substance abusers and/or reside in communities that confront this problem. Also, the face of AIDS is darkening and becoming increasingly female (Amaro, 1988; Mays & Cochran, 1988); thus, practitioners need to understand the effects and treatment of this epidemic among women of color.

Many women of color benefit from self-help groups and 12-step programs such as Alcoholics Anonymous (AA) and Narcotics Anonymous (NA). The values of many of these 12-step programs seem congruent with the experiences of many women of color. For instance, the centrality of the group parallels the collective orientation prevalent among women of color. Making amends to others tends to reinforce the interconnection between women of color and their families and communities. The emphasis on the *here and now* is also congruent with the life experiences of many low-income women of color. Lastly, the belief in a higher power is compatible with the belief in spirituality prevalent among many women of color (see Chapter 11 by Comas-Díaz, Chapter 2 by LaFromboise & colleagues, and Chapter 8 by Lewis).

The 12-step programs can serve as auxiliary treatment, but in order for them to be relevant, they must be implemented with consideration to the special racial and gender needs of women of color. For instance, some women of color feel alienated in heterogeneous racial groups in which their unique realities may be ignored. Their personal reality is plagued by the power of institutionalized racism in their lives. Many low-income women of color are suspicious of public institutions and social services as well as health professionals, because of their historical roles in the oppression and coercion of people of color. Finally, interventions for risk-taking behaviors need to be included in substance abuse treatment.

WEAVING A HEALING TAPESTRY

The contributors in this section examine critically the tenets of major therapeutic orientations and integrate these into gender, racial, and ethnocultural contexts in mental health treatment. In order to facilitate the examination of the diverse theoretical models' applicability, the contributors cover similar areas in all of the presented therapeutic orientations: the principles of each theoretical orientation, their relevance to culture and gender, their specific applicability to women of color, in addition to some of their limitations for woking with these populations. Furthermore, the contributors provide practical guidelines for the use of each therapeutic orientation, aided by clinical illustrations.

REFERENCES

Amaro, H. (1988). Considerations for the prevention of HIV infection among Hispanic women. *Psychology of Women Quarterly, 12,* 429–443.

Andersen, M. L., & Collins, P. H. (Eds.). (1991). *Race, class and gender: An anthology.* Belmont, CA: Wadsworth.

Baker, F. M. (1988). Afro-Americans. In L. Comas-Díaz & E. H. H. Griffith (Eds.), *Clinical guidelines in cross-cultural mental health* (pp. 151–181). New York: Wiley.

Brody, A. M., & Hare-Mustin, R. T. (Eds.). (1980). *Women and psychotherapy.* New York: Guilford Press.

Brody, C. M. (1987). White therapist and female minority clients: Gender and culture issues. *Psychotherapy, 22,* 108–113.

Brown, L. S. (1990). The meaning of a multicultural perspective for theory-building in feminist therapy. In L. S. Brown & M. P. P. Root (Eds.), *Diversity and complexity in feminist therapy* (pp. 1–21). Binghamton, NY: Haworth Press.

Brown, L., & Root, M. P. P. (Eds.). (1990). *Diversity and complexity in feminist therapy.* Binghamton, NY: Haworth Press.

Caetano, R. (1989). Drinking patterns and alcohol problems in a national survey of U.S. Hispanics. In D. Spiegel, D. Tate, S. Aiken, & C. Christian (Eds.), *Alcohol use among U.S. minorities* (Research Monograph No. 18). Rockville, MD: National Institute on Alcohol Abuse and Alcoholism.

Chavez, G. F., Cordero, J. F., & Becerra, J. E. (1989). Leading major congenital malformations among minority groups in the United States, 1981–1986. *Journal of the American Medical Association, 261,* 205–209.

Comas-Díaz, L. (1986). Puerto Rican alcoholic women: Treatment considerations. *Alcoholism Treatment Quarterly, 3,* 47–57.

Comas-Díaz, L. (1991). Feminism and diversity in psychology: The case of women of color. *Psychology of Women Quarterly, 15,* 597–609.

Comas-Díaz, L. (1992). The future of psychotherapy with ethnic minorities. *Psychotherapy, 29,* 88–94.

Comas-Díaz, L., & Griffith, E. E. H. (Eds.). (1988). *Clinical guidelines in cross-cultural mental health.* New York: Wiley.

Comas-Díaz, L., & Jacobsen, F. M. (1987). Ethnocultural identification in psychotherapy. *Psychiatry, 50*(3), 232–241.

DeAngelis, T. (1990, November). Race issue can hurt, help therapy conflicts. *American Psychological Association Monitor,* pp. 24–25.

De La Cancela, V., & Zavala, I. (1983). An analysis of culturalism in Latino mental health: Folk medicine as a case in point. *Hispanic Journal of Behavioral Sciences, 5,* 251–274.

Devereux, G. (1953). Cultural factors in psychoanalytic therapy. *Journal of the American Psychoanalytic Association, 1,* 629–655.

Dudley, G. R., & Rawlins, M. R. (Eds.). (1985). Psychotherapy with ethnic minorities [Special issue]. *Psychotherapy, 22.*

Escobar, J., & Randolph, E. (1982). The Hispanic and social networks. In R. Becerra, M. Karno, & J. Escobar (Eds.), *Mental health and Hispanic Americans* (pp. 41–51). New York: Grune & Stratton.

Gilbert, J. (1987). Alcohol consumption patterns in immigrant and later generation Mexican American women. *Hispanic Journal of Behavioral Sciences, 9,* 299–313.

Gould, K. H. (1985). A minority-feminist perspective on child welfare issues. *Child Welfare, 64,* 291–305.

Greene, B. (1994). Diversity and difference: The issue of race in feminist therapy. In M. P. Mirkin (Ed.), *Women in context: Toward a feminist reconstruction of psychotherapy* (pp. 333–351). New York: Guilford Press.

Harris, L. S. (1990, November). Race and transference issues in the therapeutic relationship. *Psychiatric Times: Medicine and Behavior, 7*(11), 54–55.

Herd, D. (1988). Drinking by black and white women: Results from a national survey. *Social Problems, 35,* 493–505.

Herd, D. (1989). The epidemiology of drinking patterns and alcohol-related problems among U.S. Blacks. In D. Spiegler, D. Tate, S. Aiken, & C. Christian (Eds.), *Alcohol use among U.S. minorities* (Research Monograph No. 18). Washington, DC: National Institute on Alcohol Abuse and Alcoholism.

Jordan, J. V., Kaplan, A., Miller, J. B., Stiver, I., & Surrey, J. L. (1991). *Women's growth in connection: Writings from the Stone Center.* New York: Guilford Press.

Katz, P. A., & Taylor, D. A. (Eds.). (1988). *Eliminating racism.* New York: Plenum.

Kiev, A. (1972). *Transcultural psychiatry.* New York: Free Press.

Kinzie, J. D. (1978). Lessons from cross-cultural psychotherapy. *American Journal of Psychotherapy, 32,* 510–520.

LaDue, R. A., & O'Hara, B. A. (1992, July). Documentation of critical issues related to the comprehensive Indian Fetal Alcohol Syndrome (FAS) prevention and treatment act. *Focus, 6,* 8–9.

Loring, M., & Powell, B. (1988). Gender, race and DSM-III: A study of the objectivity of psychiatric diagnostic behavior. *Journal of Health and Social Behavior, 29,* 1–22.

Lott, B. (1991). Social psychology: Humanistic roots and feminist future. *Psychology of Women Quarterly, 15,* 505–519.

May, P. A., Hymbaugh, K. J., Aase, J. M., & Samet, J. M. (1983). Epidemiology of fetal alcohol syndrome among American Indians of the Southwest. *Social Biology, 30*(4), 374–387.

Mays, V. M., & Cochran, S. D. (1988). Issues in the perception of AIDS risk and risk reduction activities by Black and Hispanic/Latino women. *American Psychologist, 43,* 949–957.

McGoldrick, M., García-Preto, N., Hines, P. M., & Lee, E. (1989). Ethnicity and women. In M. McGoldrick, C. M. Anderson, & F. Walsh (Eds.), *Women in families: A framework for family therapy* (pp. 169–199). New York: W. W. Norton.

McGoldrick, M., Pearce, J. K., & Giordano, J. (Eds.). (1982). *Ethnicity and family therapy.* New York: Guilford Press.

National Institute on Alcohol Abuse and Alcoholism. (1990, October). Alcohol and women. *Alcohol Alert, 10,* 1–4.

National Institute on Alcohol Abuse and Alcoholism. (1991, July). Fetal alcohol syndrome. *Alcohol Alert, 13,* 1–4.

National Institute on Drug Abuse. (1992). *National household survey on drug abuse population estimates 1991.* Rockville, MD: Author.

Olmedo, E. L., & Parron, D. L. (1981). Mental health of minority women: Special issue. *Professional Psychology, 12,* 103–111.

Pinderhughes, E. (1989). *Understanding race, ethnicity, and power: The key to efficacy in clinical practice.* New York: Free Press.

President's Commission on Mental Health. (1978). *Report of the Special Populations Subpanel on Women* (Task Force Reports, Vol. III). Washington, DC: U.S. Government Printing Office.

Reid, P. T., & Comas-Díaz, L. (1990). Gender and ethnicity: perspectives on dual status. *Sex Roles, 22,* 397–408.

Simons, R. C., & Hughes, C. C. (1993). Culture-bound syndromes. In A. Gaw (Ed.), *Culture, ethnicity and mental illness* (pp. 75–99). Washington, DC: American Psychiatric Press.

Sokol, R. J., Ager, J., Martier, S., Debanne, S., Ernhart, C., Kuzma, J., & Miller, S. I. (1986). Significant determinants of susceptibility to alcohol teratogenicity. *Annals of the New York Academy of Sciences, 477,* 87–102.

Spiegel, D., Tate, D., Aiken, S., & Christian, C. (Eds.). (1985). *Alcohol use among U.S. minorities* (Research Monograph No. 18). Rockville, MD: National Institute on Alcohol Abuse and Alcoholism.

Sue, S. (1988). Psychotherapeutic services for ethnic minorities: Two decades of research findings. *American Psychologist, 43,* 301–308.

Ticho, G. (1971). Cultural aspects of transference and countertransference. *Bulletin of the Menninger Clinic, 35,* 313–334.

Trimble, J. E. (1990). Prefatory notes on the enculturation of American psychology. *Focus, 4,* 1.

Walters, M., Carter, B., Papp, P., & Silvertstein, O. (1988). *The invisible web: Gender patterns in family relationships.* New York: Guilford Press.

Wilsnack, R. W., Wilsnack, S. C., & Klassen, A. D. (1984). Women's drinking and drinking problems: Patterns from a 1981 national survey. *American Journal of Public Health, 74,* 1231–1238.

7

Psychodynamic Approaches

Jean Lau Chin

When using a psychodynamic approach in psychotherapy with women of color, we need to understand how culture and gender influence the nature of psychotherapy. Cultural values and gender roles will influence what clients talk about in psychotherapy (i.e., therapeutic content). Expectations based on the sociocultural context will influence what will facilitate therapeutic change (i.e., the therapeutic method). Before work in psychotherapy occurs, however, therapists must first engage clients in a therapeutic relationship. This relationship is inherently an interpersonal process influenced by cultural values and gender-role expectations.

It is commonly known that psychodynamic psychotherapy began during the Victorian era at a time when the male perspective was especially controlling of women's lives, and in a culture that was Western and predominantly White. When a psychodynamic approach is used with women of color in the United States today, different cultural perspectives and experiences must be taken into consideration. This can occur in two ways: (1) by reconceptualizing psychodynamic psychotherapy (i.e., changing the theory to fit the population) and (2) by refining psychodynamic psychotherapy to include manifestations of culture and gender differences (i.e., adding to the theory). Both approaches are necessary to account for culture and gender differences in psychodynamic psychotherapy.

OVERVIEW OF PSYCHODYNAMIC PSYCHOTHERAPY

To change or refine the theory, we must first define what is the essence of psychodynamic psychotherapy. Given the vast psychodynamic literature, this overview will be limited to concepts that have a particular relevance for women of color. It will not address all the changes in theory and practice that have occurred since it was first conceptualized by Freud, nor will it address the disagreement among proponents about many of the earlier concepts.

Psychodynamic Content

Drive theory has been a cornerstone in understanding human development using a psychodynamic approach (Ford & Urban, 1963). Sexual and aggressive drives or instincts are viewed as present from birth and unfold as a person matures. These drives are viewed as universal and as motivating factors of human experience. Most behavior is aimed at tension or drive reduction, to bring the self into equilibrium. Intrapsychic conflicts, as viewed from a psychodynamic approach, are brought about by developmental crises or traumatic experiences. In seeking equilibrium, traumatic events are repressed and defenses are formed to resist anxiety arousing content. Conflict-laden material, therefore, tends to remain unconscious.

The purpose of psychotherapy is to bring conflict-laden material to consciousness so it can be resolved. In attempting to resolve these conflicts, psychodynamic psychotherapy emphasizes the understanding of historical events associated with conflict, developmental stages and its influence on conflict resolution, and underlying psychodynamics that give meaning to current behavior. Consequently, symbols, metaphors, and dreams in psychotherapy become important clues to the dynamic meaning and unresolved conflicts of a client.

Unresolved oedipal conflicts form the basis for neurotic conflict, and has been central to a psychodynamic approach. The oedipal complex, based on the Greek myth in which Oedipus kills his father and marries his mother, is emphasized as a crucial developmental period. Incestuous wishes in children characterize normal development between the ages of 3 and 5. In males, the threat of castration by the father figure results in the dissolution of the oedipal complex while in females, it is given up because the wish for a child (or penis envy) is not fulfilled. Early psychoanalysis considered clients with unresolved oedipal conflicts as ideal candidates for treatment.

Psychodynamic Method

"Catharsis," or the release of emotions, characterizes the psychodynamic process. The repression of emotions, key to neurotic conflict, results in maladaptive behavior patterns. The reexperiencing of repressed emotions from past conflictual relationships within the therapeutic relationship provides a corrective therapeutic experience. This is often described as a "working through" of past conflicts within the therapeutic transference. This working through also enables the client to correct past maladaptive behavior patterns and distortions that intrude from the past.

"Free association" refers to the client's verbalizing whatever is on his or her mind without screening for logic or social appropriateness. It is assumed that this uncritical attitude facilitates access to unconscious thoughts and feelings of the client. It is also assumed that this verbal method enables the client to regress to earlier developmental stages and work through conflicts experienced during that time. This process is dependent upon a client's trust in the method as leading to behavior change.

Therapist neutrality is crucial to the method because it minimizes the influence of social context and the intrusion of therapist issues into the client–therapist relationship. The therapist as a blank slate, or tabula rasa, was emphasized in the earlier literature as necessary to facilitate the development of the transference relationship.

Emphasis on interpretation rather than advice giving is key to a psychodynamic approach. Since conflicts are unconscious due to repression, the therapist role is to interpret the underlying meaning of therapeutic content. The therapeutic process is oriented toward helping the client experience repressed feelings and bring dynamic issues to consciousness. Interpretations are intended to promote insight as a means to facilitating behavior change in psychotherapy (Giovacchini, 1972).

Therapeutic Relationship

The therapeutic relationship has been differentiated to include both the real and the projected aspects of therapist characteristics (Greenson & Wexler, 1969; Langs, 1978). The real aspects form the basis for a therapeutic alliance. This is experienced as empathy between client and therapist, and has been defined as the therapist understanding the client, and in turn, by the client feeling understood. Empathy includes both affective and cognitive components. Elements of the self in the therapeutic alliance have been understood to include merging with the therapist in a primitive, infantile empathy (Kohut, 1977) and identification with the therapist.

"Transference" refers to a client's reactions to the therapist as they are determined by fantasy and unconscious factors. Viewing the therapist in terms of past relationships leads to irrational attitudes and distortions (Dewald, 1971; Giovacchini, 1972; Greenson, 1965; Langs, 1974, 1978). Earlier psychodynamic theory emphasized neurotic transferences that derived from relationships with one's parents based on unresolved oedipal relationships (Greenson, 1965). The examination of feelings associated with these prior relationships, and the working through of conflicts associated with these prior relationships experienced in the transference become the basis for changing maladaptive behavior patterns in psychotherapy. In more recent developments, object relations theory emphasizes the self as key to the transference relationship (Stolorow, Brandchaft, & Atwood, 1987). Psychotherapy is viewed as correcting failures in development of the self. Consequently, narcissistic transference and restoration of the self have become key concepts in the psychotherapeutic relationship (Kohut, 1971).

Just as clients project onto the therapist attributes associated with past relationships, therapists also project onto clients attributes associated with their own past relationships; this has been termed countertransference. While earlier psychodynamic literature considered these countertransference feelings to be undesirable, later developments emphasize the importance of therapists bringing their own feelings toward the client to consciousness, and working with them in the therapeutic relationship (Comas-Díaz & Jacobsen, 1991; Langs, 1974; Wolstein, 1983). No therapist is truly above the need to separate out the reality context from the distortions brought about by his or her own personal experiences. Moreover, the sociopolitical context of racism, sexism, and cultural stereotypes clearly set a context within the therapeutic relationship that influence a therapist's countertransference reactions.

RELEVANCE AND APPLICABILITY OF PSYCHODYNAMIC THERAPY FOR WOMEN OF COLOR

The above concepts are generally accepted as central to the practice of psychodynamic psychotherapy. Underlying assumptions predict the course of development, the nature of instinctual drives and intrapsychic conflict. Catharsis and free association, key methods in psychodynamic psychotherapy, have been more facilitative with oedipal conflicts. Neurotic problems, which represent a higher level of development, are considered more suited than other diagnostic entities for a psychodynamic approach. The emphases on universal phenomena and normative behavior influence what is expected in the transference relationship, and define criteria for selecting ideal clients. This has been criticized as restricting the approach to what have been termed YAVIS clients (i.e., young, attractive, verbal, intelligent, and successful; Toupin, 1980).

As psychodynamic theory was refined, early theorists did not emphasize cultural and gender issues as critical variables. In a homogeneous society, common dynamic themes appeared universal. In seeking a standard model of practice, cultural and gender biases resulted in psychotherapy with women of color being viewed as deviations from standard practice. Women of color often failed to meet the criteria of an ideal client, reflected in low utilization and early drop-out rates. It has, however, become increasingly clear that race, class, and culture are significant variables in the practice of psychotherapy (Acosta, Yamamoto, & Evans, 1982; Gardner, 1980; McGoldrick, Pearce, & Giordano, 1982; D. W. Sue, 1978; S. Sue, 1982; Thomas & Sillen, 1972; Yamamoto, James, & Palley, 1968).

In discussing the relevance of psychodynamic psychotherapy, this chapter addresses the "bias" against women of color, and how this should influence the evolution of psychodynamic practice. Work with ethnic minorities and the emergence of feminist thinking in the United States has forced a reconceptualization of what should be termed "standard practice" and "universal phenomena." As the United States population has become increasingly multicultural and diverse, and as feminist thinking has grown, it has become clear that psychodynamic theory erroneously conceptualized or omitted aspects of development relevant to women and ethnic minorities.

Zaphiropoulos (1982) points out that psychoanalysis ignored the dimension of culture in its theoretical conceptualizations. The emphasis on a developmental approach, dynamic constellations, and specific defenses suggested that there was a universal approach to establishing a therapeutic relationship. Chin (1987) points out how standard rules of practice are in fact culturally rooted. While most therapists are sensitive in "educating" clients to the rules prescribed for the therapeutic context (e.g., the 50-minute hour, confidentiality), most fail to see that these rules of conduct are rooted in a sociocultural context that emphasizes the importance of time and privacy. Women of color will bring different expectations to the therapeutic process. To be relevant, a psychodynamic approach must use multiple norms to interpret manifestations that arise out of culture and gender differences.

INFLUENCE OF CULTURE AND GENDER ON PSYCHODYNAMIC CONTENT

Gender roles and cultural values will influence the nature of therapeutic content. Mitchell (1974) points out that the oppression of women reflected in psychoanalysis is more an index of the condition of women at that time than of Freud's sexist position. Psychodynamic theory mirrored the Victorian era of Western culture in formulating the nature of women. The prominence of sexual themes in psychotherapy reflected social taboos against the explicit discussion of sex. Psychodynamic views of women reinforced negative views of female development, and the inferior status of women's roles prevailing in Victorian culture. Penis envy, in particular, has been criticized because the theory is based on women being viewed as anatomically deficient compared to men. The innate passivity and masochism of women described by Freud reflected a male perspective on female development. The oedipal complex reinforced the dominance of male aggression embodied in the young boy's competition with his father, and female weakness in the seduction of his mother.

Hare-Mustin (1983) reanalyzes Freud's famous case of Dora in 1900 from a feminist perspective. She criticizes Freud for failing to recognize his own countertransference, which results in the harshness and coldness with which he treats Dora. Instead of confirming the truthfulness of her complaints about her father's affair and being propositioned by a family friend, he depicts her as vengeful and noncompliant—that is, as affirming the stereotype that women are not to be believed. A key point is the inattention to the problems more prevalent in women, and how the psychological problems of women reflect societal conditions and attitudes while the solutions offered by psychotherapy reflect a sexist texture of contemporary life.

The women's movement and feminist thinking has resulted in increasing criticism of psychodynamic theory for its negative and devaluing conceptualization of feminine traits and female roles. Marecek and Hare-Mustin (1991) recount the history of the influence of feminist thinking on clinical psychology, and point out how Karen Horney and Clara Thompson presaged the feminist critiques of psychoanalysis of the 1960s and 1970s. Horney challenged the centrality of penis envy in female development, while Thompson examined cultural pressures that restricted opportunities for women and derogated women's sexuality. Westkott (1986), however, demonstrates how Horney's theory devalues women by conceptualizing feminine traits as lodged in a dependent character. Chodorow (1978) draws on object relations theory and places feminine personality development within a sociocultural context; in particular, she emphasizes that women's experiences during infancy result in greater connectedness and an identity rooted in relationships. This has been echoed by others including Miller (1976), who describes women's capacity for affiliation, and Gilligan (1982), who focuses on women's sense of responsibility for others. Gilligan postulates different but equal developmental lines for men and women, viewing masculinity as defined by separation, femininity by attachment. Miller (1986) focuses on women's psychological strengths and seeks to create a model of life that includes both female and male experience. In particular, she emphasizes issues of domination–subordination, connectedness, serving others' needs—in essence, the relational contexts and how these differentially influence psychological development for men and women. These feminist approaches have identified psychological development from a feminine perspective, and reconceptualized feminine traits in a positive and affirmative light. Most important has been the emphasis on sociocultural context, and the forces of socialization and culture that contribute to defining women's experience. As Hare-Mustin (1983) points out, little attention has been paid to differences that women experience in marriage and family relations, stresses associated with normal reproductive functions, physical and sexual abuse that serve to maintain the dominance of men, and diagnoses (e.g., hysteria) that stereotype and devalue the experiences of women.

The universality of the oedipal complex has been questioned (Yamamoto, 1982) as we have studied human development in other cultures. Yamamoto and Chang (1987) describe the Ajase complex as more syntonic with Asian culture than the oedipal complex:

In contrast to the Oedipus complex, Japanese psychoanalysts have focused upon the Ajase complex, which is based on a myth: Prince Ajase not only kills his father, as does Oedipus, but he has a very special and culturally syntonic relationship with his mother. The Indian myth of Prince Ajase reflects the intense Japanese mother–son relationship. Prince Ajase, who was destined to kill his father, becomes king. He later tries to kill his mother because she is loyal to his father, the dead king. However, Ajase is not able to accomplish this because of his guilt feelings. Apparently, as punishment for his transgressions, sores develop on his body, and an odor emanates from them so offensive that no one will come near. His mother is the only person willing to care for him. King Ajase's heart responds to this mother's display of affection and forgiveness, thus he and his mother are reunited. (Okonogi, as quoted by Tatara, 1980, cited by Yamamoto, 1982)

Unlike the Oedipus figure of Greek tradition, the Ajase figure of Buddhist tradition places emphasis on the mother–son dyad rather than the father–son dyad. Guilt feelings are raised in Ajase because of the mother's love for her son, while Oedipus', guilt feelings are due to the fear of retaliation by the "father" (Iwasaki, 1971).

Gornick (1986) points out that the typical psychodynamic therapist–client dyad emphasizes the erotic transference that characterizes the dynamic between a male therapist and female patient. This reflects the emphasis on male–female relationships in Western culture, to the relative neglect or devaluing of same-sex relationships. When other variations of the therapist–client dyad exist, different manifestations can be expected in the therapeutic relationship. Unfortunately, the concept of preoedipal maternal transference, as defined by Western culture, characterizes relationships with a maternal figure as more primitive and devaluing.

While cultures of color have also reinforced an inferior status for women, participation by women of color in feminist thinking poses additional dilemmas to those of White women. Women of color in the United States share an experience of being bicultural and of minority status. Rejection of "traditional" female roles is complicated by their association with giving up their non-Western culture. Women of color who become more liberated are often described as becoming Westernized, modernized, and so on—terms that tend to denigrate their culture of origin. Self-identity, therefore, is compromised given the association of feminine traits, cultural values, and minority status to one's sense of self. Several cultural values will be discussed to illustrate this point.

Filial Piety in Asian Cultures

Traditional Asian cultures subscribed to the Confucian view of filial piety, which valued unquestioning obedience to the parents and those in positions of authority (Tseng, 1973). While this paralleled Western culture in favoring male dominance in the social hierarchy, traditional Asian culture rigidly dictated a woman's status by the age and status of her husband within the family hierarchy. Women received greater status if they were the first wife, or wife of the eldest son. As roles of Asian women in the United States evolve, these issues become more prominent as developmental conflicts.

Asian women conforming to these roles will expect the therapeutic relationship to be hierarchical rather than equal, and the therapist to be an authority figure. Educating the client on the "rules" of catharsis or free association will be ineffective if cultural values reinforce listening in the presence of an authority figure. Miscommunication will occur if the therapist expects the client to free associate while the client expects the therapist to give advice. Each may view the other as having failed in his/her responsibility. Some therapists may perceive Asian women conforming to these roles as "too traditional" or not liberated. Therapists can utilize this expectation to facilitate the therapeutic process if interventions are framed to emphasize the benevolent authority of the therapist.

Asian women rebelling against these roles, on the other hand, may resist the authoritative nature of the therapeutic relationship. In these situations, emphasis on transcending the hierarchical relationship, a concept described by Suh (1987), will empower the client while facilitating positive self-identification. Therapists should not assume, however, that this rebellion arises from a desire to be non-Asian or to give up one's culture. A psychodynamic process must empower Asian women to face these developmental conflicts, without rejecting the Asian culture.

Machismo in Hispanic Cultures

Hispanic cultures stress the importance of *machismo* as a complex cultural value. Ignoring these realities contributes to the alienation of the client. De La Cancela (1986) describes *machismo* as a socially constructed, learned, and reinforced set of behaviors comprising the content of male gender roles in Latino society. These behaviors include stoicism, varying levels of intimacy among men, attempts to avoid shame and gain *respeto* (respect) and *dignidad* (dignity) for self and family, the displacement of stress related to economic and social factors into the interpersonal and familial sphere, and, at times, caricatured patterns of assertiveness and dominance.

Machismo has been misapplied as a concept when primarily associated with the absence of father figures in Puerto Rican families and the sexualization of women. Dynamically, it has been viewed as pathological, associated with unresolved oedipal issues, inferiority complexes, and a compensatory cult of strutting virility. It is important not to reduce the interpretation of *machismo* to an overemphasis on sexual drives. De La Cancela (1986) points to the importance of examining the context of socioeconomic oppression when working with Puerto Rican females. A Latina woman may place the burden for change on herself alone, or be angry at her mate for his oppressive behavior. Reaching out to a woman's mate by the therapist can be more facilitative to therapeutic change than supporting a Puerto Rican female client in her rebellion against her "oppressive" mate.

The virginity cult epitomized by *marianismo* serves as the cultural counterpoint to machismo and stipulates that the woman should be chaste before marriage and, when married, conform to her husband's *macho* behavior (Comas-Díaz, 1988). *Marianismo* is based on the Catholic cult of the Virgin Mary, which dictates that when women become mothers they attain the status of madonnas and, accordingly, are expected to deny themselves in favor of their children and husbands (Stevens, 1973). Latina women may face dilemmas in giving up this idealized position when in psychotherapy. More information on Latina gender roles is provided in Chapter 9 (Boyd-Franklin & García-Preto) on family therapy, in this volume.

Black Rage

With the evolution of race relations in the late 1960s, "Black rage" became a popular concept to capture the institutionalized anger of Blacks over the injustices and oppressions of slavery by Whites. This concept also became the focus of pride within the Black community, and the basis for building self-esteem eroded by a history of racism. During slavery, it was adaptive for Blacks to blunt the overt expression of affect and to employ covert channels for resisting oppression (Adams, 1976). Males were denigrated by American society and emphasis was placed on the matriarchal structure and absent father in Black families. More recently, there has been emphasis on building psychotherapeutic models for Black Americans based on competency, strengths of Black families, and resiliency of individuals (Lewis & Looney, 1983; Nobles, 1980).

For Black women, mistrust, anger, and low self-esteem is likely to characterize initial presentation in psychotherapy if the therapeutic context is perceived as "mainstream" (Jenkins, 1982; Jones & Gray, 1984). A psychodynamic approach must consider this institutionalized anger in relationship to individual aggressive drives. Struggles for positive self-esteem and identity must be weighed against the context of racism. A therapist cannot begin as a "blank screen" if he or she is to establish trust and validate the client in the therapeutic alliance. Being Black is so central to the identity of African Americans that some have recommended discussing race in the initial session to validate a significant part of the client's self-identity (Griffith, 1977; Thomas & Dansby, 1985). A Black female client may come to therapy expecting to be devalued by a White therapist, or questioning the competence of a Black therapist. The therapist using a psychodynamic approach must integrate transference issues within the context of American society.

Religiosity/Spirituality

Religion and spirituality provide philosophic guidance, social cohesiveness, and psychological support to its believers. It unites its members under a common rubric. Sometimes, the intensity of a psychodynamic approach can compete with religious and spiritual beliefs. Each holds underlying assumptions about fate, lifestyle, duty, help-seeking behavior, and so on. The emphasis on harmony in Confucian philosophy may conflict with confrontative therapeutic interventions with an Asian client. The importance of gospel music and religion as a shared social experience in the African American culture may compete with the intensity of a therapeutic alliance with an African American client. The importance of confession in Catholicism may compete with the development of transferential relationships in a Catholic Latino client. Confession can be viewed as a form of catharsis, conducted regularly, in the presence of a "blank screen" (i.e., a priest). Devout Catholics may experience conflict with the competing demands of psychotherapy or dissipate intense affect through confession before bringing dynamic issues up in psychotherapy. A client with Confucian or Buddhist values may view psychotherapy as self-indulgent.

Each of these examples point to different emphases in therapeutic content due to culture and gender differences. To avoid these potential pitfalls, therapists must utilize prevailing cultural values and roles of the client to facilitate positive growth in psychotherapy.

PROBLEMATIC CONCEPTS IN THE PSYCHODYNAMIC METHOD: ANOTHER PERSPECTIVE FOR WOMEN OF COLOR

In addition to what clients bring to the therapeutic situation, many underlying concepts of psychodynamic practice reflect the cultural values and expectations of the prevailing sociocultural context. These concepts become problematic in psychotherapy with women of color when they bias therapists toward dynamic formulations and therapeutic methods that devalue women of color or omit crucial aspects of their experience. Some problematic concepts will be discussed, together with some different perspectives held by women of color.

Individual Perspective

Importance of Self over Other

The emphasis of individual (self) over social (other) concerns is dominant in a psychodynamic approach. The importance of social and interpersonal contexts for women of color is inherent in the extended family common to cultures of color. Women's roles within the family and society emphasize nurturance, caring, and empathy. A psychodynamic approach emphasizing the importance of self over other can create intrapsychic conflict if it is perceived as dystonic with cultural roles and feminine nature.

An Asian client who is struggling with the dilemma of respecting her husband's family, or a Latina client who resents her "maternal" responsibilities, is not helped if she is encouraged simply to stand up for herself or to be herself. This may have a negative effect of encouraging rejection of her cultural roots or promoting cultural identity problems

Importance of Achieving Independence

The criterion of independence as a therapeutic outcome often violates the principle of mutual interdependence important to women of color. Separation–individuation is a developmental phenomenon defined by Mahler (1968, 1972) as deriving from an early symbiotic bond with the mother. This symbiotic bond is defined as primitive and pathological once it continues beyond its "normal" developmental period, of infancy. Separation–individuation in adulthood is often translated as independence and defined as physical separation from one's parents as at the age of 18. For women of color, in contrast, the emphasis on returning to one's family of origin and mutual interdependence is viewed as normal and represents greater self-actualization. We cannot automatically assume that a client who continues to live at home beyond the age of 18 is dependent if cultural expectations differ. Nor should we assume a pathological mother–daughter bond if a woman has a strong relationship with her mother.

Affect: Importance of Getting One's Feelings Out

The dichotomy between affect and logic is often viewed as feminine and masculine traits. Empathy, connectedness, and emotionality are more commonly associated with feminine nature. Cultures which reinforce affective styles of relating are often deemed inferior and primitive. Different values placed on overt expressiveness may result in Latina women being viewed as hysterical and Asian women as unemotional or demure.

In using a psychodynamic approach, the release of emotions (i.e., catharsis), is viewed as a necessary prerequisite to the gaining of insight. An Asian client may view catharsis as less important than the regulation of emotions or as inconsistent with her view of the ideal woman. It is important to examine how to engage her through a culturally syntonic value rather than to view this difference as a therapeutic failure. For other cultures, catharsis is a highly ritualized event within religious and social ceremonies. These differences influence greatly how a client views the therapeutic mandate. One cannot prescribe "simple" catharsis without placing it in the cultural context and role definition of the client. A client may question why it is good "to get one's feelings out." Unless this is framed in a way syntonic with the culture (i.e., as a way to learn how to regulate one's feelings), a client may be unable to share its importance in the therapeutic process.

Universality: We Are All the Same; We Are People

A psychodynamic approach often emphasizes certain phenomena as universal when in fact they are culturally specific. While there is a commonality among cultures, the relative emphasis and different values given by specific cultures are significant in understanding dynamic formulations. An intense mother–son or mother–daughter relationship, viewed as normal or valued within Asian or Latino culture, respectively, may be viewed as a pathological overattachment in Western culture, thus the differential importance in Asian cultures of the Ajase complex (described earlier) compared to the Oedipal complex. The emphasis on egalitarian relationships in Western culture appears to heighten the intensity of sibling rivalry, while the emphasis on authoritative relationships in Asian cultures appears to heighten the intensity of parent–child conflicts. The development of self-identity, understood from a White, Western perspective, often ignores the impact of race on the development of self among women of color. An emphasis on the common struggle and on universal phenomena ignores these differential values and experiences.

Psychodynamic psychotherapists select patients by comparing them with a common definition of the "ideal" client, a comparison in which women of color are found deficient. In its attempt to define a uniform model of psychotherapy to address universal criteria of psychopathology, the psychodynamic approach lacks the fluidity to be applicable to a diverse, multicultural population. Psychotherapeutic practices adapted for women of color have been described as deviations from standard practice. Differences presented by clients tend to be viewed as resistances and hindrances to psychotherapy. Symbols and metaphors used by women in psychodynamic psychotherapy are often interpreted as universal when they are, in fact, influenced by the contexts of culture and gender. These subtle cultural differences are often important in altering psychodynamic meaning. The color red, for example, is a symbol of happiness in the Asian cultures, and often worn by younger women and children to celebrate youth and beauty, yet it is often a symbol of flamboyance and hostility in Western culture. The color black has had negative connotations associated with race, depression, and denigration in Western culture while the color white has had positive associations with purity and cleanliness, yet white is generally the color used for funerals in traditional Asian culture.

Normative Behavior: Women of Color Compared to White Women

In using the principle of normative behavior, women of color are more often than not compared with White female clients as the standard. A psychodynamic approach tends to view behavior along a developmental and linear continuum. As psychopathology is conceptualized in terms of stages or levels of development, different diagnoses are viewed either as primitive or advanced. This comparative process is manifested in many facets of the therapeutic process, which emphasizes regression in the service of the ego. Women are judged in relation to men; cultures of color are judged in relation to dominant White culture. When this linear and value-laden approach is employed, women of color tend to be placed along a developmental continuum that denigrates the importance of cultural values and feminine roles. Women in general are viewed as too emotional and not logical. Asian women, compared to White women, are viewed as passive and subservient, the "good wife"; Black women as aggressive and sexualized; Latinas as emotional and hysterical.

A useful alternative conceptualization of human behavior is that of the circle. To view behavior and life cycles using a circular motif—a motif that is common in Asian and Native American cultures—we can begin to understand the fluidity of human behavior and the importance of balance and harmony in establishing psychological well-being, as, for example, in the opposing qualities of *yin* and *yang* in Asian cultures. *Yin*, the feminine properties, are always juxtaposed to *yang*, the masculine properties. As described in the *I Ching*, "One Yin and one Yang make the Tao. . . . If they repel, they are identical charges, but if they attract, one is positive and one is negative. Which is which? It does not matter" (Jou, 1984). The perspective gained from using this circular motif to represent human experience differs from cultural perspectives where confrontation and assertiveness are valued in that maintaining balance and harmony in relationships is most important.

In psychotherapy, it is important to consider how women of color differ from White women and use norms indigenous to their cultures. A Southeast Asian woman who has experienced severe trauma should be viewed in comparison with other Southeast Asian women who have experienced similar trauma. A Black woman with poor self-esteem because of her lack of vocational mobility should be assessed in relation to other Black women with similar experiences of racism. When a therapist reacts from a perspective of another culture and is "horrified" by the trauma experienced by the Southeast Asian client, or downplays the realities of racism experienced by the Black client in therapeutic sessions, the therapeutic experience is already distorted; the capacity for empathy can be lost.

An alternative formulation is to emphasize differences rather than commonality in psychotherapy with women of color. A difference perspective would not view differences in psychotherapy as instances of noncompliance and resistance, but rather would seek to understand how these differences can contribute to positive adaptations for the client. Therapeutic interventions would be reframed to fit the cultural context; differences would be viewed not as hindrances, but examined for how they might facilitate the psychotherapeutic process.

THE THERAPEUTIC RELATIONSHIP AND WOMEN OF COLOR

Transference Issues

Transference themes in psychotherapy are projections by a client of expectations and distortions based on past experience. For women of color, culture and minority-group status set a context of difference that is not "normal" and expectable in the client–therapist dyad. Projections about race and culture, therefore, will be prominent as transference themes and must be factored in as normal reality issues. Comas-Díaz and Minrath (1985) point out that the introduction of ethnic and racial factors into the therapeutic relationship seems to catalyze transference themes of self-image, race, social class, identity, and anger. To capture some transference themes common among women of color, several conceptualizations are described below.

Hierarchical Transference: Authority

For all clients, perceptions and feelings about the therapist are influenced by the authority status of the therapist. Given the importance of hierarchical relationships among women of color, they will frequently attribute greater value to the authority status of the therapist. The concept of hierarchical transference is introduced to define this phenomenon. Transference reactions with women of color will more commonly emphasize deference to authority and male figures. Women who define relationships in these hierarchical terms are more likly to view the therapist as an all-knowing advice giver, or as a wise and caring authority figure whose recommendations are to be followed.

Because the authority figure is idealized as a benevolent figure in traditional Asian culture, hierarchical transference is likely to be associated with compliance rather than rebellion, and higher expectations of cure. In an Interactive Forum on Psychotherapy with Asian Americans (Chin, Liem, Ham, & Hong, 1987), participants argued the inevitability of a hierarchical transference, and the importance of utilizing it to facilitate change in psychotherapy. Suh (1987), on the other hand, advocated the importance of transcending the hierarchical relationship in psychotherapy with Asian Americans.

Individual dynamics may be more important in deciding which approach to take, How therapists use this hierarchical transference will also determine whether it is facilitative or hindering. A woman with domineering and intrusive parents may experience this hierarchy as negative;

therapeutic analysis of the hierarchical transference and reflective interventions to promote more expanded roles is likely to be facilitative. A woman with authoritative but supportive parents may experience this hierarchy as positive; using this therapeutic alliance to promote change through authoritative directives is also likely to be facilitative. Although this hierarchical emphasis is likely to inhibit spontaneity and delay open communication in the early phases of psychotherapy, it should not be misconstrued as a communication failure.

Racial Transference: Power

With ethnic minority individuals, both therapists and clients are more likely to make attributions about one another based on past interactions with others of that racial group. Given the importance of race in the identity of ethnic minority clients, attributions and feelings about the racial background of the therapist will manifest themselves more frequently in the therapeutic relationship (Chin, 1981; Chin, 1983; Schacter & Butts, 1968). The concept of racial transference is introduced to characterize those attitudes toward the therapist related to race that have no basis in the present context. This is complicated, however, by the fact that reality-based reactions related to race often cannot be separated from non–reality-based racial transference reactions. Given the emphasis on racial differences in the United States, racial awareness is inevitable in the psychotherapeutic relationship whenever there is a non-White individual in the client–therapist dyad. Feelings about the therapist's race are likely to arise with women of color not only as a result of personal history and life circumstances, but also from the sociocultural and historical context associated with race relations in the United States.

　　The experience of the power differential in the therapeutic relationship is crucial to the concept of racial transference. Often, this involves reactions to therapist competence and authority. Women of color may experience powerlessness and helplessness vis-à-vis the therapist both as female and as non-White, especially with a White male therapist. These transference reactions are often heightened with poor women. The dynamic is complex, and it takes different forms in intraethnic dyads with women of color. While women of color are more likely to identify with a therapist of their own race and gender, this can be a positive and corrective experience for self-identity. However, some women will experience this identification negatively by devaluing the authority and competence of a non-White female therapist. The intensity of this identification process may also stir up fears of getting too close or being engulfed by a therapist of the same race and gender. Or it may result in the client feeling ambivalent about working within an intraethnic and intragender dyad (Comas-Díaz & Jacobsen, 1991).

Supporting positive identifications of race and gender in the transference is crucial when working with women of color. Empowerment by working through the racial transference is important as a therapeutic outcome with women of color. This means verbalizing the issue of race in the therapeutic relationship, and actively supporting racial identity to correct for the devaluing aspects of race in our society.

Mirror Transference: Ethnic Self/Identity

Ethnic and gender identity is intricately related to self-identity for women of color. As stated above, within the transference relationship, women of color may experience admiration or inferiority vis-à-vis the therapist. The match of the therapist–client dyad will influence greatly how this should be addressed. Cultural values, history, myths, and stereotypes will be important contextual variables that define the nature of transference phenomena. Women of color experiencing admiration with a therapist not matched for race and gender may pay the price of experiencing inferiority for their own race or gender unless this is actively addressed in the transference.

It is important to reconceptualize the concept of mirror transferences described in the literature by Kohut (1971), in which the therapist mirrors the self-identity of the client. Sometimes it is possible to validate and support the ethnic and gender identity only with a same-race/same-gender match in the client–therapist dyad. Because reality-based racial and gender issues often cannot be separated from projected distortions in the transference, it may be necessary to provide a concrete and positive role model of the same race and gender for self-identification. Conflict over ethnic identity and gender roles may also reflect the sociocultural context; differentiating these reality-based conflicts from intrapsychic conflict may be crucial to the therapist mirroring an adaptive resolution of self-identity.

The concept of a bicultural identity as opposed to acculturation into the Western world is important when working with identity issues in a therapeutic transference. The use of "splitting"—a phenomenon in which an individual behaves in two contradictory ways without consciously recognizing their inconsistency—as a defense mechanism to respond to opposing cultural prescriptions for behavior by bicultural individuals is likely to be more adapted then attempting to integrate opposing values from different cultures. Conflict with ethnic identity is likely to be part of a normal developmental phenomenon. Because gender and ethnicity are coexisting variables, clients are more likely to confuse or merge issues of power, status, and self differentiation as they occur in the transference relationship. Unless we value these cultural differences in the development of self-identity for women of color, we have but a partial understanding of mirror transferences.

Preoedipal Transference: Ethnic Gender Roles

Most cultures have been highly stratified along social class, gender, and authority lines. Most women were expected to be deferential to men in social, academic, and familial relationships. While women's roles have gained greater equality as a result of the feminist movement, this change began later for women of color. The inequality of racial and economic status characterizing the experience of women of color probably contributed to this delay.

Gornick (1986) and Gilligan (1982) have pointed out how the inequality of feminine roles in society have been recapitulated in psychodynamic models. The preoedipal or narcissistic transference, conceptualized from a male perspective, in effect renders more dominant feminine issues as less equal and more primitive than male ones. Benedek (1973) and Mogul (1982) have observed that women therapists are more likely to trigger both primitive wishes for reunion with the preoedipal mother and fears of either engulfment or abandonment by the mother. The oedipal or erotic transference of traditional psychodynamic theory essentially validates a Western male perspective. Freud's (1915) writing on the erotic transference assumes that the patient is a woman and that the analyst is a man.

In working with women of color, mother–son and mother–daughter transferences may reflect different cultural values of nurturing, filial piety, or bonding, and may represent more advanced levels of psychological development. The equating of empathic relatedness with eroticism requires that basic assumptions of normal development are reconceptualized.

This conceptualization of some specific transferences from a different perspective is intended to illustrate two points. Hierarchical and racial transferences are introduced as concepts to reflect the status differential in the psychotherapeutic relationship, which has been largely ignored in the discussion of transference. Mirror and preodipal transferences need to be reconceptualized to include more empowering and valuing notions of women. Psychodynamic psychotherapy needs to be refined to include those perspectives important in the experiences of women of color. Dichotomous perspectives brought to psychotherapy by women of color need to be examined from the client's perspective.

Therapeutic Alliance

How women of color communicate will also be manifest in the therapeutic relationship. Western values often stress getting one's point across, for example, whereas Asian values stress politeness in verbal discourse. As a result, Westerners tend to value verbal fluency while Asians tend to value not interrupting others. Therapists who fail to understand this different style of interpersonal communication are likely to face barriers in establishing a therapeutic alliance. Linguistic nuances often convey significant semantic differences in the therapeutic relationship. It has been observed (De La Cancela, 1985; Marcos & Urcuyo, 1979) how bilingual Latina clients will switch between languages in psychotherapy to express different emotional experiences and affect.

Nonverbal communication such as body language, spatial boundaries, facial expressions, eye contact, touching, and the like also have differing connotations and degrees of freedom between cultures (Hall, 1976). Cultures defined as high context cultures will rely more heavily on the nonverbal context for information than the verbal context. The therapeutic alliance will be enhanced with women of color if greater attention is paid to nonverbal, contextual communication. For an Asian client, silence cannot be interpreted as agreement if the client is not contradicting the therapist to be polite. For a Black client, silence may represent suspiciousness, and threat of challenging an authority figure.

The ability of a client to identify with the therapist is important to the establishing of a therapeutic alliance. Given the importance of race and culture in the self-identity for women of color, therapists must establish the nature of this identification when working with women of color. Some women will immediately identify with a therapist of the same race, while others may resist this identification. In any case, race is a prominent factor in the establishment of the therapeutic alliance whenever a member of the client–therapist dyad is non-White.

Whereas male status has been regarded as higher than that of female in most cultures, gender variables are likely to facilitate the therapeutic alliance. A female therapist is more likely to transcend the hierarchical relationship since her professional role is likely to supercede and be dystonic with her social role. A male therapist, on the other hand, is more likely to be confined by the hierarchical transference, since his professional role is syntonic with his social role. For female clients, establishing a more egalitarian relationship is empowering, while complying with a hierarchical relationship can be socially syntonic. For male clients, either role is likely to elicit conflict since it can represent giving up a superior male role, losing in competition with another male, or being castrated by a female. These examples illustrate the significance of gender in the therapist–client dyad in forming a therapeutic alliance.

Countertransference Issues

Just as women of color bring cultural values and biases to the therapeutic situation, so do therapists. For therapists, these values, biases, and expectations influence how therapeutic content is interpreted, choice of therapeutic method, and nature of therapeutic relationship. Given the inherent dynamics of power between client and therapist, countertransference issues will be influenced by the dynamics of culture and gender roles.

For therapists of color, these phenomena often involve overidentification with the client's experiences. The effects of racism can result in an oversensitivity to racial overtones in their interpretation of dynamic content. They may overprotect their clients against racial overtones, and avoid appropriately confronting intrapsychic dynamic issues. They may support strategies for dealing with racism when introspection and competency may be more therapeutic. The distinctions between supporting social change vs. social conformity in psychotherapy is often complicated when treating women of color. Therapists of color must guard against therapeutic interventions that promote an agenda for personal change regarding cultural and gender roles that is not the client's. In overidentifying with cultural and gender related conflicts, therapists of color can underdiagnose psychopathology. In identifying with a female victim of sexual or physical abuse, they may ignore real dynamics that contribute to dysfunctional behavior.

Therapists of color can also internalize biases and distortions related to race, culture, and gender prevalent in our society. Since most are trained in Western models of psychotherapy, they can support culturally dystonic values and strategies as therapeutic goals. For example, they may support women of color in assertively confronting their husbands; while they may view this as acculturation, liberation, and so on, such confrontation could serve to emasculate these men according to cultural norms. On the other hand, women of color may overidentify with cultural norms and support culturally prescribed gender roles, to the detriment of self-esteem and actualization.

Despite these potential pitfalls, countertransference phenomena can also be facilitative. Therapists of color may be more able to identify with women of color and their experience, thereby facilitating the development of a therapeutic alliance. They may be more sensitive to cultural nuances and meaning that may be missed by White therapists. Feelings of helplessness, rage, or alienation associated with racism or inferior status sometimes can be better understood through shared experience.

For White therapists, countertransference phenomena will often be associated with the dynamic of power and difference between client and therapist. Ethnic and/or racial differences between client and therapist often cause anxiety; therefore, it is not uncommon for White therapists to minimize cultural and gender differences when working with women of color. In an attempt to form a therapeutic alliance, White therapists may claim a commonality based on the perceived universality of wants, needs, and problems, and they may thus consider culture and gender differences irrelevant to the therapeutic relationship. Therapists with limited knowledge of a culture may rely on cultural and racial stereotypes that result in a superficial interpretation of cultural phenomena. Gaps in cultural connectedness and a common experience between client and therapist may also result in White therapists overdiagnosing psychopathology. Therapists' emotional reactions to client experiences (e.g., shock at war trauma, inquisitiveness about differing cultural norms) may cause women of color to feel misunderstood, unconnected, or alienated within the therapeutic relationship. Therapists' conscious or unconscious racism may also result in interpretations that devalue the client, stereotypic expectations of client behavior, and inappropriate displays of power by the therapist. On the other hand, some counter-transference phenomena among White therapists may be facilitative. Their wish to be perceived as liberal and able to work multiculturally may facilitate the client's feeling liked and valued in the patient–therapist dyad. Their acknowledgment of difference and ignorance of the client's culture may promote the client's feelings of safety and anonymity in the therapeutic relationship.

GUIDELINES FOR USING PSYCHODYNAMIC THERAPY WITH WOMEN OF COLOR

Reframing in the Worldview of the Client

While cultural sensitivity is emphasized in working with women of color, emphasis is often placed on the therapist learning about a client's culture. This approach tends to result in a therapist using his or her own culture as a standard of comparison. Thus the therapist may misinterpret responses by women of color that are different from what he or she would expect, and may consider them hindrances to treatment. For example, a modest Asian client or a nonverbal Black client may be viewed as a therapeutic failure when attempting to use the method of free association. From that point of view, therapists will emphasize overcoming those cultural behaviors that do not conform to standard practice. Greater cultural sensitivity would result if a perspective of positive reframing were used instead. Emphasis would then be placed on how modesty or a nonverbal style can be used to facilitate the therapeutic process. Reframing therapeutic outcomes to be syntonic with cultural values would be important. For example, encouraging a client to cooperate in achieving a therapeutic end may be more facilitative than asking her to confront a situation. Different phenomena would be interpreted as different cultural manifestations of normal development rather than as developmental failures (e.g., Ajase vs. Oedipus).

Splitting as a Useful Defense for Bicultural Individuals

Splitting has been viewed as a developmentally primitive defense, and failures in self-integration as pathological. However, women of color tend to live in bicultural environments where values and practices in both cultures can be discrepant and contradictory. It has not been uncommon for bicultural individuals to maintain separate and distinct selves syntonic with different cultures; behaviors and practice will differ depending on the cultural context. For example, a woman may be deferent with an authority figure in one context while confrontative and challenging in another. In these instances, splitting can be adaptive in enabling women of color to maintain the integrity of dual selves essential to biculturalism, and thus to avoid intrapsychic conflict.

Bicultural Identity as a Developmental Outcome

Chin (1981) describes the process of acculturation as a stressful event that influences the mental health status for women of color. Women of color are often judged in relation to a continuum of acculturation. Unfortunately, this has the net effect of implying that the desired outcome is to become Western and to give up "traditional" or "cultural" ways. As Comas-Díaz and Minrath (1985) point out, biculturalism can create exceptional strength and flexibility, but it can also create identity difficulties for women of color. It is important to emphasize bicultural identity as part of a normal developmental process in which Western and non-Western cultures are not placed on two ends of a continuum. Rather, the process of identification and adaptation with values, beliefs, and practices from two cultures can be viewed as choices necessary to achieve optimal and positive self-identity. The phenomenological experience of marginal socioethnic status for biracial individuals described by Root (1990) speaks to limitations of present models for optimal ethnic identity; she calls for the flexibility and diversity of multiple models that reach out beyond the boundaries of culture.

Women of color may present in psychotherapy with dilemmas about who they are, where they belong, and feelings of alienation. These dilemmas may be more intense for biracial individuals. While psychotherapy needs to reinforce the positive strengths of a bicultural identity, psychotherapy outcomes for those with identity problems should emphasize coming to terms with dual aspects of self-identity rather than acculturation as a means of conflict resolution.

Different versus Deviant

Psychotherapy with women of color often poses the dilemma of educating the client in the ways of Western psychotherapy versus molding psychotherapeutic practice to the ethos of the client's culture. When psychodynamic psychotherapy is viewed as involving a set of standard practices, work with women of color can be problematic. This perspective suggests that deviations or modifications of standard practice is necessary when cultural differences are encountered. If, on the other hand, psychotherapy is viewed as a culture itself, the psychotherapeutic relationship can be viewed as communicating across cultures. Wu (1987) argues for the importance of a cultural empathy that empowers the client as a partner in the therapeutic process. He underscores the importance of understanding meaning from the client's cultural perspective rather than what is currently identified as universal. Reframing psychotherapy from this anthropological perspective facilitates viewing cultural phenomena in psychotherapy as different rather than deviant.

Culturally Competent Psychotherapy

The practice of psychodynamic psychotherapy frequently emphasizes traditional practices or mainstream services. Practices designed for women of color are often described as ethnic specific. Pejorative connotations and inferior status is associated with this designation. This perspective inherently presumes that women of color will be effectively treated by traditional psychotherapy once they become "acculturated," "mainstreamed," or less ethnic. The emphasis on mainstream services ignores the perspective and context experienced by women of color. Cultural competence is a term defined by Cross, Bazron, Dennis, and Isaacs (1989) as a developmental process towards which professionals and systems ought to strive to function effectively in cross-cultural situations. Five essential elements contribute to a system's, institution's, or agency's ability to become more culturally competent. The culturally competent system would: (1) value diversity; (2) have the capacity for cultural self-assessment; (3) be conscious of the dynamics inherent in the interaction of cultures; (4) have institutionalized cultural knowledge; and (5) have developed adaptations to diversity. Each of these five elements must function at every level of the system. In applying the concept of cultural competence to psychodynamic psychotherapy, a shift in goals from mainstreaming services to multicultural perspectives for a culturally diverse population is necessary. Comas-Díaz and Duncan (1985) illustrate the use of a cultural component in an assertiveness training program to render it more culturally competent for Puerto Rican women in building self-esteem.

CLINICAL ILLUSTRATIONS

Identifying data from the following two clinical cases have been altered to protect client confidentiality. These cases illustrate the applicability of a psychodynamic approach with two women of color. The cases also illustrate some generic cultural and gender themes and how they are handled as therapeutic content and within the therapeutic relationship. Both women struggled with issues of self-identity related to gender roles. Therapeutic focus emphasized their need to define their roles as females and to be empowered within a positive bicultural context. Despite these similarities, the contrasts between the two cases are also illustrative of the individual differences within a therapeutic environment that affirms the culture of origin.

The first case involves a Chinese American immigrant couple on the verge of divorce; they were seen over a 3-year period in both individual and couples therapy. The couple had immigrated to the United States from Taiwan to further the husband's schooling. Although their marital relationship had deteriorated, they could not follow through on a divorce because of cultural taboos.

Upon initial presentation, Mrs. A. remained aloof while her husband presented her as the patient. The couple argued incessantly. Mr. A. complained of his wife's dependency, and her unwillingness to perform "wifely" duties including cooking, sex, and social entertaining. The marriage had became polarized over differences related to sex, marital roles, family obligations, work and achievement goals, and gender roles. For Mrs. A., marriage was a necessary undertaking, but symbolized many losses, including her virginity, childhood, father, homeland, and academic strivings. She had subordinated herself to her husband in the "proper role" expected of women within Asian culture; she had responded to the sexual demands of her husband, and dutifully followed him to the United States. She disliked cooking and cleaning. Mr. A. felt she should stay home; she wanted to work. He valued the importance of a social and extended family network; she did not. He willingly performed his culturally defined male roles as protector and patriarch, while she experienced her respective roles as obligations and burdens. In their marital relationship, certain traits were criticized yet accepted as characteristic of basic male and female temperament within the Asian culture. Mr. A.'s volatile temper was condoned as typically male; his dominance was criticized as controlling, yet valued as masculine and protective of women. Mrs. A.'s dependency (e.g., needing to be driven everywhere) was viewed as weak, yet typical of females.

Dynamic content focused on Mrs. A.'s poor self-esteem, issues of self-identity, and conflict over her roles as wife, female, and daughter. Throughout therapy, she struggled with her ambivalence about culturally prescribed gender roles that mitigated against her development of a positive sense of self. She resented her husband's regularly sending money to his parents; as a dutiful eldest son, yet felt guilty that she did not experience the same sense of filial piety that he did. She did not share her husband's wish to have children, yet worried that this meant she was deficient as a woman. Because she did not enjoy the roles "typically associated with" women, she struggled with the feeling that she was being "selfish" by placing herself and her needs over others, a valuation dissonant with cultural expectations.

Therapeutic outcome focused on separation and individuation. The conflicts presented by Mrs. A. often played themselves out in the conflicting contexts of greater freedom within the Western culture versus the greater obligatory demands of the Asian culture. The exposure to alternative roles for women in the United States was empowering because it offered choice. Instead of labeling these as acculturation problems or rebellion against cultural norms and supporting Mrs. A. to be more liberated and Westernized, the focus was on empowering Mrs. A. to choose roles without undermining the values of the Asian culture. Issues and therapists methods were reframed to fit the cultural worldview of Mrs. A. and to be syntonic with cultural values.

While catharsis and free association was encouraged, it was not the free expression of feelings that was stressed, but rather how the expression of feelings could enable Mrs. A. to regulate her feelings better. Free association was made culturally credible by emphasizing the therapists' role as the "knowledgeable authority figure" who would use the information prescriptively.

Therapist neutrality was not always facilitative with this couple. As a Chinese American professional woman, the therapist was a powerful transference object. Selective use of therapist self-disclosure was important in promoting therapeutic growth and self-differentiation. Mrs. A.'s questions to the therapist about her background were framed not as boundary violations or avoidance, but rather as a need to identify with the therapist as a role model to promote therapeutic growth and maturity.

Hierarchical and mirror transferences emerged within the therapeutic relationship. Mrs. A. viewed the therapist as a "wise, benevolent authority figure" (i.e., in a hierarchical regard). She played out unresolved issues with a father who had given her double messages. Mrs. A. had strong achievement strivings consistent with cultural values, yet she received strong and contradicting messages from her father to underachieve, since modesty was more befitting of an Asian female. While she excelled academically, she subordinated these strivings to remain "second best" in order to please her father and to accommodate her husband's career. Consequently, she made excessive demands upon her husband's academic excellence as befitting the ideal Asian male.

As Mrs. A. felt supported and not judged within the therapeutic relationship, she became more open in discussing her views and expectations of marriage, womanhood, and sex. She identified with the therapist, and admired her multiple roles as married woman, mother, career woman, and American-born Chinese. She talked more about the dilemmas of career versus mother roles, became more interested in the therapist's academic credentials, and shared more positive feelings about the therapist's patience, caring, and listening skills. These transference feelings enabled her to come into contact with feelings that her mother had never been a "good enough" mother. While she was angry at her father for holding her back, he was the one with whom she felt more connected. The identification with the therapist also provoked envy, fears of rejection, feelings of inadequacy, and so on; at the same time, it facilitated her acceptance of difference and validation of choice. Her admiration for the therapist's accomplishments as a professional, married, Chinese American woman and mother (i.e., mirror transference) enabled her to give up her view of women as weak and second rate, and Chinese American women as needing to fit a prescribed role. The transference facilitated many feelings associated with both paternal and maternal figures, and provided a safe and nurturing environment for self-growth and individuation. As Mrs. A. defined her own choices for self-identity, the couple agreed on an amicable divorce. At the same time, she had decided to fulfill her filial obligations to her own parents by planning for their retirement.

The second clinical example involves a Puerto Rican female married to a Chinese male who was seen in individual therapy over several years. While marital discord was also the presenting complaint, neither considered divorce as an option. Mrs. B. was characterized by her helplessness, dependency, and emotional lability, while her husband was characterized by his domineering behavior and temper outbursts. The couple argued frequently, often resulting in the husband making physical threats. Mrs. B. would seek asylum with her family.

She viewed her marriage as a permanent arrangement, and used therapy as a safe and supportive haven in which to vent potentially disruptive feelings. Consequently, therapy served a more cathartic function. She sought sympathy about her abusive, controlling, and domineering husband. As therapy progressed, it became clear that she had an investment in maintaining the marriage as status quo, and herself as the victim in her marriage. In fact, she often behaved in ways that escalated her husband's suspiciousness and anger. She would conspire with extended family members to hide information from her husband, and would justify this behavior by claiming that all men had bad tempers. The couple had evolved a cyclical pattern in their arguments, which stalemated in accusations of temperament; she was "hysterical" and he was "domineering and controlling."

While both had chosen to marry outside their culture, and had made many choices in their marriage that differed from their respective cultural norms, they had not come to terms with these decisions. Not having married a Latino male despite her family's disapproval, she was unconsciously invested in "proving" how macho he was. His temper outbursts and domineering jealousy were these proofs. She still felt compelled by her culture to be deferent to men, yet she resented this power over her. By acting out her anger in a passive–aggressive manner, she was able to maintain her image as the helpless female victim when, in fact, she exercised considerable covert control within the marriage. She was only able to define her self-identity in relation to her husband. She felt inadequate in comparison to his creative talents as an artist. Although the couple decided not to have children, she felt guilty and experienced many self-doubts about her adequacy as a female. Ambivalence about her cultural and ethnic identity, however, was not a therapeutic theme.

A "preoedipal" or narcissistic transference formed the basis for therapeutic change. This was viewed as empowering Mrs. B. through a female–female bond with the therapist. While she had defined her life in relationship to her husband and men, the transference relationship validated an empathic relatedness with a woman. Because she had chosen a Chinese therapist, it was important that the therapist did not inadvertently invalidate her Puerto Rican origins. Confrontation of her passive–aggressive behavior by a female was crucial to interrupt the maladaptive patterns she had developed within the marriage. More importantly, engaging her husband in some joint therapy sessions was crucial to maintaining his "dignity" in the face of the anger and aggression she felt. She valued and provoked his domineering and aggressive behavior to prove he was macho enough, while she was simultaneously furious at being overpowered by it. Mr. B. was able to admit how he felt emasculated by some of his wife's behavior. As the couple examined how each provoked and triggered the other to act along certain prescribed cultural and gender patterns of behavior, they were able to correct their maladaptive patterns of communication. Mrs. B. was able to accept the choices she had made in her marriage that differed from family and cultural expectations.

CONCLUSIONS

Psychodynamic psychotherapy can be relevant for women of color if we recognize the importance of cultural competence in theory and practice. We need to change the theory to fit the different perspectives brought by women of color to psychotherapy, and thus to refine the theory to include manifestations due to culture and gender differences. Understanding the influence of culture and gender on therapeutic content, therapeutic method, and the therapeutic relationship constitutes the basis for promoting cultural competence. Delineating and illustrating both problematic and useful concepts contributes to a clearer comprehension of the issues to be addressed in reformulating psychodynamic theory and practice when working with women of color.

REFERENCES

Acosta, F. X., Yamamoto, J., & Evans, L. (1982). *Effective psychotherapy for low income and minority patients.* New York: Plenum Press.

Adams, H. (1976). *The use of Gestalt therapy as an alternative treatment approach used with the Black client.* Paper presented at the First Annual Symposium for Delivery of Mental Health Services to the Black Consumer, Milwaukee, WI.

Benedek, E. (1973). Training the woman resident to be a psychiatrist. *American Journal of Psychiatry, 130,* 1131–1135.

Chin, J. L. (1981). Institutional racism and mental health: An Asian-American perspective. In O. A. Barbarin, P. R. Good, O. M. Pharr, & J. A. Siskind (Eds.), *Institutional racism and community competence* (pp. 44–55). Washington, DC: U.S. Government Printing Office.

Chin, J. L. (1983). Diagnostic considerations in working with Asian-Americans. *American Journal of Orthopsychiatry, 53*(1), 100–109.

Chin, J. L. (1987, April). *Culture and psychotherapy: Towards developing a multicultural framework.* Paper presented at the Annual Meeting of the Massachusetts Psychological Association, Boston.

Chin, J. L., Liem, J. H., Ham, M. D., & Hong, G. K. (Eds.). (1987). *Interactive forum on transference and empathy in psychotherapy with Asian Americans.* Proceedings of the conference cosponsored by South Cove Community Health Center and University of Massachusetts–Boston, Harbor Campus, Boston.

Chodorow, N. (1978). *The reproduction of mothering.* Berkeley: University of California Press.

Comas-Díaz, L. (1988). Cross-cultural mental health treatment. In L. Comas-Díaz & E. E. H. Griffith (Eds.), *Clinical guidelines in cross-cultural mental health* (pp. 335–362). New York: Wiley.

Comas-Díaz, L., & Duncan, J. W. (1985). The cultural context: A factor in assertiveness training with mainland Puerto Rican women. *Psychology of Women Quarterly, 9,* 463–476.

Comas-Díaz, L., & Jacobsen, F. M. (1991). Ethnocultural transference and countertransference in the theapeutic dyad. *American Journal of Orthopsychiatry, 61*(3), 392–402.

Comas-Díaz, L., & Minrath, M. (1985). Psychotherapy with ethnic minority borderline clients. *Psychotherapy, 22*(2), 418–426.

Cross, T. L., Bazron, B. J., Dennis, K. W., & Isaacs, M. R. (1989). *Towards a culturally competent system of care.* Washington, DC: CASSP Technical Assistance Center.

De La Cancela, V. (1985). Toward a sociocultural psychotherapy for low-income ethnic minorities. *Psychotherapy, 22*(2), 427–435.

De La Cancela, V. (1985). A critical analysis of Puerto Rican machismo: Implications for clinical practice. *Psychotherapy, 23*(2), 291–296.

Dewald, P. A. (1971). Transference. In *Psychotherapy: A dynamic approach* (pp. 196–223). New York: Basic Books.

Ford, D. H., & Urban, H. B. (1963). *Systems of psychotherapy: A comparative study.* New York: Wiley.

Freud, S. (1915). Observations on transference love. *Standard Edition, 12,* 157–171.

Gardner, L. (1980). Racial, ethnic and social class considerations in psychotherapy supervision. In A. Hess (Ed.), *Psychotherapy supervision: Theory, research and practice.* New York: Wiley.

Gilligan, C. (1982). *In a different voice.* Cambridge, MA: Harvard University Press.

Giovacchini, P. L. (1972). *Tactics and techniques in psychoanalytic therapy.* New York: Jason Aronson.

Gornick, L. (1986). Developing a new narrative: The woman therapist and the male patient. *Psychoanalytic Psychology, 3*(4), 299–325.

Greenson, R. (1965). The working alliance and the transference neurosis. *Psychoanalytic Quarterly, 34,* 155–181.

Greenson, R., & Wexler, M. (1969). The non-transference relationship in the psychoanalytic situation. *International Journal of Psychoanalysis, 50,* 27–40.

Griffith, M. S. (1977). The influence of race on the psychotherapeutic relationship. *Psychiatry, 40,* 27–40.

Hall, E. T. (1976, July). How cultures collide. *Psychology Today,* pp. 66–97.

Hare-Mustin, R. T. (1983). An appraisal of the relationship between women and psychotherapy: 80 years after the case of Dora. *American Psychologist, 38*(5), 593–601.

Iwasaki, T. (1971). Discussion, cultural aspects of transference and countertransference by G. Ticho. *Bulletin of the Menninger Clinic, 35*(5), 330–334.

Jenkins, Y. (1982). Dissonant expectations: Professional competency vs. personal incompetency. *Aware, 1*(1), 6–13.

Jones, B. E., & Gray, B. A. (1984). Similarities and differences in Black men and women in psychotherapy. *Journal of the National Medical Association, 76*(1), 21–27.

Jou, T. H. (1984). *The tao of I Ching: Way to divination.* Taiwan: Tai Chi Foundation.

Kohut, H. (1971). *The analysis of the self.* New York: International Universities Press.

Kohut, H. (1977). *The restoration of the self.* New York: International Universities Press.

Langs, R. (1974). *Technique of psychoanalytic psychotherapy* (Vol. 2). New York: Jason Aronson.

Langs, R. (1978). The patient's view of the therapist: Reality or fantasy? In *Technique in transition* (pp. 115–138). New York: Jason Aronson.

Lewis, J. M., & Looney, J. G. (1983). *The long struggle: Well-functioning working-class Black families.* New York: Brunner/Mazel.

Mahler, M. S. (1968). *On human symbiosis and the vicissitudes of individuation*. New York: International Universities Press.

Mahler, M. S. (1972). On the first three subphases of the separation–individuation process. *International Journal of Psycho-Analysis, 53*, 333–38.

Marcos, L. R., & Urcuyo, L. (1979). Dynamic psychotherapy with the bilingual patient. *American Journal of Psychotherapy, 33*, 331–338.

Marecek, J., & Hare-Mustin, R. T. (1991). A short history of the future: Feminism and clinical psychology. *Psychology of Women Quarterly, 15*, 521–536.

Miller, J. B. (1976). *Toward a new psychology of women*. Boston: Beacon Press.

McGoldrick, M., Pearce, J. K., & Giordano, J. (Eds.). (1982). *Ethnicity and family therapy*. New York: Guilford Press.

Mitchell, J. (1974). *Psychoanalysis and feminism*. New York: Pantheon.

Mogul, K. (1982). Overview: The sex of the therapist. *American Journal of Psychiatry, 129*, 1–11.

Nobles, W. W. (1980). Extended self: Rethinking the so-called Negro self concept. In R. L. Jones (Ed.), *Black psychology* (2nd ed., pp. 115–133). New York: Harper & Row.

Root, M. (1985). Resolving "other" status: Identity development of biracial individuals. *Women and Therapy, 9*(1), 185–205.

Schacter, J. S., & Butts, H. F. (1968). Transference and countertransference in interracial analysis. *Journal of the American Psychoanalytic Association, 16*, 792–808.

Stevens, E. (1973). Machismo and marianismo. *Transaction Society, 10*(6), 57–63.

Stolorow, R. D., Brandchaft, B., & Atwood, G. E. (1987). *Psychoanalytic treatment: An intersubjective approach*. Hillsdale, NJ: Analytic.

Sue, D. W. (1978). World views and counseling. *Personnel and Guidance Journal, 56*, 458–462.

Sue, S. (1982). Ethnic minority issues in psychology. *American Psychologist, 38*, 583–592.

Suh, C. (1987). *The role of the psychotherapist with Asian clients: Toward transcending the hierarchical relationship*. Paper presented at the Interactive Forum on Transference and Empathy in Psychotherapy with Asian Americans, cosponsored by South Cove Community Health Center and University of Massachusetts–Boston, Harbor Campus. Boston.

Thomas, A., & Sillen, S. (1972). *Racism and psychiatry*. New York: Brunner/Mazel.

Thomas, M. B., & Dansby, P. G. (1985). Black clients: Family structures, therapeutic issues, and strengths. *Psychotherapy, 22*(2), 398–407.

Toupin, E. (1980). Counseling Asians: Psychotherapy in the context of racism and Asian-American history. *American Journal of Orthopsychiatry, 50*(1), 76–86.

Tseng, W. (1973). The concept of personality in Confucian thought. *Psychiatry, 36*, 191–202.

Westkott, M. (1986). Historical and developmental roots of female dependency. *Psychotherapy, 23*(2), 213–220.

Wolstein, B. (1983). The pluralism of perspectives: On countertransference. *Contemporary Psychoanalysis, 19*(3), 506–521.

Wu, D. (1987). *Achieving intra-cultural and inter-cultural understanding in psychotherapy with Asian Americans*. Paper presented at the Interactive Forum on Transference and Empathy in Psychotherapy with Asian Americans, cosponsored by South Cove Community Health Center and University of Massachusetts–Boston, Harbor Campus. Boston.

Yamamoto, J. (1982). *Beyond Buddhism*. Downers Grove, IL.: Intervarsity Press.

Yamamoto, J., & Chang, C. (1987). *Empathy for the family and the individual in the social context*. Paper presented at the Interactive Forum on Transference and Empathy in Psychotherapy with Asian Americans, cosponsored by South Cove Community Health Center and University of Massachusetts–Boston, Harbor Campus, Boston.

Yamamoto, J., James, Q., & Palley, N. (1968). Cultural problems in psychiatric therapy. *General Archives of Psychiatry*, *19*, 45–49.

Zaphiropoulos, M. L. (1982). Transcultural parameters in the transference and countertransference. *Journal of the American Academy of Psychoanalysis*, *10*(4), 571–584.

Cognitive–Behavioral Therapy

Sandra Y. Lewis

> Well, chilern whar dar is so much racket dar must be something out o'kilter . . . Dat man ober dar say dat women needs to be helped into carriages, and lifted ober ditches, and to have de best place every whar. Nobody ever help me into carriages, or ober mud puddles, or gives me any best places . . . and arn't I a woman? Look at me! Look at my arm! . . . I have plowed, and planted, and gathered into barns and no man could head me—and arn't I a woman? . . . I have borne five chilern and seen 'em mos' all sold off into slavery, and when I cried out with a mother's grief, none but Jesus heard—and arn't I a woman.
> —SOJOURNER TRUTH (quoted in Beal, 1970, p. 342)

> When your race is fighting for survival—to eat, to be clothed, to be housed, to be left in peace—as a woman, you know who you are. You are the principle of life, of survival and endurance. . . . For the Chicano woman battling for her people, the family—the big family—is a fortress against the genocidal forces in the outside world. It is the source of strength for a people whose identity is constantly being whittled away. The mother is the center of that fortress.
> —MARIA VARELA (quoted in Sutherland, 1970, p. 376)

The words of Sojourner Truth and Maria Varela illustrate how life as a woman of color has long been and continues to be a complex state of being. Our gender roles are often inextricably tied to the plight of our oppressed races. As we read Sojourner Truth's comparison of her experience as a woman to what was considered an appropriate lifestyle for a woman, it becomes clear that at a societal level her experience was neither understood nor accepted as a valid female experience. Indeed, being a woman of color continues to be a blend of ethnicity and gender deserving of special consideration.

Women of color share many common bonds. Their ethnic and cultural heritage is generally one that emphasizes as key elements family (nuclear and extended), community, spirituality, and respect for authority. This ethnic cultural heritage, particularly the sense of interconnectedness with family and community and spirituality, figures prominently in understanding women of color. Our very identities, styles of coping and ways of relating are heavily influenced by our ethnic backgrounds, which most often include factors such as colonization, racism, and sexism. This makes for a quite unique and multifaceted experience, spawning a person who is equally unique and multifaceted in her needs.

The advent of this book calls forth an era in the mental health field wherein the special needs of women of color will be given much deserved attention. As we enter this era we must examine ways in which varied therapeutic approaches can be utilized to meet these needs in a culture- and gender-sensitive manner. The present chapter examines cognitive–behavioral therapy (CBT) approaches with women of color.

COGNITIVE–BEHAVIORAL THERAPY: HISTORICAL BACKGROUND AND THEORETICAL FOUNDATIONS

Historical Background

Although in the past 20 years CBT has rapidly become a widely used and accepted approach, its inception was accompanied by much debate and criticism by more traditional behavior therapists. Ledwidge (1978) likened CBT to traditional psychoanalysis. He noted that CBT focuses on modification of cognitive processes thought to mediate behavior, much like psychoanalytic approaches focus upon gaining insight as a means to behavior change. He suggested that CBT would detract from behavior therapy's good reputation, if it could not be empirically proven that CBT had greater efficacy than traditional verbal therapies.

Wolpe (1976) asserted that cognition had always been accounted for in the practice of behavior therapy. He clarified that cognitive processes are acknowledged and utilized in the behavior change process. He proposed that CBT offered a foundation for the integration of behavior therapy and psychoanalysis. However, Wilson and O'Leary (1980) offer several distinctions between these two schools of thought. They note that the focus on cognition in behavior therapy is primarily concerned with "conscious thought processes, rather than unconscious, symbolic meanings" (p. 280). They clarify that behavior therapists are concerned with "how" rather than why a client cognitively distorts. They argue that the cognitive methods of behavior therapy are "explicitly formulated and testable" (p. 280), whereas psychodynamic concepts are more vaguely conceived. Beck (1976) asserts that cognitive therapy methods are more efficient than psychodynamic approaches in terms of the length of time spent in therapy and the time needed to train the therapist.

Despite the initial criticisms and debate among behavior therapists, CBT approaches continued to grow and receive acclaim as effective treatments. Following is a description of the essential elements and basic tenets of these approaches.

Theoretical Foundations

CBT was in full swing by the mid-1970s. The works of Ellis (1970), Beck (1976), Bandura (1977), and Meichenbaum (1977) are a few examples of pioneer accomplishments in this area. Today, a large number of CBT methods and techniques have been put forward (Dobson & Block, 1988). Though somewhat varied in focus and/or method CBT approaches and techniques share some core assumptions. Dobson and Block (1988) delineate the following fundamentals of CBT:

1. Cognitive activity affects behavior.
2. Cognitive activity may be monitored and altered.
3. Desired behavior change may be affected through cognitive change. (p. 4)

In the CBT framework, cognition is viewed in three ways (Marzillier, 1980; Meichenbaum, 1986). First, there are cognitive events. These are one's conscious thoughts and images and thus are readily identifiable. Beck (1976) terms these events automatic thoughts, while Meichenbaum (1977) refers to them as the internal dialogue. Beck (1976) describes automatic thoughts as discrete, unquestioned ideas that often occur outside one's awareness. Meichenbaum (1986) noted that "internal dialogue," incorporates attributions, expectations and their concomitant emotions. Cognitive events influence our behavior, feelings and assessments of situations. They are likely to occur when one is learning or integrating a new skill; when making choices or judgments; and when anticipating or having a strong emotional experience (Meichenbaum, 1986).

Cognitive processes (Marzillier, 1980; Meichenbaum, 1986) represent the second way in which cognition is viewed in the CBT framework. They are the manner in which we process information. Cognitive processes are the "what" and "how" of selecting the information to which we attend. These processes operate as we formulate our perceptions. They are the means by which we make appraisals and assign meaning to information. Cognitive processes generally occur out of one's awareness (Meichenbaum, 1986). Beck (1976) and Beck, Rush, Shaw, and Emery (1979) speak of cognitive distortions. These writings note that when there is psychological distress, there are errors in one's reasoning ability. Thus, information is processed in a distorted manner. Beck and Weishaar (1989) explain that during times of distress one's perceptions of events become "highly selective, egocentric and rigid" (p. 23). Cognitive functions that normally operate to facilitate reality testing, concentration and reasoning are weakened. Beck et al. (1979) outline a number of cognitive distortions. Examples include arbitrary inference, drawing a specific conclusion without supporting evidence or in spite of competing evidence; and overgeneralization, making extreme rules based upon one or a few particular events, and applying them to a wide variety of situations, including dissimilar situations.

Meichenbaum and Gilmore (1984) outline a number of other cognitive processes. One of these is "metacognition," that is, our knowledge about our own cognitive processes, as well as our ability to guide and control these processes (Meichenbaum & Gilmore, 1984). This process differs from those noted above in that it is a proactive strategy: It affords us the opportunity to step back and evaluate our thinking. We become aware of the ways in which we may produce cognitive distortions, and are thus empowered to change.

Lastly, in the CBT framework, there are cognitive structures. These are deep-seated beliefs, assumptions, and schemata that function to guide screening, coding and categorizing of information (Beck et al., 1979; Meichenbaum, 1986). Cognitive structures function as templates guiding our perceptions and interpretations. Haaga and Davison (1986) note that these schemata that influence thinking patterns are likely learned early in life and may be conceived "as rules or assumptions for making sense of one's environment" (p. 250). Beck et al. (1979) note that "dysfunctional schemata" give rise to negative thinking patterns.

RELEVANCE OF CBT FOR WOMEN OF COLOR

In recent years, an increased amount of attention has been given to women's issues in the CBT and behavior therapy literature (Blechman, 1984; Davis & Padesky, 1989; Fodor, 1988; Solomon & Rothblum, 1986; Veronen & Kilpatrick, 1983; Wolfe, 1987; Wolfe & Fodor, 1975). Wolfe and Fodor (1975) and Fodor (1988) modified some theoretical foundations of CBT to address women's issues. They adapted Albert Ellis' irrational beliefs (1970) and outlined some potentially stress-inducing beliefs often developed by women in the sex-role socialization process. These include:

1. I must be loved and approved by every significant person in my life. (Wolfe & Fodor, 1975, p. 48)
2. Other people's needs count more than my own. (Fodor, 1988, p. 98)
3. It is easier to avoid than to face life's difficulties. (Wolfe & Fodor, 1975, p. 48)

4. I need a strong person to lean on or provide for me. (Fodor, 1988, p. 99)
5. I don't have control over my emotions. (Fodor, 1988, p. 99)

Wolfe and Fodor in both of these writings also offer ways of disputing the beliefs outlined above. These authors have utilized this approach in assertiveness training with women. Two examples follow:

- Disputation for Belief 1: Why would it be terrible if the other person thought I was a "bitch" or rejected me? How does that make me a worthless, hopeless human being? (Wolfe & Fodor, 1975, p. 48)
- Disputation for Belief 5: No one else can make me anxious. I make myself feel anxious by the way I view the situation. I can learn to control and change my feelings. (Fodor, 1988, p. 99)

Davis and Padesky (1989) suggest that CBT offers special advantages for women. These authors provide an in-depth discussion of the parallels and overlap between CBT and the feminist philosophy of psychotherapy, considering gender an essential variable in the therapeutic process. They (1989) argue that taking account of gender in the therapeutic process mandates knowledge of the feminist treatment approach forwarded for countering "the damaging effects of a paternalistic system" (p. 536). Davis and Padesky further support the feminist principle of an egalitarian therapeutic relationship as congruent with cognitive therapy. Beck et al. (1979) and Meichenbaum (1986) do, in fact, discuss the therapeutic relationship as a collaborative one. Therapists work to involve clients actively in the process of understanding their problems, developing skills, and trying out new behaviors and/or ways of thinking. Client–therapist discussion of alternative methods, techniques, and resources is common to both cognitive–behavioral and feminist therapies. Davis and Padesky (1989) note that this process takes the mystery out of therapy, removes the therapist from the position of the all-knowing authority and fosters the client's personal power.

Davis and Padesky (1989) acknowledge that both client and therapist operate within the broader social and political systems that support certain values, attitudes, and sex-role socialization patterns. Therapists are urged to be aware of their own belief system with respect to women and the manner in which the social context influences the female experience. Davis and Padesky (1989) offer a four-dimensional framework for conceptualizing hypotheses regarding a woman's experience. The four dimensions are: (1) ethnic/racial heritage, (2) socioeconomic status, (3) religious/spiritual affiliations, and (4) sex-role values.

They suggest that evaluation of these domains will assist the therapist in viewing a woman's belief systems. They also provide several case examples consistent with the foregoing philosophy and illustrative of therapeutic attention to the contextual experiences of women as well as content issues (e.g., physical experiences, relationships, parenting) that often arise in therapy with women.

Blechman, in editing a volume entitled *Behavior Modification with Women* (1984), indicates her intent to highlight being female as a context in bringing this project to fruition. She comments that while behaviorists have long emphasized the influence of environment upon behavior, the differences between male and female experiences have often gone without attention. Her edited volume offers chapters in which core issues in utilizing behavior modification with women, as well as behavioral and cognitive–behavioral treatment of disorders common in women, are discussed. Contributing authors (e.g., Norman, Johnson, & Miller, 1984; Padawer & Goldfried, 1984) give attention to the influence that sex-role socialization and expectancies may have upon the development and maintenance of psychological disturbance in women. Specific disorders and issues addressed include: assertiveness (Linehan, 1984); sexuality (Hoon, Krop, & Wincze, 1984); depression (Norman et al., 1984); anxiety disorders (Padawer & Goldfried, 1984); and weight disorders (Fodor & Thal, 1984). A laudable characteristic of the contributions to this volume is the authors' attempt not only to address skill deficits and problem behaviors within individuals but also have an impact on variables in the natural environmental settings (e.g., work, home) that influence treatment and generalization of treatment effects.

Solomon and Rothblum (1986) review literature relevant to understanding stress and coping in women. Specifically, they aim to highlight women's strategies for resolving stressful situations. Their review is prepared for an audience of behavior therapists. These authors discuss research outlining stressors that appear predominantly in women; stressors related to women's roles; coping strategies most often employed by women; and both the benefits and the liabilities involved in women's uses of social support systems. In their conclusion Solomon and Rothblum raise questions pertinent to the understanding and treatment of women. They question the effect that relative power may play in women's choices of coping strategies, and they acknowledge the social context of women's experiences. These authors cleverly point out that while women are socialized to have major responsibility for caretaking and nurturing, these roles are not highly valued in society. Solomon and Rothblum suggest that continuation of this pattern is likely to have a detrimental effect on women's mental health, while sparing men their share of responsibilities.

Veronen and Kilpatrick (1983) describe a stress-inoculation training program for rape victims (an issue predominant among women). Despite the societal tendency to "blame the victim" in incidences of rape, Veronen and Kilpatrick define rape broadly, to include any instance in which "a woman considers herself to have had nonconsensual sexual activity" (p. 342). The authors acknowledge that this definition relies heavily on the victim's viewpoint. However, as cognitive–behaviorists they regard this subjectivity as most appropriate, since the victim's perspective is likely to have the most profound influence on her adjustment. Veronen and Kilpatrick provide a cognitive–behavioral framework for conceptualizing the rape victim's experience as well as providing her with efficacious treatment.

Wolfe (1987) describes a cognitive–behavioral group therapy approach for women. She outlines the use of rational–emotive therapy (RET) in combination with other CBT approaches. Wolfe asserts that RET is in keeping with the guidelines of feminist therapy. The author indicates that RET provides methodology for countering the "shoulds and musts" inherent in female sex-role socialization. Other reasons cited for RET's congruence with a feminist approach are client involvement in setting therapy goals and choosing techniques, as well as the fact that RET offers women means for striving to achieve the changes necessary for an egalitarian society. An important element of groups derived from this approach is "consciousness raising." The aim here is to examine critically ways which sex-role socialization stereotypes interfere with a woman's optimal functioning. Wolfe's overall approach encourages women to become personally empowered by setting their own goals and learning to conceptualize and manage their difficulties.

Summary

While the foregoing in no way represents an exhaustive review of the literature on cognitive–behavioral approaches with women, it represents a sample of important work in this area. The examples illustrate that gender has gained an increased amount of attention in CBT as a context worthy of consideration in theorization about and treatment of mental health issues.

Advantages of CBT for Women of Color

CBT offers a number of advantages for women of color. As is discussed above, the therapeutic relationship is a collaborative one in which therapist and client work together to define problems clearly, delineate alternative solutions, and test the viability of alternatives. This approach demonstrates respect for the client and acknowledges her ability to be in control of her life and to make necessary changes. The client is not subjugated by the authority of the therapist. This kind of acknowledgement is key for women of color, who may often experience a lowering of their status due to race and gender.

CBT encourages the client to take credit for gains and successes. Clients are encouraged to reinforce themselves (Meichenbaum, 1986) when they manage problem situations. When a client encounters a setback, these are utilized as learning experiences, opportunities for growth, a chance to change or improve their strategies. This helps to protect the client from internalizing setbacks and promotes the idea that there are options. These factors can be of particular importance for women of color, who may often be confronted with limited external resources.

Lastly, within CBT approaches, emotions are interpreted as signals to problem solve (Haaga & Davison, 1986). Emotions such as anxiety, frustration, or depression become indicators alerting us to a particular issue, rather than states that overwhelm personal resources. This type of approach validates all experience as useful to one's personal growth and change process.

Possible Pitfalls of CBT for Women of Color

As noted in the opening of this chapter, the experiences of a woman of color are molded by her own unique blend of ethnicity and gender. Gender role and race/ethnic issues and beliefs are interwoven. A cognitive–behavioral therapist's failure to recognize this could hamper the use of CBT approaches with women of color. Race/ethnicity, gender, and the interaction of these must be considered in the all elements of the treatment process.

Therapists must explore their values and beliefs regarding women of color. There is a history of discriminatory practices against people of color, which forms a significant part of the societal context in which any therapy is practiced. This history has generated certain beliefs and stereotypes about women of color. Cognitive–behavioral therapists must take care to evaluate their values and beliefs for those elements that may have potentially negative influences upon the therapeutic process. Failure to do so may lead to erroneous assumptions, which in turn lead to damaging behavior on the part of the therapist that can have a negative impact on the client.

SOCIETAL CONTEXT OF CBT AND WOMEN OF COLOR

Power and CBT

The empowering nature of CBT has been highlighted throughout this chapter. For women of color CBT offers a means for recognizing, reaching, and utilizing the internal power necessary for change.

A basic tenet of CBT is that one's thinking influences one's affect and behavior. Thoughts represent one's interpretations and as such play a central role in guiding feelings and actions. Within the CBT model a factor central to change is awareness of the relationship between one's thoughts, behavior, affect, and the consequences of these. Clients are guided in understanding ways in which their appraisals and perceptions influence their difficulties. Clients learn that the ability to change their difficulties lies within them. Creating new thought patterns is a means for creating new emotional and behavioral responses. Clients become empowered when they are able to resolve problems by changing their thinking.

The goal of positive self-attribution is another empowering element of CBT. It fosters increased self-esteem and confidence in one's ability to achieve desired goals, and a sense of personal control. CBT fortifies the personal power that comes when one takes responsibility for making change happen.

Within the CBT framework, failures and/or disappointments are seen as opportunities for learning. Clients are helped to analyze these experiences systematically and generate more options. It is empowering to know that one is not "stuck" when things don't work out as expected. Furthermore, cognitive–behavioral therapists guide clients to anticipate possible problems (Meichenbaum, 1986) and prepare for these. Clients learn that problems can be managed when they arise.

While CBT can foster a sense of power through creating new perspectives, facilitating positive self-attribution, and using disappointments as opportunities for growth, one must remain aware that women of color face the societal realities of colonization, racism, sexism, and classism. These must be not only acknowledged but even confronted in the therapeutic process. In fact, a woman of color may enter therapy due to her experiences with racism and other forms of discrimination. These issues will not be eradicated through attempting to change women's perceptions of their experiences. Racism and discrimination do not originate in the thoughts of women of color. However, CBT can be utilized to facilitate a woman's coping and her ability to take action in discriminatory situations. Crucial to this process is strengthening the woman's ability to counter internalization of negative messages from the external world. Once this occurs, the woman may choose to pursue filing a grievance or taking other legal action against discriminatory practices. Therapists may be expected to explore such options with their clients and/or provide support for clients who choose these options. Such actions also serve to support the externalization of discriminatory practices and the internalization of personal worth and power. It is important to note that these ends are necessary regardless of the outcome of any grievance or legal actions.

Reality Issues and CBT

In addition to the realities of colonization, racism, sexism, and classism, women of color may also face basic survival issues such as poverty or homelessness. These or other reality issues may be presented during the process of therapy. CBT approaches such as problem solving offer a means of focusing on such urgent issues. This approach capitalizes on empowering elements of CBT, in that a number of alternatives are generated, emotions are utilized as signals, and setbacks are treated as catalysts for personal growth. There is recognition that any of a client's experiences can foster her growth and personal empowerment.

APPLYING CBT WITH WOMEN OF COLOR: GUIDELINES AND CLINICAL ILLUSTRATIONS

The field of CBT offers a wide range of approaches and techniques. Included in this range are assertiveness skills training and cognitive restructuring. These are elaborated below with special attention to their application with women of color. Since spirituality tends to play a major role in the lives of women of color, an approach combining spirituality and CBT is also described. In the elaboration of these clinical approaches, the focus will be upon two groups, Puerto Rican women and African American women.

Earlier in this chapter I discussed Wolfe and Fodor's work on adapting the theoretical tenets of CBT to correspond to women's issues. While these beliefs may be common to some women of color, there are a number of other beliefs that are shared by some African American women and that have developed out of a combination of racial and gender socialization experiences. These are as follows:

1. Life is a struggle. Everything I do must involve struggle.
2. I must be strong and unemotional and do everything.
3. Showing emotions means I'm "weak," "falling apart," or "breaking down."

Countering these beliefs facilitates a woman's development of more encouraging, supportive, and empowering ways of thinking and behaving. This can be accomplished by sharing alternative ways of viewing experiences and helping women formulate positive self-statements and beliefs that support these alternatives. It is useful to assess the woman's experience for the presence of examples, beliefs, and so on that counter the above stress-inducing beliefs. Following are some ways of countering these beliefs:

- Alternative Belief 1: Life often presents us with challenges. I can use the skills I have to meet these challenges and learn new skills from handling tough situations. Challenges are opportunities; I deserve some ease in my life and I can make that happen.
- Alternative Belief 2: It's okay to say no; I can take a break when I feel tired. Showing emotions can be a show of strength/assertiveness/comfort with myself. Why is it necessary to be all things to all people? Other people can be responsible for themselves. It's okay to get help.

- Alternative Belief 3: How does crying inhibit one from taking action? I am in control of my emotions. I can release my emotions in ways that help me feel better and take action.

These alternatives may be utilized in conjunction with other interventions such as those in the following descriptions. Thorough and continuous assessment of each client's needs will facilitate determination of the most appropriate combination of interventions.

Assertiveness training for women has been given a good deal of attention in the field of CBT. Comas-Díaz and Duncan (1985) describe an assertiveness training program utilized with Puerto Rican women who had recently relocated to the mainland, United States. These authors were apt to point out that while assertiveness is valued and useful in the United States, it is often discouraged within Puerto Rican culture, particularly among women. Thus, any assertiveness training with Puerto Rican women must address its dissonance with Puerto Rican cultural values and practices (Comas-Díaz & Duncan, 1985). The training program described by Comas-Díaz & Duncan, (1985) addressed this issue. Participants developed appropriate assertive responses while adhering to cultural norms such as respect for one's elders and responsibility to one's family. In addition, this program addressed issues related to minority status in the United States. Assertiveness as related to issues of sexism, racism and discrimination was included in the training.

Comas-Díaz and Duncan (1985) were careful to teach women to examine the consequences of being assertive versus being nonassertive. Specific examples were utilized from the women's cultural and familial contexts, through which they were able to evaluate potential consequences of asserting or not asserting themselves. This provided the women with the information necessary to make reasonable choices about their behavior, which is crucial given that women are sometimes more highly valued when they are passive and are often punished rather than rewarded for the behaviors encouraged by assertiveness training programs (Fodor, 1988).

Cognitive restructuring refers to the process of helping clients delineate and change dysfunctional thoughts and thought patterns. Important elements of this process are to decrease self-punitive behavior while increasing those thoughts which facilitate better coping and management of problem situations. For women of color it may also be useful to capitalize upon those cultural values and practices that facilitate personal empowerment. Following is a case example of an African American woman, Barbara, that illustrates this approach. All identifying data have been changed to protect the client's confidentiality.

Barbara presented in tears with her 13-year-old son, who was quite oppositional. Each time she described her son's refusal to listen to her she became tearful. Her attempts to engage him in dialogue were met with withdrawal or verbal hostility. Upon exploring their relationship, Barbara revealed feeling helpless (e.g., "I don't know what to do"; "I have tried ..."; "I can't ..."). Due to a long-term illness and childhood memories of an abusive father, she did not employ corporal punishment. She preferred verbal reasoning and other forms of punishment (e.g., taking away privileges). However, she was ineffectual at enforcing punishments and rules. During discussion, she revealed her perception that her long history of illness and childhood memories of family troubles had left her feeling inadequate as a person and as a parent. At times she had found strength (i.e., perseverance) through prayer.

Her use of prayer was encouraged, and it was pointed out that her difficulty enforcing rules gave her son permission to break rules. Examples of her adequacy as a mother and a person were highlighted, and we developed firm disciplinary statements and measures for use with her son. During therapy sessions, I modeled ways of interacting with her son as a firm yet caring authority figure. As Barbara took on this posture at home, her son's behavior improved. Each time she reverted to her nonassertive behavior, his oppositionality increased. Setbacks were predicted and normalized. Biblical scriptures and prayer were used as a means of helping her cope with and learn from setbacks. As she became aware of the interactional patterns, more comfortable with her new stance as a caring yet firm authority figure, and her self-esteem improved, she was more competent in her parenting and her son's behavior greatly improved.

Lastly, I will describe an approach I have developed and utilized with African American women that translates CBT into a spiritual system of beliefs and practices incorporating cultural concepts and values common to women of African descent. Since spirituality is central in the lives of many African American women, a psychospiritual approach such as this is often perceived as congruent with their lifestyle, values, and personal practices or rituals. This approach is also in keeping with the African concept of oneness of psyche/mind and spirit. Nobles (1980) notes that religion was so interwoven into the natural fabric of everyday life that many African tribes had no word for religion in their language.

Paralleling CBT, many spiritual beliefs and practices adhere to the idea that our thoughts influence our experiences (behavioral, emotional, etc.). Spiritual practices such as prayer, meditation, visualization, and affirmations mirror the imagery techniques and positive self-statements of CBT. However, these spiritual practices add the element of belief in a higher and supernatural power which is most often an integral part of the cultural experience of African American women. "Prayer changes things" is a common expression within many sectors of the African American community. Meditation is viewed as a form of prayer. It can be useful during meditations or discussions to incorporate gospel music, African drumming, or other music common to African American women's cultural experience.

My psychospiritual approach has been implemented in a small group format as half- or full-day workshops/retreats. This format is consistent with African cultural values, which encourage community unity, networking, and support. Mbiti (1969) summarizes this value in the expression, "I am because we are; and because we are, therefore, I am" (p. 108).

As a group leader I define myself as a guide and collaborator. Each woman expresses her goal and any concerns regarding the process are explored. Concerns are viewed as opportunities for learning and growth, as are setbacks in CBT approaches.

The day begins with meditations and/or visualizations aimed at relaxation and creating a comfortable safe space in which to explore one's inner world and work towards one's goal(s). A subsequent imagery exercise helps participants create a "guide" to whom they can turn for support or information throughout the group process. Images and ideas included in this exercise are based on shared cultural experiences. Africa is offered as a place participants may choose to go to meet with their "guide." The concept of a "guide" is likened to cultural traditions of ancestors being available for support in spirit—whether they are alive or not—and to historical figures such as Harriet Tubman serving as role models of accomplishment. The African concept of oneness among humans and other life forms is also utilized to describe the various forms spiritual guidance may take (Mbiti, 1969). A "guide" might be an historical figure, a minister, a grandparent, the voice of wisdom, or it might take the form of a tree or an animal. Music that incorporates nature sounds (e.g., birds, ocean) also support this concept.

Discussion follows each exercise, wherein core beliefs and feelings are revealed. Interactions between these beliefs, feelings, and behavior are noted. The core belief that consistently arises is "Life is a struggle; everything I do must involve struggle." The women discuss how the history of African American people's struggle for abolition of slavery, desegregation of schools, equal rights, and so on fostered an expectation of struggle in all aspects of their lives. They often note that this idea was supported through messages from their families as well as the experiences of their families. Women often perceive their strength and personal power as existing because they are struggling with many problem situations. Personal power and capability are reframed as existing within us whether or not we have problems. An ending meditation, described below, is conducted to help solidify this reframing.

Cognitive structures (i.e., core organizing principles or core beliefs) are also addressed through an imagery exercise that facilitates talking to "the child within" the adult. If needed, participants are instructed that they can utilize their guides for spiritual support during this exercise. This particular exercise allows participants to begin pinpointing those life experiences that lead to their development of some limiting beliefs.

The group process ends with an imagery exercise designed to have participants experience their personal power. If they choose to do so, they may imagine experiencing their personal power in a problem situation.

Participants are encouraged to sense their personal power whether or not they develop a potential solution to the problem in that particular visualization. They are reminded that their "guides," the knowledge they have obtained from the day, and their personal power are always available to them. Thus, if a resolution is not obtained by the end of our time together, they have the resources they need to reach a resolution.

As a final exercise, we join hands in our "sisterhood circle." This symbolizes the resources we have obtained from our community support that remain available to us even when we are apart. During the circle, personal power is also reaffirmed, sometimes through repetition of affirmations.

Upon follow-up, most women reveal that the psychospiritual process aided their movement through difficult or stagnant situations. However, more importantly, participants reveal a stronger sense of personal power and an ability not only to manage difficulties but also to experience accomplishment with joy and ease. It is important to note that some of the cultural concepts included in this approach may be shared by other women of color. Thus, with some adaptations, this approach may prove equally beneficial to other groups.

CONCLUSION

Psychotherapy with women of color presents a complex set of variables for mental health professionals. The interaction between gender roles and culture must be taken into account. The foregoing chapter has illustrated some of what CBT can offer women of color. Elements such as the collaborative relationship between client and therapist, the goal of positive self-attribution regarding therapeutic gains, and emotions as signals to problem solve have been highlighted as empowerment tools inherent in this theoretical approach. Specific details are provided regarding CBT as a means of empowering women of color to address the emotional challenges of their inner world as well as to utilize CBT approaches to address their outer realities, such as issues of poverty and racism. The need to address the disparity between cultural values and skills sometimes taught within CBT techniques has been discussed. A psychospiritual approach for African American women, which translates CBT into a culturally appropriate therapeutic strategy, illustrates one way cultural values can become an integral part of the healing, learning, and growing process in psychotherapy for women of color.

REFERENCES

Bandura, A. (1977). *Social learning theory.* Englewood Cliffs, NJ: Prentice Hall.
Beal, F. M. (1970). Double jeopardy: To be black and female. In R. Morgan (Ed.), *Sisterhood is powerful* (pp. 340–353). New York: Random House.

Beck, A. T. (1976). *Cognitive therapy and the emotional disorders.* Madison, CT: International Universities Press.

Beck, A. T., Rush, A. J., Shaw, B. F., & Emery, G. (1979). *Cognitive therapy of depression.* New York: Guilford Press.

Beck, A. T., & Weishaar, M. (1989). Cognitive therapy. In A. Freeman, K. M. Simon, L. E. Beutler, & H. Arkowitz (Eds.), *Comprehensive handbook of cognitive therapy* (pp. 21–36). New York: Plenum Press.

Blechman, E. A. (Ed.). (1984). *Behavior modification with women.* New York: Guilford Press.

Comas-Díaz, L., & Duncan, J. W. (1985). The cultural context: A factor in assertiveness training with mainland Puerto Rican women. *Psychology of Women Quarterly, 9*(4), 463–476.

Davis, D., & Padesky, C. (1989). Enhancing cognitive therapy with women. In A. Freeman, K. M. Simon, L. E. Beutler, & H. Arkowitz (Eds.), *Comprehensive handbook of cognitive therapy* (pp. 535–557). New York: Plenum Press.

Dobson, K. S., & Block, L. (1988). Historical and philosophical bases of the cognitive–behavioral therapies. In K. S. Dobson (Ed.), *Handbook of cognitive–behavioral therapies* (pp. 3–38). New York: Guilford Press.

Ellis, A. (1970). *The essence of rational psychotherapy: A comprehensive approach to treatment.* New York: Institute for Rational Living.

Fodor, I. G. (1988). Cognitive behavior therapy: Evaluation of theory and practice for addressing women's issues. In M. A. Dutton-Douglas & L. E. Walker (Eds.), *Feminist psychotherapies: Integration of therapeutic and feminist systems* (pp. 91–117). Norwood, NJ: Ablex.

Fodor, I. G., & Thal, J. (1984). Weight disorders: overweight and anorexia. In E. A. Blechman (Ed.), *Behavior modification with women* (pp. 373–398). New York: Guilford Press.

Haaga, D. A., & Davison, G. C. (1986). Cognitive change methods. In F. H. Kanfer & A. P. Goldstein (Eds.), *Helping people change.* New York: Plenum Press.

Hoon, E. F., Krop, H. D., & Wincze, J. P. (1984). Sexuality. In E. A. Blechman (Ed.), *Behavior modification with women* (pp. 113–142). New York: Guilford Press.

Ledwidge, B. (1978). Cognitive behavior modification: A step in the wrong direction? *Psychological Bulletin, 85,* 353–375.

Linehan, M. M. (1984). Interpersonal effectiveness in assertive situations. In E. A. Blechman (Ed.), *Behavior modification with women* (pp. 143–169). New York: Guilford Press.

Marzillier, J. S. (1980). Cognitive therapy and behavioral practice. *Behaviour Research and Therapy, 18,* 249–258.

Mbiti, J. S. (1969). *African religions and philosophies.* Garden City, NY: Anchor Books.

Meichenbaum, D. (1977). *Cognitive behavior modification: An integrative approach.* New York: Plenum Press.

Meichenbaum, D. (1986). Cognitive-behavior modification. In F. H. Kanfer & A. P. Goldstein (Eds.), *Helping people change.* New York: Plenum Press.

Meichenbaum, D., & Gilmore, J. B. (1984). The nature of unconscious processes: A cognitive behavioral perspective. In K. S. Bowers & D. Meichenbaum (Eds.), *The unconscious reconsidered* (pp. 273–298). New York: Wiley.

Nobles, W. (1980). African philosophy: Foundations for Black psychology. In R. Jones (Ed.), *Black psychology* (2nd ed., pp. 23–36). New York: Harper & Row.

Norman, W. H., Johnson, B. A., & Miller, I. W. III. (1984). Depression: A behavioral–cognitive approach. In E. A. Blechman (Ed.), *Behavior modification with women* (pp. 275–307). New York: Guilford Press.

Padawer, W. J., & Goldfried, M. R. (1984). Anxiety-related disorders, fears and phobias. In E. A. Blechman (Ed.), *Behavior modification with women* (pp. 341–372). New York: Guilford Press.

Solomon, L. J., & Rothblum, E. D. (1986). Stress, coping, and social support in women. *Behavior Therapist, 9,* 199–204.

Sutherland, E. (1970). An introduction. In R. Morgan (Ed.), *Sisterhood is powerful* (pp. 376–379). New York: Random House.

Veronen, L. J., & Kilpatrick, D. G. (1983). Stress management for rape victims. In D. Meichenbaum & M. Jaremko (Eds.), *Stress reduction and prevention.* New York: Plenum Press.

Wilson, G. T., & O'Leary, K. D. (1980) *Principles of behavior therapy.* Englewood, Cliffs, NJ: Prentice-Hall.

Wolfe, J. L. (1987). Cognitive behavioral group therapy for women. In C. M. Brody (Ed.), *Women's therapy groups: Paradigms of feminist treatment* (pp. 163–173). New York: Springer.

Wolfe, J. L., & Fodor, I. G. (1975). A cognitive/behavioral approach to modifying assertive behavior in women. *Counseling Psychologist, 5*(4), 45–59.

Wolpe, J. (1976). Behavior therapy and its malcontents: II. Multimodal eclecticism, cognitive exclusivism, and "exposure" empiricism. *Journal of Behavior Therapy and Experimental Psychiatry, 7,* 109–116.

9

Family Therapy: The Cases of African American and Hispanic Women

Nancy Boyd-Franklin
Nydia García-Preto

The field of family therapy has grown considerably in the last 30 years. Since the late 1970s, underlying assumptions based on gender have been questioned (McGoldrick, Anderson, & Walsh, 1989), and within the last 10 years the field has begun to explore ethnic, cultural, and racial differences in therapy (McGoldrick, Pearce, & Giordano, 1982). In applying family therapy concepts to African American and Hispanic families, authors such as Bernal (1982), Hines and Boyd-Franklin (1982), Boyd-Franklin (1989), Falicov (1982), and García-Preto (1982) have demonstrated the importance of understanding and respecting cultural differences when engaging families in therapy.

African culture, brought by slaves to the Caribbean islands, Central America, and parts of South America, has influenced the culture of some Hispanics and accounts for similarities between African Americans and some Hispanics. Both African American and Hispanic cultures are based in extended familial systems, where kinship is not limited to marriage and blood but includes ties of mutual obligations to good friends, godparents, and close neighbors. The informal adoption of children within these extended systems is another pattern common to both groups, wherein the person who does the caretaking may not be the biological mother but is referred to as "mother."

In both cultures women play pivotal roles in the family and have caretaking responsibility. In the United States, a significant percentage

Portions of this chapter are reprinted from the following previously published material: García-Preto (1982); copyright 1982 by The Guilford Press; reprinted by permission. García-Preto (1990); copyright 1990 by Haworth Press; reprinted by permission.

of both groups face similar problems of lower socioeconomic status and poverty. Many African American and Hispanic women have little education, occupy substandard housing, and carry the burden of the family alone on their shoulders. Most also work outside the home, regardless of whether they are married or live with a partner, and depend on other females in the extended family system for support and for help with caretaking chores.

For both groups the family is the principal source of support, and in times of crisis it is where women and other family members go for help. Therefore, family therapy lends itself in a very positive way to the treatment of African American and Hispanic women and their families.

This chapter will begin by presenting a brief overview of some of the most widely used models of family therapy and their applicability to African American and Hispanic women. A section on each group will then focus more specifically on the role and cultural context of women in African American and Hispanic families and how family therapy interventions can challenge inequalities in gender arrangements and yet retain respect for the culture.

CAUTION AGAINST STEREOTYPING

Before beginning our discussion of the different schools of family therapy and the cultural values of African American and Hispanic women, it is very important that therapists view this material as a "cultural lens" that must be adjusted with each new client and family. There is a great deal of diversity among African American women and their families, based on socioeconomic level, geographic area, age, education, skin color, and so on. Similarly, "Hispanic" is an adjective describing many nationalities, including people from Puerto Rico, Cuba, Mexico, Santo Domingo, El Salvador, Nicaragua, Colombia, Peru, Argentina, Ecuador, Chile, Guatemala, Venezuela, or Spain.

SOCIETAL CONTEXT

Before we explore the specific cultural and racial issues for women from both of these ethnic groups, it is necessary first to put this exploration within a broader contextual framework. This chapter will explore the specific impact of racism on the socialization of men and women within African American families. It is important to recognize, however, that many African American and Hispanic women are affected by the racist and sexist views of gender roles that have been prevalent within the dominant culture. For example, African American women who raise children alone may be subject to the pejorative, "blame the victim" mentality with which some service providers approach single-parent families, and Hispanic women may face therapists who are very judgmental of what to them are culturally accepted sex-role practices. Within the field of family therapy, a gender bias exists that has often viewed traditional African American and Hispanic mothers as "enmeshed" or "overinvolved." The changing social, political, and economic realities in this country also create changes and role strain for many African American and Hispanic women. It is very important that clinicians be helped to understand the norms within each cultural and racial group, as well as understanding the complex intragroup diversity that exists. These issues will be explored in more detail in a later section of the chapter.

It is also important to note that women may label similar experiences differently. For example, some African American women, when confronted with situations that have elements of racism and sexism, may respond by viewing the situation through the lens of race. This is often confusing to White therapists who are more sensitized to gender biases.

FAMILY THERAPY MODELS

Of the family therapy models that have emerged in recent years, perhaps the most useful in working with African American and Hispanic women is the structural family therapy model. This model of treatment, originally designed for work with inner-city African American and Hispanic families by Minuchin (1974), Haley (1976), and Aponte (1976), is problem-focused and prescribes a very active role for the therapist, who produces change in the family by exploring and reforming structural patterns. Women are helped to redefine their roles and shift responsibilities in relationship patterns with men, children, or other family members.

The Bowenian school of family therapy, based on the work of Murray Bowen (1976, 1978), although not originally designed for African Americans or Hispanics, may be very useful. Its intergenerational approach to treatment—consistent with most African Americans' and Hispanics' own views of their families—can help in identifying key members of the extended family. It allows women to identify other family members as supports, as people from whom they are emotionally cut off, as prototypes they would like to emulate, and as people from whom they want to differentiate.

Bowenians such as Guerin (1976) and McGoldrick and Gerson (1985) have provided a tool known as the genogram, or family tree, which can be very useful in diagramming complex extended family relationships. A word of caution is necessary about using this tool, however. Although the Bowenian model encourages therapists to collect a great deal of historical family data and draw the genogram in initial family sessions, it is wise to wait until rapport has been established before collecting extensive data with African Americans because of the legacy of racism and the suspicion with which many approach treatment. Similarly, although some Hispanics are more trusting of "doctors," they will have difficulty revealing family information without trust. Also, clients want to focus on the present problem; extensive history taking will make them feel unheard and not understood.

The strategic and paradoxical schools are the third major area of the family therapy field. The work of Haley (1973), Papp (1981), Watzlawick (1978), and Madanes (1981) are examples of this model. Change is produced through the strategic use of paradoxical interventions with families such as techniques of "prescribing the symptom," reframing, and so on. Family therapists must apply this model with caution because of the hesitancy that African American and Hispanic women may bring to therapy. Many are put off by paradoxical models initially because they are perceived as tricks. However, the use of metaphors, a technique that these models employ to introduce new information, can be very helpful in highlighting cultural differences with Hispanics because they often use metaphoric language, expressions termed *indirectas*. *Indirectas* are cutting statements with double meanings meant to address conflicts or situations indirectly that are difficult to confront directly, and are also used as sexual and romantic innuendos.

The Multisystems Model of Family Therapy with African American and Hispanic Women

The multisystems model of family therapy (Boyd-Franklin, 1989) incorporates family therapy techniques of the above schools and applies them in a culturally sensitive manner to the treatment of women and their families. It requires flexibility and challenges therapists to expand their model far beyond that of the traditional nuclear family.

A family therapist in the multisystems model must have the flexibility to intervene on an individual, family, or extended family level. Because of the cultural role that religion has played for African American women, church family members may be involved; similarly, with Hispanic women the role of the spiritist, *santera*, or *curandera* may need to be considered. Therapists working with inner-city families may need to intervene in other systems that can become very intrusive and may wield a great deal of power in the lives of these families, systems such as schools, courts, police, housing agencies, child welfare agencies or the welfare department, and so on. The child welfare department, for example, has the power together with the family court to remove a child from his or her family, to determine custody decisions, and to petition the courts for termination of parental rights. Since these different agencies do not communicate with one another and may work at cross purposes, the family therapist may have to empower an African American or Hispanic family to clarify agency roles, set limits, and draw boundaries. Many therapists working with inner-city families intervene to facilitate meetings with family members and representatives of different agencies and devise with the family a common plan in their best interest.

Therapists working with African American and Hispanic families cannot be narrow-minded in the type of therapy they pursue. It is important to maintain a family-systems focus, whether one is working with an individual woman or an extended family network. The next section will look at the many different levels of family interventions with African American and Hispanic women and their families. We can now proceed to explore the ways in which African American and Hispanic women present in family therapy. The first of these, and the most common, involves family therapy with one person.

Family Therapy with One Person

Despite the "resistance" to therapy by many people of color, women are often the first to seek therapy. They may later bring into therapy husbands, boyfriends, lovers, children, or extended family. Also, a growing number of African American and Hispanic single women seek therapy for themselves. Family therapy concepts and techniques are often useful in working with an individual because of the strong extended-family ties of many African American and Hispanic women. In this model of "family therapy with one person," derived from the Bowenian school and developed and elaborated by McGoldrick and Gerson (1985), a genogram or family tree is drawn and blood and nonblood significant relationships are explored with an individual in therapy.

Many African American and Hispanic women find it helpful to explore how relationships in their family of origin are being replicated in their relationships with men and/or with their own children. Through "coaching" (Bowen, 1978), women can be taught how to explore intergenerational conflicts and issues inhibiting individual and family functioning. Strategies are then formulated to guide them in relating deliberately and consciously, and, when appropriate, to change their pattern of relating to significant family members. In other situations, the therapist may arrange sessions with extended family members in order to help a woman resolve conflicts. This form of therapy may lead to couples therapy with a lover or spouse.

Couples Therapy

The term "couples therapy" is used rather than "marital therapy" because it is more inclusive. For example, in our own practice, we have treated unmarried couples with relationship difficulties, couples who seek premarital therapy, and many couples who seek traditional marital therapy. This term does not include the growing number of lesbian women of color who enter treatment with their lovers.

African American and Hispanic women may seek help as a result of very painful couple relationships. Commonly, a woman will request couples therapy and later report her partner's refusal to participate. In that case, we encourage the woman to come for herself so that the therapist can help the woman to become more assertive and discuss strategies for reaching out to the man. Since in our experience African American and Hispanic men are often hesitant about therapy, the therapist may need to reach out to engage them in treatment. If the woman has initially been seen alone, the therapist needs to spend some time alone "joining" with the man early in their first session.

Divorce Therapy

There are an increasing number of African American and Hispanic families who seek therapy when they feel that divorce is inevitable. The therapist, as divorce mediator, may help families negotiate the complex decisions involved in dissolving a marriage or a long-term relationship. Couples may also indirectly seek divorce therapy. African American and Hispanic couples are far more likely to come in for treatment for their children. A child who is caught in the middle between two angry parents may be the initial identified patient. The next two major sections of this chapter will explore the issues first for African American women and then for Hispanic women and their families.

AFRICAN AMERICAN WOMEN

Extended Family Patterns

In order to understand the cultural context of African American women fully, a therapist must recognize that they are often raised in complex extended families in which mothers, fathers, aunts, uncles, grandmothers, grandfathers, brothers, sisters, cousins, and so on may have played an important role in child rearing and family life. Also, because of the practice of incorporating nonblood relatives into the family, many African American women also have strong ties to their godmothers and godfathers, "church family," former babysitters, and others. This is extremely important information because a therapist must first know who the client includes in her "family" and understand these complex relationships in order to identify who should be included in the family therapy process (Billingsley, 1968; Boyd-Franklin, 1989; Hill, 1972; Hines & Boyd-Franklin, 1982).

Religion and Spirituality

Most people enter therapy when they are experiencing pain, but African American people, particularly women, have traditionally drawn on their spiritual strength in times of pain or trouble. A working understanding of the cultural values and the psyche of African American women and their families is dependent upon the therapist's awareness of the importance of spirituality in their lives. Some African American women have strong ties to a particular religion or church group, while others have a deeply ingrained belief in God and a spiritual orientation to the world. It is also important to recognize that the African heritage does not draw the Western dichotomy between the psyche and the spirit. Therefore, forms of therapy that do not acknowledge and discuss a spiritual component will not be effective with a large percentage of African American women.

In addition to the issue of belief systems, it is important for a therapist to be aware of the special significance of the "church family." For many African American women, ministers, ministers' wives, deacons, deaconesses, and "brothers" and "sisters" in the church are an integral part of their extended family and constitute a traditional support system that may provide "counseling" in times of trouble. Therapists can draw upon these resources to find support for African American women and their families (Boyd-Franklin, 1989).

The Impact of Racism on Socialization and Gender Roles

There are many variations of socialization patterns and gender roles among African American families. These differences may be related to socioeconomic and educational levels, geographic area, religion, age, and so forth. The therapist must understand the tremendous impact that racism and oppression has had on family and gender socialization practices.

Many African American parents feel a need to prepare their children for the realities of racism. Although African American men and women are both historical victims of racism, racism has manifested itself differently toward each, which has led to contrasting socialization and gender roles. Ever since the days of slavery, a fear of Black men has had direct impact on socialization practices. Conscious of the image of aggression particularly associated with African American males by many in "mainstream" America, many Black parents experience a great deal of fear which permeates certain aspects of child rearing and leads to an emphasis on discipline in the household. This discipline—which may be seen as harsh to therapists from other cultures—is regarded by some African American parents as a way of protecting children from the harsh sanctions of social systems (e.g., schools and police) against misbehavior.

The fear of aggression discussed above has severe repercussions. Starting from an early age—when African American males' behavior is often seen as threatening in school—they have higher dropout rates, experience discrimination in employment, and are at greater risk for drug addiction and crime. Male–female relationships as well as socialization patterns in many African American families have been skewed because men have had far more difficulty finding jobs than women, and women were frequently only able to obtain low-level positions. Many African American women are more educated than men. Because of the large number of African American men who are involved with drugs, incarcerated, or who have been victims of homicide, more African American women survive into the adult years than men.

African American families have developed coping strategies for dealing with racism. Families, particularly mothers, in some African American homes are very protective of their male children. In many of these families, it is said that they "raise their daughters but love their sons." This can create gender-role patterns that are quite different from those of other cultures. Many African American women from an early age carry adult responsibility for care of the younger children and become "parental children." Because of role flexibility in African American families, boys can also serve as parental children, unlike in Hispanic families, for example, where only female children can serve this role.

Parent–Child Relationships

Parent–child relationships are complicated by extended family patterns. A young African American girl may have many "mothers" and "fathers." In some families, for example, where there are multigenerational patterns of teenage pregnancy, a girl may grow up with her biological mother in a sibling relationship, particularly if the mother is 16 or younger, and the grandmother is "mama." Therefore, it is very important to find out who the biological parents are and also to ask the crucial question, "Who raised you?" Moreover, because of the pattern of informal adoption or taking in children among African American families, many women report that they were raised by different extended family members over time (Billingsley, 1968; Boyd-Franklin, 1989; Hill, 1972, 1977).

Mother–Daughter Relationships

The pattern of extended family relationships for African American women discussed above gives rise to complicated mother–daughter relationships. In some families, there is a very strong bond between mothers, daughters, and often grandmothers. In others, relationships with a biological mother may be conflictual, if the daughter was raised by grandmothers, aunts, godmothers, and so on, each of whom may have been "mama" in different ways and at different times. This factor is compounded by "family secrets" that often arise around parentage issues, wherein children are often not told of their parentage. Therefore, women may be sorting out complex relationships and feelings for the first time in therapy.

Father–Daughter Relationships

One of the most complicated relationships that many African American women bring into therapy is their connection (or lack thereof) with their fathers. Some African American women struggle with memories of very conflictual relationships between their parents, others report having grown up in "single-parent families" or extended families with few men, many have very ambivalent relationships with their fathers. In some families, the role of provider may have fallen to the mother because of a father's trouble maintaining employment.

The number of African American families affected by divorce is increasing, as it is for all American families. Many African American women report a yearning for closeness with their fathers that they have never truly experienced. Many report that their lack of role models for healthy male–female relationships impacts their own adult male–female relationships.

Male–Female Relationships

As has been demonstrated above, for a variety of reasons, including racism and discrimination, it is a serious error for therapists from other cultures to assume that gender roles are the same for African American women as they are for themselves. Society is more threatened by African American men and has blocked access to areas of societal success. African American women have been granted "limited access." Thus, they are often better educated and earn more money than men, a situation that can create a power disparity in male–female relationships. The tensions of living and working in a racist society and those of raising and protecting children create additional pressures on male–female relationships for African Americans. These issues have been explored more fully in the section on couples therapy.

Racism and the Responses of African American Families to Therapy

Before we discuss family therapy with African Americans in detail, another cultural reality must be addressed, that is, the attitude toward therapy in the African American community. In general, therapy has been viewed as something for "crazy" or "sick" people by many African Americans. Even more significantly, women particularly see therapy as something for "weak" people (Boyd-Franklin, 1989).

Grier and Cobbs (1968) have also discussed the resistance with which African Americans approach therapy. Many have a suspicion of White institutions and bring to therapy a "healthy cultural paranoia" that nevertheless has serious implications for family therapy. Families may be sensitive to people "prying into their business," and children are often taught that family problems are "nobody's business but our own." As mentioned previously, attempts to collect family history, genograms, and data are often counterproductive with African American families until trust between the therapist and the family has been established.

Therapists trained to work with clients who come for help need to approach therapy differently for families who are not self-referred, and who may thus come into treatment with little knowledge, many misconceptions, or no belief in therapy. It is important for therapists to ascertain how clients were referred and what they know about therapy. The first step in the treatment process is joining with each family member and engaging each in therapy. Therapists need to adopt a problem-solving model in the first session. This will help build credibility with the family for both the therapist and the treatment process. This joining and trust building must take place before history taking. With these cultural realities as guidelines, we can now discuss specific models of family therapy and their relevance for the treatment of African American families (Boyd-Franklin, 1989).

Family Therapy and Extended Family Therapy Involvement

There are an increasing number of African American families who are now being seen in family therapy in which a mother, father, and children, or a single parent and children are seen for treatment. Often mothers bring the family into treatment. In many families, the mother is the "gatekeeper" for the family and decides who comes in for the treatment. As mentioned previously, families frequently come into treatment with the child as the identified patient.

In many African American families, family structures are as they appear and the therapist can apply the more "traditional" structural or Bowenian family treatment approaches. Appearances may be misleading, however. In many of these families a grandmother, grandfather, aunt, boyfriend or father may be a crucial player in the family drama but may never have been involved in the treatment process. It is very important for family therapists to reach out to these key extended family members through phone calls, letters, and home visits.

Women, especially grandmothers, play central and powerful roles in African American families. As stated earlier, a grandmother may function as "big mama." Often one important level of the treatment process involves helping the women in the family to renegotiate their maternal roles and to clarify their different functions so that family members don't remain in a self-defeating cycle of conflicting and inconsistent messages. These patterns are particularly problematic for children who sense conflict between adults and begin to act out.

As stated above, an African American child may be informally adopted by members of her extended family. Often as a girl begins to grow up, at the age of preadolescence—age 11 or 12—she begins to wonder more about her biological family. This can create a problem in which "secrets" exist about maternity as well as paternity. A teenage girl may begin to act out in adolescence when she senses a "toxic family secret" that has never been discussed. The therapist then needs to help the family clarify the young woman's roots. When confronting this issue it is important for therapists to meet first with the adults involved and gain their trust in order to allow a more in-depth discussion of these "secrets," particularly because many African American families believe that there are certain things that one does not discuss with children.

The following case example illustrates many of the issues discussed in this chapter. It demonstrates how family therapy with one person can expand to include sessions with other family and extended family members, how multigenerational "secrets" can become toxic simply because they are never discussed, and how a multisystems model of therapy based on empowerment can produce change. For so many African American women this process involves helping them to differentiate from their family of origin while also staying connected in a more appropriate way. The data identifying the clinical cases have been altered to protect clients' confidentiality.

Case Example

Sarah was a 36-year-old single parent, mother, and grandmother. She sought therapy because of severe depression and the dilemma common to many African American women, of being overwhelmed by extended-family demands.

The therapist chose a Bowenian "family therapy with one person" model to help Sarah differentiate herself within both her family of origin and her household. The therapist, overwhelmed with the number of people in Sarah's life, clarified these complex relationships by helping Sarah to draw a genogram. (An example of a genogram is provided later in this chapter in the discussion of Mrs. Vazquez.)

Sarah, the oldest of four siblings, had always been a "parental child" in her family of origin and had carried this pattern into the next generation with her own family. Her sister, Cathy (34), who had two children (age 11 and 7), were currently living with Sarah as a result of eviction and presented a considerable financial and emotional burden. Her brother Chris died at 14 through random violence. Her youngest sister, Bonnie (16), was very close to Sarah's children and had been raised as their cousin. Sarah's mother, Emma, a needy, dependent women, suffered from chronic depression and had been hospitalized for a suicidal gesture 10 years earlier after Chris's murder. Sarah's father, Edward, was an active alcoholic. As a child Sarah often mediated fights between her parents and intervened when her father beat her mother. Her parents had been separated for 19 years.

Sarah expressed a great deal of concern and a sense of hopelessness about her daughters Susan (20, with a 4-year-old son), and Sandy (15), as well as her sister Bonnie. Sandy was repeating the pattern of staying out late and acting "boy crazy" set by her older sister. Bonnie habitually "ran away from home" (to Sarah's house) after fights with her own mother, and often was a truant.

The therapist worked with Sarah first to prioritize her concerns. Sarah stated that she had felt especially overwhelmed since her sister and her two children had moved in. The therapist helped Sarah to role play and, through a technique known as "coaching," Sarah was able to set limits for her sister and to give her one month to find a new living arrangement. It actually took four months for Cathy to find a new apartment.

During this same period, Bonnie and Sandy were suspended from school for "playing hookey" together. Bonnie had been suspended many times and Sarah was afraid that she was "leading Sandy down the wrong path." With the therapist's help, Sarah identified two problems: her own need to take charge of parenting Sandy, and her stepping in to parent Bonnie because of her own mother's inability to do so.

Sarah also confronted the very painful issue of multigenerational teenage pregnancy, a pattern that had begun with Sarah's mother and had become a "toxic family secret" because it was never discussed. Sarah was very concerned that her daughter and her sister would become pregnant as she had, and felt as powerless to stop them as her own mother had felt with her.

With the therapist's help, Sarah planned two different family sessions. Sarah brought in her daughters first. Sarah began by saying that she was very concerned for Sandy, and, with the therapist's support, was able to talk about her own experience growing up and how she could see herself in Sandy. Both girls expressed surprise at Sarah's revelations of her own experiences.

Sarah then spoke to Sandy about her truancy, grounding her for a month, and telling her they would go together to speak to Sandy's principal the following day. The therapist talked with Sarah and Susan about the need to "tighten up" on Sandy as they were often "too easy on her." Susan told Sandy that she wished their mother had done this for her. With the therapist's encouragement, Sarah asked Sandy what her concerns were. Sandy stated that her mother didn't like her friends and didn't want her to be with them. What emerged was that Sarah didn't feel that she knew Sandy's friends. They agreed that after the month's grounding, Sandy would begin to bring her friends home and Sarah would contact some of their parents.

Sarah also had a meeting with her therapist, her mother, and her sister Bonnie. Sarah told her mother that although she loved her and her sister, she couldn't take on the burden of raising her sister. The therapist talked to Bonnie and her mother about a referral for family therapy for them, a process recommended by Sarah.

The many levels of individual and family therapy continued for another year while the therapist worked with Sarah on consistent parenting and setting limits with her family and extended family members. Sandy began to "straighten out" as Sarah set clear limits and consequences for her.

Gradually, the therapist began to shift the focus to Sarah individually. As Sarah let go of the tremendous demands, she found that she was very lonely and isolated. As a girl she had made many friends in a local church but had felt "shunned" after her daughters were born. With the therapist's help, she was able to find a new church and joined the choir. Sarah, who as a nurse's aide at a hospital, told the therapist of her "lost dream" of getting her nursing degree and began to achieve that goal at a local college.

She met a man on her job who began to drive her home, and she began to question the messages which she had received all of her life that "Black men ain't no good." Her new "friend" was in fact very good to her and she struggled with the issue of her own entitlement.

The Role of the Family Therapist in Working with African American Women and Their Families

The process of therapy with African American women and their families requires flexibility in terms of role and use of self. First, the role of the therapist is a very active one, both in therapy and in outreach to extended family members and outside systems. Secondly, the therapist must be conscious of the fact that she or he is *the* therapeutic instrument and must learn to use him- or herself in the treatment process. These families are very sensitive to therapists conveying respect or condescension and acceptance or judgment. Likewise, the therapist needs to recognize the concept of "vibes" in the treatment of African American families (Boyd-Franklin, 1989). Given the legacy of racism in this country, a therapist's approach is a very important "vibe."

White therapists working with African American families need to raise the issue of race early in the treatment process. This gives the family permission to discuss any issue with the therapist. Black therapists need to realize that the healthy cultural suspicion of African American families can apply to them also. Families will often test a therapist to see if she or he is "for real." Often families will challenge an African American therapist on the issue of being different or having "made it." It is very important that therapists be true to themselves when working with African American families. With these families the important issue is often who you are as a person, rather than your credentials or what you know (Hunt, 1987).

HISPANIC WOMEN

Hispanic women tend to occupy the central position in their families. They carry the responsibility of keeping the family together by providing the caretaking and nurturance needed to maintain relationships in what are usually extended systems of kinship (Bernal, 1982; Falicov, 1982; García-Preto, 1982). They are also expected to mediate conflicts between family members and to prevent confrontations. Often, when they marry, it is their obligation to bring the two families together and avoid conflict with in-laws. In a cultural context that expects the family to solve most problems, women primarily assume the responsibility of helping individuals under stress.

Although fulfilling these roles can make women feel strong, worthwhile, and wise, these expectations may also lead women to feel so much pressure that they begin to experience resentment. In a culture that tends to give women much less freedom than men, they usually have difficulty confronting their spouses or other family members. Instead, it is common to express resentment through somatic complaints, depression, or emotional outbursts (Abad & Boyce, 1979; Torres-Matrullo, 1976). Assuming that the role expectations she values are dysfunctional, or that the woman is enmeshed (Minuchin, 1974), however, would be too simplistic and devaluing. This formulation usually leads to viewing the woman's behavior as pathological, and does not take into consideration that even though expectations for mutual aid in Hispanic families can sometimes lead to overfunctioning and self-sacrifice, the support and acceptance provided is also very healthy and nurturing, as well as reassuring and validating. Interventions that aim at separation, independence, and autonomy—goals that are based on European American values—may not be as effective with Hispanics, who are more likely to value interdependence, mutuality, and reciprocity. A more effective approach would be for clinicians treating Hispanic women to ask questions about the role they have in their families, and about their level of satisfaction and dissatisfaction. This information will help clinicians engage the women in clarifying what they want to change in their relationships and to identify who else in the family should be included in the therapy process.

Belief in Spirituality

Hispanics in general tend to emphasize spiritual values and are willing to sacrifice material satisfaction for spiritual goals. They do not usually differentiate between psyche and spirit, and when problems are perceived as nonphysical they are usually categorized as spiritual. Examples of spiritual problems are guilt, shame, sin, and disrespect for elders or for family values (Padilla, Ruiz, & Alvarez, 1975). In these cases, the family will probably suggest a visit to the clergy and/or the folkhealer.

Women usually are more involved than men in the church and are more likely to go to the clergy and to suggest it as a solution for handling emotional distress to others in the family. There is also a significant probability that Hispanics will consult a spiritualist. This person, usually a woman, may be a spiritist (medium), a *santera*, or a *curandera* (folkhealer) who is believed to have special powers and the ability to intervene, or be in contact with the spirit world. It is not unusual for Hispanic women to consult more than one spiritualist while also attending therapy.

Clinicians should be careful not to alienate women in therapy by rejecting this belief in spiritualism or by downgrading its importance.

Spiritual healers, unlike many mental health professionals, take into account the family situation and cultural milieu when evaluating and treating behavior (Sager, Brayboy, & Waxenberg, 1972). Rejecting the belief, or not being aware that a spiritualist is being consulted, creates triangles in the therapeutic process that can work against the process of change or cause women to leave therapy. The goal for clinicians is to acknowledge the ways in which the spiritualist tries to alleviate anxiety and focuses on change by helping women gain control of their lives, and by positive reframing of dysfunctional behavior (Delgado, 1978).

Gender Roles

Hispanic women often find themselves in cultural paradoxes. From an early age they receive conflicting messages about their identity. On the one hand, they are considered to be morally and spiritually superior to men, while on the other they are expected to accept male authority. This is reinforced by the concept of *marianismo*—stemming from the cult of the Virgin Mary—that considers women morally and spiritually superior to men and, therefore, capable of enduring all suffering inflicted by men (Stevens, 1973).

Also implicit in the concept of *marianismo* is women's repression or sublimation of sexual drives and consideration of sex as an obligation. The cultural message is that if a woman has sex with a man before marriage, she will lose his respect, he will not marry her, and she will bring dishonor to herself and to her family. Traditionally, the line separating *doñas* (a respectful term for Mrs.) from *putas* (whores) has been quite clear: no sex before marriage and afterward an accepting attitude without much demonstration of pleasure.

Another sex-role characteristic of some Hispanics is *hembrismo*, which as described by Comas-Díaz (1989),

> literally means femaleness, and adds to the complexity and paradoxical nature of Hispanic gender roles. *Hembrismo* connotes strength, perseverance, flexibility, and an ability for survival. However, it can also translate into the woman's attempt to fulfill her multiple role expectations—in other words, the superwoman working the *doble jornada* (or double day, i.e., working both at home and outside the home). This situation can generate stress and emotional problems for the woman behaving in the hembrista fashion. Likewise, many Hispanic women may present to treatment with symptoms of *marianista* behavior at home and *hembrista* behavior at work. (p. 35)

Although her role as wife is not as romanticized as that of mother, it is also important. Traditionally, she must be respectful of her husband and his family, an expectation eloquently defined by a Puerto Rican client as "respect between husband and wife means that as a wife you must be loving, considerate, and never have negative thoughts about me." Women are expected to be submissive and passive in comparison to men. However, while overtly supporting their husband's authority, wives usually assume power in the house.

The support that women provide for each other enables the culture to maintain certain gender roles, such as not expecting husbands to perform household tasks or help with child rearing. Without the extended family to offer this support, a woman is likely to experience her situation as unbearable and begin to demand her husband's help. He may resent it and become distant and argumentative, or turn to drink, gambling, or affairs. Without relatives or friends to intervene in the arguments and to advise the spouses to respect each other, serious difficulties may develop (García-Preto, 1989).

Parent–Child Relationships

Marianismo is reinforced by the acclaim that the culture gives to motherhood. Motherhood has been romanticized in Hispanic cultures in their literature and their music, and the association made between mothers and the Virgin Mary is so strong that the mere mention of the word mother tends to evoke an almost religious response. Having children also raises the status of women in society and is a rite of passage into adulthood, which elicits respect from family members and friends. Mothers are glorified when they put their children's welfare above everything else and protect them. This sacrificial role is reinforced by the admiration of society. Feeling pressured and obligated to sacrifice themselves to be good mothers, women may assume positions of martyrdom in the family. Keeping the family together becomes their devotion, their cross to bear (García-Preto, 1990).

This central position yields them a degree of power that is reflected in the alliances mothers often build with children against authoritarian fathers who are perceived as lacking understanding of emotional issues. Relationships between sons and mothers in particular are close and dependent, and it is not uncommon to see a son protecting his mother against an abusive husband. A family therapist working with this type of family may want to intervene by helping the son to separate from the mother. The woman in turn may be labeled passive and manipulative. The problem, however, is not the closeness between the mother and son, since strong loyalty ties between children and mothers are within the cultural norm among Hispanics, but the lack of power women in these positions experience. Rather than trying to separate mothers and sons, a more useful approach would be to empower women to stop the abuse. It would also be important to challenge the dependence that mothers foster in sons, and to address the alienation that is often created between fathers and children when men are uninvolved or abusive at home. Mothers and daughters also have close relationships, but these are more reciprocal in nature. Mothers teach their daughters how to be good women who deserve the respect of others, especially males, and who will make good wives and mothers. It is usually daughters who take care of their elderly parents and who take their mothers into their homes when they are widowed. In turn, older women will help out at home, enabling their daughters to attend school or work.

Relationships between Hispanic women and their fathers vary depending on the family structure. In families where fathers assume an authoritarian position there tends to be more distance and conflict. While attempting to be protective, they may become unreasonable, unapproachable, and highly critical of their daughters' behavior and friends. On the other hand, in families where fathers are more submissive and dependent on mothers to make decisions, they may develop special alliances with their daughters, who in turn assume a nurturing role toward them. With the increasing number of Hispanic families being headed by single women, however, common scenarios are for fathers to be absent and distant, or for daughters and sons to grow up having memories of their fathers' violent, abusive, and addictive behavior.

Changing Gender Roles and Male–Female Relationships

Most Hispanic women, especially in this country, are also expected to work to help support the family; otherwise they may be dependent on the welfare system. Most are not well educated, and tend to occupy the lowest paid, unskilled blue collar and service occupations. They are also more frequently heads of families than other women. Wilson (1987), in a demographic overview about women and poverty, found that 26.4% of Hispanic women live below the poverty line. Many work as domestics in order to obtain legal status, leaving their children in their countries of origin until they can establish themselves here and can afford to send for them.

Obviously, it would be a mistake to assume that all Hispanic women in the United States are poor, uneducated, in low-paying jobs, and unmarried. It would also be erroneous to assume that all Hispanics are recent immigrants, since many, especially in the Southwest and California, have lived in this country for generations. Their ancestors were here before the United States became a nation, and many of them identify more readily with the dominant culture than with their Spanish or Latin heritage. Others such as Puerto Ricans also differ from other Hispanic immigrants in that they are United States citizens. However, when they arrive on the "mainland" they are generally perceived as second-class citizens by the overall society, and experience as much prejudice and hardship as any other Hispanic immigrant group. Poverty and racism are the two major factors adversely affecting the Puerto Rican immigrant's quality of life in the continental United States.

Traditional sex roles are also undergoing change among Hispanics in the United States. The pressures of economic survival in this country, as well as the type of skills that are marketable, have caused a role reversal among many low-income Hispanic immigrants, since it is often easier for the women to obtain employment in the United States, by selling their sewing and domestic skills, than it is for the men (Comas-Díaz, 1989).

This situation can present problems for men because it challenges their basic role as provider and protector of the family. At a deeper level, they may also fear that women who work outside the home run a greater risk of being seduced and of having affairs, an act that would threaten the innermost core of any Hispanic "*macho*" (García-Preto, 1989). The potential for conflict is certainly less when couples are well educated and when the man is employed and earning more than the woman. Although in most cases wives who work continue to respect their husbands' authority as the head of the household, they may feel more independent and self-confident.

If the husband is not able to regain his dominant position through employment, he may experience panic, confusion, and a sense of emasculation. The wife may develop contempt for a spouse in this position or experience pain, helplessness, and compassion for him, since women are aware of the extreme prejudice and racist attitudes that most Hispanic men face in this society, especially when they are uneducated, cannot speak the language, and cannot pass for white. For Hispanic women caught in this conflict, understanding the problem from a gender and power perspective may be difficult. Instead, helping them see how the balance in their relationship has been affected by the process of cultural transition would be more helpful.

Although this role reversal situation can create marital and family problems, adjusting to a new culture demands change from individuals. Cultural transition, states Comas-Díaz (1989),

> also tends to give individuals a certain plasticity, particularly within their gender roles. In a study of sex roles among Hispanics in the United States, Canino (1982) found that on the surface, both husband and wife espoused traditional attitudes. However, when couples were interviewed more extensively and were observed during actual decision making, most of the couples shared the decision-making process. Most of the couples studied by Canino were Puerto Ricans, but her findings seem relevant to other Hispanic populations as well. Falicov (1982) reports that while in some Mexican American families the husbands are domineering and patriarchal, others are submissive and depend upon their wives to make major decisions, while still other families have an egalitarian power structure. (p. 36)

Family Therapy with Hispanic Women

A family therapy approach to treatment with Hispanic women makes sense in that it considers the problems they present in the context of the family, and takes into account the larger systems affecting their lives. Taking a genogram of the family will help the therapist obtain a history of migration. It is important to know how long the family has lived in the United States, what country they came from, the reason for migration, who migrated first, who is here and who remains behind, and at what point the family is in the process of cultural transition. It is also important to know what their social status was in their country of origin, and to what extent their status has been affected by the migration.

In most cases, low-income Hispanic women who come to family therapy are referred by other agencies, and the problems presented are child focused. They are usually alienated from their families, or have no extended family nearby, and find themselves isolated. With Hispanic women, it is essential for therapists to spend a significant period of time forming an alliance by engaging them as adults, as women. They may tend to personalize relationships more than other groups because many Hispanics find it difficult for cultural reasons to confide in a therapist who is strictly professional, perceiving this as too distant for trust. While they may also mistrust anyone who acts in too friendly a manner and view that person as not serious enough to be a professional, the therapist's sharing personal thoughts and revealing something about her or his own family helps win trust.

In therapy, Hispanic women often complain about their husband's drinking, abusive behavior, and general absence from the home. They find it difficult, however, to complain about their husbands and are highly ambivalent about accusing them. On the one hand, they feel disloyal, and on the other, they feel betrayed. Often, they try to justify the husband's behavior by saying that he is basically a good human being and that his behavior is caused by the alcohol, the lack of job opportunities, the friends, or, in general, the way of life in this country. They may have attempted to change the situation at home by threatening to leave their husbands. Their lack of resources, however, makes carrying out this threat difficult. Since they are unable to change the situation at home, they experience themselves as failures. Their relatives and the other women in the community often advise them to be strong and accepting. This advice reflects the cultural belief that it is the woman's role to hold the family together. There is a tendency among Hispanics to admire a woman who "carries the cross" (García-Preto, 1989), or bears her difficulties with resignation.

The case of Mrs. Conde illustrates the bind in which some of these women find themselves.

During the past 5 years, Mrs. Conde, a Mexican-American woman, has come to therapy on different occasions when the situation at home has reached a crisis. In therapy, she claims to feel embarrassed about coming with the same problem and not taking steps to change it. She wants to do things by herself but feels helpless. She wants to leave her husband and her family of origin for a place where she can live in peace with her children. She holds back for fear that she will not be able to handle the children, especially her son, alone. She would prefer to stay home and help her husband. She does not want to talk about him behind his back, but he refuses to seek help.

Women like Mrs. Conde often drop out of therapy when the crisis is over and return when another crisis arises.

Often women will ask therapists to convince their partners to come to therapy. The therapist should assess the situation carefully before interpreting the request as manipulative. Hispanics who ask an outsider to intervene in this fashion usually feel powerless and embarrassed. They tend to view authority figures as influential and this type of request as legitimate. Pushing the woman to do the convincing herself may alienate her and result in her withdrawal from therapy. In some cases, a call from the therapist will prove more effective because of the cultural roles of respect for authority. Every effort should be made to include the husband in therapy by appealing to his sense of responsibility and to his traditional role as head of the family. The following case (from García-Preto, 1982, p. 182) illustrates this situation.

Mr. and Mrs. Arce, a working-class couple in their mid-40s, were referred to therapy by a local Puerto Rican community agency. Both parents worked in factories in an urban setting, and had been living in the United States for 10 years. Mr. Arce was clearly the main provider financially, and Mrs. Arce was overwhelmed with all the responsibilities of home and child care. They were having difficulties managing their children, especially a 12-year-old son. Therapy focused on helping the parents set clear limits and provide a reward system for their children. The parents appeared distant and angry and had difficulty working together. In the first session the therapist, a Puerto Rican woman, commented that they seemed to be having difficulties and that she sensed tension between them. They denied any difficulty in their relationship, and quickly agreed on needing to be more clear with their son about expectations, and more consistent in limit setting.

The next therapy session was attended by Mrs. Arce alone. She stated that her husband had refused to come. He did not believe in therapy and was angry with her for seeking help. It was her fault, he felt, that the children were disobedient and disrespectful. She went on to complain about his lack of interest in her, his absence from the home, and his outbursts of anger. She wanted the therapist to call her husband and ask him to come to therapy. Although Mrs. Arce was beginning to question the fairness of her burden, she was not ready to confront his authority and to go against his wishes.

The therapist called Mr. Arce and told him that his absence had shown how much his wife needed his help to discipline the children and that in order to help his son he needed to be present. Mr. Arce attended the next session where his traditional role in the family was supported, and his boundaries regarding intimate matters respected. When the husband presented his work schedule as an obstacle in continuing attending sessions, the therapist suggested making a home visit at a convenient time for them as a way to relieve their burden. The strategy was an attempt at further engagement by joining them in their dilemma, and showing a more personal interest in their lives. In the privacy of their home they were able to perceive the therapist as part of their support system. The therapist supported the wife by involving the husband in the family as a father. Involving the father in therapy expanded the context to parenthood, and helped take some of the blame from Mrs. Arce, who had assumed responsibility for all their children's problems. Uniting them as parents strengthened generational boundaries and had a positive effect on the children's behavior. By showing a personal interest in their lives the trust level was heightened, enabling them eventually to share more about their relationship.

Regardless of the therapist's ability to engage Hispanic couples in therapy, it is usually extremely difficult and embarrassing for them to talk about sexual problems and physical abuse, especially with a woman. Talking about issues concerning lack of respect, jealousy, and problems with in-laws is easier. In situations where women are adapting to the dominant culture faster than men, the men should be encouraged to move forward by finding programs where other Hispanic men are learning English and seeking job training. Asking couples to visualize a future together may help them see the present as a transition in their lives.

Engaging them in discussions that force them to reflect on cultural contrasts and on what they see as positive and negative about each culture may lead them to ways of relating that take from the old and the new. The idea that to make it in this country both men and women have to struggle together is generally accepted by Hispanics and can be used to join the couple in a more egalitarian relationship. After all, they chose to come to this country because they wanted to improve their situation (García-Preto, 1989). Comas-Díaz (1989) has found that challenging traditional dysfunctional roles is easier to accomplish with couples who are working on coping with cultural differences than those who remain in a culturally homogeneous environment. She also finds that the value of *hembrismo* can provide an archetype for changing sex roles.

If the man refuses to come in, the woman may be coached to mobilize the extended family for support. Helping them make connections with relatives, friends, or community supports may be their therapist's most crucial task. In cases where the extended family is not available or supportive, the therapist may help to break the cycle by mobilizing external systems such as welfare, child care facilities, and women's self-help groups to support the woman. The therapist's willingness to meet the woman's request for concrete services and to act as her advocate is an important vehicle for establishing a trusting relationship (García-Preto, 1982).

When children demand independence and challenge their mother's authority, Hispanic women experience these actions as rejections and feel anxious about the children's need for separation. If the marriage is not a good one, the prospect of spending more time alone with her husband makes the situation worse. Reframing their need to protect and take care of their children as necessary and positive helps to engage them in the task of teaching children to be more independent and responsible. Emphasizing that, in the United States, parents need to teach their children to be independent and assertive in order to confront the challenges they face in school and at work addresses some of the cultural differences that cause conflict when children acculturate faster than their parents. Because Hispanic mothers have the responsibility of raising respectful and obedient children, they are blamed, and tend to blame themselves, when there are problems.

Hispanic mothers are especially worried about protecting their daughters' virginity. It is their responsibility to teach their daughters how to protect themselves from men who are viewed as being interested primarily in sex, and trying to get whatever they can from women, but marrying only virgins. It is generally considered shameful for women to lose their virginity and a peril to their future, since a woman's honor and place in society depends so much on whether or not she is a virgin. Discovering that they have failed to do this can produce a crisis of sufficient magnitude to bring the family to therapy. The following case (from García-Preto, 1990, p. 15) illustrates this situation.

Mrs. Vazquez, a 38-year-old, divorced Puerto Rican mother, came to therapy with her daughter, Carmen (15). She lived with Carmen, her younger daughter Maria (12), and a 67-year-old paternal aunt. She had divorced her alcoholic husband when Carmen was 7, and had returned to a graduate school of social work on a part-time basis while continuing to work as a post office clerk. (The Vazquez family's genogram is presented in Figure 9.1.)

The referral to therapy was made by a school counselor after reading a letter that Carmen had written in which she threatened to run away from home and to kill herself. The reasons she gave were her mother's strict rules and recent threats of rejection. When the therapist first met them, the expressions of hurt, shame, and sadness in their faces were signals that the conflict had to do with issues of sexuality. The situation was familiar because she had seen so many Hispanic families in which mothers and daughters present a similar picture after the discovery is made that the daughter is no longer a virgin. This reaction seems to be more pronounced in families where daughters acculturate faster than mothers, complicating the usual conflicts caused by generational differences between parents and children during adolescence (García-Preto, 1988).

Her reaction was typical of Hispanic mothers in that they tend to experience their daughters' experimentation with sex as a betrayal rather than as the result of a developmental need (García-Preto, 1990). Carmen's inability to express anger toward her mother is also not uncommon, since in Hispanic cultures there is a strong expectation for children to revere mothers. This is particularly true when, as in Mrs. Vazquez's case, mothers sacrifice their lives for the welfare of the children.

In therapy, the therapist was able to help Mrs. Vazquez explain how she was trying to protect Carmen from further disgrace by keeping her close to

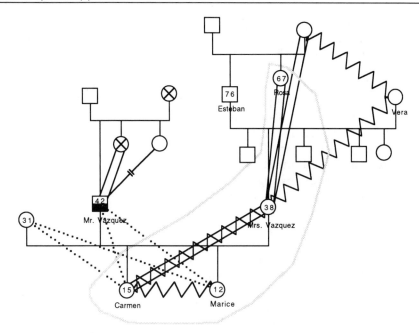

FIGURE 9.1. The Vazquez family genogram. In this type of genogram, squares designate males and circles females. A horizontal line connecting a square and a circle indicates a marital liaison. Offspring are drawn on vertical lines descending from the marital line, in chronological order, beginning with the oldest on the left. An X inside a circle or square indicates that a person has died, and a half-blackened figure indicates drug or alcohol abuse. (See McGoldrick & Gerson, 1985, for a detailed discussion of genogram symbols.)

home. The only solution she saw was for her daughter to stay away from boys, and to finish school. She thought that with an education she could at least take care of herself financially, since her chances of finding a good man were now lessened. She felt personally rejected by her daughter's action, and was in turn rejecting Carmen, but was determined to do whatever possible to protect her from further risk.

By framing Mrs. Vazquez's need to protect her daughter as positive and caring, the therapist was able to engage her in looking at other ways of helping her daughter become more independent. At the therapist's urging, she was able to encourage Carmen, who was much more acculturated to this society than her mother, to talk about how she found Mrs. Vazquez's cultural premise about sexual behavior antiquated and not relevant to her experience. Mrs. Vazquez had difficulty hearing her daughter's perspective without feeling personally attacked and rejected, yet was able to be more accepting when it was suggested that the conflicts and differences they were expressing about sexuality were inevitable since they had grown up in such different cultures. In a similar way, Carmen was able to experience her mother as less rejecting and to understand Mrs. Vazquez's behavior as an attempt to take care of her. She reassured her mother that she was not thinking of hurting herself or running away but was afraid of losing her love. Mrs. Vazquez was able to tell Carmen that she would always love her, but that she was having difficulty trusting her.

The value of rebuilding mutual trust among broken and dysfunctional relationships has been emphasized by Boszormenyi-Nagy and Spark (1973). Bernal (1982) has found that helping Hispanic families who have migrated to the United States reconnect family ties is vital to their growth. This is especially true with Puerto Ricans because of the back and forth migration that often leads to repeated cutoffs and breaks in the family system. Sometimes discussing the family's migratory process will clarify conflicts caused by contrasts between cultural values.

The structural approach to family therapy has been used to engage Hispanic women and their families effectively in a personal and trusting relationship (Minuchin, Montalvo, & Guerney, 1967). The emphasis that the approach places on engaging the family in such a relationship is a reason for its success with Hispanics. Some other reasons for its success, according to Canino and Canino (1980), are that it uses the family and extended family as integral components of the therapy; it considers stressful external life events like migration, poor housing, and unemployment as part of the family's context and, therefore, as contributors to the development and maintenance of symptomatic behavior; it is present, concrete, and goal oriented, factors that have been found successful with low-income groups.

SUMMARY

This chapter discusses the relevance of the family context in the treatment of women of color, presenting different aspects of family therapy with African American and Hispanic women. It explores many of the cultural factors that are unique to both groups and the effects of racism on African American women. It is hoped that therapists will use this information to aid their work and expand their thinking. As stated above, it is crucial to be willing to learn from each new family and thereby to avoid unnecessary stereotyping.

REFERENCES

Abad, V., & Boyce, E. (1979). Issues in psychiatric evaluation of Puerto Ricans: A sociocultural perspective. *Journal of Operational Psychiatry, 10*(1), 28–39.

Aponte, H. (1976). Underorganization in the poor family. In P. J. Guerin (Ed.), *Family therapy: Theory and practice.* New York: Gardner Press.

Bernal, G. (1982). Cuban families. In M. McGoldrick, J. K. Pearce, & J. Giordano (Eds.), *Ethnicity and family therapy.* New York: Guilford Press.

Billingsley, A. (1968). *Black families in White America*. Englewood Cliffs, NJ: Prentice-Hall.

Boszormenyi-Nagy, I., & Spark, G. (1973). *Invisible loyalties: Reciprocity in intergenerational family therapy*. New York: Harper & Row.

Bowen, M. (1976). Theory in the practice of psychotherapy. In P. J. Guerin (Ed.), *Family therapy: Theory and practice*. New York: Gardner Press.

Bowen, M. (1978). *Family therapy in clinical practice*. New York: Jason Aronson.

Boyd-Franklin, N. (1989). *Black families in therapy: A multisystems approach*. New York: Guilford Press.

Canino, G. (1982). Transactional family patterns: A preliminary exploration of Puerto-Rican adolescents. In R. E. Zambrana (Ed.), *Work, family and health: Latina women in transition* (pp. 27–36). New York: Fordham University, Hispanic Research Center.

Canino, I., & Canino, G. (1980). The impact of stress on the Puerto Rican migrant: Some treatment considerations. *American Journal of Orthopsychiatry, 50*(3), 232–238.

Comas-Díaz, L. (1989). Culturally relevant issues and treatment implications for Hispanics. In D. R. Koslow & E. Salett (Eds.), *Crossing cultures in mental health*. Washington, DC: Society for International Education Training and Research (SIETAR).

Delgado, M. (1978). Folk medicine in Puerto Rican culture. *International Social Work, 21*(2), 46–54.

Falicov, C. (1982). Mexican families. In M. McGoldrick, J. K. Pearce, & J. Giordano (Eds.), *Ethnicity and family therapy*. New York: Guilford Press.

García-Preto, N. (1982). Puerto Rican families. In M. McGoldrick, J. K. Pearce, & J. Giordano (Eds.), *Ethnicity and family therapy*. New York: Guilford Press.

García-Preto, N. (1988). Transformation of the family system in adolescence. In B. Carter & M. McGoldrick (Eds.), *The changing family life cycle*. New York: Gardner Press.

García-Preto, N. (1990). Hispanic mothers. In Ethnicity and mothers [Special issue]. *Journal of Feminist Family Therapy, 2*(2), 1–65.

García-Preto, N., McGoldrick, M., Hines, P. M., & Lee, E. (1989). Ethnicity and women. In M. McGoldrick, C. M. Anderson, & F. Walsh (Eds.), *Women in families: A framework for family therapy*. New York: W. W. Norton.

Gomez, A. G. (1982). Puerto Rican Americans. In A. Gaw (Ed.), *Cross-cultural psychiatry*. Boston: John Wright.

Grier, W., & Cobbs, P. (1968). *Black rage*. New York: Basic Books.

Guerin, P. (1976). *Family therapy*. New York: Gardner Press.

Habach, E. (1972). Ni machismo, ni hembrismo [Neither *machismo*, nor *hembrismo*]. In *Coleccion: Protesta*. Caracas, Venezuela: Publicaciones EPLA.

Haley, J. (1973). *Uncommon therapy: The psychiatric techniques of Milton H. Erickson*. New York: W. W. Norton.

Haley, J. (1976). *Problem-solving therapy*. San Francisco: Jossey-Bass.

Hill, R. (1972). *The strengths of black families*. New York: Emerson-Hall.

Hill, R. (1977). *Informal adoption among Black families*. Washington, DC: National Urban League Research Department.

Hines, P., & Boyd-Franklin, N. (1982). Black families. In M. McGoldrick, J. K. Pearce, & J. Giordano (Eds.), *Ethnicity and family therapy*. New York: Guilford Press.

Hunt, P. (1987). Black clients: Implications for supervision of trainees. *Psychotherapy, 24*(1), 114–119.

Madanes, C. (1981). *Strategic family therapy.* San Francisco: Jossey-Bass.

McGoldrick, M., Anderson, C. M., & Walsh, F. (Eds.). (1989). *Women in families: A framework for family therapy.* New York: W. W. Norton.

McGoldrick, M., & Gerson, R. (1985). *Genograms in family assessment.* New York: W. W. Norton.

McGoldrick, M., Pearce, J. K., & Giordano, J. (Eds.). (1982). *Ethnicity and family therapy.* New York: Guilford Press.

Minuchin, S. (1974). *Families and family therapy.* Cambridge, MA: Harvard University Press.

Minuchin, S., Montalvo, B., Guerney, B. G., Jr., Rosman, B. L., & Schumer, F. (1967). *Families of the slums.* New York: Basic Books.

Padilla, A. M., Ruiz, R. A., & Alvarez, R. (1975). Community mental health services for the Spanish speaking/surnamed population. *American Psychologist, 30*, 892–905.

Papp, P. (1981). Paradoxes. In S. Minuchin & C. Fishman (Eds.), *Family therapy techniques.* Cambridge, MA: Harvard University Press.

Sager, C., Brayboy, T. L., & Waxenberg, B. R. (1972). Black patient–white therapist. *American Journal of Orthopsychiatry, 8*(3), 128.

Stevens, E. (1973). Machismo and marianismo. *Transaction-Society, 10*(6), 57–63.

Torres-Matrullo, C. (1976). Acculturation and psychopathology among Puerto Rican women in mainland United States. *American Journal of Orthopsychiatry, 46*(4), 710–719.

Watzlawick, P. (1978). *The language of change.* New York: Basic Books.

Wilson, J. (1987). Women and poverty: A demographic overview. *Women and Health, 12*, 21–40.

10

Feminist Approaches

Oliva M. Espín

It is a rather pervasive belief among some White feminists and some people of color that feminism does not have anything to offer women of color and that consequently women of color would not benefit from a feminist approach to therapy. The assumptions made and the arguments advanced by these people are that most women of color in the United States come from poor or working-class backgrounds and are, more often than not, preoccupied by immediate issues of survival. Thus, goes this line of reasoning, issues related to women's rights are secondary to the pressing needs of everyday life. Feminism is perceived from this perspective to be the concern of White, middle-class, educated women intent on reaching economic and political parity with men of their social class and race.

Regrettably, there is much that could be said about the insensitivity, racism, and classism of feminists in psychology (e.g. Brown, 1990; Espín & Gawelek, 1992) and of the women's movement in general (e.g. Anzaldúa, 1990; hooks, 1984). I would contend that the nearsightedness of White feminists as to the possibilities of the movement and the far-reaching consequences of its ideas is very much to blame for the narrowness of some definitions of feminism and for the movement's goals being perceived as limited and exclusionary. As Gloria Anzaldúa (1990), bell hooks (1984), Audre Lorde (1984), and other feminists of color (e.g., Combahee River Collective, 1979) have stated, White middle-class women do not "own" feminism, nor is feminism irrelevant to the experiences of women of color. Rather, the oppression of women of color in a White-dominated society takes on specific characteristics related to both gender and race (e.g. Anzaldúa, 1990; Hurtado, 1989; Joseph & Lewis, 1981; Lorde, 1984). These characteristics are molded by forces that multiply and reinforce each other, as well as by the particular situation of men of color in this society.

White racism combines with sexism in unique ways to influence the oppression of women of color. The poverty and lack of education and resources that many women of color suffer from are a consequence of centuries of racist denial of the opportunities this country is supposed to provide for all of its citizens. Poor and working-class women of color and their children, as we know, are at the bottom of the social and economic pyramid in this country. Racism influences the experiences of women of color directly. Sexism is also a powerful force in their lives.

When "being a man" is defined by White upper-middle-class opportunities and standards that are unattainable by most men of color, the expression of manhood becomes distorted. For poor and working-class men of color, asserting dominance over women and children may be nothing but a last desperate gesture to "prove their manhood" in a world that both expects all men to achieve a certain success and systematically destroys the chances of some men to achieve that position. Domineering, aggressive, and sometimes violent behavior towards women on the part of these men may be understood as this desperate gesture. However, this understanding does not in any way diminish or justify the suffering it causes women and their children. The oppression to which all women are subjected in one form or another is intensified in the case of poor and working-class women of color by the oppression of these men.

The fewer outlets there are in the world at large for men of color to assert their domination and "masculinity" through economic, political, educational, or professional roles, the more they will turn to the territory of personal relationships and the family as the arena where they can, in fact, dominate and "prove" that they are indeed "real men" like the White men who deprive them of opportunities.

Women and children then become suitable recipients for the displaced anger of oppressed men. Violence takes many forms: incest, rape, wife beating. It is not unusual to hear supposedly "enlightened" persons defending the violent behavior of men of oppressed groups on the grounds that their only outlet is to beat their wives. Even if the displacement is understandable in individual cases, to accept and justify it is to condone injustice and another form of violence against women (Espín, 1984).

As a reaction to the oppression experienced by these men, women of color may subordinate their needs even further. Root's (1992) analysis of the impact of trauma on personality helps us understand the experiences of different groups of women. She expands the conventional notion of trauma to include not only direct trauma, but also indirect and insidious trauma. She believes that women are more prone to suffer indirect trauma because of their tendency to empathize with others and their suffering. Thus a woman of color is bound to feel empathy for the pain suffered by men of color due to discrimination and racism. This type of reaction may be seen by White feminists as a "proof" that women of color continue to be "male identified," thus failing to recognize that it is a consequence of empathy and identification with the trauma suffered by others.

Not as unfortunate as his poor counterpart, the middle-class, professional man of color strives for what should "legitimately" be his, "as a man," without any more understanding than White males about the fact that what men perceive as their "legitimate" right frequently impinges on the rights of the women closest to them. Thus it can be asserted that in a world where male dominance is expected, rewarded, and approved of, middle-class men of color are as likely as middle-class White men to act from a patriarchal perspective, and to become abusive, domineering, and oppressive to women in their lives.

In fact, although negative reactions to the feminist movement as arrowly defined by the interests and experiences of White women are indeed justified (e.g., hooks, 1984), a lot of the opposition to feminist ideas on the part of men of color is nothing but a reaction by yet another group of men to women's efforts to change their subservient position. Because the feminist movement is indeed guilty of racism, the sexism that is as prevalent in communities of color as in the dominant White society hides insidiously behind a cloak of ethnic loyalty.

While affirmative action efforts to enable some men of color to become "more like White men" may reduce certain gaps between these groups of men, thus creating a trend towards equalization, these efforts tend to have the opposite effect on real equality for women. For example, it is common knowledge that when non-White men begin to emulate White men, they often pressure non-White women to become more "like White women," which in this society is still interpreted as meaning "more like a middle-class, suburban, presumably idle housewife," precisely the trap that White middle-class women have been trying to escape. There is nothing surprising about this trend among young middle-class men of color. The standards for the "good life" in this country have been defined in terms of the White middle and upper classes, so it is understandable that young people of color who are professional and/or middle-class would aim to achieve that lifestyle for themselves. However, for young women of color, emulating those standards means that at some point in the future they are likely to find themselves in the situation from which many White middle-class women are still trying to extricate themselves. Assuming that at least superficial "equality" could be achieved on the basis of these standards and that the state of the economy and social climate would allow it, one could predict a situation in the future in which middle-class women of color could find themselves in positions that would again be belittled by society, because being a middle-class, suburban, presumably idle housewife may not be appreciated by society at large by the time they achieve this status. (Espín, 1979).

For the young ethnic minority woman who is in the process of obtaining a college degree, the lifestyle associated with the middle-class, suburban housewife may be a great temptation, with little consideration given to possible future disadvantages. However, most professional, middle-class women of color do not hold too many fantasies about the promises of a housewife role.

Women of color who are professional and/or middle class encounter both racism and sexism in their daily lives. The sense of responsibility for their less fortunate sisters and brothers is an inherent component of the lived experience of these women. Their access to middle-class professions and lifestyles adds specific circumstances that need to be negotiated in their daily lives (e.g., Combs, 1986; Trotman, 1984).

For the woman of color of all socioeconomic classes, an understanding of the oppression men of color experience in the world at large creates a double-bind. Wanting to support and understand those men, including their own brothers, fathers, and sons, they can feel trapped in situations of domination, abuse, and oppression at the hands of the men in their lives just as White middle-class women do, even though their experiences may appear to be so different. On the other hand, the experiences of women of color remain in the end vastly different from those of White women (e.g., Greene, 1986; Hurtado, 1989). Just the fact that White women partake of White privilege (McIntosh, 1988; Rave, 1990; Spelman, 1988) creates profound psychological and material differences between these groups of women.

WOMEN OF COLOR AND MENTAL HEALTH

Anyone who has a sense of the connections between life stress and mental health understands that "mental health" is not an exclusively intrapsychic and individual/existential concept. To be subjected to the constant stresses of racism and sexism has a definite impact on a person's mental health. Attempts at restoring a person's well-being (or "mental health") that do not include a consideration of all stressors in a person's life are obviously doomed to failure.

Root's (1992) discussion of insidious trauma, which "includes but is not limited to emotional abuse, racism, antisemitism, poverty, heterosexism, dislocation, ageism" is relevant here. The effects of insidious trauma are cumulative and are often experienced over the course of a lifetime. Needless to say, women of color are subject to different degrees of insidious trauma throughout their lives. According to Root, the exposure to insidious trauma activates survival behaviors that might be easily mistaken for pathological responses when their etiology is not understood. Misdiagnosis of pathology can be a consequence of lack of understanding of the impact of insidious trauma on women who have lived their lives under the impact of racism, heterosexism, or class discrimination. An additional effect of insidious trauma caused by negative social stereotypes is their self-fulfilling influence.

For those women of color who are lesbians, the experience of being a woman of color is compounded by conflicting loyalties and additional tasks in the development of their identity as women of color and as lesbians, which could be additional sources of insidious trauma (see Greene, Chapter 14, this volume; Espín, 1987a; Greene, 1986).

The above discussion illustrates some of the life situations women of color may bring to the therapeutic context that resemble "typical" situations presented by White women to White feminist therapists. It also points to some of the unique stressors characteristic of the experience of being a woman of color.

From its beginning, feminist therapy has been concerned with the psychological effects of social forces. Although its focus has mostly been the impact of everyday sexism on the lives and mental health of women rather than the combined effect of racism and sexism, the fact that it emphasizes the social construction of women's psychology and the necessity of attending to the social world in order to understand and restore the integrity of the psychic world gives it a unique perspective. To acknowledge the impact of social forces on mental health makes feminist therapy uniquely suited to the needs of women of color rather than foreign or irrelevant to those needs. As Comas-Díaz (1987) states, "defined as a set of political, economic and social values which support balanced power relations between the sexes, feminism is potentially relevant to all women. However, in order to be effective with Hispanic women (and other women of color), this perspective needs to be culturally embedded" (p. 40).

An examination of the principles of feminist therapy and their possibilities for becoming more directly "culturally embedded" and sensitive to differences among women is in order at this point.

DEFINING FEMINIST THERAPY

Feminist criticism of psychotherapy prompted a reevaluation of the field in the early 1970s. The result of this reevaluation was the development of feminist therapy. Feminist therapy challenges the authoritarian, patriarchal approaches of traditional psychotherapy that tend to reinforce women's sense of dependency and inadequacy, to treat women's unhappiness as pathology and illness, and to make adjustment to traditional roles the goal of treatment for women. Feminist therapists attempt to reconceptualize the goals of therapy and the role of the therapist in order to make the therapy process compatible with the new theories of women's psychology and the goals of the women's movement. Feminist therapy is distinguishable not only from the traditional, more or less sexist forms of therapy, but also from a nonsexist approach to therapy. The distinctive feature of feminist therapy is the analysis of the social, political, and economic oppression that affects women individually and as a group. This analysis informs the therapist's understanding of women's psychological development and the therapeutic process (Donovan & Littenberg, 1981).

A crucial aspect of the work of the feminist therapist is in helping clients distinguish the situations in their lives for which they are personally responsible from circumstances and intrapsychic attitudes that reflect broader social problems. In feminist therapy it is as important to help clients to set goals and develop skills to make appropriate individual changes as it is to validate the client's experiences of frustration or powerlessness and to encourage the client to meet with others who suffer from similar problems (Donovan & Littenberg, 1981; Espín, 1985; Greene, 1986):

> The explicit commitment to feminist values as a basis for conceptualizing therapy is what distinguishes feminist therapy from other forms of therapy. Simply to be non-sexist and to attempt modification of existing approaches is inadequate. What is necessary is a critical recognition of sociocultural agents and factors as generating emotional distress in women, and the development of special expertise in working with women's issues and concerns. (Faunce, 1985, p. 1)

As Faunce also maintains, "Important is the philosophy that determines the attitudes with which techniques are used and theories supported" (1985, p. 1). Moreover, one of the most basic principles of feminist philosophy is that *the personal is political*. In simple terms, this means that the individual experience expresses the collective situation while, at the same time, "a feminist perspective . . . regards the individual's behavior as best understood by examining the social structure." (Comas-Díaz, 1987, p. 52). This postulate that the personal is political has profound implications for the work of the feminist therapist because it presupposes that changes in the lives of women necessitate changes in the basic structure of society. Feminist therapists believe that therapy is not value-free and that the therapist has to understand and acknowledge her values. This means that the therapist has to be aware and struggle against her own sexism, racism, classism, and heterosexism. The feminist therapist is aware of the fact that there are no individual solutions for social, moral, and political problems that are at the root of her clients' distress. Thus she recognizes the need to join others to work for social change and the importance that such activity has for her clients' validation and empowerment (Donovan & Littenberg, 1981). As a consequence, from a feminist point of view, "in both therapy and politics, transformation means finding a way to give voice to the unheard, to embody the invisible" (Hill, 1990, p. 57). Because women of color are the most invisible and unknown among women (Espín, in press), it is relevant to examine what a feminist approach to therapy can offer them.

Guidelines for Feminist Therapy

Although total agreement on the theory and practice of feminist therapy has not been achieved yet, Butler (1985) offers a set of guidelines that distinguish a feminist therapy approach from other approaches to therapy:

1. *Recognition of women's oppression based on gender, race, and class.*

   The basis for feminist therapy is a recognition of the harmful effects of the sexist society in which we live. Real oppression of women based on gender as well as class and race is the basis for the conflicts, low self-esteem, and powerlessness reported by many women who seek therapy. (Butler, p. 33)

2. *Relevance of the sociocultural context.*

   Feminist therapy explores with clients the inherent contradictions in the pre-scribed social roles for women. Rejected is the medical model of psychiatry, which locates the source of human conflict within the individual, that is, in a vacuum, with no relationship to the socioeconomic system within which we live. Emphasized is a sociocultural and systems approach to psychological growth and change. (pp. 33–34)

3. *Focus on women's empowerment.*

   Feminist therapists support women in an exploration of their inner resources and capacity for nurturance and self-healing. They encourage the process of individual goal-setting and support those client goals that transcend traditional sex-role stereotyping. They encourage the exploration of various lifestyles and sexual orientations and support the acquisition of skills for self-directed and interdependent living. (p. 34)

4. *Diverse therapeutic modalities.*

   Feminist therapy distinguishes itself from traditional therapies by its nonsexist frame of reference. Feminist therapists utilize appropriate existing therapeutic modalities and develop new techniques compatible with the underlying phi-losophy of feminist therapy. (p. 35)

5. *Demystification of power in the therapeutic relationship.*

   Feminist therapists work on demystifying the power relationship inherent in any therapeutic situation. Doing so requires a feminist therapist to be open about her own values and attitudes. (p. 35)

6. *The therapist and other women as role models.*

   Feminist therapy affirms that matching women clients with women therapists is often the most therapeutic choice for women. Feminist therapists use both individual and group approaches to therapy. Affirmed, in particular, is the value of an all-women's group therapy model. The group model enables women to (1) validate each other's strengths; (2) develop mutual support systems; (3) break down their isolation from each other; and (4) help each other perceive various possibilities for growth. (p. 36)

7. *The therapist's ongoing self-examination and reflection on her values.*

Feminist therapy requires that a therapist (1) conduct an ongoing evaluation of her practice, (2) make provision in her practice for low-income clients, (3) examine her lifestyle and values as they relate to her therapeutic approach, (4) identify with the goals and philosophy of feminism, and (5) examine her own race, class, and sexual orientation as they may lead to therapeutic blind spots with clients. (p. 37)

8. *Encouragement of growing experiences in addition to therapy.*

Feminist therapists acknowledge that therapy per se is not a cure-all, and they encourage women to consider other avenues for growth and support instead of or in addition to therapeutic experience. (p. 37)

I believe that these guidelines coincide with what women of color would need from the therapeutic relationship. In particular, it is relevant that they emphasize the importance of empowerment, choice, and active social action as healing factors that would foster mental health for all women.

Positive Contributions of Feminist Therapy to the Mental Health of Women of Color

Feminist therapy's central tenet of the importance of sociocultural factors in the psychology of all women is its most obvious positive contribution to the effective delivery of mental health services for women of color.

Of particular relevance for women of color seeking psychotherapy is that a central focus of feminist therapy is to empower women. "Empowerment is usually understood as the process of helping a powerless individual or group to gain the necessary skills, knowledge or influence to acquire control over their own lives" (Smith & Siegel, 1985, p. 13). It is clear that women of color need to be empowered individually and as a group, and it is also clear that such empowerment will be psychologically healing and validating. Several authors who have discussed the empowering effects of feminist approaches to therapy with women of color (Comas-Díaz, 1987; Mays & Comas-Díaz, 1988; Solomon, 1982) state that feminist approaches help women of color to acknowledge the deleterious effects of sexism, racism, and elitism; to deal with negative feelings imposed by their status as ethnic minorities; to perceive themselves as causal agents in achieving solutions to their problems; to understand the interplay between the external environment and their inner reality; and to perceive opportunities to change the responses from the wider society.

Although consideration of life choices for women is not limited to reproductive issues, these issues constitute an extremely important component of women's life choices. Thus, another positive contribution of a feminist approach to therapy with women of color derives from the feminist conceptualization of reproductive choice. In terms of both access to birth control and abortion as well as the right to be protected from forced sterilization, feminist positions reaffirm women's right to control their own bodies. For all women of color, the access to safe abortion and birth control and the governmental funding of such programs is of primary importance, but perhaps even more so is the issue of forced sterilization for poor ethnic minority women. Regrettably this is an issue that has not attracted as much attention from White feminists, although it has been of primary importance for women of color (Davis, 1981).

The issue of forced sterilization has galvanized the energy of women of color, but so have other issues that have prompted them to become involved in social action. Housing and the homeless, neighborhood safety, pregnant teenagers, educational opportunities, drugs, the AIDS crisis, and violence in the family are examples of some of the issues that have served as catalysts for the involvement of women of color in social change projects. Because, as feminists maintain, the psychological effects of oppression have their roots in the social world, and the psychological healing of women does not occur only through a focus on the intrapsychic, changing the conditions of oppression under which women live is both a promoter and a consequence of psychological healing. For women of color, involvement in social action represents a form of empowerment, a productive expression of anger, and a way of testing their inner strength and resources. Involvement in social action becomes a powerful antidote to the helplessness engendered by oppressive social conditions. Thus feminist therapy's encouragement of participation in activities outside therapy provides a support that is uniquely relevant for women of color.

Women of color, by virtue of their constant exposure to instances of racism and sexism, are frequently in touch with their anger. Since the acknowledgment and expression of angry feelings is seen as contradicting the cultural image of the "good" woman, women of color find their femininity questioned when they express their justified anger.

One of the contributions of feminist therapy to the treatment of women is the validation of women's anger and the facilitation and management of that anger as a source of strength in oppressive social contexts. In feminist therapy, women of color can find their anger validated, examine their experience of anger, learn to manage it, and circumvent depression through freedom to express anger in productive action both in their personal lives and in their social worlds. For women to be able to express anger in articulate and appropriate verbalizations and confrontations is one of the goals of feminist therapy (Burtle, 1985). However, this presupposes a therapist who is able to deal with her own anger and with expressions of anger directed at her. This issue is particularly poignant when the therapist is a White woman, because the anger of the woman of color can become threatening to the therapist or evoke feelings of guilt in her that would not be productive for the client.

Contradictions in Feminist Therapy with Women of Color

It is rather ironic that a theory that evolved from the awareness that sociocultural factors are essential determinants in the psychology of women has been so slow to extend its own major insight to sociocultural factors other than gender, thus excluding the experiences of the vast majority of women who are not White, and in that process excluding the impact of sociocultural factors other than gender, (e.g., race, class, and ethnicity) on the lives of all women, including White women (Espín & Gawelek, 1992; Spelman, 1988). Recent theoretical efforts at correcting this distortion within feminist psychology (e.g. Ballou, 1990; Brown, 1990; Espín & Gawelek, 1992) are still not widespread. Most therapists, regardless of their race, ethnicity, or class, continue to be trained in theories that are presented as universally valid (Greene, 1986), even though these theories are based on the specificity of life conditions of a mostly middle-class, White, Western, heterosexual male population. Bradshaw (1990) provides an example of this bias in her discussion of Masterson's theory, and accurately describes the "racism cloaked in psychological jargon" (p. 75) present in so many theories. Thomas and Sillen (1972) provide innumerable examples of racist biases in both theory and practice.

Theories of psychological development and psychopathology have been notorious for their neglect of cultural variability as well as gender issues. Most psychological theory is literally European American in its perspectives and conceptions of human nature. Psychology's preoccupation with scientific objectivity has divorced it from an understanding or description of human experience in its fullness and has limited it to data that is mostly based on the experience of White European American men. Data on White women or ethnic minority people of both sexes have mostly either been excluded as "nuisance variables" or included only as "difference" and more often than not understood as deficiencies. Basically psychology has understood human diversity from two diametrically opposed perspectives. Either differences among people are a reflection of abnormalities or deficiencies, in which case efforts should be made to change the individuals and make them healthy. Or these differences are regarded as dictated by nature rather than as a result of the sociocultural context, so that there is no need for any intervention. (Espín & Gawelek, 1992; Fine & Gordon, 1989). Current feminist psychological theory has not fully escaped this bias and unfortunately is also encumbered by the scientific paradigm of psychology:

> Most feminist therapists and theoreticians, although trained in traditional systems and theories of personality and psychotherapy, have been quick to identify the masculinist biases inherent in other theories and practices that are associated with them. Many have also been able to cull out the heterosexist and homophobic biases. But the subtle aspects of racist and classist assumptions have been less visible and less salient to many white feminist therapists who have benefitted from privilege of race and class. (Brown, 1990, p. 4)

Thus, tendency to overgeneralize from data and information gathered from the experience of White women continues for the most part unchallenged, rendering women of color invisible yet one more time and limiting the development of a theory that should and could render them more visible (Brown, 1990; Espín, in press; Greene, 1986).

In spite of this limitation, I still believe that feminist therapy has a lot to offer to women of color and their mental health, particularly if White therapists take seriously their own White privilege and actively engage in antiracist self-education in this area (Katz, 1978; McIntosh, 1988; Rave, 1990).

THEORY AND PROCESS IN FEMINIST THERAPY WITH WOMEN OF COLOR

By definition the therapist in a feminist approach to therapy is a woman who is a feminist, but nothing much is said in feminist therapy's theory about the sociocultural background of the therapist, such as her race, ethnicity, class, and so on.

I would like to propose that the best form of therapy for women of color is a feminist ethno-specific approach. By a feminist ethno-specific approach I mean a therapeutic context in which the therapist is a woman from the same ethnic/racial background as the client. I am fully aware of the small numbers of feminist therapists who are women of color and thus of the difficulties involved in implementing this approach. Nevertheless, I would like to explain my rationale for stating that feminist ethno-specific therapy is the best approach to psychotherapy with women of color.

As feminist therapists maintain, the similarities in life experience between therapist and client provide a unique—perhaps the only—context in which women can feel both nurtured and empowered in therapy (e.g., Eichenbaum & Orbach, 1984; Gilbert, 1980; Kaschak, 1981). Arguments about the absolute importance of a woman therapist for women also provide the justification for the importance of cultural specificity in therapy. In spite of some contradictory information (Brody, 1984), it seems that the advantages of same gender as well as same culture/ethnicity/race between therapist and client are evident. I believe that these advantages are that (1) the therapist can understand the culture/ethnicity/race (and the language: Espín, 1987b) of the client from first-hand experience; (2) the therapist can serve as a more adequate and effective role model for the client because a therapist from the same ethnic/racial group can, just through her presence, raise the client's consciousness as to what a woman of that background can accomplish; (3) the therapeutic relationship can be more equalized because therapist and client share the same culture/ethnicity/ race, thus the balance of power in the therapeutic context, rather than reproducing the inequalities of the world at large, better approximates the feminist philosophy of therapy; and (4) the therapist is more likely to be invested in the client's success in therapy and life.

Obviously there are also some pitfalls to this approach, such as the danger of overidentification of therapist with client, which could lead to excessive expectations or impatience about the client's progress and the danger of other countertransferential reactions evoked in the therapist that may interfere with the therapy and that could be triggered precisely by the similarity between the two parties involved. These dangers, however, are present in all feminist therapy by the very fact that both parties in the dyad are women. As Rave (1990) aptly puts it, White racism and privilege are still present in therapy when both parties involved are White women because these forces are an inescapable component of all of our lives, not just the lives of those who are "different."

In spite of my belief that a feminist ethno-specific approach would be best suited to therapy with women of color, the reality is that the number of feminist therapists of color is so small that most women of color who seek out a feminist therapist will find themselves in therapy with a White woman. Good therapy provided in the woman of color client/White therapist dyad could be a tool for further understanding about differences and bridging gaps between races, classes, and so on for both therapist and client. On the other hand, this dyadic context could place the client in the position of "teaching" about culture, ethnicity, class, or race to the therapist, once again depriving the client from fully receiving what she needs. This dyad obviously involves the dangers of transferential/countertransferential reactions inherent in all therapy. In addition, it reproduces power differentials inherent in this society and thus a specific set of conflicts that exist prior to and outside the therapy. Once again the client finds herself in a context in which the White woman (this time as her therapist) has more power than her, thus defeating the possibility of empowerment that feminist therapy is supposed to offer all women (Gilbert, 1980; Kaschak, 1981). In this dyadic context it is essential that the therapist "[acknowledge] the deleterious effects of sexism and racism" (Comas-Díaz, 1987, p.41) on the life of her client and that these be addressed within the context of the therapy as well as acknowledged in the world at large, or else the therapy will be doomed to failure or fall short of what it should offer the client.

In those rare instances when the therapist is a woman of color and the client a White woman, another set of possibilities and pitfalls can become part of transference and countertransference. A case example presented later on in this chapter illustrates this point.

Comas-Díaz and Jacobsen (1991) offer a rather encompassing and clear framework for understanding the different shapes that transferential and countertransferential reactions can take in cross-cultural contexts. Their framework is applicable to the varying compositions of the therapeutic dyad that may be found in feminist therapy.

CLINICAL ILLUSTRATIONS

It is sometimes naively assumed by people not involved in feminist therapy that these therapists spend their time "preaching feminism," rather than doing therapy per se. It is also assumed that feminist therapists attribute all psychological conflicts to the social context and pay little attention to intrapsychic individual conflicts. Rather than disputing these assumptions, I will refer the reader to authors who have described feminist therapy and its applications in detail (e.g., Comas-Díaz, 1987; Espín, 1985; Gilbert, 1980; Greene, 1986; Kaschak, 1981) and will devote the rest of this chapter to clinical illustrations of feminist therapy with women of color. One vignette addresses the therapeutic dyad where the therapist is a woman of color and the client is White. This example was chosen because it illustrates poignantly some of the issues encountered when feminist therapy is done in a cross-cultural context. Details of the cases that are irrelevant to the illustration of a feminist approach to therapy have been omitted. All names as well as other identifying information have been modified.

Case 1: Amalia

Amalia was a 37-year-old Latin American woman who was an undocumented immigrant. She was in a cohabitating relationship with a working-class White man who was a car mechanic. Amalia had one son from a previous union who was 10 years old, and a son and a daughter, ages 5 and 3 respectively, from her present union. She had been taking some English as a Second Language (ESL) classes at a community center, and one of her teachers there referred her to me for therapy because she was apparently depressed. We agreed on a fee that was affordable for her and acceptable to me and began to work steadily on her feelings of depression, although she frequently missed sessions.

Soon after we started working together, Amalia told me that Mike did not know she was in therapy and that he was abusive toward her and the

children, particularly her older son. He could become violent when his wishes
and commands were not followed. Because of her immigration status and her
lack of education and English, it was clear that she could not afford to leave
him. But more importantly, the thought that he did not have the right to be
violent and domineering had not ever crossed her mind. When I shared with
her that I did not like to see her trapped in this situation and that I would
never tolerate that treatment from any man, she was extremely surprised, and
her facial expression showed vividly how startled she was at my comment.

Amalia's father had been violent with her mother and the children, and
so had Amalia's previous mate. Her only sister was also in an abusive marriage,
and she believed all her brothers and other men she knew beat their wives as
a matter of course. I explained to her that although I believed she probably
was describing a reality, I thought this was a sad reality and one that should
be changed. She commented at this point that she had heard some White
American women say that but had never heard another Latina woman say
that it was not right for a man to beat his wife. She expressed her excitement
at the possibility of rebelling against Mike's violent treatment without having
"to become too Americanized." I, in turn, was surprised at her response,
because I do not believe that wife abuse is specific to Latino culture and because
up to that point I had interpreted her submission to his violence to be a result
of her violent family history and her economic and legal situation. It had not
occurred to me to interpret it as an expression of her fear of becoming too
acculturated into American values.

During the next few sessions Amalia became very inquisitive about my
opinions on violence against women. She obtained a phone number from me
and went as far as contacting a shelter for battered women that serviced mostly
a Black and Latino population—then she got pregnant by Mike for a third
time. I continued to work with her through her pregnancy, and during that
time explored with her her unconscious motivation to become pregnant at a
time when she was beginning to question her relationship with Mike. During
her pregnancy Amalia continued taking ESL classes and also started training
as a beautician, which she had almost finished by the time her baby was born.
Her therapy sessions became more regular during her pregnancy, and the
violence at home subsided considerably to the point where Mike was directing
almost no violence against her and much less toward the children. She took
advantage of this more calm environment to convince Mike that she ought to
settle her immigration status legally, particularly considering that she now had
three American children. Mike, who had more or less opposed this move by
telling her that it was not necessary, agreed to it now, probably because she
was more firm in expressing her wishes about this and other matters at home.
When the baby was born, Amalia decided to terminate therapy because the
beautician courses, the baby, and her other obligations already demanded
100% of her time.

Case 2: Camila

Camila came to the United States from South America with her family when
she was 15. The family had decided to migrate because of political changes in

her country. When she started therapy 3 years later Camila was studying at a university and had recently become sexually involved with an Irish American woman in her dorm. Her grandmother, who was still living in her country of origin, had been more important to her as a maternal figure than her own mother. However, her grandmother was very opposed to Camila's lesbian relationships, which had started right before she immigrated to the United States.

She came to therapy wanting to speak in Spanish because, according to her, "her problems were in Spanish," and she also wanted a feminist therapist who would not reject her lesbianism. She actually was not sure that such a therapist really existed because she thought all feminist therapists were White, and she had been in therapy for a short period of time with a Latino man, at the insistence of her family. This therapist had been intent on convincing her that her attraction to women was transitory and that she should try to get sexually involved with men. Camila, who is rather smart and to the point, told him that perhaps he should encourage his heterosexual female clients to get involved with women as a transitory stage too, and left the therapy.

She was very pleased to see that rather than trying to encourage her to change her sexual orientation, I was interested in ways of helping her be happier in her relationships by choosing more appropriate partners (the woman with whom she was involved was an active alcoholic). We worked intensely on self-esteem issues and also on her relationship with her grandmother, her parents, and her partners. She worked in therapy on and off for about 7 years, coming to see me when she needed immediate help and taking extended "breaks" from the therapy when things were going well. When Camila finally terminated her therapy, she went back to her country for an extended visit with her grandmother. Her partner for the last two years, a Jewish woman she had met through their common interest in music, was coming to stay at the grandmother's home for part of the visit, at grandmother's invitation.

Case 3: Eileen

Eileen sought out a feminist therapist in order to deal with some relationship difficulties that she thought needed a feminist approach. She was 35, White, upper middle class, the third in a family of three daughters, and a college professor, teaching German literature at a prestigious university. Her father was an executive for a powerful international company he had worked for all his life. He was very successful, and the family lived in comfort. Her mother was a homemaker. Her two older sisters were married to very successful White men. Eileen had been involved in several relationships with Latino and Black men, much to the disgust and opposition of her parents, who believed that her teaching career had made her "too liberal." All the relationships had ended with the men leaving after many verbal fights in which they all said in one form or another that she was too needy. Although it was very clear that her parents had been cold and emotionally abusive throughout her childhood and continued to be as verbally abusive to her as she and her lovers were to each other, she insisted that they were good parents and she alone was to blame for her incapacity to sustain good relationships.

In her view, her choice of men of color as sexual partners was not an issue that needed to be discussed. She "just fell in love with the individuals" and was surprised that I could be "prejudiced like her parents in assuming that she should be with White men only." While agreeing that race should not be a factor against choosing a partner, I continued to question her pattern of always being involved with men of color and choosing me as a therapist, considering that there are so many more White women who are feminist therapists. Her response was always that she did not have "any of those prejudices" and "did not pay attention to a person's race or ethnicity" in choosing friends, lovers, or a therapist.

After some time in which she did not make much progress in therapy, she started referring to her father's questioning of my competence on a regular basis. Although she knew I also taught at a university, we had never discussed my education. Eventually, she directly asked about my credentials as a therapist, but immediately made a comment about not wanting to know that I had "too many degrees" or "too many years of experience" because then I "might be too good for her." When I confronted her with the implied racism in this statement and the implied self-deprecatory meaning of it, she denied that any of those interpretations were true.

Later in the therapy, when she finally started acknowledging the cold and verbally abusive atmosphere in which she had grown up, she mentioned in passing several novels about Black families she had read in the course of her education. In these novels, family members were loving and supportive of each other, in spite of the fact that they were poor. She added that when she had first read these novels, as an adolescent, she had wished her father was not successful in his business; perhaps if they were poor, the family would be more loving.

This revelation brought on the unraveling of an elaborate fantasy that her relationships with men of color would be warmer and better than her sisters' marriages. Eventually, she was able to confront the role her fantasy about the warmth and loving characteristics of people of color had had in her choice of a Latina woman as her therapist. From that she went to a full acknowledgement of her emotional deprivation during childhood and her feeling that she would never be good enough because "no White person could really be loving enough." All she could hope for was that her therapist or her lovers, as people of color and thus able to love, could provide all the warmth and love she craved and was incapable of giving. At the same time that she held this over-idealized image of people of color, she also held strong racist views. Like her parents, she assumed that neither her therapist nor her lovers "were fit to lick her boots" (her father's words) and was intent on defeating her therapy and her relationships to prove this point. This was yet another effort to "prove" to herself and others that her parents were right and thus "good."

Needless to say, there were other issues in Eileen's therapy that have been left out of this account. The point I want to make by presenting this case vignette is that cross-cultural feminist therapy contexts present unique challenges. Because Eileen's issues expressed themselves in a rather strong fashion, they were more clearly observable. The powerful unconscious forces involved in cross-cultural therapy are made more obvious in Eileen's story precisely because these issues express themselves dramatically in this case, and also because the usual cross-cultural pattern in feminist therapy of White therapist/woman of color client is reversed. But I believe that some variation of these issues is always present in cross-cultural therapy contexts. I believe that it is impossible to live in a racist society such as ours and not have those forces be present in the therapy room, even when client and therapist share the experience of being female.

The strong tenet of feminist therapy that sexism always creeps into the therapy context when the therapist is male and the client is female is paralleled by the differences in race/ethnicity/class between client and therapist in feminist cross-cultural therapy. It would be naive to believe that the racism of White feminist therapists will never creep into their therapy with women of color clients. The cross-cultural context lends itself to the expression of these feelings and patterns in as powerful a way as the cross-gender therapy context (Comas-Díaz & Jacobsen, 1991). This is the reason why I believe that a feminist ethno-specific approach provides the best alternative for women of color, in spite of the fact that I am well aware of the limitation that the small numbers of feminist therapists of color impose on this possibility.

Since most women of color seeking feminist therapy will probably be in therapy with White women therapists, it is incumbent on the White feminist therapist to be aware, educated, and actively involved in dealing with the influence of racism in her life in order to counter the existence of these forces in herself and in her therapy with women of color.

THE TAPESTRY OF THERAPY WITH WOMEN OF COLOR

The case vignettes presented above provide an illustration of how feminist concerns are present in therapy with women of color, even when the focus seems to be on ethnocultural issues, and how ethnocultural issues are present even when the focus appears to be more on feminist concerns. In other words, all the threads of the social context are interwoven in the tapestry of therapy, and it is essential for good therapy that attention be paid to all of them.

For example, in Amalia's case, the effect of acculturative stress was expressed through her concern about becoming "too Americanized." This concern was an important factor in how she perceived and tolerated the expression of anger in herself and violent behavior on the part of others. While preventing the abuse of women is usually defined as a feminist concern, Ho (1990) warns us not to interpret and/or justify violent behavior towards women in ethnic minority communities under the guise of cultural traditions: "Violence hurts victims physically regardless of cultural heritage and customs" (Ho, 1990, p. 147), and thus abusers "should not be allowed to use their cultural background as an excuse for their abusive behavior" (p. 146).

Amalia's family background, her fear of the effects of acculturation, and her tenuous legal status combined to create a situation of helplessness that, although to some extent specifically female, was also amplified by stressors shared by both females and males in her legal, social, and acculturative situation. In disclosing my unwillingness to tolerate violence in my life, I apparently modeled for her the possibility of refusing to tolerate violence and still remain faithful to Latino culture. Feminist therapy's emphasis on the relevance of appropriate therapist disclosure provided a vehicle for an apparently successful intervention. At the same time, the ethnospecific context of the therapy was essential for Amalia's acceptance of the relevance of the therapist's position for her own life as a Latina. It was the combination of both perspectives that produced an enhancement of Amalia's life situation and mental health.

With Camila, the open exploration of sexuality, in Spanish, also provided a form for the resolution of her ambivalence. In her previous experience, every Latino person (e.g., grandmother, psychiatrist) was rejecting of her lesbianism, and her sexuality could only be expressed in an English-speaking context where other aspects of her self-esteem were endangered (Espín, 1987a). The encouragement of individual goal setting and transcendence of traditional sex-role stereotypes that are characteristic of a feminist perspective were, in her case, strengthened by the support of a Latina therapist who could accept Camila's sexuality and discuss it positively in Spanish from within the same cultural context in which she felt nurtured and supported in all other aspects of her life. The presence of this role model provided her with options she would not have been aware of otherwise.

In Eileen's case, the intermingling of the ethnocultural and feminist themes presented itself in a more subtle, and even confusing, form. However, the same themes of racism, classism, and need for acknowledging the diversity of women's experiences that are usually identified as issues for women of color were clearly present in the therapy of this White upper-middle-class woman. The equalization of power in the context of her therapy operated under some peculiar conditions. Had I been more aware of the existence of issues of race and class as a significant factor in her life, rather than assuming that they were not as relevant for a White upper-middle-class woman, Eileen's therapy would probably have progressed more rapidly. Moreover, had I not taken at face value her apparent lack of racism and prejudice, we would have been able to uncover the elaborate fantasies that precluded her involvement in realistic relationships and disguised her intense self-denigration and self-hatred at a much earlier stage in her therapy.

CONCLUSION

Let me conclude by saying that I do not see a feminist approach to therapy as something that can be used by a therapist for one patient and then not used for the next, according to the patients' needs. The preceding discussion of the case vignettes serves to illustrate this perspective. I believe that when a therapist has a feminist analysis of the social world and thus a feminist understanding of women's life experiences, there is an inherent feminist approach to her therapy as well as to her own life. Consequently, she will approach the therapy of all her clients from this vantage point. By the same token, when a therapist has an analysis and understanding of the impact of racism, social class, privilege, and sexual orientation as factors in the construction of personality, it is impossible and ineffective to approach any client without this perspective.

I will go so far as to assert that a therapist who does not have an analysis of the social world could not be a good therapist. That analysis includes an understanding of the impact of oppression due to gender, race, ethnicity, class, sexual orientation, disability, and age (and, conversely, of the impact of privilege on the lives of those who do not belong to oppressed groups in these categories). I believe that this analysis and awareness are as essential for good therapy as knowledge of psychological theory or practical therapeutic skills. Indeed, to espouse a theory or use a skill without understanding its embeddedness in the social context in which it was developed can, in fact, be dangerous and unethical (Katz, 1985).

Thus a therapist who has a feminist philosophy of treatment and who actively seeks to assist her women of color clients in their healing and empowerment will always, in one form or another, be doing feminist therapy, regardless of what the specific focus of the therapeutic work is at any given time.

REFERENCES

Anzaldúa, G. (Ed.). (1990). *Making face, making soul—Haciendo caras: Creative and critical perspectives by feminists of color.* San Francisco: Aunt Lute Foundation.

Ballou, M. B. (1990). Approaching a feminist principled paradigm in the construction of personality theory. In L. S. Brown & M. P. P. Root (Eds.), *Diversity and complexity in feminist theory* (pp. 23–40). New York: Harrington Park Press.

Bradshaw, C. K. (1990). A Japanese view of dependency: What can Amae psychology contribute to feminist psychology and therapy? In L. S. Brown & M. P. P. Root (Eds.), *Diversity and complexity in feminist therapy* (pp. 67–86). New York: Harrington Park Press.

Brody, C. M. (1984). Feminist therapy with minority clients. In C. M. Brody (Ed.), *Women therapists working with women: New theory and process of feminist therapy* (pp. 109–115). New York: Springer.

Brown, L. S. (1990). The meaning of a multicultural perspective for theory building in feminist therapy. In L. S. Brown & M. P. P Root (Eds.), *Diversity and complexity in feminist therapy* (pp. 1–21). New York: Harrington Park Press.

Burtle, V. (1985). Therapeutic anger in women. In L. B. Rosewater & L. Walker (Eds.), *Handbook of feminist therapy* (pp. 71–79). New York: Springer.

Butler, M. (1985). Guidelines for feminist therapy. In L. B. Rosewater & L. Walker (Eds.), *Handbook of feminist therapy* (pp. 32–38). New York: Springer.

Comas-Díaz, L. (1987). Feminist therapy with Hispanic/Latina women: Myth or reality? *Women and Therapy, 6*(4), 39–61.

Comas-Díaz, L. & Jacobsen, F. M. (1991). Ethnocultural transference and counter-transference in the therapeutic dyad. *American Journal of Orthopsychiatry, 61*(3), 392–402.

Combahee River Collective. (1979). A Black feminist statement. In Z. Eisenstein (Ed.), *Capitalist patriarchy and the case for socialist feminism* (pp. 135–139). New York: Monthly Review Press.

Combs, H. G. (1986). The application of an individual/collective model to the psychology of Black women. In D. Howard (Ed.), *The dynamics of feminist therapy* (pp. 67–80). New York: Haworth Press.

Davis, A. (1981). *Women, race and class.* New York: Vintage Books.

Donovan, V. K., & Littenberg, R. (1981). Psychology of women: Feminist therapy. In B. Harber (Ed.), *The women's annual: 1981* (pp. 211–235). Boston: G.K. Hall.

Eichenbaum, L., & Orbach, S. (1984). Feminist psychoanalysis: Theory and prac-tice. In C.M. Brody (Ed.), *Women therapists working with women: New theory and process in feminist therapy* (pp. 46–55). New York: Springer.

Espín, O. M. (1979). The needs of Third World/minority women in historically white universities. *Debate and Understanding No. 5* (pp. 27–31). Boston: Boston University Martin Luther King Jr. Center for Academic Services and Minor-ity Affairs.

Espín, O. M. (1984). Cultural and historical influences on sexuality in Hispanic/ Latina women: Implications for psychotherapy. In C. Vance (Ed.), *Pleasure and danger: Exploring female sexuality* (pp. 149–163). London: Rutledge & Kegan Paul.

Espín, O. M. (1985). Psychotherapy with Hispanic women: Some considerations. In P. Pedersen (Ed.), *Handbook of cross-cultural counseling and psychotherapy* (pp. 165–171). Westport, CT.: Greenwood Press.

Espín, O.M. (1987a). Issues of identity in the psychology of Latina lesbians. In Boston Lesbian Psychologies Collective (Ed.), *Lesbian psychologies: Explora-tions and challenges* (pp. 35–55). Champaign, IL: University of Illinois Press.

Espín, O. M. (1987b). Psychological impact of migration on Latinas: Implications for psychotherapeutic practice. *Psychology of Women Quarterly, 11*(4), 489–503.

Espín, O. M. (in press). On knowing you are the unknown: Women of color constructing psychology. In J. Adleman & G. E. Enguídanos (Eds.). *The significance of racism in the psychology of women.* NY: Haworth Press.

Espín, O. M., & Gawelek, M. A. (1992). Women's diversity: Ethnicity, race, class and gender in theories of feminist psychology. In M. Ballou & L. S. Brown (Eds.), *Personality and psychopathology: Feminist reappraisals* (pp. 88–107). New York: Guilford Press.

Faunce, P. S. (1985). A feminist philosophy of treatment. In L. B. Rosewater & L. Walker (Eds.), *Handbook of feminist therapy* (pp. 1–4). New York: Springer.

Fine, M., & Gordon, S. M. (1989). Feminist transformations of/despite psychol-ogy. In M. Crawford & M. Gentry (Eds.), *Gender and thought: Psychological perspectives* (pp. 146–174). New York: Springer.

Gilbert, L. A. (1980). Feminist therapy. In A. M. Brodsky & R. Hare-Mustin (Eds.), *Women and psychotherapy* (pp. 245–265). New York: Guilford Press.

Greene, B. A. (1986). When the therapist is white and the patient is Black: Considerations for psychotherapy in the feminist heterosexual and lesbian communities. In D. Howard (Ed.), *The dynamics of feminist therapy* (pp. 41–65). New York: Haworth Press.

Hill, M. (1990). On creating a theory of feminist therapy. In L. S. Brown & M. P. P. Root (Eds.), *Diversity and complexity in feminist therapy* (pp. 53–65). New York: Harrington Park Press.

Ho, C. K. (1990). An analysis of domestic violence in Asian American communities: A multicultural approach to counseling. In L. S. Brown & M. P. P. Root (Eds.), *Diversity and complexity in feminist therapy* (pp. 129–150). New York: Harrington Park Press.

hooks, b. (1984). *Feminist theory: From margin to center.* Boston: South End Press.

Hurtado, A. (1989). Relating to privilege: Seduction and rejection in the subordination of white women and women of color. *Signs: Journal of Women in Culture and Society, 14*(4), 833–855.

Joseph, G. I., & Lewis, J. (Eds.). (1981). *Common differences: Conflict in Black and White feminist perspectives.* New York: Anchor.

Kaschak, E. (1981). Feminist psychotherapy: The first decade. In S. Cox (Ed.), *Female psychology: The emergent self* (pp. 387–401). New York: St. Martin Press.

Katz, J. (1978). *White awareness: Handbook for anti-racism training.* Norman, OK: University of Oklahoma Press.

Katz, J. (1985). The socio-political nature of counseling. *Counseling Psychologist, 13*(4), 615–624.

Lorde, A. (1984). *Sister outsider.* Freedom, CA: Crossing Press.

Mays, V., & Comas-Díaz, L. (1988). Feminist therapies with ethnic minority populations: A closer look at Blacks and Hispanics. In M. A. Dutton-Douglas & L. E. Walker (Eds.), *Feminist psychotherapies: Integration of therapeutic and feminist systems.* (pp. 228–251). New Jersey: Ablex.

McIntosh, P. (1988). *White privilege and male privilege: A personal account of coming to see correspondence through work in Women's Studies* (Working Paper No. 189). Wellesley, MA: Center for Research on Women, Wellesley College.

Rave, E. J. (1990). White feminist therapists and antiracism. In L. S. Brown & M. P. P. Root (Eds.), *Diversity and complexity in feminist therapy* (pp. 313–326). New York: Harrington Park Press.

Root, M. P. P. (1992). The impact of trauma on personality: The second reconstruction. In L. S. Brown & M. Ballou & (Eds.), *Personality and psychopathology: Feminist reappraisals* (pp. 229–265). New York: Guilford Press.

Smith, A. J., & Siegel, R. F. (1985). Feminist therapy: Redefining power for the powerless. In L. B. Rosewater & L. Walker (Eds.), *Handbook of feminist therapy* (pp. 13–21). New York: Springer.

Solomon, B. B. (1982). The delivery of mental health services to Afro-American individuals and families: Translating theory into practice. In B. A. Bass, G. J. Wyatt, & G. J. Powell (Eds.), *The Afro-American family: Assessment, treatment and research issues.* New York: Grune & Stratton.

Spelman, E. V. (1988). *The inessential woman: Problems of exclusion in feminist thought.* Boston: Beacon Press.

Thomas, A., & Sillen, S. (1972). *Racism and psychiatry.* New York: Brunner/Mazel.

Trotman, F. K. (1984). Psychotherapy of Black women and the dual effects of racism and sexism. In C. M. Brody (Ed.), *Women therapists working with women: New theory and process of feminist therapy* (pp. 96–108). New York: Springer.

11

An Integrative Approach

Lillian Comas-Díaz

THE NEED FOR INTEGRATION

The need for integration of numerous psychotherapeutic techniques is emerging as a trend in the delivery of mental health services. For example, the Society for the Exploration of Psychotherapy Integration (SEPI) established the *Journal of Psychotherapy Integration* to increase understanding of the processes of change and improve the effectiveness of psychotherapy based on integrative approaches to the field (SEPI, 1991). Similarly, Okun (1990) advocates integration and pluralism in psychotherapy. She argues that the clinician needs to find multiple ways to treat clients by selecting methods from different theoretical schools. This pluralistic approach affords flexibility, helping the practitioner to be a more effective healer. Moreover, it has been argued that the future of psychotherapy will witness a consolidation of traditional orientations, a receptive stance toward pluralism, a focus on interventions for specific clinical problems, an application of findings from cognitive science, plus an integration of psychotherapy and pharmacology (Goldfried & Castonguay, 1992).

Effective mental health treatment for women of color requires such an integrative and comprehensive perspective. This chapter presents an integrative approach developed specifically for treating women of color that reconciles psychotherapeutic process variables with the dual (gender and race) and multiple group membership of women of color. It addresses the effects of minority group membership on women of color in a manner that effectively constitutes a psychotherapeutic decolonization. The integrative approach acknowledges the confluence of the therapist's and the client's realities. Given that such confluence is accentuated within the dyadic encounter, the therapeutic relationship is presented as an illustration of the integration of essential process variables into a gender-, ethnicity-, and race-informed clinical work. Furthermore, the chapter discusses the woman of color's sense of self and its relevance to treatment. Vignettes illustrate the application of the integrative approach. Clinical material has been altered to protect confidentiality.

For women of color the integration further requires combining traditional psychotherapeutic models with sociocultural (Comas-Díaz & Minrath, 1985), ethnoracial, and gender contexts. Similarly, in discussing the efforts to develop a culturally sensitive clinical curricula, Myers, Echemendia, and Trimble (1991) assert that the ultimate goal is to train cross-culturally competent clinicians who use an integrative approach. The reality of belonging to more than one minority (i.e., being a woman and an ethnic minority) is a paramount consideration within the integrative approach. Consequently, the experiences of racism, sexism, identity, conflict, oppression, cultural adaptation, environmental stressors, plus internalized colonization prevalent among and specific to many women of color, constitute critical considerations in the delivery of relevant psychotherapeutic services.

COLONIZATION, DECOLONIZATION, AND *CONSCIENTIZAÇÃO*

The integrative approach is conceptualized as a therapeutic decolonizing and empowering perspective that is aware of ethnicity, race, and gender. The metaphor of colonization is preferred to that of oppression because people of color in the United States are obliged to adapt to the norms of the dominant culture. Such adaptation involves an inevitable sacrifice in the level of connection to one's culture of origin. Additionally, outright racism and stereotypes further aggravate the identity conflicts involved in making this sacrifice. Members of the society such as White women, gays and lesbians, the elderly, the disabled, and many other minorities experience discrimination and oppression. However, only people of color have been historically colonized and are still being subjected to a form of neocolonialism by virtue of their race and color, and regarding women, by virtue of their combined race and gender. Contemporary political oppression is compounded in the minds of people of color by history, which includes the North American legacy of the American Indian genocide, the United States' enslavement of African Americans, its imperialistic and annexationist relationship with Mexico, its past colonial relationship with Hawaii and the Philippines, in addition to its contemporary colonization of Puerto Rico, plus its conflictual and consequent ambivalent relationship with Asians due to World War II and the Korean and Vietnam wars.

These historical lessons figuratively color the relationship between mainstream group members and people of color, resulting in the creation of a racial collective consciousness (and unconsciousness). This racial collective unconsciousness affected by such things as the fact that during World War II, those U.S. populations from countries that were our political adversaries—Germany, Japan, and Italy—only the Japanese Americans were interned and not German Americans nor Italian Americans. The racial visibility of people of color facilitates their becoming a target for projections of national hate. Similarly, the fear of the enemy extends to those biracial persons who were products of interracial unions during foreign wars (Root, 1990). Consequently, as highly visible minorities, people of color have been historically designated as savages, slaves, conquered enemies—in sum, colonized people.

The inferior and negative designations of people of color appear to remain immutable in the collective unconscious of many North Americans. Moreover, as an imperialistic nation, the United States has a history of discouraging racial intermarriage between mainstream group members and conquered/colonized individuals. Antimiscegenistic thought and White supremacist tendencies have historically opposed mixed-race marriages in the United States (Root, Chapter 16, this volume). Furthermore, when intermarriage occurs, the first generation offspring are labelled people of color, identified with the racial/ethnic group of lower status (Root, 1992). The result is that color becomes the sign of the colonized. This sign is so powerful that it bonds together people of color. Race is the greatest identifying characteristic in a racist environment, transcending gender, sexual orientation, and class identities (Almquist, 1989), and subordinating such identities to the condition of being colonized.

Many women and men of color experience contemporary colonization, which compounds their marginality. For the colonized individual, colonization often results in alienation, victimization, self-denial, assimilation, strong ambivalence, and a fundamental need for change (Memmi, 1965). These dynamics mediate the relationship between colonized and colonizer. Colonized individuals are not only exploited and victimized for the benefit of the colonial power, but also serve as the quintessential scapegoats. For instance, many young African Americans fear being the victim of racial genocide (Turner & Darity, 1973). The perspective of blaming the victim so prevalent in social analyses of the realities of women of color is also reminiscent of this scapegoating. Women of color have often been blamed for their family ills and stresses, which are in fact caused by institutional racism (Greene, 1990). However, the colonized condition involves more than the dynamics of dominance and subordination, power and powerlessness, aggression and identification with the aggressor; it involves a systematic negation of the colonized, resulting in pervasive identity conflicts for the person of color (Fanon, 1967).

For women of color, the status of being colonized involves the added negation of their individuality by their being subjected to sexual–racial objectification. Women of color are stripped of their humanity, denied their individuality, and devalued. As female colonized entities, women of color are often perceived as part of the bounty conquered by the colonizer. Historically, conquered males have been killed while conquered females have been raped, enslaved, and sexually subjugated. The contemporary versions of these dynamics follow these gender lines. On the one hand, men of color often struggle with unemployment and underemployment (which has led to widespread substance abuse) and intraracial murder. On the other hand, conquered women of color suffer from sexual objectification and subjugation. The mythology of the sexual personae of women of color ranges from oversexuality and asexuality on one polarity, to creation (e.g., the concept of *marianismo*, in imitation of the Virgin Mary's long-suffering chastity, or mother earth) and destruction (e.g., the Dragon Lady, dark Lilith, the Queen of Sheba) on the other. The interested reader can see Comas-Díaz and Greene's chapter on professional women in this volume for a fuller discussion of the sexual–racial objectification of women of color (Chapter 13).

The context of colonization often leads to a contradiction whereby in order to liberate herself, the woman of color must resist a tendency in herself that derives from her female oppression—her dualistic and dichotomous mode of thinking (women are good; men are bad, or vice versa; Downing & Roush, 1985), in addition to a dualistic thinking due to her racial oppression (Black is bad; White is good, or vice versa). Moreover, the woman of color needs to confront her internalized negative self-image. This process is particularly complex because women of color in the United States reside in the colonial nation, which augments their internalization of colonization. Such colonization in the belly of the beast profoundly affects the colonized's sense of self. The decolonization involves a paradox for women of color because by being part of the colonial nation, their alienation from others and from themselves is pervasive. Thus, the boundaries between the colonizer and colonized become blurred, often giving birth to depersonalization and ambivalence. The ambivalence is further accentuated by the idealized White middle-class female standard.

The dynamics of liberation and decolonization involve a three stage process: (1) recovery of the self; (2) achievement of autonomous dignity; and (3) action toward fundamental change of self and/or the colonial condition (Memmi, 1965). The integrative approach mirrors this process by helping women of color recover and reclaim the self through increasing positive self-attribution and self-esteem; achieve autonomous dignity through self-efficacy, self-mastery, and self-determination; and transform themselves and their situation by developing a critical consciousness (*conscientização*).

Conscientização is a critical element in the psychotherapeutic decolonization of women of color. According to Paulo Freire (1967, 1970) *conscientização* involves an awakening of consciousness, a change of mentality involving a realistic awareness of one's locus in nature and society; the capacity to analyze critically its causes and consequences, comparing it with other situations and possibilities; and action of a logical sort aimed at transformation. In other words, it involves the awareness and restoration of dignity and self-perception by recognizing the ability to transform one-self and one's world. On an applied level, the process of psychotherapeutic decolonization for women of color involves the following processes:

1. Recognizing the systemic and societal context of colonialism and oppression, thus, becoming aware of the colonized mentality.
2. Correcting cognitive errors that reinforce the colonized mentality, for example, working through dichotomous thinking (superior–inferior, the colonized is good, the colinizer is bad, etc.) and acknowledging ambivalence (toward self and others).
3. Self-asserting and reaffirming racial and gender identity, as well as developing a more integrated identity.
4. Increasing self-mastery and achieving autonomous dignity.
5. Working toward transformation of self and/or the colonized condition (e.g., improving the condition of women, men, and children of color).

Recognizing the systemic context is a prerequisite for the decolonization process because of the colonization's detrimental effect of negating women's multiple identities. Developing a contextual understanding of the colonized condition facilitates the awareness of the colonized mentality. A foundation of the colonized mentality is dichotomous thinking. Conscientization can lead to polarization—us against them, Black against White. Hence, the integrative approach facilitates acknowledging that ambivalence toward oneself or one's race is an adaptive reaction to colonization. Indeed, ambivalence about being a woman of color is an appropriate reaction to culturally sanctioned bigotry (Rosewater, 1990). Ambivalence can also be perceived as a strategy of resistance against colonization. Consequently, self-assertion and reaffirmation of multiple identities not only empower women of color, but also facilitate the development of a more integrated and less dysfunctionally fragmented sense of identity.

Psychotherapeutic decolonization further attempts to increase awareness of and differentiation between external and internalized colonization. For instance, the integrative approach helps clients to differentiate between the external basis of colonization and their individual attribution of personal adequacy or inadequacy. It addresses and corrects cognitive errors that maintain the colonized mentality (see Lewis' discussion of cognitive–behavioral approaches, Chapter 8, this volume). Similarly, it attempts to decolonize and empower women of color within their personal spheres so that they can make informed decisions. Increasing options as well as the perception of options for women of color helps to encourage their personal control and self-mastery. Self- and collective mastery are central to achieving autonomous dignity whereby women of color define themselves independent of the colonizer's idealized White female standard. Additionally, decolonization addresses the colonized group's need for fundamental change, by helping women to become aware of their capacity to shape their environments. Although decolonization requires transcending the individual, the decision for sociopolitical action needs to be articulated by the woman herself. Although it is important for the conscientization to include activism, such activism should not replace therapy by having the clinician act solely as a sociopolitical advocate and reformer. Moreover, many women of color may decide not to choose sociopolitical action because of their own personal, developmental, ethnic, socioeconomic, and geopolitical perspectives. Instead, they may focus on personal and/or family transformation. For example, an American Indian woman may decide that transformation involves the decolonization of her children through her parenting skills, and not necessarily through sociopolitical action. Similarly, an undocumented Latina may choose to help refugees with their adjustment needs over becoming politically active, due to fears of being deported.

THE THERAPEUTIC RELATIONSHIP

The therapeutic relationship is the crux of psychotherapy. Within the process of conscientization, Freire (1970) argues that dialogue involves the encounter between individuals, mediated by the world, in order to name the world, transform it, and subsequently achieve significance as humans. Consequently, in the decolonization process, the therapeutic relationship functions as a dialogue that facilitates the process of critical consciousness. Thus, the integrative approach focuses on the therapeutic relationship as a central component of treatment. It acknowledges the confluence of both the therapist's and the client's realities. Such confluence is galvanized within the therapeutic dialogue.

The therapeutic relationship has been identified as a critical variable in working with people of color (Jenkins, 1990), as well as working with women (Jordan, Kaplan, Miller, Stiver, & Surrey, 1991; Kaplan, 1979). Successful clinical work with women and men of color depends on the therapist's skill in establishing and managing the therapeutic relationship (Jenkins, 1990). It also depends on the therapist's self-awareness and understanding of how ethnocultural and racial factors (Jones, 1985), in addition to gender factors (Bernardez, 1987; Brown, 1990; Jordan et al., 1991) affect both therapist and client.

Clinical work tends to provide a fertile ground for the manifestation of ethnocultural and racial factors in the therapeutic process (Comas-Díaz & Griffith, 1988). These manifestations involve the conscious and/or unconscious acknowledgment of clients' and therapists' feelings and attitudes about their own ethnoracial and cultural identities, as well as conscious and unconscious messages about racial, ethnic, and cultural differences that may be conveyed in the therapeutic dyad (Comas-Díaz & Jacobsen, 1987;

Jones, 1985; Lorion & Parron, 1985; Riess, 1971). Moreover, Jackson (1976) asserts that individuals' racial history provides the perceptual framework for how they experience reality. Similarly, the therapist's racial and sociocultural reality tends to create a filtering process that may inhibit the therapist's understanding of cultural diversity and may result in a desire to work with clients who are culturally similar to the therapist (see Vasquez, Chapter 10, this volume). Indeed, empirical research has documented the existence of ethnoculturally stereotyped attitudes toward culturally different clients on the part of therapists (Wampold, Casas, & Atkinson, 1981).

Gender factors also tend to evoke conscious and unconscious reactions in the therapeutic dyad (Bernardez, 1987; Kaplan, 1979). Thus, clinicians need to examine their own bias in working with women of color. The interaction of gender, racial, and ethnocultural roles may facilitate the clinicians' projection of negative images. For example, Lopez (1989) asserts that gender stereotyping among clinicians leads them to bias information selectively according to the way they imagine their clients' social identities and to what they attribute their behaviors, thus affecting clinical judgments of diagnosis and treatment.

The powerless position in society of women of color may tend to evoke negative social images in the therapist. The inherently unequal power dynamics within the therapeutic relationship may reinforce this powerless position. Among the different therapeutic dyads, the woman of color client and White male clinician dyad may replicate the woman of color's societal powerlessness; that is, it is the dyad most likely to encounter therapeutic failure (Wilkinson, 1980). The power differential between the therapist and client needs to be examined and addressed in order to minimize the replication of societal inequities within the therapeutic dialogue.

The therapeutic dyad could potentially mirror the colonizer–colonized relationship. The therapist–client relationship can be aggressive–passive, leader–led, dominant–submissive, and any number of other polarities (Brown, 1974). Furthermore, it can be reified at the expense of the less powerful member of the dyad (Brown, 1974). Although therapists with an empowering framework are cognitively aware of these issues, unconsciously or preconsciously they may project onto women of color their own ambivalence or internalized tendency to dominate (if they belong to the dominant group) or oppression (if they are oppressed by virtue of gender, sexual orientation, age, etc.). Internalized domination in therapists of the mainstream group may create a sense of entitlement to physical and interpersonal space, an overconfident sense of being right or having all the answers, and a superiority to others who do not share their good fortune (Brown, 1993). Even progressive and well-meaning therapists experience internalized domination because the domination itself is so pervasive a phenomenon (Brown, 1993).

Establishing a therapeutic relationship with a woman of color is in part a function of how she will allow the therapist to enter her life. Women of color have diverse perceptions of mental health and illness and diverse expectations of both treatment and clinicians, and these affect the therapeutic relationship. Moreover, such factors as the gender, ethnicity, race, culture, class, sexual orientation, and age of the therapist, as well as nonspecific factors such as the therapist's attitude toward women of color, can significantly affect the therapeutic relationship. For example, LaFromboise, Trimble, and Mohatt (1990) assert that when clinicians understand and respect the American Indian worldview this helps the development of a therapeutic relationship with American Indian clients.

The therapeutic relationship with a woman of color needs to be reexamined in order to accommodate the worldviews of both the client and the therapist. Its reexamination includes the recognition of specific dyadic variables. The integrative approach closely examines the dyadic variables of empathy, intuition, and attributions of "the Other."

Dyadic Variables in the Therapeutic Relationship

As an interpersonal construct, empathy includes both affective and cognitive components (Jordan, 1991). The affective component involves feelings of emotional connectedness to and a capacity to take in and contain the feelings of the client (Kaplan, 1991), which is similar to a subjective and phenomenological experience of being like the client. On the other hand, the cognitive component involves an intellectual understanding of the client, similar to witnessing the client's experience (Kleinman, 1989). Kaplan (1991) observes that the cognitive component follows a different and contradictory course from that of the affective component. She argues that the affective component tends to facilitate identification of the self with the other, whereas identity tends to remain differentiated in the cognitive empathy.

Empathy in a cross-cultural context raises the question of how empathic a therapist can be in an interethnic dyad without having experienced the client's ethnocultural and gender-related reality. For instance, how much can a White therapist empathize with an African American client? Similarly, the question of how much a White woman therapist can empathize with an African American woman client is not less provocative. The experience of being a woman is diverse and White women's experiences do not necessarily translate into the experiences of women of color. Furthermore, the question of how much an African American female therapist can empathize with an African American female client is determined by a number of factors including but not limited to age, class, and sexual orientation.

Within the cross-cultural encounter, clinicians may be able to empathize at a cognitive level, but not necessarily at an affective level. In cognitive empathy therapists can study the client's culture and confer with colleagues who share the client's cultural background. Kleinman (1989) has termed his concept *empathic witnessing*, where the therapist recognizes his or her ethnocultural ignorance of the client's reality and reaffirms, through empathic witnessing, the client's experience and reality. The emergence of empathy for the emotional experience of the culturally different client may be difficult (Sager, Brayboy, & Waxemberg, 1972), and recognizing this difficulty is a useful component of managing the therapeutic relationship within the integrative framework.

Another important dyadic variable the integrative approach to mental health treatment with women of color explores is intuition. Given the diverse realities that the therapist must examine, intuition becomes a guide for understanding. Indeed, intuition is a clinical compass in the confusing land of cross-cultural encounters. Intuition informs the inner processes and provides information beyond the particular information that is verbally communicated (Butler, 1992). As an illustration, it has been argued that the technical aspects of cross-cultural psychotherapy necessarily needs to include the recognition of nonverbal communication and sensitivity to the subjective aspects of the client's life (Kinzie, 1978). The clinical use of intuition is consistent with the reliance on internal cues, hunches, and vibes as a means of problem solving prevalent among many women of color (Butler, 1992). Consider the ethnocultural dynamics present in the following intragender and intraethnic therapeutic dyad.

Rosa, a Chicana graduate student, was referred by her university counselor for intensive psychotherapy. Rosa was experiencing concentration and attention problems coupled with anxiety about not being able to successfully complete her studies. She felt that she did not belong in an Ivy League environment. Rosa was a nontraditional student: she was the mother of two, a woman in her forties, who had a history of community work in the barrio before going back to college to obtain a master's in Social Work. After an initial assessment the university counselor referred her to a Mexican American female practitioner. During the first session, Rosa behaved appropriately to the context; that is, she was articulate, demonstrated insight into her problems, and expressed an interest in continuing therapy. However, the therapist intuitively sensed a barrier coming from Rosa, which created a distance in the treatment. This barrier continued and during the third session the clinician verbally acknowledged its presence. Rosa also acknowledged the barrier. Although she recognized the facilitative effects of their common gender, ethnoracial, and age identities, she also admitted to feeling ambivalent about it. Indeed, ambivalence is a typical ethnocultural reaction to the intraethnic therapeutic dyad (Comas-Díaz & Jacobsen, 1991). Rosa also expressed concern at the therapist's assumed affluent socioeconomic class background. The class issue was both an external experience (Rosa was from a low socioeconomic background) as well as a symbol of her inner reality (she felt excluded from her family of origin and within her significant relationships). The clinician's direct eliciting of the client's nonverbal behavior initiated a discussion of Rosa's self-disclosed marginality problem. The therapist's intuition regarding Rosa's distance catalyzed the unfolding of an issue central to the client's emotional structure and prevented a premature treatment termination.

Attribution of the other is another dyadic variable relevant to the therapeutic relationship with women of color. This variable refers to the process whereby an individual's attribution of people of different ethnocultural backgrounds helps the person to ethnoculturally define his or her own concept of self. For instance, Kovel (1984) asserts that Europeans' fantasies about Africans and American Indians helped the former to define themselves. Similarly, Jenkins (1985) has argued that for White Americans, people of color may be a cultural representation of the polar opposite. The other facilitates a dichotomous thinking and objectification, where difference is defined in oppositional terms. According to Collins (1991), the dynamics of color and racial projection create a dramatic polarity, the projection of the "not-me." She argues that the other gains meaning only in relationship to the counterpart. Thus, the member of an ethnic minority stops being an individual person, and instead his or her goal is defined by being the other, thereby deriving self-esteem from the White person's attributions (Fanon, 1967).

For women of color, the experience of being the other, may be quite intense and poignant. Collins (1991) believes that maintaining images of African American women as the other provides ideological justification for race, gender, and class oppression. This justification can be generalized to women of color, in that they are seen as outsiders whose experiences and traditions may be too alien for the mainstream individual to comprehend (Lorde, 1984). Women of color are doubly marginalized because they represent the other's other (Comas-Díaz, 1991). For instance, women in the general population are described as the other for men because they are defined with reference to men and not the other way around (de Beauvoir, 1961). Consequently, women of color are doubly marginalized because they are the other for White women and other for the men of color (Comas-Díaz, 1991).

It is crucial to understand the relationship between self and other. According to Rosewater (1990), understanding otherness involves acknowledging the delicate balance between the universality of oppression and the uniqueness of an individual woman's experience. She further asserts that while a therapist who has experienced oppression can empathize with a client's experience of oppression, their experiences of oppression are not necessarily interchangeable:

A Jewish female therapist was working with an American Indian woman. The therapist, a Holocaust survivor, had deep empathy for her client's generational history of ethnic oppression. However, by equating the Jewish genocide with the American Indian genocide, the therapist was negating her client's specific reality of being an American Indian woman who struggles with contemporary racism, oppression, imperialism, colonialism, and sexism. The client terminated treatment during the assessment stage, complaining that the therapist did not understand what it is like to belong to a community that is killing itself with alcohol.

APPLICATION OF THE INTEGRATIVE APPROACH

The integrative approach stipulates that culture is not the only internal representation (Gehrie, 1979) but that gender and race, in addition to their interaction, also provide a unique internal representation for women of color in our society. Furthermore, the integrative approach postulates that clinicians themselves have internal representations that are manifested through ethnocultural and gender-based countertransference (Comas-Díaz & Jacobsen, 1991).

The integrative approach requires that clinicians examine how their own realities and internalizations interact and affect their work with women of color. For example, therapists from the dominant group need to examine their internalized domination through an "antidomination" training. To be effective, an antidomination training requires both didactic (cognitive) information and experiential (affective) involvement (Brown, 1993).

The gender and race/ethnicity interaction can complicate, and sometimes actually hinder, the process and outcome of treatment with women of color. Both variables and their interactive effects on client and therapist need to be seriously considered at all stages of treatment. The ethnicity or gender of a woman of color can potentially obscure issues relevant to the other if the clinician overemphasizes one of these. It has been argued that failure to examine gender dynamics in mental health treatment tends to support traditional sexism that still operates in society (Papp, 1988), as well as in communities of color.

The integrative approach with women of color considers the utilization of diverse therapeutic orientations and modalities tailored to the needs of women. For example, the conceptualization and understanding provided by psychodynamic theories, combined with the reduction of dysfunctional behaviors by cognitive–behavioral modalities, are added to a feminist perspective, which are then integrated into a contextual framework. However, as the previous chapters in this section have demonstrated, the diverse theoretical orientations need to be modified to the specific needs of the woman of color. Furthermore, the integrative approach advocates the need to respect the culture of the woman, while simultaneously challenging dysfunctional responses that are culturally sanctioned.

In addition to being flexible and pluralistic, the clinician working within the integrative approach needs to work simultaneously at several levels—affective, cognitive, behavioral, and systemic. The recognition and utilization of the client's strengths (for recovery of the self) constitute a central tenet in the integrative approach. Similarly, the clinician needs to be aware of special issues relevant to the woman of color's sense of self. Being cognizant of these special issues is important because they tend to surface during mental health treatment. Because of the diversity of women of color, these issues may be more relevant for some women than for others. Nevertheless, there are three areas that I believe are relevant to the sense of self of many women of color: the concept of womanhood, identity conflicts, and the spiritual self.

THE WOMAN OF COLOR'S SENSE OF SELF

Womanhood

The concept of womanhood among women of color offers paradigms that are at variance with those of women from the mainstream group. Women of color are not perceived as being like other women, instead, they are perceived as fragmented or hybrid women: African American women, Latina American women, American Indian, Asian American women, and so on. Thus, treatment requires an examination of the woman's perception of what it is like to be a hybrid entity. The client may or may not initially share this self-image with her therapist, however, eliciting and addressing this issue legitimizes the influence of gender and ethnoracial issues in the client's concept of womanhood.

The experiences and definitions of womanhood among women of color are diverse. Many women have an extended, collective, and contextual definition of themselves. The extended self is validated only by its functioning in relationship and in harmony with the collective whole (Nobles, 1980). Women of color tend to define themselves as females in the contexts of family, group, community, and even universe. They often perceive themselves as individuals within a collective and nonlinear context, and therefore their relationships to others—family, community, and universe—are central to their well-being and sense of continuity. The extended self values interdependence among individuated group members, with an emphasis on collective responsibility (Greene, 1990; McGoldrick, García-Preto, Hines, & Lee, 1989; Nobles, 1980). This extended self is an adaptive mechanism of people in an antagonistic colonized condition. Within hostile racial environments the extended self often protects the group by subordinating the individual's needs to those of the collective.

The family roles of women of color illustrate their experiences of womanhood. Women of color have traditionally formed the center of complex extended families (Boyd-Franklin, 1991; García-Preto, 1990). As females, they are often expected to be strong and to take care of themselves emotionally as well as to take care of the emotional needs of significant others (McGoldrick et al., 1989; Reid, 1989). They are also expected to be resilient (LaFromboise, Heyle, & Ozer, 1990), self-sufficient, reliant, and competent at taking care of others (García-Preto, 1990; McGoldrick et al., 1989; Robinson, 1983). Consequently, family therapy is highly relevant to the special needs of women of color (Boyd-Franklin & García-Preto, Chapter 9, this volume) and congruent with their concept of womanhood.

The experiences of womanhood of many women of color are consistent with the self-in-relation model of female development. This theory postulates that women tend to develop and organize their sense of identity, find meaning, achieve a sense of coherence and continuity, and are motivated in the context of their interpersonal relationships (Jordan & Surrey, 1986). The self-in-relation model is also applicable to women of color, but with considerable modifications and expansions. For example, this theory seems to focus on the mother–daughter dyad to the exclusion of other relationships (Lerner, 1988). Motherhood or mothering is a central aspect of the experiences of womanhood for many women of color, but the mother–daughter relationship is different from that of mainstream women. In an analysis of the legacy of racism and sexism in the lives of African American mothers and daughters, Greene (1990) posits that racial and sexual socialization involves the maternal communication of what it is like to be an African American woman in American society. Specifically, it consists of understanding the expectations of African Americans as well as of White individuals, developing coping mechanisms to deal with such expectations, and examining critically the accuracy of disparaging messages from the mainstream culture. Similarly, among some Latinas, mother–daughter relationships tend to be more reciprocal than mother–son relationships in that mothers expect daughters to assume more responsibility than the sons, a dynamic that often results in more egalitarian relationships between mothers and daughters (García-Preto, 1990). Frequently, Latina mothers pity their daughters because as females they will experience multiple types of oppression. Often, the mechanisms against gender oppression (to bear the cross) that traditional Latina mothers teach their daughters is to accept their cross (submit) (García-Preto, 1990) or to attack with the cross (rebel).

The heritage of women of color working outside the home also influences their experiences of womanhood. Many women of color, as children, played a parental role in their families, partly because of sociocultural norms (Boyd-Franklin, 1991), but also because their mothers were working. Being a parental child tends to reinforce a sense of self-reliance prevalent among women of color. Women of color communicate to their daughters (verbally, nonverbally, or both) not to depend solely on their male counterparts for economic sustenance.

This heritage of females working is closely connected to the concept of womanhood for women of color. When mothers work outside the home, extended family members are often actively involved in child rearing, particularly the grandmother. Although clinical lore identifies the mother–daughter dyad as a central one for mainstream woman, the relationships of woman of color to grandmothers, fathers, siblings, grandfathers, and extended family and friends also have prominent stature in their lives. Among many people of color, the grandmother is a pivotal figure with enormous power and influence, and because human longevity is being further extended, grandmothers will continue to have an active and central role in families of color (Comas-Díaz, 1992). The figure of the grandmother appears to be neglected in the mainstream women's mental health literature. For example, in her review of the Walters, Carter, Papp, and Silverstein (1988) book on gender patterns in family relationships, Travis (1991) asserts that although the volume is cogent and insightful, it is missing sections on grandmothers and sisters.

The grandmother–granddaughter dyad differs from the mother–daughter dyad. Although there are several similar parenting elements, the grandmother–granddaughter relationship seems to empower women of color in a unique manner. The grandmother is often the bearer of and linkage to the woman's ethnoracial heritage. The intensity of this dyad can strengthen the affiliation to her ethnoracial group by reinforcing transgenerational ties. The grandmother often helps to shape the granddaughter's gender and ethnoracial identity by transmitting to her a sense of historical continuity, providing a comprehensive context to her existence.

The experiences of womanhood of women of color often result in a combination of instrumentality (masculine) and expressiveness (feminine). Their highly relational mode is the backdrop for such combined instrumentality and expressiveness. For example, African American women are often instrumental in that they must perform multiple roles (mothers, daughters, partners, etc.) in the social and emotional support they provide for their families (Ridley-Malson, 1983). The heritage of slavery, oppression, and participation in the labor force appears to have forced African American women to find instrumental ways of reconciling their multiple roles (Gump, 1980; Reid & Comas-Díaz, 1990; Tucker, James, & Turner, 1985). Moreover, an investigation studying androgyny among African American women found that the majority of the research participants reported androgynous sexual identities, but had traditional beliefs about the female role in the family (Binion, 1990). Furthermore, research has suggested that African American females tend to favor more masculine qualities than White women do (Brown, Fee-Fulkerson, Furr, Ware, & Voight, 1984; Mason & Bumpass, 1975), and Latinas tend to endorse more masculine qualities than White women, though less than African American women (Pugh & Vasquez-Nutall, 1983). Thus, in order to carry the emotionally and physically tasks of taking care of significant others, many women of color need to combine instrumentality with the standard female quality of expressiveness.

Clinical Applications

The experiences of womanhood by woman of color have several clinical implications. Therapeutic interventions geared to increase a woman's independence from the context of her ethnic group may prove to be unsuccessful. A clinician's attempts to help a client individuate, if it is at the expense of her family or group's needs can be counterproductive. However, a compromise can be made to help the woman function with some degree of autonomy within the family and group context, while extending her self-definition.

A therapeutic technique congruent with a woman of color's sense of womanhood is to utilize narratives in treatment. Storytelling by the client is a technique that addresses the development of identity as a life story construction (Howard, 1991). It can be combined with what McGill (1992) calls the "cultural story," which refers to an ethnocultural group's origins, migration, and identity. At the family level, the cultural story is used to tell where the ancestors came from, what kind of people they were, what issues were important to them, and what lessons have been learned from their experience. At an ethnic level, McGill (1992) further postulates that cultural stories tell the group's collective story of how to cope with life and how to respond to pain and problems. According to Stone (1988), family stories define the sense of the unique nature of families and the individual's own place in them, by providing inspiration, warnings, and cherished values. These tasks are very relevant to the special needs of women of color. Discussing family stories involving female protagonists can build and enhance self-esteem among women of color.

Asking women of color about their mothers' stories can be another helpful clinical technique. For example, Virginia Satir (quoted in Hare-Mustin, 1990) says that the most telling question she asks in a clinical interview is the nature of the woman's relationship with her mother. Similarly, in working with women of color I often ask them about the lives of their mothers, their surrogate mothers, and other females they know. Although I do not provide specific guidelines, I often explore how the woman would describe these female figures to a stranger, her recollections of them when they were her age, how they exhibited gender and cultural roles, and how they dealt with sexism, racism, and oppression. This line of questioning can unfold identity conflicts, generational issues, developmental stages, and gender and ethnoracial expectations. If the woman does not have a strong identification with female family members, I ask her about other important people in her life (female or male). Often, we discuss the history, art, and mythology in a client's ethnocultural heritage. As an illustration, True (1990) reports the use of culturally relevant myths as a therapeutic tool in helping Asian women deal with psychological distress.

Clinical work can help some women of color understand that willingly or unwillingly they are a link to a generational pattern (Greene, 1990). The sense of being the next in a series of the women who preceded her can give the woman of color a different perception of herself and others. Such historical context often offers a comprehensive framework for the woman's internal representation. Similarly, ethnocultural factors outside the woman's control influence the shaping of her internal reality (Brown, 1990). Understanding this interplay, helping women of color to accept their generational legacy, and aiding them to break away from dysfunctional generational cycles can be empowering and therapeutic (Greene, 1990).

Treatment modalities such as family therapy (Boyd-Franklin & García-Preto, Chapter 9, this volume) and group therapy seem to be consistent with womanhood as felt by women of color (Boyd-Franklin, 1991; Chan, 1987; Hynes & Werbin, 1977). A racially homogeneous group provides opportunities to examine and separate dysfunctional behaviors that are idiosyncratic to an individual from those that are culturally embedded. The interested reader can see Melba Vasquez' chapter (Chapter 4, this volume) on Latinas for a discussion of a group therapy from a Latina perspective. LaFromboise, Berman, and Sohi's chapter (Chapter 2, this volume) describes groups tailored for therapy with American Indian women. They posit that using special themes such as self-esteem or assertiveness training could prove helpful. Hardy-Fanta and Montana (1982) describe a group therapy model for Latina adolescents. The content themes that emerged during the group sessions were cultural adjustment, Latino and American gender roles, sexuality, self-esteem, and generational conflict.

A racially and ethnically heterogenous group can address the commonalities and differences among women of color. For example, Lanktree, Comas-Díaz, and Crayton (1983) describe the process of a multi-ethnic (African American, Latino, and White) women's clinical group. Content analysis of the group themes revealed an increased awareness of sex-role stereotypes, an understanding of ethnocultural and racial factors contributing to their problems in functioning, an increased sense of autonomy from their mental health problems, and development of an increased mutual support and empathy for other women.

Identity Conflicts

Cultural pluralism is a salient factor in the identity formation of women and men of color (Comas-Díaz & Minrath, 1985). Being a woman of color means facing some inherent cultural conflict, as people of color tend to be bicultural and/or multicultural (Smith, Burlew, Mosley, & Whitney, 1978). Women of color navigate between two major cultural seas, the mainstream culture and the ethnic minority culture, seas fed by many rivers (sexual orientation, age, class, etc.). Such a journey requires an attempt to cope with and integrate different perceptions, values, and behaviors (Dreyfuss & Lawrence, 1979). The attempt at integration is manifested through a dual or multiple set of distinct responses according to context (Chestang, 1976). Although biculturalism and multiculturalism can provide exceptional strength and flexibility, they can also cause strain, stress, and identity confusion (Pinderhughes, 1982).

"You are what you were," states Levine (in Swartz, 1983) while discussing the impact of culture on psychotherapy. These words gain even more intensity for women of color, where the colonized condition creates identity conflict, precluding self-affirmation. Another special issue for many women of color is conflict within their multiple identities. The extended and contextual self-definition of women of color may cause identity conflicts (Reid, 1988). Indeed, identity conflicts are common among women of color, given the visible contrast between self and the other when they compare themselves with the majority White society (see Chin, Chapter 7, this volume). Feeling different often results in alienation and loneliness, as Ramirez (1991) describes. He further asserts that the majority society puts pressure on ethnic minorities to conform to unrealistic and capricious ideals, resulting in people of color having to abandon their individuality and the self-rejection this entails. Consequently, among many ethnic minority groups, personal and group identity is a psychological minefield (Swartz, 1983). Indeed, conflict over one's ethnic identity is likely to be part of normal development for women of color (Chin, Chapter 7, this volume).

Identity for women of color is indeed a complex issue. Identity conflicts have been recognized as a main complaint of many women of color in psychotherapy (Jones & Gray, 1984). Likewise, cultural and racial identity issues have been identified as crucial elements of mental health treatment with people of color (Atkinson, Morten, & Wing, 1979). In discussing identity and psychotherapy, Helms (1985) reviews different models of identity formation among people of color. She states that most of these models describe stages of ethnic minority identity development in which the attitudes toward self and others change. On a continuum of identity integrations, these stages and attitudes are: (1) the precultural awakening stage, consisting of low esteem for one's self and minority reference group; (2) the transitional stage, characterized by withdrawal, conflicts between self-depreciation and self-appreciation, and cultural reassessment; (3) the immersion–emersion stage, characterized by self-appreciation and by interpersonal relationships limited to the client's cultural group members; and (4) the transcendental stage, characterized by internalization of one's own cultural identity with improved self-esteem.

Research has demonstrated that the development of racial identity is related to self-esteem, affective state, and self-efficacy (Helms, 1990). The stages of racial identity formation are frequently manifested during mental health treatment. Thus, this is a crucial element in the process and outcome of mental health treatment for women of color. For example, Helms' (1990) research has indicated that racial identity attitudes have more impact on the therapeutic process than the racial makeup of the therapeutic dyad. Furthermore, she found that clients' racial identity attitudes are more related to their satisfaction than to the therapist's level of cultural sensitivity. These findings underscore the importance of identity issues in the mental health process.

Ethnoracial identity formation among women of color is additionally influenced by gender factors, among them societal standards of female beauty. In U.S. society the ideal of female beauty is a White standard. This standard negatively affects the self-esteem of women of color who do not resemble it. For instance, among women of African descent, skin color and other physical features connote different levels of attractiveness that garner more or less approval from mainstream society, and that can generate resentment from other women of color, in addition to other conflicts. (For an extended discussion of this topic, see Chapter 5 by Janet Brice-Baker on Jamaican women and Chapter 1 by Beverly Greene on African American women in this volume.) The issue of physical attractiveness is also extended to other women of color. For example, Carla Bradshaw illustrates how racial characteristics and gender issues affect self-esteem among Asian American women (Chapter 3, this volume), while Maria Root discusses this issue among women of mixed racial background (Chapter 16, this volume).

Clinical Applications

The integrative approach to mental health can provide a receptive forum for women of color to express their conflicted identity issues. It can facilitate acceptance of the aspects of self that are race- and gender-based first by conveying that racial, ethnocultural, and gender issues are important. The affirmation of a complex identity facilitates its working through and resolution. Such a therapeutic task can be reached through formally assessing identity issues. Part of this task is provided by ethnocultural assessment. As described by Jacobsen (1988), ethnocultural assessment is a practical diagnostic and treatment tool that considers several stages that may have contributed to the development of the client's ethnocultural identity. The first stage—ethnocultural heritage—involves obtaining a history of the client's ethnocultural heritage while the second—family myth—focuses on the circumstances that led to the client's (and her family's) ethnocultural translocation(s). The third stage—posttransition analysis—is based on the client's intellectual and emotional perception of her family's ethnocultural identity in the host society since the translocation. The fourth stage—self-adjustment—considers the client's own perceived ethnocultural adjustment in the host culture as an individual, distinct from the rest of her family. The last stage—transference and countertransference—calls for consideration of the therapist's ethnocultural background to determine specific areas of real or potential overlap with the client's background.

　　　　Gender issues also need to be integrated into the assessment process. Brown (1986, 1990) recommends that the clinician observe and interpret behaviors of the client through the lens of a heightened awareness of culturally determined norms and roles for each gender. More specifically, she recommends that clinicians familiarize themselves with scholarship and research on gender and its relation to clinical judgments of mental health. As an illustration, Brown (1986) suggests the gathering of contextual information such as age cohort, the nature of religious beliefs, the family's ethnic history and the client's level of awareness of it, number of generations removed from the time of immigration, the client's language(s) and those spoken by the family, family history and the symbolic meaning of the client's name, family roles of women and men, parental class background and education, the level of appreciation of children (including the client); the presence of physical and sexual abuse, and other details.

Spirituality

Spirituality has a central role in the lives of many women of color. Spirituality provides a sense of oneness and harmony which permeates the universe, wherein all elements are bonded together, while at the same time each one has its own niche (Brown, 1982). Many traditional societies such as American Indian, Latin American, and African assume an ecological–ethical universe in which all creatures are ethically required to live in an understanding of, respect for, and harmony with other creatures (Brown, 1989).

The spirituality of many people of color includes a belief in the cyclical nature of existence, where life is a cycle of becoming to which individual development is the transforming key (Comas-Díaz, 1992). The dynamic development of the self through spiritual, physical, social, and emotional modes is central to the spiritual transformation. For instance, the spiritual realm affects the emotional state, which in turn affects the physical condition and vice versa. Some people of color may expect a clinician to also engage in spiritual transformation (LaFromboise, Trimble, & Mohatt, 1990).

In times of crisis or conflict, women of color may immerse themselves in their ethnocultural traditions, particularly spiritual beliefs, as a source for reawakening personal strength. By reaffirming the traditions of their ethnic culture, women of color tap into culturally consistent coping mechanisms as sources of strength (LaFromboise, Trimble, & Mohatt, 1990), obtaining a sense of personal power (Boyd, 1990). For many women of color, defining their sense of self through spiritual rituals and traditional customs is paramount to developing a stronger sense of self, both individually and collectively. For example, the process of retraditionalization among American Indian women relies on the use of cultural beliefs, customs, and rituals as an effective means of overcoming problems and achieving self-determination (LaFromboise, Heyle, & Ozer, 1990).

Many women of color turn to spirituality for support and solace (Berman, 1989; Binion, 1990; Boyd-Franklin & García-Preto, Chapter 9, this volume; LaFromboise, Heyle, & Ozer, 1990, LaFromboise, Berman, & Sohi, Chapter 2, this volume). Spirituality can provide emotional support for the oppressed (Kiev, 1972) and colonized. Some women may manifest their spirituality through formal participation in an organized religion: among African American women, for example, church participation may be an organizing force in their lives (Greene, Chapter 1, this volume). Other women may not belong to an organized religion, but their spiritual beliefs are central to their worldview. The reality of many women of color involves the belief in a higher/supernatural power (Lewis, Chapter 8, this volume).

A strong spiritual and religious orientation has been a central force in the lives of African American women (Boyd-Franklin & García-Preto, Chapter 9, this volume). Greene (1990) suggests that within this context, African American women may exercise leadership roles and use their talents in ways that are not open to them in mainstream society, but that are encouraged in African American churches.

There is a resurgence of spirituality among women (and men) in the general population (Ostling, 1991). They are looking for spiritual connections beyond the confines of ordinary Western monotheism. This spirituality highlights principles that emphasize the feminine. For example, there has been growing interest in spiritual practices that are goddess oriented, or that promote a female and earth-centered style of worship, rather than specific bodies of liturgy (Weinraub, 1991). Similarly, the feminist movement has also recognized the importance of spirituality in women's lives. For example, Conarton and Silverman (1988) state women go through a spiritual development phase, during which they develop healing or spiritual abilities generally associated with the feminine. This phase, they argue, also integrates the masculine or instrumental aspect with the feminine or intuitive and expressive aspect. The spiritual self of many women of color is consistent with this concept of womanhood, because in their cultures femininity integrates expressiveness and instrumentality.

Clinical Applications

The spirituality of women of color has several clinical implications. Spirituality in itself is closely associated with being balanced, harmonious, and psychologically healthy. Being psychologically healthy implies interdependence of mind and body, as well as of person and group. Maintenance of well-being depends on the interaction of physical and psychological elements, in accordance with the belief of many people of color that physical and psychological health are interrelated. Consequently, illness can develop when a harmonious balance is disrupted. According to some spiritual beliefs, illness can be the result of a transgression, or flaw in a person's existential condition. Brown (1989) states that healing such an illness is based on the action of a spiritual guide who mediates between the source of the transgression and the suffering individual in order to restore balance. Consequently, spiritual leaders, members of the clergy, and folk healers are relied on to repair spiritual imbalance.

Spiritual healing is often a female role in the cultures of many people of color (Espin, 1984; Greene, 1991). Spiritual healers often enjoy great power within their communities. Historically, spiritual healing has been a means of empowerment for women (Bourguignon, 1979). Similarly, many Latinas gain power through their roles as folk healers—the *curanderas, espiritistas,* and *santeras* (Comas-Díaz, 1988). In a study of Latina healers, Espin (1984) found that these women were transformed by virtue of their healing powers, from powerless members of the family (due to gender-role expectations) to the most powerful ones.

Adjustments need to be made while delivering clinical services to women who are highly spiritual. For example, Jones (1991) observes that because some people of color attribute causation to spiritual forces rather than personal and social ones, this may result in a tendency to externalize the causes of problems, leading to the perception that they deny personal responsibility. He asserts that such externalization may represent a belief system and not necessarily an evasive problem-solving strategy. In any case, addressing the spirituality of women of color is extremely important in the integrative approach. As an illustration, Lewis (Chapter 8, this volume) offers a cogent discussion of the integration of cognitive–behavioral approaches with the spiritual beliefs of women of color.

CLINICAL ILLUSTRATION

The following is a clinical case illustrating the use of the integrative approach in the mental health treatment of a woman of color.

Presenting Problems and Identifying Data

Anita is an African American woman who was referred to mental health treatment by her internist. She suffered from anxiety, which became acute after she got stuck in the elevator at her workplace. Her internist prescribed Xanax, leading to some relief of her symptoms. However, two months after the elevator incident she experienced a fear of falling when she approached the electric escalators in the subway, and this fear terrified her. Thinking that Anita's acrophobia had been generalized and was contaminating other situations, her internist recommended mental health treatment. When she entered treatment, Anita was very adamant that she only wanted short-term treatment. She presented as a self-reliant woman for whom receiving mental health treatment was incongruent with her self-definition.

Anita was 32 years old, married, with two children, a 6-year-old girl and a 3-year-old boy. Her husband, also 32 years old, worked as a paralegal. They had been married for 11 years. Anita considered her marriage as a good one, and her husband was supportive of her. She worked as a secretary in a law firm, and she felt that she had job security. Anita was raised in the Baptist faith and attended church regularly.

Short Treatment for Acrophobia

Given Anita's request and the urgency of her phobic symptoms, the clinician decided to begin mental health treatment immediately, after a brief diagnostic assessment. The treatment consisted of systematic desensitization, to which Anita responded extremely well. Her positive response to treatment facilitated the development and solidification of the therapeutic relationship. The treatment was designed to be consistent with the strength of Anita's self-reliance. However, during treatment, her husband was laid off from his job, and consequently she became depressed. In view of the change in her clinical presentation, the therapist and Anita modified the treatment contract and began a more comprehensive assessment and treatment.

Assessment: Gender and Ethnoracial Considerations

Anita was the second of four children. Her older sister died of a fall at age 6. The circumstances of the accident were unclear. Anita remembered only that she had been playing with her sister before she died. After the death of her sister, Anita became the parental child, having to take care of her two younger brothers. Her parents owned a small grocery store where they both worked. The paternal grandparents were immigrants from Barbados who appeared to have fulfilled the immigrants dream. In other words, they worked hard and bought the grocery store and Anita's father inherited it. Her paternal grandmother was a quadroon (a racially mixed person with at least one immediate Black ancestor, that is, having one-fourth Black ancestry). Anita's maternal grandmother was an American Indian of the Cherokee nation, while her grandfather was African American. In describing her family's background, Anita proudly referred to it as her rainbow heritage. Her childhood was punctuated by another major incident when she was 12. This was when her father had a serious business setback, lost the grocery store and went bankrupt, and began to drink heavily. As a result, her family experienced financial stress throughout her adolescence and early adulthood. Two months prior to this traumatic event, Anita went through menarche. Afterwards, she developed an "omen formation" (an attempt to control traumatic evens by assuming responsibility for the situation) by associating her menarche with the trauma (believing her menarch caused it), and thus taking responsibility for the trauma. This omen formation was a cognitive distortion (or error) that needed to be addressed in therapy.

Anita had then attended secretarial school, relinquishing her desire to become a lawyer. She remembered having to work and study full time in order to make ends meet and to help her family financially. Anita and her husband married after she completed secretarial school. However, she continued to help her parents out financially.

Mother's Story

During the assessment the clinician asked Anita about her mother's story. Anita was hesitant and later stated that she and her mother were not close.

She said that her deceased sister had been her mother's favorite. She also felt that her mother secretly, blamed her for her sister's death. On the other hand, Anita was able to acknowledge that she was her father's favorite, who, in turn, had been his mother's favorite. When asked to elaborate, she responded that she looked physically like her paternal grandmother. Exploration revealed that Anita felt that her skin color (very light-skinned or high yellow) was another source of conflict between her and her mother. Her mother's skin was several shades darker than Anita's, and Anita was profoundly ambivalent about her light skin. On one hand she liked and enjoyed the privileges of being light (a typical response to internal colonization, and an adaptive mechanism in a racist environment), but, on the other hand, she felt guilty and ashamed at not being Black enough.

While telling her mother's story, Anita interrupted it and told her paternal grandmother's story instead. The major themes in her depiction of her grandmother conveyed an admiration for and identification with her grandmother's self-reliance, perseverance, and overall strength, plus a strong belief in spirituality. Her grandmother belonged to a Barbadian spiritual Baptist church, was a recognized healer, and was a powerful woman within her community.

Treatment

Due to the wealth of information gathered in the ethnocultural and gender-informed assessment, the clinician decided to complete a family cultural transitional map (see Ho, 1987, for a discussion of this tool) and a genogram with Anita (see Figure 11.1), as part of her treatment.

The use of the genogram with this client helped her to connect the development of depression with her husband's loss of employment. In other words, Anita's husband's loss of employment was reminiscent of when her father lost his business, triggering a major loss for Anita, since he had become an alcoholic. Another learned family script for Anita was that when her oldest daughter reached age 6 she would die. As we can see from the genogram, at the time of treatment Anita's oldest daughter was 6. However, it appeared that Anita additionally had identified herself with her deceased sister in that she developed acrophobia after being stuck in the elevator. In other words, her fear of heights seemed to be a metaphor for her own fear of dying of a fall (as her sister had). Further exploration of this issue revealed that did Anita feel somewhat responsible for the death of her sister.

Anita had not completed her mourning process. Grief work therefore focused on reframing her situation. This work consisted of helping Anita grieve her sister's death and the emotional loss of her father due to alcoholism. Cognitive restructuring was utilized to help her cope with her guilt. Family sessions were held to encourage and reinforce Anita's current support system. Additionally, she was encouraged to use the supportive network of the Baptist church, while therapeutic decolonization work involved an appreciation and mobilization of Anita's own resources. Within this context, the treatment emphasized the recognition and utilization of Anita's strengths, such as her cognitive capabilities, her emotional resources, a solid sense of self, and her strong racial and ethnic identity (her proud rainbow heritage).

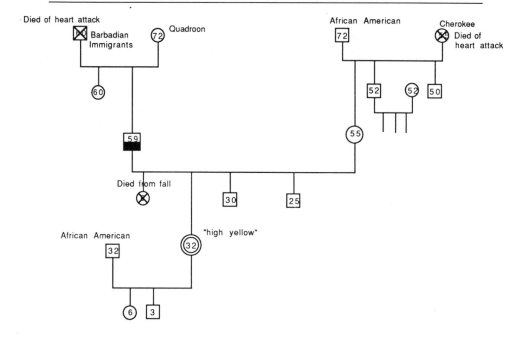

FIGURE 11.1. Anita's genogram. In this type of genogram, squares designate males and circles females. (The circle within a circle indicates the index person, Anita.) A horizontal line connecting a square and a circle indicates a marital liaison. Offspring are drawn on vertical lines descending from the marital line, in chronological order, beginning with the oldest on the left. An X inside a circle or square indicates that the person has died, and a half-blackened figure indicates drug or alcohol abuse. (See McGoldrick & Gerson, 1985, for a detailed discussion of genogram symbols.)

During treatment Anita was able to identify feelings of abandonment that she experienced when her mother was grieving for her sister. She also expressed resentment at her mother for not being there when Anita's father emotionally abandoned her due to his alcoholism. Anita began to address in treatment her strong ambivalence toward her mother. A relevant piece of information was revealed in using the genogram, which was that her mother's position in her family had been similar to Anita's; she was the parental child to two younger brothers. Additionally, at the time of therapy her mother was of the same age that Anita's maternal grandmother had been when she died of a heart attack. This situation produced anxiety in the mother, which seemed to affect the mother–daughter relationship profoundly.

The therapy helped Anita understand her mother's role in a contextual and historical basis. She was also able to appreciate her mother's strengths, understand her limitations, and recognize her own link in the generational chain. This work coincided with a visit from her mother. A single dyadic session consisting of Anita and her mother helped Anita significantly. One important message that Anita took from this session was that in order to nurture others one needs to nurture oneself. Indeed, after this session, a dialogue developed between Anita and her mother, focusing on how to parent Anita's daughter in the context of racism and sexism. Like Anita's mother,

her daughter had dark skin, and thus, as a light-skinned woman, Anita's own experience with racism had been different from her mother's and from how her daughter's would be. Another relevant issue addressed during the mental health treatment was Anita's dysfunctional need to be in control while under stress. As indicated previously, Anita had developed omen formation connecting her menarche with the loss of her father's business and his subsequent alcoholism. She felt that her becoming a woman through menarche (the omen) had led to the loss of her family's security and happiness. This is a version of a common psychological defense mechanism, in this case reinforced by a belief in supernatural causation ("If I had not started menstruating, my family would still be secure and happy."). Cognitive restructuring was done to address her cognitive distortions.

Anita's need for control and her overresponsibility were initially presented as examples of her strengths; however, it was then thought that they could be interpreted as one of the dynamics characteristic of Adult Children of Alcoholics (ACOA). Her father's alcoholism and its impact on Anita was further discussed. Exploration revealed that Anita was ambivalent about her father. In fact, she had previously idealized him and after his alcoholism, she had buried him, that is, removed him completely from her conscious life. Within this context, Anita was referred to an ACOA women's group. However, the clinician overlooked Anita's need to be in a racially homogeneous group. After attending a few sessions, Anita left the group, charging that one of the White women insulted her by saying that she could pass (i.e., could be mistaken for White). This issue had a profound effect on the therapeutic relationship afterward.

The Therapeutic Relationship

The therapeutic relationship was a significant variable in Anita's treatment. As indicated earlier, the initial stages of the therapeutic relationship were characterized by Anita's assertive behavior, manifested in her asking for a short-term treatment for her phobia. The therapist, a Latina, interpreted this request as an example of Anita's strong sense of herself, as being decisive and reliant, and communicated this to the client. The success of the cognitive behavioral techniques helped to develop and cement the therapeutic alliance. Anita developed a transferential reaction to her therapist based on her relationship with her paternal grandmother, in fact saying to her, "You remind me of my grandmother." The clinician interpreted this as a positive ethnocultural identification (Comas-Díaz & Jacobsen, 1987) and as an illustration of a positive therapeutic alliance. This alliance faciliated the clinician's negotiation of the change in treatment plan with the client.

As part of the comprehensive assessment, the clinician examined the potential areas of overlap and conflict in the therapeutic relationship, focusing on ethnoracial and gender considerations. This examination yielded some significant similarities. Both therapist and client were women of color, with a range of ethnicities in their heritages. The therapist had personal knowledge of people of Anita's socioeconomic background. Additionally, both women were ACOAs, and each with a grandmother exerting a positive influence in their lives. These commonalities helped in the development of affective empathy. The commonalities enhanced the development of credibility and trust, thus cementing the therapeutic alliance. However, the same commonalities raised issues over the development of ethnocultural countertransferential reactions prevalent in intraracial and intragender therapeutic dyads. Some of these reactions include overidentification, an "us and them" mentality, cultural myopia, and an overinvolved level of anger, hope, and despair (Comas-Díaz & Jacobsen, 1991). Although most therapists tend to work with clients like themselves, the ethnocultural countertransferential reactions need to be monitored at different levels. Given that every culture has its own unique form of the unconscious (Hall, 1982), ethnocultural and racial factors often become targets for projection (Comas-Díaz & Jacobsen, 1991). Within this clinical example, the ethnocultural countertransferential reactions focused on the nondifferentiation of identity within the therapeutic dyad (Kaplan, 1991), thus resulting in overidentification. A systematic examination of these issues, as well as consultation with a colleague, helped the clinician to manage her countertransference.

The management of the therapeutic relationship was crucial in Anita's treatment. One therapeutic task was to address Anita's inability to recognize ambivalence. The recognition of ambivalence is part of the therapeutic decolonization process facilitated by the integrative approach. Anita's inability to tolerate her own ambivalence had interfered with her primary relationships and impeded her mourning process. Another therapeutic task was to express anger in a functional manner. When Anita was referred to the racially heterogenous ACOA group, she felt that the therapist had not protected her from the White woman's accusation of being able to pass. Even though the referral was for auxiliary care, Anita felt abandoned by her therapist. The therapist helped Anita to express her anger and disappointment with her. She devised a way to validate Anita's feelings and at the same time not abandon her by becoming guarded or defensive. The therapeutic relationship was also presented as a model for her relationship with her mother, who had inadvertently neglected Anita's needs.

Another turning point in the therapeutic relationship and thus in treatment, was when the therapist suggested the possibility of using hypnosis for Anita's inability to remember her sister's death. The client took the suggestion seriously and, through a systematic review of her options and consequences, decided not to go through the hypnosis. This review process empowered Anita to make a relevant decision for herself and facilitated the completion of mourning her sister's death.

Treatment Termination

Anita was in therapy for $1^{1}/_{2}$ years. Major therapeutic themes involved her sense of self, relationships with significant others, her multiple losses, and her diverse contextual roles. At the time of terminating treatment Anita was not suffering from acrophobia or depression. She had broken a dysfunctional female generational pattern and had lifted the burden of a complicated bereavement. At that time Anita was working on her family's genealogy and was planning to develop a family tree—a genealogy book for her daughter. This appeared to illustrate the unfolding of Anita's transformation and decolonization.

CONCLUSION

In this chapter I have presented an integrative approach to the mental health treatment of women of color. This approach acknowledges the complexity, paradoxes, and heterogeneity present among women of color. It involves the integration of mainstream mental health treatment with the dual and multiple minority group membership of women of color. The integrative approach recognizes the dynamic interaction of women's gender and ethnoracial realities, connecting women's inner experience with their contextual colonial reality. The therapeutic relationship is viewed as an essential process variable, addressing the interaction of gender and ethnoracial factors of both client and therapist. The integrative psychotherapeutic approach involves pluralism, flexibility, and the therapeutic recognition of the strengths prevalent among women of color. It provides a contextual framework for working clinically with women of color.

ACKNOWLEDGMENTS

The author gratefully acknowledges the comments made by Laura S. Brown and Gwendolyn P. Keita on earlier versions of this chapter. Thanks are also extended to Iris Zavala-Martínez and Frederick Jacobsen.

REFERENCES

Almquist, E. (1989). The experience of minority women in the United States. In J. Freeman (Ed.), *Women: A feminist perspective* (4th ed., pp. 414–445). Mountain View, CA: Mayfield.

Atkinson, D. R., Morten, G., & Wing, S. D. (1979). *Counseling American minorities: A cross-cultural perspective*. Dubuque, IA: William & Brown.

Berman, J. S. (1989). A view from rainbow bridge: Feminist therapy meets Changing Woman. *Women and Therapy, 8*, 65–78.

Bernardez, T. (1987). Gender based countertransference of female therapists in the psychology of women. *Women and Therapy, 6*, 25–39.

Binion, V. J. (1990). Psychological androgyny: A Black female perspective. *Sex Roles, 22*, 487–507.

Boyd, J. (1990). Ethnic and cultural diversity: Keys to power. In L. S. Brown & M. P. P. Root (Eds.), *Diversity and complexity in feminist therapy* (pp. 151–167). New York: Haworth Press.

Boyd-Franklin, N. (1991). Recurrent themes in the treatment of African Americans. *Women and Therapy, 11*, 25–40.

Bourguignon, E. (1979). *A world of women: Anthropological studies of women in societies of the world.* New York: Praeger.

Brown, D. (1989, May 19). *Theories of illness, diagnosis, and healing.* Paper presented at the conference "Psychotherapy of Diversity: Cross-cultural Treatment Issues," sponsored by Harvard Medical School, Boston, MA.

Brown, D., Fee-Fulkerson, K., Furr, S., Ware, W. B., & Voight, N. L. (1984). Locus of control, sex role orientation, and self-concept in Black and White third and sixth-grade male and female leaders in a rural community. *Developmental Psychology, 20,* 717–721.

Brown, J. E. (1982). *The spiritual legacy of the American Indian.* New York: Crossroad.

Brown, L. S. (1986). Gender-role analysis: A neglected component of psychological assessment. *Psychotherapy, 23,* 243–248.

Brown, L. S. (1990). The meaning of a multicultural perspective for theory-building in feminist therapy. In L. S. Brown & M. P. P. Root (Eds.), *Diversity and complexity in feminist therapy* (pp. 1–21). Binghamton, NY: Haworth Press.

Brown, L. S. (1993). Anti-domination training as a central component of diversity in clinical psychology education. *Clinical Psychologist, 46,* 83–87.

Brown, P. (1974). *Toward a Marxist psychology.* New York: Harper-Colophon Books.

Butler, J. P. (1992). Of kindred minds: The ties that bind. In M. Orlandi (Ed.), *Cultural competence for evaluators: A guide for alcohol and other drug abuse prevention practitioners working with ethnic/racial communities* (pp. 23–54). Rockville, MD: Office for Substance Abuse Prevention, U.S. Department of Health and Human Services.

Chan, C. S. (1987). Asian American women: Psychological responses to sexual exploitation and cultural stereotypes. *Women and Therapy, 6,* 33–38.

Chestang, L. (1976). The Black family and Black culture: A study in coping. In M. Sotomayor (Ed.), *Cross-cultural perspectives in social work practice and education.* Houston: University of Houston Graduate School of Social Work.

Collins, P. H. (1991). *Black feminist thought: Knowledge, consciousness, and the politics of empowerment.* New York: Routledge.

Comas-Díaz, L. (1988). Mainland Puerto Rican women: A sociocultural approach. *Journal of Community Psychology, 16,* 21–31.

Comas-Díaz, L. (1991). Feminism and diversity in psychology: The case of women of color. *Psychology of Women Quarterly, 15,* 597–609.

Comas-Díaz, L. (1992). The future of psychotherapy with ethnic minorities. *Psychotherapy, 29,* 88–94.

Comas-Díaz, L., & Griffith, E. H. E. (Eds.). (1988). *Clinical guidelines in cross-cultural mental health.* New York: Wiley.

Comas-Díaz, L., & Jacobsen, F. M. (1987). Ethnocultural identification in psychotherapy. *Psychiatry, 50,* 232–241.

Comas-Díaz, L., & Jacobsen, F. M. (1991). Ethnocultural transference and countertransference in the therapeutic dyad. *American Journal of Orthopsychiatry, 61,* 392–402.

Comas-Díaz, L., & Minrath, M. (1985). Psychotherapy with ethnic minority borderline clients. *Psychotherapy, 22* (Suppl.), 418–426.

Conarton, S., & Silverman, L. (1988). Feminine development through the life cycle. In M. A. Dutton-Douglas & L. E. Walker (Eds.), *Feminist psychotherapies: Integration of therapeutic and feminist systems* (pp. 37–67). Norwood, NJ: Ablex.

de Beauvoir, S. (1961). *The second sex.* New York: Bantam Books.

Downing, N. E., & Roush, K. L. (1985). From passive acceptance to active commitment: A model of feminist identity development for women. *Counseling Psychologist, 13,* 695–709.

Dreyfuss, B., & Lawrence, D. (1979). *Handbook for anti-racism.* Norman, OK: University of Oklahoma Press.

Espín, O. M. (1984, August). *Selection of Hispanic female healers in urban U.S. communities.* Paper presented at the annual meeting of the American Psychological Association, Toronto.

Fanon, F. (1967). *Black skin, White masks.* New York: Grove Press.

Freire, P. (1967). *Educação como prática da liberdade* [Education as a practice of freedom]. Rio de Janeiro: Paz e Terra.

Freire, P. (1970). *Pedagogy of the oppressed.* New York: Seabury Press.

García-Preto, N. (1990). Hispanic mothers. *Journal of Feminist Family Therapy, 2,* 15–21.

Gehrie, M. J. (1979). Culture as an internal representation. *Psychiatry, 42,* 165–170.

Goldfried, M. R., & Castonguay, L. G. (1992). The future of psychotherapy integration. *Psychotherapy, 29,* 4–10.

Green, R. (1991). Culture and gender in Indian America. In M. L. Andersen & P. H. Collins (Eds.), *Race, class, and gender: An anthology* (pp. 510–518). Belmont, CA: Wadsworth.

Greene, B. (1990). What has gone before: The legacy of racism and sexism in the lives of Black mothers and daughters. *Women and Therapy, 9,* 207–230.

Gump, J. (1980). Reality and myth: Employment and sex role ideology in Black women. In F. Denmark & J. Sherman (Eds.), *The psychology of woman.* New York: Psychological Dimensions.

Hall, E. T. (1981). *Beyond culture.* Garden City, NY: Anchor Books.

Hardy-Fanta, C., & Montana, P. (1982). The Hispanic female adolescent: A group therapy model. *International Journal of Group Psychotherapy, 32,* 351–366.

Hare-Mustin, R. (1990). [Review of *Don't blame mother: Mending the mother–daughter relationship,* by Paula Caplan]. *Psychology of Women Quarterly, 14,* 143–145.

Helms, J. E. (1985). Cultural identity in the treatment process. In P. Pedersen (Ed.), *Handbook of cross-cultural counseling and therapy.* Westport, CT: Greenwood Press.

Helms, J. E. (Ed.). (1990). *Black and White racial identity: Theory, research and practice.* Westport, CT: Greenwood Press.

Ho, M. H. (1987). *Family therapy with ethnic minorities.* Newbury Park, CA: Sage.

Howard, G. S. (1991). Culture tales: A narrative approach to thinking, cross-cultural psychology, and psychotherapy. *American Psychologist, 46,* 187–197.

Hurtado, A. (1989). Relating to privilege: Seduction and rejection in the subordination of white women and women of color. *Signs, 14,* 833–855.

Hynes, K., & Werbin, G. (1977). Group psychotherapy for Spanish-speaking women. *Psychiatric Annals, 7,* 52–59.

Jackson, G. G. (1976). The African genesis of the Black perspective in helping. *Professional Psychology, 7,* 292–308.

Jacobsen, F. M. (1988). Ethnocultural assessment. In L. Comas-Díaz & E. H. E. Griffith (Eds.), *Clinical guidelines in cross-cultural mental health* (pp. 135–147). New York: Wiley.

Jenkins, A. H. (1985). Attending to self-activity in the Afro-American client. *Psychotherapy, 22*(Suppl.), 335–348.

Jenkins, A. H. (1990). *Dynamics of the relationship in clinical work with African-American clients. Group, 14*(1), 36–43.

Jones, B. E., & Gray, B. A. (1984). Similarities and differences in Black men and women in psychotherapy. *Journal of the National Medical Association, 78,* 21–27.

Jones, E. E. (1985). Psychotherapy and counseling with Black clients. In P. Pedersen (Ed.), *Handbook of cross-cultural counseling and therapy* (pp. 173–179). Westport, CT: Greenwood Press.

Jones, J. M. (1991). Psychological models of race: What have they been and what should they be? In J. D. Goodchilds (Ed.), *Psychological perspectives on human diversity in America* (pp. 3–46). Washington, DC: American Psychological Association.

Jordan, J. V. (1991). Empathy and self boundaries. In J. V. Jordan, A. G. Kaplan, J. B. Miller, I. P. Stiver, & J. L. Surrey, *Women's growth in connection: Writings from the Stone Center* (pp. 67–80). New York: Guilford Press.

Jordan, J. V., Kaplan, A., Miller, J. B., Stiver, I. P., & Surrey, J. L. (1991). *Women's growth in connection: Writings from the Stone Center.* New York: Guilford Press.

Jordan, J. V., & Surrey, J. L. (1986). The self-in-relation: Empathy and the mother–daughter relationship. In T. Bernay & D. W. Cantor (Eds.), *The psychology of today's woman: New psychoanalytic visions.* Hillsdale, NJ: Analytic Press.

Kaplan, A. G. (1979). Toward an analysis of sex-role related issues in the therapeutic relationship. *Psychiatry, 42,* 112–120.

Kaplan, A. G. (1991). Female or male therapists for women: New formulations. In J. V. Jordan, A. G. Kaplan, J. B. Miller, I. Stiver, & J. L. Surrey, *Women's growth in connection: Writings from the Stone Center* (pp. 268–282). New York: Guilford Press.

Kiev, A. (1972). *Transcultural psychiatry.* New York: Free Press.

Kinzie, J. D. (1978). Lessons from cross-cultural psychotherapy. *American Journal of Psychotherapy, 32,* 510–520.

Kleinman, A. (1989, May 19). *Culture, suffering and psychotherapy.* Paper presented at the conference "Psychotherapy of Diversity: Cross-cultural Treatment Issues," sponsored by the Harvard Medical School, Boston.

Kovel, J. (1984). *White racism: A psychohistory.* New York: Columbia University Press.

LaFromboise, T. D., Heyle, A. M., & Ozer, E. J. (1990). Changing and diverse roles of women in American Indian cultures. *Sex Roles, 22,* 455–476.

LaFromboise, T. D., Trimble, J. E., & Mohatt, G. V. (1990). Counseling intervention and American Indian tradition: An integrative approach. *Counseling Psychologist, 18,* 628–654.

Lanktree, C., Comas-Díaz, L. & Crayton, C. (1983). *Effects of a multi-ethnic group on the sex roles and attitudes of its members.* Unpublished manuscript, Yale University, Psychiatry Department.

Lerner, H. G. (1988). *Women in therapy.* New York: Jason Aronson.

Lopez, S. (1989). Patient variable biases in clinical judgment: Conceptual overview and methodological considerations. *Psychological Bulletin, 106,* 184–203.

Lorde, A. (1984). *Sister outsider: Essays and speeches.* Trumansburg, NY: Crossing Press.

Lorion, R. P., & Parron, D. L. (1985). Countering the countertransference: A strategy for treating the untreatable. In P. Pedersen (Ed.), *Handbook of cross-cultural counseling and therapy*. Westport, CT: Greenwood Press.

Mason, K. O., & Bumpass, L. L. (1975). United States women's sex role ideology. *American Journal of Sociology, 80*, 1212–1219.

McGill, D. W. (1992). The cultural story in multicultural family therapy. *Families in Society, 73*, 339–349.

McGoldrick, M., García-Preto, N., Hines, P. M., & Lee, E. (1989). Ethnicity and women. In M. McGoldrick, C. M. Anderson, & F. Walsh (Eds.), *Women in families: A framework for family therapy* (pp. 169–199). New York: W. W. Norton.

McGoldrick, M., & Gerson, R. (1985). *Genograms in family assessment*. New York: Norton.

Memmi, A. (1965). *The colonizer and the colonized*. Boston: Beacon Press.

Myers, H. F., Echemendia, R. J., & Trimble, J. E. (1991). The need for training ethnic minority psychologists. In H. F. Myers, P. Wohlford, L. P. Guzman, & R. J. Echemendia (Eds.), *Ethnic minority perspectives on clinical training and services in psychology* (pp. 3–11). Washington, DC: American Psychological Association.

Nobles, W. (1980). Extended self: Rethinking the so-called Negro self-concept. In R. H. Jones (Ed.), *Black psychology*. New York: Harper & Row.

Okun, B. F. (1990). *Seeking connections in psychotherapy*. San Francisco: Jossey-Bass.

Ostling, R. N. (1991, May 6). When God was a woman. *Time, 137*, 73.

Papp, P. (1988). Couples. In M. Walters, B. Carter, P. Papp, & O. Silverstein (Eds.), *The invisible web: Gender patterns in family relationships* (pp. 200–249). New York: Guilford Press.

Pinderhughes, E. (1982). Afro-American families and the victim system. In M. McGoldrick, J. K. Pearce, & J. Giordano (Eds.), *Ethnicity and family therapy* (pp. 108–122). New York: Guilford Press.

Pugh, C., & Vasquez-Nutall, E. (1983, April). *Are all women alike? Reports of white, Hispanic and Black women*. Paper presented at the meeting of the American Personnel and Guidance Association, Washington, DC.

Ramirez, M., III (1991). *Psychotherapy and counseling with minorities: A cognitive approach to individual and cultural differences*. New York: Pergamon Press.

Reid, P. T. (1988). Racism and sexism: Comparisons and conflicts. In P. A. Katz & D. A. Taylor (Eds.), *Eliminating racism* (pp. 203–221). New York: Plenum.

Reid, P. T., & Comas-Díaz, L. (1990). Gender and ethnicity: perspectives on dual status. *Sex Roles, 22*, 397–408.

Ridley-Malson, M. (1983). Black women's sex roles: The social context for a new ideology. *Journal of Social Issues, 39*, 101–113.

Riess, B. F. (1971). Observations of the therapist factor in interethnic psychotherapy. *Psychotherapy: Theory, Research and Practice, 8*, 71–72.

Robinson, C. R. (1983). Black women: A tradition of self-reliant strength. In J. H. Robbins & R. J. Siegel (Eds.), *Women changing therapy: New assessment, values, and strategies in feminist therapy* (pp. 135–144). Binghamton, NY: Haworth Press.

Root, M. P. P. (1990). Resolving the "other" status: Identity development of biracial individuals. *Women and Therapy, 9*, 185–205.

Root, M. P. P. (1992). Reconstructing the impact of trauma on personality. In L. S. Brown & M. Ballou (Eds.), *Personality and psychopathology: Feminist reappraisals* (pp. 229–265). New York: Guilford Press.

Rosewater, L. B. (1990). Diversifying feminist psychotherapy and practice: Broadening the concept of victimization. *Women and Therapy, 9,* 299–311.

Sager, C. J., Brayboy, T. L., & Waxemberg, B. R. (1972). Black patient–White therapist. *American Journal of Orthopsychiatry, 42,* 24–27.

Smith, N. D., Burlew, A., Mosley, M. E., & Whitney, W. (1978). *Minority issues in mental health.* Reading, MA: Addison-Wesley.

Society for the Exploration of Psychotherapy Integration. (1991). The inaugural issue [Special issue]. *Journal of Psychotherapy Integration, 1.*

Stone, E. (1988). *Black sheep and kissing cousins: How our family stories shape us.* New York: Penguin Books.

Swartz, J. (1983, May). Ethnic stereotypes may be therapy tools. *American Psychological Association Monitor, 14*(5), 22.

Travis, C. B. (1991). [Review of *The invisible web: Gender patterns in family relationships*]. *Psychology of Women Quarterly, 15,* 179–180.

True, R. H. (1990). Psychotherapeutic issues with Asian American women. *Sex Roles, 22,* 477–486.

Tucker, C. M., James, L. M., & Turner, S. M. (1985). Sex roles, parenthood, and marital adjustment: A comparison of Blacks and Whites. *Journal of Social and Clinical Psychology, 3,* 51–61.

Turner, C., & Darity, W. (1973). Fears of genocide among Black Americans as related to age, sex, and religion. *American Journal of Public Health, 63,* 1029–1034.

Walters, M., Carter, B., Papp. P., & Silverstein, O. (1988). *The invisible web: Gender patterns in family relationships.* New York: Guilford Press.

Wampold, B. E., Casas, J. M., & Atkinson, D. R. (1981). Ethnic bias in counseling: An information processing approach. *Journal of Counseling Psychology, 28,* 498–503.

Weinraub, J. (1991, April 28). The new theology: Sheology. *The Washington Post,* pp. F1, F6.

Wilkinson, D. Y. (1980). Minority women: Social–cultural issues. In A. Brodsky & R. Hare-Mustin (Eds.), *Women and psychotherapy: An assessment of research and practice* (pp. 285–304). New York: Guilford Press.

12

Psychopharmacology

Frederick M. Jacobsen

The treatment of women of color with psychotropic medications is a topic that has been studied surprisingly little. Although women of color now comprise a significant and increasing portion of the total population of women in the United States, as a group minimal attention has been paid to their biologically based psychological needs. In fact, although 70% of all psychoactive medications are prescribed to women (Ogur, 1986), the overlap of gender and ethnoracial factors are rarely taken into consideration in research concerning psychotropic medications. A review of the drug outcome studies published in 1991 in two major U.S. psychiatric journals (the *American Journal of Psychiatry* and the *Archives of General Psychiatry*) found that while gender of research subjects was reported in 94% of studies, it was analysed in only 57%, and race/ethnicity were reported in only 18% of studies and analysed in only 12% (Turner, 1992). Similar findings were presented by the Institute of Medicine (1993), underscoring the underrepresentation and exclusion of people of color and other minorities as research subjects in clinical drug trials. Currently, federal legislation is mandating the inclusion of women and minorities as research participants in clinical studies.

The purpose of this chapter is to discuss the clinical management of the psychopharmacologic treatment of women of color within a sociocultural and gender-sensitive context. In conjunction with the larger goals of this book, this chapter represents an effort to describe briefly the current theoretical and clinical knowledge regarding the practice of clinical psychopharmacology with women of color. I will review the history of psychopharmacologic treatment of women of color, briefly describe the few areas investigating the factors influencing the biological basis of psychopharmacology with this population, consider some of the dynamic issues surrounding prescription of psychotropic medications to its members, and finally offer some practical suggestions regarding evaluation and treatment. Where specific case illustrations are presented, identifying data have been altered to protect the confidentiality of the patients.

HISTORICAL ASPECTS

Historically, North American racism has played a significant role in the delivery of mental health services to people of color (Willie, Kramer, & Brown, 1973). Studies have documented that people of color with mental health problems have been more likely to be misdiagnosed and to receive psychopharmacologic treatment than psychotherapy. For example, Flaherty and Meaer (1980) reported a greater use of medications and restraints in people of color than in Whites in an inpatient hospital setting. Similarly, Loring and Powell (1988) empirically found that the sex and race of the patient and of the psychiatrist influence the diagnosis made of major depression and undifferentiated schizophrenia even though clear-cut diagnostic criteria for these diseases exist. The results of Loring and Powell's study indicate that race and gender interact with diagnosis in a complex way, leading to misdiagnoses by practitioners relying soley upon clinical judgments. These findings also raise concerns about proper treatment, since the prescription of psychoactive medications for depressive disorders differ from those used to treat schizophrenia. Additionally, racial and gender stereotypes may operate in the variety of clinical judgments that go into diagnosis. López (1989) states that patient variables such as gender, race, and class, contribute to bias in diagnosis such as overpathologizing, minimizing (inappropriately judging symptomatology as normative for members of a group), overdiagnosing, and underdiagnosing (inappropiately avoiding application of a diagnosis as a function of group membership).

As a consequence of injustices ascribed to the racial and gender power imbalances present in many segments of the health care establishment, there is a perception among many ethnic minorities that psychopharmacologic treatment has been employed somewhat punitively to people of color, and specifically to women of color. Many women of color, particularly African Americans, face racism within the medical establishment (White, 1990). For example, Martin (1987) presents evidence that African American women are treated with less respect by nurses and doctors than are White women. She found that African American women who exhibited "inappropriate" and "resistant" behavior while in labor reported being sedated and restrained, while White women who slap or bite medical personnel did not incite repraisal. Within this framework, Angela Davis (1990) urges us to contextualize African American women's health in relation to the prevailing political conditions. She argues that the interaction of oppressive forces such as racism, sexism, and economic injustice makes ill health inevitable for African American women. This situation is frequently applicable to other women of color as well.

Unfortunately, public attitudes towards mental health treatment have lagged far behind the tremendous advances in our knowledge of the biology of mental illness, and treatment, particularly psychopharmacologic, is still widely regarded as stigmatizing (Freedman & Stahl, 1992), if not dangerous or harmful. Such perceptions have been mythologized by popular movies such as *One Flew Over the Cuckoo's Nest*, in which a misunderstood Native American is held in an abusive, repressive White-run psychiatric hospital and is overmedicated. Similarly, psychopharmacology has been perceived by many women of color as a means to silence their complaints (L. Comas-Díaz, personal communication, May 1993).

The combinations of the harsh realities of well-intentioned but often underfunded treatment programs, the health insurance industry's outrageous discrimination against "mental illness," with lower reimbursement rates applying even to diseases of an undeniably physical nature such as manic-depression and schizophrenia, and the frequent sensationalist presentations of the media with respect to mental health treatment, have left many women of color with a deep suspicion regarding the use of psychotropic medications that may even surpass the generally negative attitude toward psychopharmacologic treatment held by the larger North American society.

Psychosocial Aspects of Psychopharmacologic Research

It is an unfortunate, dismaying, and disheartening fact that most psychopharmacologic research has been conducted in men, even when investigating medications that are used to treat illnesses which are much more common in women (such as depression). In lower animals as well as humans, research on the pharmacologic responses of females has been ignored or avoided due to a number of different factors. First of all, there is the widespread concern among investigators that women's medication responses tend to be inherently unstable due to hormonal and chemical fluctuations associated with the menstrual cycle, pregnancy and lactation, menopause, and so on. In effect, the profound physiological changes associated with the female gender have been used by a predominantly male-dominated scientific establishment to disqualify their significance in both research and clinical practice, even though women have constituted a majority of the general population for decades. It was not until 1990 that the National Institutes of Health began seriously considering how to approach these issues by developing an Office of Research on Women's Health.

Pharmacologic research using women of childbearing ages has been avoided due to fears that potential intrauterine exposure to medications carries a significant (and avoidable) risk of future malpractice suits, regardless of whatever preventative medicolegal protective measures are adopted

(Jacobsen, 1993). However, the General Accounting Office (1992) released a study examining the policies and practices of including women in clinical studies by private drug companies. In response, the Food and Drug Administration (FDA) has lifted the ban on women's participation in most drug safety test and is requiring companies to analyze results by sex (Hilts, 1993). The FDA has also stated that there are ways to protect the fetus and to include women in the studies (Hilts, 1993). Unfortunately, such fears may continue given the pervasive socially destructive climate of litigiousness perpetuated by some lawyers in the United States over the past two decades. Although progress is being made, it is unclear if the studies will meaningfully analyze the interaction of gender and race. The problem of a lack of psychopharmacologic data on women of color is ultimately multidetermined and related to larger societal problems.

ETHNORACIAL EFFECTS IN PSYCHOPHARMACOLOGY

Only a small number of studies have investigated potential ethnoracial differences in basic or clinical psychopharmacology. Moreover, this research has been complicated by the fact that the broadly described groups in the United States that are usually studied (e.g., Asians, Hispanics/Latinos) are composed of multiple subgroups (Japanese versus Chinese versus Filipino; Mexican versus Caribbean versus South Americans; etc.), which may differ significantly among themselves in numerous genetic and environmental characteristics potentially influencing psychopharmacology and response. However, the studies that have been performed have often revealed significant differences in drug metabolism of and/or clinical response to psychotropic medication in people of color as compared with Whites (Lin, Poland, & Nakasaki, 1993). Unfortunately, few studies have investigated the potential psychopharmacologic differences between women of color and White women, or between women of color and their male counterparts (e.g., Goldberg, Schooler, Davidson, & Kayce, 1966; Raskin & Crook, 1975).

There is, however, a substantial body of biological and psychosocial evidence to support the conclusion that non-Whites should not be assumed to have identical responses to psychotropic medications as Whites (Lin, Poland, & Nakasaki, 1993; Mendoza, Smith, Poland, Lin, & Strickland, 1991). Unfortunately, the data from different studies are frequently not directly comparable nor consistent, and since gender effects are generally not taken into account in these studies, any conclusions drawn must be rather cautious. Broadly summarized and somewhat oversimplified with a few examples, the evidence supporting ethnoracial differences in psychopharmacology comes from the areas detailed below.

Genetic Differences in Liver Function and the Metabolism of Psychotropic Drugs

Multiple studies have documented ethnoracial differences in a variety of liver enzymes whose function may directly or indirectly effect the metabolism of specific psychotropic agents. For example, a majority of Chinese and Japanese have some variation in the forms of liver enzymes that are involved in the metabolism of alcohol, leading to an increased sensitivity and potentially heightened toxicity to alcohol (Lin, Poland, Smith, Strickand, & Mendoza, 1991; Yoshida, 1993). The fact that Native Americans have found to have aberrant metabolism of alcohol may contribute to their increased rate to alcoholism (Yoshida, 1993). Such increased sensitivity may also increase potentially negative interactive effects of alcohol with other psychotropic agents.

In some cases, ethnoracial differences in psychopharmacologic activity are directly measureable. For example, in comparisons of the best-studied class of antidepressants—the tricyclic antidepressants—African Americans tend to attain higher blood levels than Whites when taking identical doses of tricyclics (Strickland et al., 1991; Silver, Poland, & Lin, 1993). Asians have also been reported to metabolize tricyclic antidepressants at a slower rate than Whites (Rudorfer, Lane, Chang, Zhang, & Potter, 1984; Silver et al., 1993) and therefore also tend to attain higher blood levels of tricyclic antidepressants than Whites. In both African Americans and Asians, this tendency towards higher blood levels means that the "standard" doses required for optimal treatment may be quite different from the doses published in the general literature and taught in the medical schools. However, even when broadly described ethnoracial group differences in blood levels of psychotropics exist, there is often a significant degree of overlap among different groups and there is not infrequently a large amount of individual variability in such physiological parameters.

Differences in Clinical Responses to Specific Psychotropic Drugs

In addition to the sometimes measureable differences in physiological parameters between different ethnoracial groups, there may be differences in clinical responses to psychotropic medications. For example, African Americans tend to respond better and faster than Whites to tricyclic antidepressants, but also tend to develop more toxic side effects than Whites (reviewed in Strickland et al., 1991; Silver et al., 1993). Asians and Asian Americans may require lower doses than Whites for therapeutic response to neuroleptics, tricyclic antidepressants (Silver et al., 1993), lithium (Strickland, Lawson, Lin, & Fu, 1993), and benzodiazepines, (Lin, Poland, Fleishaker, & Phillips, 1993) and like African Americans, may also be more susceptible to side effects than Whites (Lin et al., 1991; Lin, Poland, & Nakasaki, 1993). Unfortunately, research efforts in this area are just beginning and the studies that have been performed have focused almost exclusively upon men or have not analyzed gender differences.

Psychosocial Factors Influencing Psychotropic Drug Metabolism and/or Response

1. Diet and nutritional factors can effect an individual's response to psychotropic medications through changes in metabolic activity (Clark, Brater, & Johnson, 1988), how the drugs are distributed in the body (leaner individuals will tend to accumulate smaller amounts of fat soluble drugs over time), and so on. Additionally, the consumption of certain types of food favored by specific ethnoracial groups may have profound effects on the activity of psychotropic medications. One example of such dietary factors are Fava beans—a type of broad bean which are most frequently included in the diet of southern Italians and other Mediterranean peoples—which may trigger a potentially lethal high blood pressure reaction in individuals being treated with antidepressants of the monoamine oxidase inhibitor class, due to the bean's high content of the chemical dopamine (a brain neurotransmitter). It is probably not trivial that in a country populated by almost innumerable ethnoracial groups, "unusual" (i.e, nonmainstream WASP) dietary supplements, spices, and foodstuffs may have psychopharmacologic effects that are rarely recognized or even considered. Even more common—and insidious—negative influences on both mental health and psychopharmacology are seen in the poor nutrition and dietary habits associated with poverty, alcoholism, and drug abuse, which tend to be disproportionately overrepresented in the ethnic and racial minority populations in the United States.

2. Differences in consumption of cigarettes, caffeine, alcohol, herbs, and other psychoactive substances may directly influence both psychotropic drug metabolism and/or response. Smoking cigarettes, for example, may increase the levels of certain medications in the blood and thereby alter their effects in the brain. Although frequently ignored even in otherwise well-designed culturally sensitive psychopharmacologic studies, the effects of nonprescribed psychoactive substances should be taken into consideration, since certain groups of women of color are more likely than White women to be exposed to such substances. For example, African Americans as a group tend to smoke more than Whites (Wynder, 1979), a trend that may have increased during the 1980s as advertising launched campaigns particularly targeting ethnic minority groups. There has also been a striking increase in cigarette smoking among women in recent years. If current trends of smoking continue, by the late 1990s women will smoke at higher rates than men (U.S. Department of Health and Human Services, 1992).

In this regard, it is important to note that cigarette smoking has also tended to be associated with consumption of several other addictive substances such as caffeine and alcohol (Wynder, 1979), which may further adversely affect a woman's mental health, as well as altering the effects that psychotropic medications have upon the brain and nervous system. These interactive relationships are rarely recognized or questioned by either patients or their health care providers, and research on them is just beginning.

Another example of the consumption of psychoactive substances is the use of herbal medicines. It has been reported that traditional herbal medicines continue to be extensively used by Asians, African Americans, and Hispanics/Latinos in the United States (Smith, Lin, & Mendoza, 1993). The interactions of herbal and psychotropic drugs have not been well studied, but they are likely to cause or intensify side effects if they contain an atropine-like substance that is known to produce anticholinergic effects (Chien, 1993; Smith, Lin, & Mendoza, 1993). Similarly, Smith and associates (1993) recommend that clinicians routinely elicit patients' use of herbs, and that if an herb–drug interaction is suspected, then the active ingredients of the herbs should be investigated.

3. Differences in sleep or activity/rest patterns such as the habit of afternoon napping (*siesta*) may alter an individual's nocturnal sleep pattern in a variety of ways (timing of sleep onset, duration of sleep, continuity of sleep, etc.). Such alterations represent changes in the functioning of the brain control center for sleeping and the biological clock (the hypothalamus), which in some cases may trigger other neurophysiologic events that influence behavior. For example, daytime napping tends to be associated with the secretion of the pituitary hormone prolactin, which is otherwise not usually present during the daytime (Parker, Rossman, & Vander Laan, 1973) and may reflect changes in the activity of the neurotransmitter serotonin. Ultimately, such changes in serotonergic activity may be associated with profound changes in neurobehavioral functioning, including changes in mood, appetite, level of anxiety, and so on, as seen in the following example. Identifying data have been altered for confidentiality reasons.

A 40-year-old Puerto Rican woman was accustomed to staying up until at least 2 a.m. each night and taking a afternoon break from work each day to nap for several hours. Having lived in Madrid for many years following her university education, Rodriga D. moved to the United States in search of economic opportunity. Accepted for work as a translator by a Washington, D.C. agency, Ms. D.'s African American supervisor was alarmed by her excessive caffeine consumption, irritability, and occasional falling asleep on the job in the early afternoons. Neuropsychiatric evaluation revealed a long-standing Delayed Sleep Phase Syndrome, which had apparently not been dysfunctional in her cultures of origin but which was difficult to treat pharmacologically.

4. Differences associated with evironmental or geographical effects, such as exposure to toxins/pollutants in the air, soil, or water, the intensity and duration of sunlight or temperature effects, may have dramatic effects on neurobehavioral functioning. Although any individual—regardless of race or gender—residing in a particular area would be exposed to the local environmental, the resultant psychopharmacologic effects may in some instances be more prevalent for specific ethnoracial groups. For example, impoverished African Americans and Hispanics/Latinos living in major U.S. cities are more likely than Whites to reside in high population density dwellings having significant amounts of "noise pollution." Studies have demonstrated that repeated uncontrollable exposure to noise can ultimately lead to central nervous system changes closely resembling those characteristic of mood and anxiety disorders (Breier, 1989).

5. Differences in exposure to psychological "stress" may be associated with significant functional alternations in the release of the "fight or flight" neurohormone adrenaline. Increased levels of adrenalin in the blood stimulate an increased production and release of the stress hormone cortisol. Cortisol has wide-ranging effects throughout the brain and body, effecting cognitive and emotional functioning, and physiological processes such as sleep, appetite, immunity, sexual function, and so on. Acting through this neurohormonal system, exposure to psychological stress can ultimately lead to central nervous system changes closely resembling those characteristic of mood and anxiety disorders (Breier, 1989). In the United States women of color confront stresses both overt and and insidious (Root, 1992) related to the racism and sexism inherent in the society (see Comas-Díaz, Chapter 11, this volume). In their societally designated roles women are subject to interpersonal violence, harassment, sexual discrimination, poverty, and inadequate access to health care more frequently than men (Rodin & Ickovics, 1990). Taken together, the multiple stresses encountered by women of color place them at greater risk than most other groups in U.S. society for developing psychophysiologic disorders (e.g., depression, eating disorders) that may require consideration of psychopharmacologic treatment. As an illustration, there is an increasing vulnerability among women of color to developing eating disorders due to pressures from mainstream standards, in addition to sociopolitical and economic factors (Root, 1990).

GENDER EFFECTS IN PSYCHOPHARMACOLOGY

When considering the ethnoracial factors potentially effecting psychopharmacology, it should be remembered that the differences listed above may be further complicated or even magnified when the critical variable of gender is added. Significant differences in drug metabolism of and/or clinical response to psychotropic medication have been found in numerous studies contrasting women to men (Hamilton & Parry, 1983; Dawkins &

Potter, 1991; Yonkers, Kando, Cole, & Blumenthal, 1992). However, these studies have been performed mainly with White research participants rather than with ethnic minorities, so that we can do little more than to try to extrapolate the potential significance of the findings to women of color.

Gender effects in psychopharmacology may occur for a variety of reasons, including the fact that reproductive hormones such as estrogen and progesterone may change the rates of absorption of different medications or cause changes in the activity of liver enzymes that metabolize many of the psychotropic medications (Yonkers et al., 1992). Moreover, estrogen and progesterone often have dramatic psychotropic effects in their own right that in my experience tend to be ignored by physicians. Estrogens and other steroids found in oral contraceptives may also be particularly likely to interact with psychotropic medications (Hamilton & Parry, 1983) and thereby change the way a female patient responds to the primary psychotropic medication. I have found that the potential interactive effects of "nonpsychiatric" medications that nonetheless have psychotropic activity are generally given short shrift or ignored entirely by most physicians.

Other physiological parameters effecting a medication's activity, such as the volume of distribution of the medication in the body, may also be more subject to fluctuations in women of reproductive ages, since the increase in water retention occuring premenstrually may lead to a larger volume of blood circulating in the body and thereby potentially dilute the effects of a fixed-dose medication. To further complicate matters, as with ethnoracial determinants of drug metabolism, many of the studies investigating gender effects are contradictory and final guidelines must await carefully controlled studies on individual psychotropic medications.

Although a complete review of racial and gender differences in response to psychotropic medications is beyond the scope of this chapter, the following table provides a summary listing of the classes of the most commonly prescribed psychotropic medications for which clinically relevant ethnoracial and/or gender differences have been reported. Table 12.1 divides psychoactive medications into broad categories, and since many of the individual members of a particular class of drug (e.g., tricyclic antidepressants), may not have been adequately assessed for ethnic, racial, or gender differences, the entire class is given a positive designation if differences have been described for any class member.

A broad but practical interpretation of the information presented in Table 12.1 is that people of color may be likely to vary in psychopharmacologic response when compared with Whites, and that these potential differences may be complicated further when gender factors are taken into consideration.

Given this degree of potential variability in psychotropic response, any characteristic of a medication offering enhanced precision of usage may be considered as conferring a relative advantage. The use of blood levels, for example, may be quite helpful in determining a relative probability of whether the medication is likely to be in a therapeutic versus subthera-

TABLE 12.1. Examples of Psychotropic Medication Differences by Race, Gender, and Blood Level

Medication	Ethnoracial differences	Gender differences	Blood levels useful?
Antidepressants			
Tricyclic antidepressants	Yes	Yes	
Imipramine (Tofranil), desipramine (Norpramin, etc.), clomipramine (Anafranil)			Yes
Nortriptyline (Pamelor, Aventyl)			Yes
Amitriptyline (Elavil)			Conflicting data
Doxepin (Adapin), protripyline (Vivactil), amoxapine (Asendin), etc.			No
Serotonin reuptake inhibitors	No	No	No
Fluoxetine (Prozac), sertraline (Zoloft), paroxetine (Paxil), fluvoxamine (Luvox)			
Monoamine oxidase inhibitors	Probably	Insufficient data	Probably not
Phenelzine (Nardil), tranylcypromine (Parnate), isocarboxazid (Marplan), deprenyl (Eldepryl)			
Other antidepressants			
Bupropion (Wellbutrin)	No	No	Yes
Trazodone (Desyrel)	No	No	No
Venlafaxine (Effexor)	Insufficient data	No	Insufficient data
Nefazodone (Serzone)	Insufficient data	No	Insufficient data
Mood stabilizing agents			
Lithium (Eskalith and others)	Yes	Yes	Yes
Valproate (Depakote)	Possibly	Possibly	Yes
Carbamazepine (Tegretol)	Yes	Yes	Yes
Antipsychotic agents			
Phenothiazines	Yes	Yes	Possibly
Chlorpromazine (Thorazine), perphenazine (Trilafon), trifluoperazine (Stelazine), thioridazine (Mellaril), etc.			
Nonphenothiazines	In some cases	In some cases	In some cases
Haloperidol (Haldol), thiothixene (Navane), molindone (Moban), loxapine (Loxitane), pimozide (Orap)			
Atypical neuroleptics			
Clozapine (Clozaril)	Yes	Yes	Yes
Risperidone (Risperdal)	Insufficient data	Insufficient data	Unclear

TABLE 12.1. (Continued)

Medication	Ethnoracial differences	Gender differences	Blood levels useful?
Antianxiety agents			
Benzodiazepines Diazepam (Valium), alprazolam (Xanax), lorazepam (Ativan), chlordiazepoxide (Librium), etc.	Yes	Yes	No
Buspirone (BuSpar)	No	No	No
Hydroxyzine (Atarax)	No	No	No
Hypnotic agents			
Benzodiazepines Flurazepam (Dalmane), triazolam (Halcion), quazepam (Doral), temazepam (Restoril), etc. (see also benzodiazepine antianxiety agents)	Yes	Yes	No
Imidazopyridine Zolpidem (Ambien)	Insufficient data	Insufficient data	No
Stimulant and anorectic agents			
Methylphenidate (Ritalin)	Insufficient data	Insufficient data	No
Amphetamines	Insufficient data	Insufficient data	No
Fenfluramine (Pondimin)	Insufficient data	Insufficient data	No

Note. Brand names are listed in parentheses.

peutic (or toxic) range. However, it should be noted that blood levels of psychotropic medicatons may be available but not necessarily clinically useful. This is the case because while medical laboratories will gladly measure the blood levels of almost any psychotropic medication, many of the psychotropics do not have blood level ranges with demonstrated clinical significance. A practical guideline to follow is that when using psychotropic medications (e.g., tricyclic antidepressants, antipsychotics) to which, in documented studies ethnic minority individuals tend to respond at lower blood levels than Whites, blood levels should be obtained where practical.

ETHNOCULTURAL EXPRESSIONS OF ILLNESS

The ways in which individuals from different ethnic or cultural groups express themselves are likely to have a tremendous effect on how they are evaluated and treated in a medical context. It has been reported, for example, that certain ethnic groups are more likely to describe physical pain as being severe, while other groups are more likely to minimize pain (Zborowski, 1969). It is not difficult to conclude that such differences may lead to potential differences in the types or amounts of analgesics prescribed to the individuals. Such subjective differences between ethnoculturally diverse groups may be magnified when describing characteristics more difficult to quantify, such as "psychic pain." Considering the paradigm of depression, for example, many White Anglo-Saxon Protestants may be more likely to express sadness, guilt, and elation while many African Americans may be more likely to express somatization, negativism, irritability, and suspiciousness (Harwood, 1981). There are ethnic differences in terms of response to stress; for instance, many Irish may suffer silently and minimize their symptoms, while some Puerto Rican females may respond with physical symptoms combined with anxiety and depression (Jalali, 1988).

Confronted with such wide ranges of emotional expression, stable characteristics become exceedingly important in order to facilitate apppropriate treatment. Asking about specific physical processes can therefore be a valuable tool for beginning to sort out different types of psychopathology, as indicated by the fourth edition of the *Diagnostic and Statistical Manual of Mental Disorders* (American Psychiatric Association, 1994). However, while questions regarding the exact time of sleep onset, number and duration of nocturnal awakenings, presence of day naps, and so on are pieces of information that may be more easily quantifiable and less subjectively variable, one must remain ever alert to the ethnocultural and gender expressions of illness in order to understand fully the problem (Comas-Díaz & Griffith, 1988), as well as to be able to emphathize with the patient's experience and maintain compliance with a treatment contract.

PSYCHODYNAMICS OF PSYCHOPHARMACOLOGY FOR WOMEN OF COLOR

Given the large number of women of color in the United States it is appalling how little has been researched or written about their psychopharmacology, much less the psychodynamics of prescribing psychoactive medications. In fact, there is a dearth of literature in this area, so that much of what follows is necessarily derived from clinical experience. When evaluating or treating women of color it is important to not let the characteristic of race or ethnicity overshadow the fact that the individuals being treated are first of all *women*. Women are subject to certain illnesses and conditions at much greater rates than men, such as depression, anxiety disorders, eating disorders, sexual abuse, domestic battering (see Kanuha, Chapter 15, this volume), certain types of post-traumatic stress disorders, reproductive cycle syndromes, and so on. However, as other chapters in this book delineate, the characteristic of being a woman *of color* is likely to place them at even greater risk for the development of certain types of psychopathology.

In the past, I suspect that many women of color suffered quietly or at best received inadequate attention from family practitioners, internists, or clergy when afflicted by even the most commonplace maladies, such as mood and anxiety disorders. The women of color receiving the most psychotropic attention were those who were so overtly and dramatically ill as to enter into an inpatient health care system (e.g., schizophrenics, manic-depressives, and substance abusers). With the educational efforts of the past decade, mood, anxiety, eating, and substance-abuse disorders are being increasingly recognized in the general population, and larger numbers of women of color are seeking and receiving treatment for the first time. Paradoxically, however, women of color may still be less likely to receive adequate evaluation for psychotropic medications, even when their presenting symptoms are recognized (or recognizeable) by health providers. This can occur due to the increasing societal attention paid to the adverse psychosocial events triggering the illnesses, which may in some cases actually divert attention from the underlying physiological processes. Moreover, it is not uncommon, for example, that African American, Latinas, and Native American women feel patronized by a health care system that tends to portray them as either "victims" or "perpetrators" of societal ills such as drug abuse, crime, and so on, rather than as individuals. On the other hand, some groups—such as Asian Americans—have a tendency to "delay and underutilize" psychiatric care (Lin, Innui, Kleinman, & Womank, 1982) leading to an "invisibility" of their problems.

Owing to these factors, some women of color may be suspicious regarding the consideration or suggestion of psychotropic medication, feeling that this type of drug may be used as a punishment for complaining, "being bad," or, in effect, being non-White. Many non-Whites have a deep-seated distrust of cross-ethnocultural dyadic provider–patient relationships (Comas-Díaz & Jacobsen, 1991), which cannot be ignored if treatment is to proceed successfully. Due to ignorance, diffidence, or the experience of being punished for being assertive ("uppity") many women of color may be less likely than their White counterparts to ask questions of the physician about alternative treatments. These difficulties may be compounded by the perception of the physician (regardless of race or gender) as an authority figure and member of the power establishment who should not be questioned and who, by virtue of the stigma attached to mental illness, may actually be feared. Unfortunately, in some cases the prescription of psychotropic medications has been a way for physicians at once to fulfill a medical role as a caretaker while at the same time silencing complaints.

Adding to the complexity of these problems is the fact that some ethnic minority individuals fail to remain in treatment for an adequate duration of time, thereby perpetuating inadequate treatment. Asian Americans and Hispanics/Latinos, for example, have been reported to be less likely than Whites to seek mental health treatment (Snowden, 1988) and somewhat more likely to drop out of treatment earlier after initial entry into the treatment system (Baekelund, 1975). This dropping out is more likely to occur if the treatment is perceived as not being culturally relevant. In order to promote better treatment outcomes for women of color, it is therefore critical to include ethnocultural and gender-specific contexts when considering different aspects of psychopharmacologic treatment.

PRACTICAL CONSIDERATIONS IN TREATMENT

Treatment should be considered to be a two phase process. In the evaluation phase it is critical to define clearly the presenting complaint and the parameters of the evaluation and treatment. A full discussion of these issues with the referral source should be considered an essential component of the evaluation. The following case study illustrates the importance of examining why the patient is being referred for evaluation/treatment.

An Employment Assistance Program (EAP) counselor referred a 26-year-old African American female for medication evaluation due to the suspicion of a depressive disorder. The identified patient's supervisor (a White woman) had ordered her to consult with the EAP (a White male) in order to comply with the procedures involved in terminating employees. In the discussion of the case with the psychiatrist (a White male), the EAP counselor failed to mention the forced nature of the consultation, which contributed to the patient's strong oppositon to the referral. As is all too frequently the case, Ms. Brown had also been simultaneously referred for counseling to a therapist (an African American female) who, given the historico-political context of medicating women of color, believed that psychotropic medications were generally not only unnecessary but also frequently harmful. Part of the psychodynamics of the referral evolved into an "us against them" (Comas-Díaz & Jacobsen, 1991) situation. Obviously, the hurdles involved in trying to carry out a psychopharmacologic evaluation in such a situation are substantial but unfortunately not uncommon (Jacobsen, in press).

Ms. Brown's symptoms of depressed mood, lack of energy, early morning awakening, and concentration and attention problems were classic symptoms of depression. However, it was her irritability that was causing major problems at work, particularly with her supervisor. The psychopharmacologist's first task was to develop an alliance with Ms. Brown by providing her with factual information about depression. After this educative stage, the psychopharmacologist invited her to negotiate the treatment by presenting her with several pharmacologic options and enlisting her cooperation. It was during this stage that the psychopharmacologist realized the enforced nature of the referral. This issue was addressed by developing a comprehensive treatment plan involving Ms. Brown's therapist and a significant other, in this case, her mother (with

Ms. Brown's authorization). Ms. Brown was given a trial of antidepressant medication, and after 3 weeks on the medication her symptoms subsided. She was able to function at work and the threat of being fired was lifted.

The issue of long-term medication maintenance also needed to be negotiated with Ms. Brown due to her fear of being considered sick, which was being operationalized by taking medications. This was a complex situation because Ms. Brown's family background reinforced her not taking medications even though she had suffered numerous past depressive episodes. Furthermore, as indicated previously, her therapist was initally skeptical and suspicious about the politics of prescribing medication to women of color. Notwithstanding these difficulties, the psychopharmacologist was able to collaborate with the therapist, who was impressed by the positive effects of the medication. This collaboration followed an empowering approach within a psychopharmacologic–psychotherapeutic concurrent model. Within this approach, emphasis is given to the therapeutic relationship in the form of a therapeutic triangle and to education as a emancipatory psychosocial method aimed at helping the patient manage her situation in a self-affirming manner (Comas-Díaz & Jacobsen, in press). In conclusion, Ms. Brown was seen in short-term psychotherapy for 3 months and continued in psychopharmacologic treatment thereafter, being seen by the psychopharmacologist once every 6 weeks.

A full neuropsychiatric evaluation should be considered for women of color in order to avoid missing some unexpected details that might impact on the treatment (Vega, 1993). As part of this evaluation it may be helpful to perform an ethnocultural evaluation (Jacobsen, 1988). The ethnocultural evaluation explores the biopsychosocial heritage of the patient including specific ethnoracial origins that, as described above, may influence illness presentation as well as response to psychopharmacologic treatment. When possible, gathering data from other relatives may be useful to help flush out parts of the personal and extended family history that may be unknown to or denied by the patient. The assessment should also include detailed inquiry regarding possible physical and emotional traumas, which tend to occur at higher rates in women of color (McGrath, Keita, Strickland, & Russo, 1990). Culturally validated and gender-sensitive psychological or neuropsychological testing should be considered in any assessment in which the diagnosis is unclear, or to help with formulating treatment plans.

With many women of color it is important to ask about home remedies, herbal medicines, vitamins, and the use of over-the-counter medications. Similarly, the patient may have her own ideas of the etiology of her symptoms, which will also reflect upon her acceptance of treatment. It is extremely important to elicit the patient's understanding of her symptoms, and, whenever possible, to present the psychopharmacologic treatment as congruent to her worldview. Consider the following case study.

A Mexican immigrant woman was seen in a psychopharmacologic consultation. Her main complaint was that her heart was about to get out of her chest.

She was referred by her primary physician after all of her physical exam results were negative. An assessment revealed that Ms. Flores, a secretary in a law firm, was preoccupied by relatives left behind in Mexico, particularly her 15-year-old son. The apparent precipitating event was a case being handled by her boss that involved a 15-year-old Salvadoran male who killed another man during a drunken argument. Ms. Flores became very anxious, fearing that her son might be in a similar situation back home. Ms. Flores' interpretation of her symptoms was that they were caused by *susto* (fright). Susto is a folk illness charaterized by anorexia and various painful sensations brought on by traumatic experiences such as witnessing a death (Kiev, 1968; Simons & Hughes, 1993). Exploration revealed that without medical consultation Ms. Flores had been taking an antidepressant that can be purchased over the counter in Mexico and was being sent to her by her relatives for treatment of her *susto*. Many Latin American countries have a wider range of over-the counter and traditional medications than the United States (National Coalition of Hispanic Health and Human Services, 1988). This antidepresant was exacerbating Ms. Flores' anxiety reaction. The prescription of an anxiolytic medication and the recommendation of tapering off her antidepressant was presented within the context of treating her *susto*.

Once the evaluation process has been completed, if a medication trial is deemed appropriate, then explicit instructions regarding the use of the medication along with education regarding side effects should be given before pharmacologic treatment is initiated. This educational phase should be considered to be an integral part of the treatment, since it helps to engage the patient and increases the likelihood of her following through on treatment recommendations. As in the evaluation phase, it is frequently helpful to include significant others in this educative phase. Establishing an open rapport with the patient and significant others is important since both parties must feel comfortable in contacting the prescribing physician in the event of unexpected adverse events, which are not uncommon with psychotropic medications. Otherwise, the all-too-common scenario of the patient arriving at an appointment having discontinued treatment earlier may occur.

Many members of ethnic minority groups in the United States are often unwilling to relinquish to medical personnel complete control over the care of a patient, even in acute care settings (Clark, 1983). For some women of color treatment is a family affair. Due to the collective orientation prevalent among many people of color (Ho, 1987), individual illness is actually considered an illness affecting all family members. For example, it is common among some Latinos to involve the whole family in the treatment process (Canino & Canino, 1982). Moreover, Ramos-McKay, Comas-Díaz, and Rivera (1988) argue that among Puerto Ricans, sharing medications among significant others and relatives is a common practice. Among Latinos, relatives sometimes give each other medications that were prescribed for and helpful to them, reasoning that the medication will also help the identified patient (National Coalition of Hispanic Health and Human Services Organizations, 1988).

Because of the differences in metabolism of drugs mentioned earlier, ethnic minority women should probably be started at or below the standard lowest initiating dose for psychotropics and only gradually increased based upon clinical response and side-effects profile. Polypharmacy, the use of more than one medication, should be avoided whenever possible because the use of multiple medications may dramatically increase the complexity of the resulting pharmacologic picture due to potentially negative interactive effects. Since, however, there are no psychotropic medications that are universally effective and without side effects, it should be noted that the avoidance of polypharmacy is an ideal that may often not be attainable in the real world due to variability in response, side effects, and so on. Moreover, not all cultures regard polypharmacy as undesireable. For example, polypharmacy is widely practiced and accepted in many Asians countries (Chien, 1993).

Once started on psychotropic medications, the person of color may find treatment complicated by a faster or greater development of side effects than the physician is accustomed to hearing from the White patient. The emergence of adverse effects may be due not only to the physiological differences in psychotropic drug metabolism mentioned earlier, but may also be influenced by psychological factors described above. Careful monitoring for the emergence of psychosomatic effects should therefore be considered an integral and continuing component of prescribing psychotropic medications.

In summary, there are many complex factors contributing to the psychopharmacology of women of color, almost all of which are poorly researched or only beginning to be explored. Given the ethnocultural population shifts occuring in the United States and the rapid advances being made in the neurosciences and psychopharmacology, however, we are hopeful that more attention will be paid to this area in the future.

REFERENCES

American Psychiatric Association. (1994). *Diagnostic and statistical manual of mental disorders* (4th ed.). Washington, DC: Author.

Baekelund, F., & Lundwall, L. (1975). Dropping out of treatment: A critical review. *Psychological Bulletin, 82,* 738–783.

Breier, A. (1989). Experimental approaches to human stress research: Assessment of neurobiological mechanisms of stress in volunteers and psychiatric patients. *Biological Psychiatry, 26,* 438–462.

Canino, G., & Canino, I.A. (1982). Culturally syntonic family therapy for migrant Puerto Ricans. *Hospital and Community Psychiatry, 33,* 299–303.

Chien, C.-P. (1993). Ethnopsychopharmacology. In A. Gaw (Ed.), *Culture, ethnicity and mental health* (pp. 413–430). Washington, DC: American Psychiatric Press.

Clark, M. M. (1983). Cultural context of medical practice. *Western Journal of Medicine, 139,* 806–810.

Clark, W. G., Brater, D. C., & Johnson, A. R. (Eds.). (1988). *Goth's medical pharmacology* (12th ed.). St. Louis, MO: C.V. Mosby.

Comas-Díaz, L., & Griffith, E. H. E. (Eds.). (1988). *Clinical guidelines in cross cultural mental health.* New York: Wiley.

Comas-Díaz, L., & Jacobsen, F. M. (1991). Ethnocultural transference and counter-transference in the therapeutic dyad. *American Journal of Orthopsychiatry, 61,* 392–402.

Comas-Díaz, L., & Jacobsen, F. M. (in press). Psychopharmacology for women of color: An empowering approach. *Women and Therapy.*

Davis, A. Y. (1990). Sick and tired of being sick and tired: The politics of black women's health. In E. C. White (Ed.), *The Black women's health book: Speaking for ourselves.* Seattle, WA: Seal Press.

Dawkins, K., & Potter, W. Z. (1991). Gender differences in pharmacokinetics and pharmacodynamics of psychotropics: Focus on women. *Psychopharmacology Bulletin, 27,* 417–426.

Flaherty, J. A., & Meaer, R. (1980). Measuring racial bias in inpatient treatment. *American Journal of Psychiatry, 137,* 679–682.

Frank, E., Kupfer, D. J., Perel, J. M., Cornes, C., Jarrett, D. B., Mallinger, A. G., Thase, M. E., McEacharan, A. B., & Grochocinski, V. J. (1990). Three-year outcomes for maintenance therapies in recurrent depression. *Archives of General Psychiatry, 47,* 1093–1099.

Freedman, D. X., & Stahl, S. M. (1992, Fall). Pharmacology: Policy implications of new psychiatric drugs. *Health Affairs,* pp. 157–163.

General Accounting Office. (1992, October 29). *Women's health: FDA needs to ensure more study of gender differences in prescription drug testing.* (GAO/HRD-93-17), Washington, DC: Author.

Goldberg, S. C., Schooler, N. R., Davidson, E. M., & Kayce, M. M. (1966). Sex and race differences in response to drug treatment among schizophrenics. *Psychopharmacologia, 9,* 31–47.

Hamilton, J., & Parry, B. (1983). Sex related differences in clinical drug response: Implications for women's health. *Journal of the American Medical Women's Association, 38,* 126–132.

Harwood, A. (Ed.). (1981). *Ethnicity and medical care.* Cambridge, MA: Harvard University Press.

Hilts, P. J. (1993, March 24). F.D.A. ends ban on women in drug testing. *New York Times,* p. F8.

Ho, M. H. (1987). *Family therapy with ethnic minorities.* Newbury Park, CA: Sage.

Institute of Medicine, National Academy of Sciences. (1993, March 24–25). *The legal and ethical issues relating to the inclusion of women in clinical studies* (Workshop presented at Georgetown University). Washington, DC : Author.

Jacobsen, F. M. (1988). Ethnocultural assessment. In L. Comas-Díaz & E. E. H. Griffith (Eds.), *Clinical guidelines in cross-cultural mental health.* New York: Wiley.

Jacobsen, F. M. (1993): Medicolegal issues in outpatient psychopharmacology. *Rx for Risk, 5*(5), 1–4.

Jacobsen, F. M. (in press). *Psychoactive medications in mental health practice: A handbook for therapists.* New York: Wiley.

Jalali, B. (1988). Ethnicity, cultural adjustment, and behavior: Implications for family therapy. In L. Comas-Díaz & E. E. H. Griffith (Eds.), *Clinical guidelines in cross-cultural mental health* (pp. 9–32). New York: Wiley.

Kiev, A. (1968). *Curanderismo: Mexican American folk psychiatry*. New York: Free Press.

Lin, K., Innui, T. S., Kleinman, A., & Womank, W. (1982). Sociocultural determinants of the help-seeking behavior of patients with mental illness. *Journal of Nervous and Mental Disease, 170,* 78–85.

Lin, K.-M., Poland, R. E., Fleishaker, J. C., & Phillips, P. (1993). Ethnicity and differential responses to benzodiazepines. In K.-M. Lin, R. E. Poland, & G. Nakasaki (Eds.), *Psychomarmacology and psychobiology of ethnicity* (pp. 91–105). Washington, DC: American Psychiatric Press.

Lin, K.-M., Poland, R. E., & Nakasaki, G. (Eds.). (1993). *Psychopharmacology and psychobiology of ethnicity*. Washington, DC: American Psychiatric Press.

Lin K., Poland, R. E., Smith, M. W., Strickand, T. L., & Mendoza, R. (1991). Pharmacokinetics and other related factors affecting psychotropic responses in Asians. *Psychopharmacology Bulletin, 27,* 427–439.

López, S. (1989). Patient variable biases in clinical judgment: Conceptual overview and methodological considerations. *Psychological Bulletin, 106,* 184–203.

Loring, M., & Powell, B. (1988). Gender, race, and DSM-III: A study of the objectivity of psychiatric diagnostic behavior. *Journal of Health and Social Behavior, 29,* 1–22.

Martin, E. (1987). *The woman in the body: A cultural analysis of reproduction*. Boston: Beacon Press.

McGrath, E., Keita, G. P., Strickland, B. R., & Russo, N. F. (1990). *Women and depression: Risk factors and treatment issues*. Washington, DC: American Psychological Association.

Mendoza, R., Smith, M. W., Poland, R. E., Lin, K, & Strickland, T. L. (1991). Ethnic psychopharmacology: The Hispanic and Native American perspective. *Psychopharmacolgy Bulletin, 27,* 449–461.

National Coalition of Hispanic Health and Human Services Organizations. (1988). *Delivering preventive health care to Hispanics: A manual for providers*. Washington, DC: Author.

Ogur, B. (1986). Long day's journey into night: Women and prescription drug abuse. *Women and Health, 11,* 99–115.

Parker, D. C., Rossman, L. G., & Vander Laan, E. F. (1973). Sleep-related nychtemeral and briefly episodic variation in human plasmaprolactin concentrations. *Journal of Clinical Endocrinology and Metabolism, 36,* 1119–1124.

Ramos-McKay, J., Comas-Díaz, L., & Rivera, L. (1988). Puerto Ricans. In L. Comas-Díaz & E. E. H. Griffith (Eds.), *Clinical guidelines in cross-cultural mental health* (pp. 204–232). New York: Wiley.

Raskin, A., & Crook, T. H. (1975). Antidepressants in Black and White inpatients. *Archives of General Psychiatry, 32,* 643–649.

Rodin, J., & Ickovics, J. R. (1990). Women's health: Review and research agenda as we approach the 21st century. *American Psychologist, 45,* 1018–1034

Root, M. P. P. (1990). Disordered eating in women of color. *Sex Roles, 22,* 525–536.

Root, M. P. P. (1992). Reconstructing the impact of trauma on personality. In L. S. Brown & M. Ballou (Eds.), *Personality and psychopathology: Feminist reappraisals* (pp. 229–265). New York: Guilford Press.

Rudorfer, M. V., Lane, E. A., Chang, W. H., Zhang, M., & Potter, W. C. (1984). Desipramine pharmacokinetics in Chinese and Caucasian volunteers. *British Journal of Clinical Pharmacology, 17,* 433–440

Silver, B., Poland, R., & Lin, K.-M. (1993). Ethnicity and the pharmacology of tricyclic antidepressants. In K.-M. Lin, R. E. Poland, & G. Nakasaki (Eds.), *Psychopharmacology and psychobiology of ethnicity* (pp. 61–89). Washington, DC: American Psychiatric Press.

Simons, R. C., & Hughes, C. C (1993). Culture-bound syndromes. In A. Gaw (Ed.), *Culture, ethnicity and mental illness* (pp. 75–99). Washington, DC: American Psychiatric Press.

Smith, M., Lin, K.-M., & Mendoza, R. (1993). "Nonbiological" issues affecting psychopharmacotherapy: Cultural considerations. In K.-M. Lin, R. E. Poland, & G. Nakasaki (Eds.), *Psychopharmacology and psychobiology of ethnicity* (pp. 37–58). Washington, DC: American Psychiatric Press.

Snowden, L R. (1988). Ethnicity and utilization of mental health services: An overview of current findings. In *Proceedings: Oklahoma Mental Health Research Institute, Professional Symposium* (pp. 227–238). Oklahoma City: Oklahoma Mental Health Research Institute, 227–238.

Strickland, T. L., Lawson, W., Lin, K,-M., & Fu, P. (1993). Interethnic variation in response to lithium therapy among African-American and Asian-American populations. In K.-M. Lin, R. E. Poland, & G. Nakasaki (Eds.), *Psychopharmacology and psychobiology of ethnicity* (pp. 107–121). Washington, DC: American Psychiatric Press.

Strickland, T. L., Ranganath, V., Lin, K.-M., Poland, R. E., Mendoza, R., & Smith, M. W. (1991). Psychopharmacology and considerations in the treatment of Black American populations. *Psychopharmacology Bulletin, 27,* 441–448.

Turner, S. M. (1992). Socioecologic issues in psychopharmacology: A methodologic critique. In *Interethnic psychopharmacology—Current pharmacogenetic, pharmacokinetic, and diagnostic considerations.* Washington, DC: American Psychological Association.

U.S. Department of Health and Human Services. (1992). *Women's health issues.* Washington, DC: Author.

Vega, S. (1993, August). Neuropsychological assessment of women of color. In H. Coons & A. M. Austria (Chairs), *Clinical assessment in women's health: From research to practice.* Symposium presented at the annual meeting of the American Psychologic Association, Toronto.

White, E. C. (Ed.). (1990). *The Black women's health book: Speaking for ourselves.* Seattle, WA: Seal Press.

Willie, C. V., Kramer, B. M., & Brown, B. S. (Eds.). (1973). *Racism and mental health: Essays.* Pittsburgh: University of Pittsburgh Press.

Wynder, E. L. (1979). Interrelationship of smoking to other variables and preventative approaches. In M. E. Jarvik, J. W. Cullen, E. R. Gritz, T. M. Vogt, & L. J. West (Ed.), *Research on smoking behavior* (pp. 67–85). Rockville, MD: Department of Health, Education, and Welfare.

Yonkers, K. A., Kando J. C., Cole J. O., & Blumenthal, S. (1992). Gender differences in pharmacokinetics and pharmacodynamics of psychotropic medication. *American Journal of Psychiatry, 149,* 587–595

Yoshida, A. (1993). Genetic polymorphisms of alcohol-metabolizing enzymes related to alcohol sensitivity and alcoholic diseases.

Zborowski, M. (1969). *People in pain.* San Francisco: Jossey-Bass.

III

THE LABYRINTH OF DIVERSITY: SPECIAL POPULATIONS OF WOMEN OF COLOR

Overview: Connections and Disconnections

Lillian Comas-Díaz
Beverly Greene

ARIADNE AND THE LABYRINTH OF DIVERSITY

In Greek mythology, Adriadne wove a thread that guided Theseus through the labyrinth where he killed the Minotaur, finding his way back by following the thread (Hamlyn, 1963). We use the concept of labyrinth as a symbol of the enigmatic diversity of women of color. A successful journey into the labyrinth of diversity requires the combination of guidance (Ariadne's feminine thread) with instrumental behavior (Theseus' strength). Solving the labyrinth's mystery involves a recognition of the connections and disconnections present among the special groups of women of color.

The first section in this volume focused on what individual women in an ethnic group share, while this section explores some of the things that make their lives dissimilar, through the examination of special populations. The contributors in this section offer guidelines on how to address the mental health needs of special groups of women of color. The diverse experiences and needs of women of color are compounded by the multiple and interactive effects of racism, sexism, classism, ageism, heterosexism, ethnocentrism, ablism, and xenophobia. Some of the special groups represented in this section include professional women, lesbians, battered women, mixed-race women, and Southeast Asian refugee women. Although this list is not exhaustive, it offers an introductory look at some of the diverse concerns of women of color.

341

THE DIALECTIC OF CONNECTIONS AND DISCONNECTIONS

Diversity among women of color creates a tension between what connects them and what separates them. Women are brought together by their similarities and divided by their differences (Cole, 1986). Within this framework, many members of special populations of women of color share commonalities with other groups of women. The challenge therefore is to build upon the connections while recognizing the differences. However, this challenge remains unfullfilled. We can see this in the case of women of color with professional status. Professional women of color have much in common with their White counterparts, such as being subjected to sexist oppression and subordination in a White patriarchal system. Both groups also share concerns about the glass ceiling phenomenon, equal pay for equal work, maternal leave, and others. Notwithstanding these commonalities, coalitions between the two groups have produced ambivalent results (Comas-Díaz, 1991). For instance, in the area of women's rights, White mainstream feminists have been responsive to the call of diversity in membership but have neglected a thorough analysis of race, gender, and class in feminist thinking, a phenomenon that has been described as inclusion without influence (Uttal, 1990). Similar dynamics are often present in the attempts at forging alliances between professional mainstream women and women of color with professional status. Lillian Comas-Díaz and Beverly Greene expand on these issues in their chapter on professional women (Chapter 13).

Like professional women, lesbian women of color are members of multiple groups. Although being a member of multiple groups can be advantageous, it can also increase stress and marginality. A lesbian of color is in triple jeopardy due to the combination of being a woman, a person of color, and a lesbian (Kanuha, 1990). Having multiple-group identity does not necessarily increase the total level of support and solidarity provided to the woman by her groups. Sometimes the diverse groups conflict in their priorities, goals, causes, and perceptions of one another. For lesbians of color there is the additional stress of managing homophobia and sexism from the dominant and ethnic minority groups and racism from the gay and lesbian communities. Beverly Greene's chapter expands on these issues (Chapter 14).

Being victims of violence is considered to be a serious cause of mental health problems for women (Koss, 1990). Women of color often live in extremely stressful, antagonistic, and even hostile environments (Anderson, 1991). Many women of color belong to a low socioeconomic class and face survival and environmental stressors that significantly affect their daily lives. As an illustration, Fuchs (1990) coined the term "ethno-underclass" to describe poor African Americans, American Indians, Puerto Ricans, and Mexican Americans who are chronically isolated from the mainstream. Concerns about concrete matters, such as employment, housing, and food, as well as concomitant issues of personal safety, violence, sexual abuse, and physical health may emerge during mental health treatment. These environmental and concrete limitations are often compounded by the racism, sexism, and classism that many women of color encounter, in addition to the heterosexism and homophobia that lesbians of color experience.

Women of color who have escaped the limitations of poverty may still be affected by the environment created by poverty because they belong to a community that struggles with survival issues. Many women of color experience victimization. Their victimization is direct or indirect, the result of what Pinderhughes (1982) identifies as the victim system of racism and oppression, where limitations in resources lead to stress, impairment in growth, destabilization of communities, and thus more powerlessness. A person who is subjected to a great deal of racist treatment can be afflicted by powerlessness, learned helplessness, depression, anxiety, and even post-traumatic stress disorder (Melba Vasquez, Chapter 4, this volume). Hamilton (1989) also says that for victims of discrimination the processes of denial or suppression are often similar to those in posttraumatic stress disorder (PTSD), in which emotional flooding and disorganized behavior can be triggered by subtle clues, reminders, or even mini-instances of what has been suppressed. This situation is exacerbated for women of color, who confront societal barriers due to the inferior status assigned to both their gender and their ethnicities.

Women of color may be exposed to what Root (1992) calls insidious trauma. She believes that this type of trauma includes the cumulative effect of racism, sexism, dislocation, and other types of oppression. Moreover, sexual and physical victimization are so prevalent among women in the general population that it has been postulated that they are normative aspects of female development (Hamilton & Jensvold, 1992). As both females and people of color, women of color become an easy target for victimization and oppression. Many women of color are oppressed by their own communities as well as by the dominant group. Lorde (1984) asserts that African American women are exposed in African American communities to sexual hostility and violence against them and their children. The discussion of domestic violence by Valli Kanuha (Chapter 15, this volume) further illustrates some of these issues for women of color.

The diversity among women of color extends to political contexts. Historical and sociopolitical variables significantly contribute to the dynamics of multiple group membership for women of color. For instance, the history of slavery and the unpredictability of life after emancipation, the consequent oppression, and the need to reaffirm identity have had an overwhelming impact on many African Americans' senses of self (Pinderhughes, 1976). For many women of African descent, the legacy has resulted in serious negative sexual stereotyping (on African American women see Beverly Greene, Chapter 1; on Jamaican women see Janet K. Brice-Baker, Chapter 5). Similarly, being a mixed-race woman has specific connotations in North American society. Moreover, the number of mixed-race individuals is increasing. Maria P. P. Root's chapter on mixed-race women highlights some of the unique issues for these populations (Chapter 16).

Another example of differing historical and sociopolitical variables is the status of the political relationship between the United States and the country of origin of some women of color. Sensitive clinical work with women of color requires a contextual understanding of the effects of both international and national politics on people of color. For instance, as a highly heterogeneous group, Asian Americans have experienced the different effects of political variables. A poignant example is the forced internment of Japanese Americans when the United States and Japan became political adversaries during the World War II. Internment camps constituted just one of the many effects of political forces on this ethnic minority group.

The history of immigration provides yet another source for the diversity of women of color. Immigration is a central experience in the lives of many women of color, particularly Asians and Hispanics/Latinas. Immigration with its attendant ethnocultural translocation may affect individuals and their families, regardless of generational status or how far back the immigration occurred (Jacobsen, 1988). Being a refugee is a crucial element of a woman of color's psychology. Refugee women are often disconnected from their original countries with little hope of returning and/or being reunited with loved ones. There is also diversity among the experience of refugee groups. For instance, while Cubans are frequently accorded the status of political exiles, Salvadorans during the 1980s were not granted political refugee status and so had to enter the United States illegally (García & Rodríguez, 1989; Leslie & Leitch, 1989; Vargas, 1984). These different circumstances and the often serious needs of refugee populations dictate different psychotherapeutic interventions. Issues of loss, security, trauma, post-traumatic stress disorder, victimization, physical illness, culture shock, language proficiency, rape-related issues, and environmental problems affect women differently according to the circumstances of their ethnocultural translocation. The chapter on Southeast Asian American refugee women by Liang Tien (Chapter 17, this volume) discusses some of these issues in detail.

INCLUSION AND EXCLUSION

Unfortunately, several special populations of women of color such as substance abusers, the disabled, the aged, the homeless, Latina and Haitian refugees, and many others are not addressed in this volume. These populations haved unique needs that require special attention in their mental health treatment. The older woman of color is in fact receiving attention in the mental health literature. In reviewing the economic, psychological, and cultural dimensions of the aging process for women of color, Padgett

(1988) concludes that researchers and clinicians need to address the shorter life span in this population, the reality of quadruple jeopardy (being old, poor, female, and of minority status), and the adaptive advantages minority women may have in dealing with aging. Aging may also affect women of color differently according to their ethnicity and race. For example, Zuniga (1984) found that the themes prevalent among elderly Latina women were: (1) the sacrifices they made as mother and grandmother; (2) the changing cultural arena that presents them with unexpected issues that conflict with their cultural stances as a cohort group; (3) the combined sexism and racism they experienced and its effects, which continue to place them in vulnerable situations; and (4) service delivery issues that encumber culturally appropriate interventions. Of course, not all elderly women of color share these issues.

The contributors in this section present the issues of special populations of women of color and discuss their mental health implications. As in the other sections of this book, the contributors here offer practical guidelines for the clinical care of women in these populations. It is beyond the scope of this volume to address all special groups of women of color, but we hope that the five groups described here will provide an introduction to the complex diversity of women of color, their strengths, and their hardships.

REFERENCES

Anderson, L. P. (1991). Acculturative stress: A theory of relevance to Black Americans. *Clinical Psychology Review, 11*, 685–702.

Cole, J. B. (1986). Commonalities and differences. In J. B. Cole. (Ed.), *All American women: Lines that divide, ties that bind* (pp. 1–30). New York: Free Press.

Comas-Díaz, L. (1991). Feminism and diversity in psychology: The case of women of color. *Psychology of Women Quarterly, 15*, 597–609.

Fuchs, L. H. (1990 *The American kaleidoscope: Race, ethnicity, and the civic culture.* Middletown, CT: Wesleyan University Press.

García, M. O., & Rodríguez, P. F. (1989). Psychological effects of political repression in Argentina and El Salvador. In D. R. Koslow & E. Salett (Eds.), *Crossing cultures in mental health* (pp. 64–83). Washington, DC: Society for International Education Training and Research (SIETAR).

Hamilton, J. A. (1989). Emotional consequences of victimization and discrimination in "special populations" of women. In B. Parry (Ed.), *Women's disorders.* Philadelphia, PA: W. B. Saunders.

Hamilton, J. A., & Jensvold, M. (1992). Personality, psychopathology, and depressions in women. In L. S. Brown & M. Ballou (Eds.), *Personality and psychopathology: Feminist reappraisals* (pp. 116–143). New York: Guilford Press.

Hamlyn, P. (1963). *Greek mythology.* London: Westbook House.

Jacobsen, F. M. (1988). Ethnocultural assessment. In L. Comas-Díaz & E. H. Griffith (Eds.), *Clinical guidelines in cross-cultural mental health* (pp. 135–147). New York: Wiley.

Kanuha, V. (1990). Compounding the triple jeopardy: Battering in lesbian of color relationships. *Women and Therapy, 9,* 169–184.

Koss, M. P. (1990). The women's mental health research agenda: Violence against women. *American Psychologist, 45,* 374–380.

Leslie, L. A., & Leitch, M. L. (1989). A demographic profile of recent Central American immigrants: Clinical and service implications. *Hispanic Journal of Behavioral Sciences, 11,* 315–329.

Lorde, A. (1984). *Sister outsider: Essays and speeches.* New York: Cross Press.

Padgett, D. (1988). Aging minority women: Issues in research and health policy. *Women and Health, 14,* 213–225.

Pinderhughes, C. (1976). Black personality in American society. In M. Smythe (Ed.), *The Black America reference book.* Englewood Cliffs, NJ: Prentice-Hall.

Pinderhughes, E. (1982). Afro-American families and the victim system. In M. McGoldrick, J. K. Pearce, & J. Giordano (Eds.), *Ethnicity and family therapy* (pp. 108–122). New York: Guilford Press.

Root, M. P. P. (1992). Reconstructing the impact of trauma on personality. In L. S. Brown & M. Ballou (Eds.), *Personality and psychopathology: Feminist reappraisals* (pp. 229–265). New York: Guilford Press.

Uttal, L. (1990). Inclusion without influence: The continuing tokenism of women of color. In G. Anzaldúa (Ed.), *Making face, making souls—Haciendo caras: Creative and critical perspectives by feminists of color.* San Francisco: Aunt Lute Foundation.

Vargas, G. (1984, Autumn). Recently arrived Central American immigrants: Mental health needs. *Research bulletin* (pp. 1–3). Los Angeles: Spanish-Speaking Mental Health Research Center.

Zuniga, M. E. (1984). Elderly Latina mujeres: Stressors and strengths. In R. Anson (Ed.), *The Hispanic older woman.* Washington, DC: National Hispanic Council on Aging.

13

Women of Color with Professional Status

Lillian Comas-Díaz
Beverly Greene

The presence of women of color in professional settings has been aided by federal legislation and affirmative action policies forbidding discrimination in employment practices on the basis of race, color, sex, religion, or national origin (Romero & Garza, 1986). The ongoing influx of White women and people of color into managerial and other professional ranks traditionally dominated by White males is changing the face of American professions. It is estimated that by the year 2000, the majority of the American labor force will be comprised of White women and men and women of color (Henry, 1990).

Women of color with professional status are increasing their presence in the labor force. However, they face a complex discouraging reality: racism, sexism, few role models and mentors, isolation, competing personal and career demands, and shifting social norms and expectations (Farrant & Williams, 1990). Many women of color who are professionals are caught in a conflicting web of expectations from their own communities and from the dominant culture, which make life far more complex than simply being a professional woman or a woman of color would make it (Gilkes, 1982). For instance, they may become a hyphenated creation, such as the African American woman administrator, who has a place in the organizational structure, but lacks guaranteed security and significant power (Epstein, 1987). The lack of these things creates a paradox for women of color with professional status. For instance, they are expected to perform well, but without real power are unlikely to succeed; their lack of success may then be interpreted as a lack of quality in their work, which—reflecting their disappointment and frustration—may even become inferior over time.

Although gains have been made since the Civil Rights and the Women's Liberation movements, women of color with professional status encounter conflicting messages in the workplace (Alexander, 1990). On one hand, their extraordinary strength and stamina are demonstrated in their attainment of professional positions, usually over enormous obstacles. On the other hand, the need to manage their lives effectively as women of color in a White male culture places them at risk of stress (Bell, 1990). Succeeding this environment requires specialized coping and adaptation skills (Denton, 1990). The stress of adapting increases their vulnerability to health and mental health problems. Their professional status may make them more vulnerable to depression, anxiety, and other stress–related reactions, psychosomatic disorders, and addictive behaviors.

We recognize a wide diversity among women of color with professional status, however, in this chapter the concentration is on those factors that appear to be common to most of these women. We present ethnocultural factors that both facilitate and impede their success in professional positions. We discuss the discriminatory double bind of racism and sexism (and heterosexism for some women) in its manifestations of tokenism and stereotyping. The coping styles of women of color, both functional and dysfunctional, are examined. Their special mental health needs are identified and treatment implications are presented. There is a growing yet limited professional and empirical literature on this population, and we have complemented it with what is available in the popular literature, anecdotal data, and our own clinical experience. Clinical and anecdotal data have been altered to protect confidentiality.

THE PRESENCE OF WOMEN OF COLOR IN THE PROFESSIONAL WORKPLACE: ETHNOCULTURAL FACTORS

The mental health needs of women of color with professional status are determined by the interaction of several variables such as gender, race, sexual orientation, sociohistorical influences, political forces, and psychological factors. Before addressing the mental health needs of this population, we believe that it is crucial to frame the ethno- and sociocultural context of these women's realities, especially as it relates to their presence in the workplace.

That women of color in the work environment face significant obstacles is paradoxical because women of color have a long heritage of work outside the home, mainly for reasons of economic survival (Reid & Comas-Díaz, 1990). For example, African American women were brought to the United States to labor and to produce children who would be laborers. And to this day, they have worked outside the home and have often been the sole wage earners in times of high unemployment (Greene, 1992; Hines & Boyd-Franklin, 1982). The majority are raised with the expectation that whether single or married, childless or not, they will have to work most of their adult lives (Lerner, 1973; Reid, 1988).

The gender roles of many women of color also tend to facilitate their presence in the professional arena. African American and American Indian women tend to be relatively adaptable and flexible in their gender roles (Binion, 1990; LaFromboise et al., 1990). LaFromboise et al. (1990) assert that American Indian women are seen as less threatening to the dominant culture than American Indian men. Their traditional flexibility in gender roles may have facilitated a readiness to take on work roles within the dominant society that American Indian men would be offended by or unwilling to perform. African American family structures tend to have flexible gender roles (Binion, 1990), which may have helped facilitate African American women's entry into the workplace. Additionally, women who personally or generationally experience the effects of immigration, such as many Latinas and Asians, tend to develop more dynamic, flexible, and adaptive gender roles (Comas-Díaz, 1989; McGoldrick, García-Preto, Hines, & Lee, 1989). Such adaptability and flexibility can also be transferred into the workplace. Like Native American women, many women of color may exhibit behaviors that are considered less threatening, compared to their male counterparts, thus facilitating their education and achievement (Farrant & Williams, 1990). For instance, other cultural values that stress female subordination and lack of assertiveness mean that they do not threaten the status quo the way men of color may. The relatively easier access that women of color have to the mainstream is evident on each of the different steps of the professional ladder, from education, obtaining a job, to achieving some degree of professional advancement.

The value that many people of color place on education tends to facilitate the presence of woman of color in the professional arena. For many people of color education is a means of survival and progress within the mainstream society (Gilkes, 1982; McGoldrick, Pearce, & Giordano, 1982). In fact, many African American families tend to invest in educating their daughters, occasionally at the expense of their sons, as a means of keeping African American women away from domestic work, which is viewed as a position of sexual vulnerability (Epstein, 1973). Indeed, the definition of African American womanhood tends to integrate the concepts of work, achievement, and independence (Giddings, 1984).

Many Latinos transmit the role of aspiring to a good education to their offspring (McGoldrick et al., 1982). Latinas have achieved a pivotal role in the development of their communities (Almquist, 1989). Many have focused on education as a tool for the development of the Latino community. Similarly, many Asian American women are highly educated and have a high rate of labor force participation (Woo, 1989). However, they are overrepresented in low-paying and blue-collar positions without benefits such as health and pension (Woo, 1985). Those Asians who follow the philosophy of Confucius believe that education is the only route to success (Loo, 1988; Rigdon, 1991). Asian American women may be encouraged to obtain an education and achieve so as not to shame their families (Loo, 1988). Likewise, women from India who have a professional status are considered an asset to their husbands (Jayakar, Chapter 6, this volume). In sum, for many women of color, education is very often considered a portal to success in the United States (Williams, 1990).

A difference in the level of fear of success between some women of color and their White counterparts may be another facilitative variable in the former's attaining professional status. The fear of success syndrome consists of female anxiety and guilt about competence and success (Horner, 1972). In this syndrome, women equate success or the wish for it with loss of femininity and attractiveness, loss of significant relationships, and loss of health and overall functioning (Person, 1982). We believe that the fear of success is a complex and contextual issue, and thus that the characteristics that White women manifest as a result of it may not be the same for women of color. The combination of internal barriers and external obstacles blocking the path of achievement takes on a different configuration among women of color vis-à-vis their perception of success. Among many women of color, work and success are not necessarily connected to femininity or attractiveness, nor is the acceptance of significant others conditional on their achievement. However, some women of color also receive the conflictive message that they can educate themselves out of a husband.

The heritage of work among women of color and the strong connection to the fate of their ethnoracial group, often provide a backdrop for striving, competence, and success, thus making the fear of success not a significant factor for this population. Even if women of color do experience it they often do not have the financial option of staying at home, and so they become successful, although they may end up feeling guilty about it.

Another factor that has contributed to the presence of women of color in the professional arena is their strength in the face of adversity. Endurance, resilience, self-reliance, and tenacity have been characteristic of many women of color in the United States (LaFromboise et al., 1990; Loo, 1988; McGoldrick et al., 1989; Robinson, 1983). These traits can certainly help to sustain them in the face of the vicissitudes they confront in a professional setting.

Conversely, there are ethnocultural factors that tend to impede women of color's entrance and advance into professional work. Women have been socialized into placing the needs of others (particularly significant others) before their individual needs. Therefore, they tend to subordinate their own needs, and if they assert them they may be labeled by others as selfish. As an illustration, "contrary" is a term frequently used in African American culture (Christian, 1985) to denote woman's attempts at self-definition in her own culture and in the face of race, class, and gender definitions of the mainstream society as well. A woman is perceived as contrary if she makes her own self-development or her own needs a priority, ahead of the many needs of her family or the African American community, and is dismissed as irrational (Mays & Comas-Díaz, 1988).

There are other aspects of the socialization of women of color that tend to impede their access to professional careers. For some women of color, ambition may be necessary but is not considered a desirable female trait. For example, among some Asians, ambition was traditionally considered heroic in a man, but wicked and depraved in a woman (Loo, 1988). Similarly, some women of color are expected to know their place, namely to be subordinate to others, particularly men, and this can conflict with their ability to be assertive and to promote themselves in the professional arena. For example, Castro (1990) posits that many Asians value humility and thus, have difficulty being assertive in the workplace.

Regardless of the ethnocultural factors facilitating or hindering the presence of women of color in the professional arena, once they arrive at the workplace they encounter another variable in their path: the discriminatory double bind of racism and sexism, and for lesbians, heterosexism.

RACISM AND SEXISM: DOUBLE BIND IN THE WORKPLACE

Professionals are the elite of our society's work force. Their prestige is partly due to the fact that they are highly educated, derive fulfillment from their work, and enjoy a relative high degree of autonomy compared to nonprofessionals. However, Kaufman (1989) argues that women of color with professional status do not enjoy these advantages to the same extent as their male or White female counterparts do. She posits that even when women are willing and able to make the commitment to a professional career, most find themselves in subsidiary positions in prestigious professions or in positions that do not accord them the autonomy, prestige, or pay that other professionals receive. Furthermore, Kaufman states that African American women (and we believe this assertion extends to other women of color as well) are more likely to fit this pattern than White women. Women of color tend to be heavily concentrated in the lower-paying specialties, in the female-dominated professions, serving other people of color, poor, and/or working-class people in the public sector (Sokoloff, cited in Kaufman, 1989). Although the disparity between White women's and African American women's incomes appears to be disappearing, according to 1989 and 1990 Census Bureau figures (Vobejda, 1991a), women of color still face harder circumstances than women from the mainstream society. For example, Vobejda (1991a) states that African American women are more likely than White women to support a household on a single income, and that they work slightly more hours than White women.

For women of color, obtaining a formal education and achieving a professional status is not the end of their vocational journeys. Many women of color with professional status may be confronted with situations in which few or no women of color preceded them and where they remain unwelcome. These women may face tremendous isolation and despair, while being told that they have somehow made it (Greene, 1992). Attaining and maintaining a professional position may involve more than learning the "games mother never taught you." This phrase, coined by Harragan (1977), asserts that in order to survive and advance in the business world (and in other professional settings), women need to learn the games and rules of business that have been designed by and for White men. However, even if many women of color learn to play the games their mothers never taught them, their behaviors are often interpreted differently, and institutional barriers will prevent them from becoming successful players in the game of professional advancement.

As discussed earlier, many women of color who are professionals are caught in a conflicting web of expectations that is far more complex than that of simply being a professional or a woman of color (Gilkes, 1982). Women of color must overcome the difficulties any professional faces, such as obtaining academic degrees, meeting professional standards, and meeting licensing requirements, but in systems and institutions in which they are often unwelcome. Additionally, they share many of the specific concerns of men of color, such as racial discrimination in hiring and professional advancement (Leggon, 1980). They also share many of the problems White professional women face, such as sexual harassment, problems obtaining maternity leave, equal pay for equal work, the "mommy track" (the creation of separate and unequal tracks, one for exclusively career-oriented women, as opposed to the other for those who seek to blend career and parenting; see Schwartz, 1989), and the impact of these factors on professional advancement. Hence, professional women of color should not be subsumed under the rubric of professional people of color, nor under the rubric of professional women alone.

In addition to the difficulty of achieving professional status in a discriminatory work environment, professional status in itself does not appear to be an antidote to the venom of discrimination in society at large. One of the few empirical investigations on the mental health needs of professional women of color was conducted by Amaro and her associates (1987). These researchers studied the family and work predictors of psychological well-being among a sample of affluent professional Latina women. They found psychological distress ("How often do you feel depressed?") to be significantly related to the experience of discrimination, which was reported by more than 82% of the sample.

Regardless of their employment status (self-employed or salaried) women of color working in professional settings face special situations related to their double minority status. One of these is the problem of tokenism: the issue of whether or not a person is a "token," performance pressure, and possible retaliation from those who perceive the person as a token.

Tokenism

In an era of declining support for affirmative action policies revealed by such things as reverse discrimination lawsuits and financial constraints (cited as the reason for not meeting minority quotas), why and how women and people of color have been professionally advanced has become an issue of public discussion (Romero & Garza, 1986). According to Greider (1991), whenever people are losing their jobs and socioeconomic decline is visible, it is often easier to blame the troubles on racial minorities—especially those who have made some advancement—than it is to confront the political leaders who are responsible. Women of color may be particularly targeted by such scapegoating, because of their dual "categories," gender and race, and long-standing negative stereotypes about women and people of color. This double discrimination in the professional domain takes its form in claims of tokenism.

Being the only woman of color (or one of the very few) in a professional setting means becoming a token, a symbol of how women of color do, a role model for all women of color. Often, a token position is designed to give affirmative action credibility to an institution. As a double minority, a woman of color can be perceived as a double token—filling two affirmative action categories (female and race/ethnicity) in a single person (Wyche & Graves, 1992). Although many of the professional women of color may not experience direct blatant discrimination on the job, there is a tendency to question their qualifications by presuming that their gender and race and not their merit got them the position or gave them an advantage.

In a poignant discussion of tokenism among women in the corporate world, Kanter (1977) observes that it is the proportionally small numbers of women, rather than femaleness per se, that breeds the dynamics of tokenism. She states that the charge of tokenism, like powerlessness, sets in motion self-perpetuating cycles that reinforce the low numbers of women in professional settings and maintains the perception of them as tokens.

Being hired as a token, or being perceived that way by coworkers is a form of racism because it implies that the woman of color with professional status in not qualified for her position. Although women of color get attention and heightened visibility by being tokens, and thus the token does not have to work hard to be noticed, paradoxically, the woman of color has to work extraordinarily hard to have her achievements noticed. According to Kanter (1977) the presence of a token causes members of the dominant group to become more aware of their commonality, and to preserve their commonality they try to keep the token slightly outside. This has detrimental consequences for the token, such as loneliness and alienation. Indeed, many of the women that Kanter studied had higher turnover and failure rates than their male counterparts.

Being a token means encountering special pressures. As an illustration, women of color may alternate between being showcased (being highly visible) and being invisible. They may be showcased by their employers as documentation of conforming to affirmative action policies, but also as proving that by hiring a woman of color they have progressive attitudes and are above prejudice. In other words, showcasing a professional woman of color may be an example of being politically correct. However, being showcased can affect negatively the performance of the professional woman, as we see in the following vignette.

Maria, an American Indian woman, was repeatedly asked to represent her department during interagency meetings. The majority of these meetings had nothing to do with Maria's actual position in the agency. When she complained about the inordinate time spent attending these meetings, her supervisors replied that her department needed minority representation and that she was the only person of color. After 6 months, Maria was formally counseled by her immediate supervisor because of a decrease in her work productivity. Consequently, Maria felt that by being showcased at the expense of her work, she was indirectly penalized for being a woman of color in a professional setting.

The converse dynamic of a token's visibility is invisibility. The heightened awareness of hiring women of color who are professionals can paradoxically result in making them invisible. Castro (1990) investigated the tokens' invisibility in a study on the multicultural labor force in the United States conducted by Rutgers University. The study found that White women and women of color suffer from an invisibility syndrome, in which White male managers commonly tend to ignore them in meetings and thus overlook their contributions.

Tokens tend to perform their jobs under public and symbolic conditions different from those of the members of the majority group. The token visibility phenomenon makes women of color public figures, at times causing them to lose their individuality and privacy. Because their lives are put in the limelight, their work and behavior are more closely scrutinized than that of other employees. Their mistakes and intimate relationships also become public knowledge (Kanter, 1977). Women of color may feel that their freedom of action is restricted and that they have less independence than members of the dominant group.

Being a symbol or a representative of all women of color, of all persons of color, of all African Americans (Latinos, Asian Americans, American Indians, etc.) can be potentially draining (Wiltz, 1991). For example, in discussing the dilemmas faced by African American women in leadership positions, Dumas (1980) states that these women are torn between their symbolic image to others in the organization and their own professional tasks and goals. Regardless of their professional expertise, women of color may be asked to provide an ethnic minority perspective, or a woman's perspective, or both. The extended symbolic consequences of their behavior are powerful for many of these women, who have real reasons to feel that their performance could affect the prospects of other women and men of color in the professional setting. Indeed, the existence of successful ethnic minority role models can help to counteract racist opinions that people of color cannot succeed (Williams, 1990). Although some women of color may embrace this symbolism and decide to represent some or all people of color, they may do so at the expense of their own individual needs. They may also make themselves easy scapegoats in this regard. For example, women of color may be punished if what they say makes those in power uncomfortable or contradicts their view of themselves as liberal minded.

Tokenism can also involve not being taken seriously at work, resulting in being assigned tasks below one's capacity, bearing minimal responsibilities, or being placed in a dead-end job. For example, Jenkins (1985) argues that for African American women, significant barriers in the labor market often relegate these women to marginal positions within the workplace, threatening their well-being.

Tokenism may afford an initial access to professional positions for women of color. However, being perceived as a token also entails a denial of the woman's capabilities. For instance, many majority group members often attribute people of color's successes to luck or other situational factors, while attributing failures to laziness, stupidity, or other internal factors (Weitz & Gordon, 1993). Likewise, professional women of color carry the burden of needing to prove that their achievement is more than the result of affirmative action policies. As Carter (1991) asserts, some individuals suspect that all people of color with professional status achieved their status because of affirmative action policies, and not because of their merit. He terms this suspicion the "qualification question."

Paradoxically, if women of color become too successful, they run the risk of being penalized. This penalization is translated into retaliation by the members of the dominant group. Kanter (1977) argues that when a token does well enough to out-perform members of the dominant group, it cannot be kept a secret, since the token's behavior is public and therefore it is more difficult to avoid being publicly humiliated by a colleague from the dominant group. On the other hand, the woman's success may be kept conspicuously secret or minimized. It may be hard for some women of color to maintain the fine balancing act between doing well and doing too well, thus generating peer resentment.

The culture within professional settings appears to have institutionalized a practice to impede women of color from becoming too successful (i.e., more successful than members of the dominant group). The glass ceiling phenomenon is an illustration of such a practice. Women and ethnic minorities encounter an invisible barrier that limits their advancement toward upper management in organizations in the United States. The phrase "glass ceiling" refers to a barrier so subtle that it is transparent, yet so strong that it prevents women and people of color from moving up in the management hierarchy (Morrison & Von Glinow, 1990; Wiltz, 1991).

Stereotyping: Objectification Based on Gender and Race

Ingrained cultural conditioning socializes men to think of women in terms of stereotypes. As Lott (1991) argues, expectations of status and power are embedded in gender. These stereotyped attributions are carried into the workplace. For example, Harragan (1977) argues that many men have had no prior experience in dealing with women as autonomous individuals; instead, in the workplace they assign them the stereotyped role of mother, sister, daughter, wife, mistress, prostitute, or nurturer of some kind (nurse, teacher, etc.). Empirical research seems to corroborate some of these notions. As an illustration, McKenzie-Mohr and Zanna (1990) found that men previously identified as strongly gender schematic were found more often than other men to have sexual feelings about a woman in a professional situation after being exposed to nonviolent pornography.

Most women of color have been socially and legally perceived as paradigmatic sex objects in the United States. As an illustration, hooks (1981) argues that African American women have been the recipients of White male misogyny, and White women defended against it by the denying and/or justifying African American women's scapegoating. Additionally, African American women have been portrayed in the literature and media as being mammies or matriarchs, or as sexually promiscuous, castrating, or masculinized females (Carey, 1990; Gilkes, 1982; Greene, 1990, 1994; McGoldrick et al., 1989). This type of stereotyping has serious implications for African American women who are assertive and/or are in authority positions.

Latinas may tend to be stereotyped into the madonna/whore or Virgin Mary/Eve complex (Almquist, 1989; Comas-Díaz, 1989; Espín, 1986). On the one hand they are perceived as being overly sexual, promiscuous, sexually available (whore), and self-serving temptresses (Eve), while on the other, they are perceived to be virginal, chaste, sexually repressed, altruistic, martyred, and madonna-like woman (Virgin Mary) (Almquist, 1989; Espin, 1986). This type of objectification, reinforced in the popular media, makes it difficult for some males to take Latinas who have professional status seriously.

Asian American women are stereotyped as being submissive, shy, quiet, gentle, unassertive (Chow, 1989; McGoldrick et al., 1989), but also sexually attractive and available (Chan, 1987). There are also the more specific stereotypes of them as sexually exotic and eager to please (geisha) (Chan, 1987), as monstrously threatening (dragon lady) if they are too strong and assertive, or as gender neutral (i.e., as a sexless worker bee) (Loo, 1988; True, 1990). Furthermore, True (1990) states that due to the persistence of stereotyping Asian American women as hardworking and uncomplaining handmaidens, they are often exploited in their work. The sexual and racial stereotypes often affect the peer relationships of professional women of color, for example, a Chinese American woman developed a confrontational interpersonal style with her colleagues because she was tired of being perceived as a China doll.

American Indian women are the most invisible women of color (Almquist, 1989). They represent perhaps the least researched group of people in the United States (Snipp, 1990). According to Allen (1986), self-image constitutes the central issue with which American Indian women must come to terms. She argues that negative images of American Indians in the media and educational materials profoundly affect American Indian women's sense of self, how they behave, and how they relate to others. Nonetheless, some American Indian women in professional settings may attempt to embody exotic and mythical images for the benefit of coworkers. Although there is wide diversity among American Indian women, members of mainstream society often stereotype them as the American Indian princess or Pocahontas figure (Green, 1976). Seeing an American Indian women as a Pocahontas involves attributing to her courage, resourcefulness, and a devotion to Whites that historical accounts ascribe to this historical figure (Stevens, 1950). Conversely, a different stereotype involves assuming that American Indian professional women are too culturally committed, making their priorities the family and the cultural group as opposed to the job (Teresa LaFromboise, personal communication, 1992). This stereotype implies that American Indian women may not be properly committed to their professional work, and thus, should not be taken seriously. There are of course other stereotypes of American Indian women with professional status resulting from an objectification based on race and gender.

RELATIONSHIPS: SELF IN CONTEXT

In the general population, women tend to define themselves in terms of their relationships to others (Miller, 1986), and women of color also define themselves in these terms. As an illustration, professional women of color may define themselves as members of a community of women, as people of color, as women of color in White society, as members of a professional group, as professional women, and so on. Their multiple sources of identity can generate quite a bit of cultural, personal, and professional confusion.

The management of differing demands from the majority culture and an ethnic minority culture may result in bicultural stress (Bell, 1990). Additionally, participation in a profession entails complex directives to support the norms and values of the dominant society (Gilkes, 1982). Professionals are expected to behave according to the needs and values of mainstream society (Rueschemeyer, 1972). For many women of color this expectation may be paradoxical and conflictual. For some professional women, the intrinsic political sensitivity of an ethnic minority identity is not conducive to a full commitment to the values of the dominant society (Gilkes, 1982).

The professional woman of color may encounter paradoxes within her relationship to her ethnoracial community as well. For example, she may be dually perceived by her community. On one hand, she may be seen as a role model to be emulated and thus, pressure may be placed on her to return to her community part of what she has received without a realistic understanding of the demands of her work. She may be asked to participate in community agencies, volunteering in churches or schools, being on the boards of nonprofit organizations that are helping her ethnic minority community, and others. Many professional women of color feel a deep commitment toward their communities (Almquist, 1989; Gilkes, 1982), which may be related to a sense of responsibility toward their less fortunate sisters and brothers (Espín, Chapter 10, this volume).

The more successful women of color become in a professional context, the more alienated they may feel from their ethnic and racial communities. They can be perceived as having a bourgeois "oreo" image (i.e., black on the outside, white on the inside), of having forgotten their roots and thus being sellouts. Some community members may receive the women's success with envy and question how ethnic they really are. Ethnic professional women are perceived to have entered a Mephistophelean bargain of selling their souls to the White establishment in order to be successful. Her community's perception of a successful professional woman of color may oscillate between regarding her as a community heroine and as a traitor, or as both (Comas-Díaz & Jacobsen, 1991).

The other face of Janus (a Roman god who has two faces looking in opposite directions) is the woman of color who identifies herself as special and exceptional as a reaction to internalized racism or to the internalization of a negative self-image. Some people of color internalize racism and when successful their identification with the dominant group leads to a desire to leave and/or denigrate their own ethnic group (Greene, 1992). It is a psychological defense mechanism against racism that causes them to see their professional status as evidence that they are innately superior to and an exception to the stereotypes of less fortunate members of their racial group. It must be noted that the woman of color believes that the stereotypes of her group are true and that she must distance herself from the group in order to distance herself from the stereotypes. Additionally, the successful professional woman may have to cope with multigenerational guilt and the resultant conflicts. For example, Lerner (1988) argues that mainstream women who experience privileges and challenges, that separate them from female traditions of the past, tend to develop multigenerational guilt. She asserts that for these women multigenerational guilt has to do with a sense of the hardship, deprivation, and unfulfilled longing of previous generations of women in their families. We believe that multigenerational guilt can be compounded among women of color with professional status who have trauma in the generational history of their families. The diverse perceptions of self and others in the wake of trauma in previous generations often carry serious emotional consequences.

Interpersonal Relationships

Women of color with professional status face a dilemma in their interpersonal relationships. If they seek the support of White women coworkers for instance, they may encounter a conflict. Indeed, such relationships can be quite complex. They share the common denominator of being women with professional status with White women. There is the negative impact of sex-role stereotypes, the realities of gender discrimination, the impact of situational and contextual factors that affect women in a male dominated arena (Kanter, 1977), and there are others. However, racial and ethnic differences may interfere in the development of an enduring solidarity between mainstream women and women of color (Almquist, 1989). Many women of color question the sincerity of White women's solidarity or their capacity for and commitment to rectifying racial and gender injustices of the society (LaRue, 1970). For example, although White women share gender oppression with women of color, this commonality does not make White women immune to being ethnocentric or even racist. In fact, many women of color experience racism rather than sexism as the greater barrier to opportunity in their lives. Moreover, some women of color may feel that they are betraying their ethnic group if they reveal secrets of sexism from men of their own ethic group. Within this context, many women of color have been taught that personal disclosure outside their ethnic and cultural community is synonymous with treason (Boyd, 1990). Consequently, the emphasis on conciousness raising and sharing of experiences with White women may produce conflicts with the cultural norms of some women of color. Furthermore, if women of color form alliances with White women, many fear that their ethnic and racial concerns will be minimized (Barret, 1990; Greene, 1994), ignored, or misunderstood (Comas-Díaz, 1991). Moreover, it has been shown that, when in conflict, women of color tend to put racial loyalty over gender loyalty (Painton, 1991). Furthermore, many women of color will empathize with the pain experienced by men of their ethnic group due to racial discrimination in the workplace, without necessarily implying that they are male-identified (Espín & Gawalek, 1992).

For some women of color, such as African American women, the capacity to be friends with White women often corresponds to sociopolitical and historical developmental stages. For instance, many women of color have been measured by the idealized and stereotyped standard of White beauty (Greene, 1990, 1992). For many, the inability to meet this standard has negatively affected their self-esteem. The history of slavery, as well as racism within both the abolitionist and suffrage movements, may still be responsible for barriers impeding the development of true solidarity between African American and White women (Weems, 1991). Another area of conflict in women of color's relationships with White women is competition in the workplace. For instance, it seems that there is an increased frequency of women sabotaging female coworkers in the workplace (Mathias, 1991). According to Barber and Watson (1991), women's expectations of carrying on the female tradition of being care-takers and having sensitivity toward other women (as opposed to men) do not prepare them for female sabotage in the workplace.

Women of color tend to expect support from other women of color with professional status, and often report feelings of isolation if such support is absent. Clinical and anecdotal evidence points to the need for professional women to be in contact with other women of color with professional status (Denton, 1990; Lykes, 1983). As an illustration, Denton (1990) researched the bonding and supportive relationships among African American professional women. She found two major types of supportive relationships: (1) other-related relationships, where women's bonds emphasize the provision of support; and (2) self-enhancing relationships, where women's bonds are reciprocal and oriented towards self.

Female–male relationships among women of color with professional status can be intricate. However, the solidarity among people of color may break down along gender lines. Many men of color may engage in sexism in an effort to enhance male power or appear to ignore gender differences when characterizing the experience of people of color (Reid, 1988). In discussing male and female power issues within an organizational setting, Melia and Lyttle (1986) assert that not only do White men join ranks against a woman when male identity is on the line, but African American men will sometimes join ranks with White men against African American women. Additionally, men of color in the professional arena may feel resentful and envious of the women's perceived advantage of being a double minority. Just as shared gender oppression does not preclude White women from being racist, shared racial oppression does not preclude men of color from being sexist. The work environment seems to reinforce this dynamic by placing women of color in competition against men of color.

Romantic relationships, not surprisingly, are central to the lives of many women of color who are professionals. In the aforementioned research on Latina professional women, Amaro and her associates (1987) found that marital status was not associated with psychological distress, but instead was associated with personal life satisfaction. In other words, Latina professional women with romantic partners were more satisfied with their personal lives than those who did not have romantic partners.

The reality that many women of color generally are more educated and have better jobs than men of color may further aggravate problems between them. This situation is accentuated for African American women who outnumber African American males by at least 1.5 million (Census

Bureau, quoted in Vobejda, 1991b). In explaining this situation, Joyce Ladner (in Vobejda, 1991b) identifies the combined effects of joblessness, low skill level, lack of education, substance abuse, alcoholism, and imprisonment as factors reducing the pool of African American men who would be able to earn a living and support a family. Moreover, Hines and Boyd-Franklin (1982) state that African American women are keenly aware that they outnumber their male counterparts. These authors further argue that African American women may feel empathy for their husbands' frustration with a racist society and thus have difficulties holding them responsible for negative behavior.

Other women of color are also affected by a demographic lack of available men of color. Our society's focus on class differences makes relationships with men from a lower socioeconomic stratum more difficult. Many men of color do not want to marry a woman who is more educated or makes more money. As an illustration, American Indian women with a university education have limited chances for marrying within their ethnic group because American Indian men without college education will seldom marry a university graduate (LaFromboise et al., 1990). Thus, the heterosexual woman of color usually faces limited options. She may marry "down" by pairing with a man who has less formal education or makes less money, she may marry out of her ethnic group in order to have a partner comparable to her level of education and achievement, she may remain single, or she may share a man with another woman. Similar problems affect lesbian women of color with professional status (Greene, Chapter 14, this volume).

Balancing Family, Community, and Work

Balancing career and family demands is difficult for the general population of professional women. For example, an investigation exploring how women in academic medicine balance career and family responsibilities found they believe that motherhood slows the progress of their careers (Levinson, Tolle, & Lewis, 1989). The 1992 Women in Science issue of *Science* (AAAS, 1992) finds the glass ceiling, a lack of mentors, subtle obstacles and unconscious assumptions (e.g., that women will not have the same level of success as men), as well as family pressures to be obstacles for women in science. Professional women outside of academia also face difficulties in balancing their careers with their family lives (Trochet, 1991). However, most women of color with professional status have always had to balance family and work needs, but in addition they face specific expectations and demands from their ethnoracial communities. There is the clear and explicit expectation, as we mentioned before, that those who have some measure of success need to help to bring others along. This may further impinge on financial and emotional resources in a way that it does not for White women (Greene, 1990, 1992). These issues are ignored when the personal and professional demands of women are discussed. As an illustration, the 1992 Women in Science issue excluded women of color in their feature on women scientists. However, the 1993 Women in Science issue (AAAS, 1993) has presented some scientists who are women of color and addressed some unique concerns that they face, such as high visibility, loneliness, being outsiders, and their commitment to work towards helping other people of color.

In general, women of color tend to face a significant degree of stress related to their multiple roles and demands (Watts-Jones, 1990). Although some women of color may find support from their families and significant others, still, balancing multiple roles and conflicting demands can cause a lot of stress. A poignant example is the ambivalence that many women of color with professional status have about hiring domestic help (who would usually be other women of color). On the one hand they may feel that they need help, but on the other, they feel that hiring a woman of color for domestic help is exploitative.

Women's occupational stress affects family life and may test the quality of marital and parental relationships (Nieva & Gutek, 1981). There are different stressors associated with the different family options. For example, if the professional woman of color decides to enter an interracial, interethnic romantic liaison, she must face several issues. McGoldrick and García-Preto (1984) assert that interracial couples are more vulnerable to being alienated from both racial groups, not to mention their respective families, and may be forced into social isolation. A similar situation is faced by interracial lesbian couples, who may be isolated within the lesbian community as well as their respective ethnoracial communities and families (Greene, Chapter 14, this volume).

Single mothers with professional status also face serious difficulties in balancing work and family. Although many single women of color may have some support system available for raising their children, the reality of family obligation still falls squarely on their shoulders. This reality involves financial concerns, the immediate need of being both mother and father to their children, and numerous others.

COPING

Stress is endemic to women of color with professional status who face the combined effects of racism and sexism (Denton, 1980), the pressure to perform, the strain in interpersonal relationships, and the task of balancing multiple roles and demands. Professional women of color encounter specific circumstances that must require negotiation on a daily basis (McCombs, 1986; Trotman, 1984). For instance, Wiltz (1991) observes that a woman who hears cutting racial remarks about her patients, students, clients, or customers will need to decide whether to confront them or let them slide. She also says that the constant need to monitor one's responses can be a strain on the professional woman of color. Many women in this population indicate that they have a heightened sensitivity in their reactions to racism and sexism. Some of their coping styles are functional, while others may be dysfunctional (Greene, 1992).

Linking Professional Aspirations with Community Needs

Women of color with professional status tend to be very resourceful. They have had to work doubly hard to have their achievements recognized, and continue to do so. Women of color have usually overcome significant socioeconomical and cultural barriers even before achieving their professional status. A study of ethnic minority high school valedictorians conducted by psychologist Terry Denny and educational researcher Karen Arnold (in Moses, 1991) found that these individuals often face economic, family, and cultural pressures. According to the study, these students often lack the types of resources that White middle-class students typically have. For example, many of the students of color had to juggle getting a degree with helping to support their poor or dysfunctional families; many lived at home for financial and cultural reasons, while others had difficulties fitting in, in predominantly White institutions. The valedictorian students that became successful by completing college were described as having determination, persistence, self-sufficiency, and effective interpersonal skills (Moses, 1991).

Many successful professional women confront obstacles early in their careers and continue to cope with limitations specific to women of color. However, many of them are creative in integrating their professional aspirations with the needs of their communities. For example, women in the professional world are advised in the popular literature to gain recognition through outside exposure, such as self-promotion, being active outside their organizations, serving on high-profile boards and committees, winning awards for community services; and so on (Fox, 1991).

Resourceful women of color have responded to this challenge by linking professional aspirations with the needs of their communities. Some of them successfully shape their careers while responding to the ethnic minority community's survival and its aspirations for change. For instance, in discussing the professional identity and community commitment of African America women, Gilkes (1982) states that successful and activist professionals have made a conscious linkage between their work and the troubles of the African American community. Gilkes concludes that community commitment does not necessarily conflict with professional ideals if success is defined in terms of community achievement and positive evaluation by sympathetic colleagues.

Being the Conscience of the Organization

Some women of color may feel ambivalent about working in a primarily White professional setting. One strategy for coping with this ambivalence is to take responsibility for raising consciousness of their peers regarding race and gender (Peterson, 1990). Likewise, partly because of the symbolic nature of their presence in professional settings, women of color may adopt the role of being the conscience of the organization. This task entails voicing gender, racial, and ethnic issues within the professional context. As an illustration, in higher education, ethnic minority faculty members are more likely to research minority issues than White faculty members (Graves, 1990). Thus, the interest and motivation to examine race, ethnicity, and gender within the mainstream professional arena usually comes from women of color.

Women of color with professional status often acquire an activist role in order to challenge discrimination and oppression. This may be both an externally imposed role and a self-imposed role. Playing the conscience of the organization may be adaptive; however, it may also result in "too much of a good thing." Playing the conscience of the organization may result in the woman of color being identified solely with race and gender issues. Thus, she may be marginalized and pigeonholed into being the woman of color, where her contributions in other areas are ignored and/or dismissed (Sanders & Mellow, 1990). If she then reacts to such limitation, she could be further stereotyped as being an ungrateful, angry, and hypersensitive minority member. Although some members of the dominant group prefer to have others take care of their conscience, the presence of a woman of color in such a role can make others uncomfortable or even angry. Therefore, this role is often emotionally and physically depleting to the woman of color. Notwithstanding the activist role, many women of color do want to be accepted as members of a group but also as distinct individuals (Comas-Díaz, 1991).

Exaggerating the Need to Prove Competence

One reaction that women of color may experience, as a result of the stressors of professional status, is the exaggerated need to prove their competence. This need extends to more than working extraordinarily hard. For example, an African American woman in an office setting may be assumed to be the secretary, not the executive (Reid & Comas-Díaz, 1990). Having to constantly face the negative assumptions and prejudices engendered by affirmative action policies and by racial and gender prejudices, women of color may experience the increased stress of performance pressure resulting from having continuously to prove competence. A variant of the need to prove competence is the constant justification of being the professional. Women of color know that by virtue of their race and gender, their professional status and expertise may be ignored or minimized. Some of them may use coping styles that potentially can alienate them from their peers.

Another variant of proving competence is the superwoman syndrome. Conarton and Silverman (1988) argue that achieving White women very often attempt to be superwomen in that they try to become superior males and females simultaneously. For some women of color this dynamic is magnified by the attempt to compensate for their dual lower status of gender and race or by their being made to feel that this compensation is necessary. For other women of color being a superwoman is part of their cultural heritage and a result of their resistance to oppression and domination (Kanuha, Chapter 15, this volume). For example, among many African American women, the term superwoman describes what they have always had to do under extraordinary circumstances (Carey, 1990). However, being a superwoman can also cause stress. According to Conarton and Silverman (1988) more often than not, superwomen do not acknowledge their limitations and do not seek mental health treatment, unless problems are quite severe. When they do seek treatment, it is often with great shame and a sense of being a failure.

Expressing Anger

Anger and rage directed at racial inequities are central issues for people of color (Watson, 1989). The continued challenge of being caught in a system that undervalues their contributions is a constant burden for women of color and generates anger. Many women of color experience frequent anger at their exposure to the double bind of racism and sexism (Loo, 1989), and if they confront the problem its reality may be denied, thus intensifying the rage.

Bernardez–Bonesatti (1978) has argued that women's problems with the expression of anger are related to the development of dysfunctional behaviors such as depression, self-destructiveness, problems in sexual functioning, and others. It has been argued that a woman's image of herself as a nonaggressive person is often so salient that she will become depressed or anxious when she discovers that she has had angry feelings (Cidylo, 1990). Bernardez–Bonesatti (1978) further asserts that problems expressing anger are central to understanding women's difficulties in creative and active pursuits.

Women of color experience difficulties in expressing their anger similar to those of mainstream women, in addition to their multidimensional societal subordination. However, the management of anger among women of color with professional status becomes a dilemma, taking a different course from White women's anger. For the woman of color, to fight back openly may result in her becoming the target of institutionalized racism designed to keep her in her proper place by means of rules and regulations

(Boyd, 1990). Women of color may also be provoked into expressions of anger so as to confirm the stereotype of the angry minority and perhaps to discredit their complaints. Moreover, the expression of anger by women of color is often viewed as aggressive or potentially violent, while for White women the same behavior is seen as assertive (Almeida, 1993).

Dealing with anger in a covert manner therefore has been a necessary adaptive skill among many women of color. However, adaptive behaviors can have a costly, exacting high price (Pinderhughes, 1989). The use of behaviors such as opposition, passive aggression, manipulation, and dependency constitute reactive rather than active behaviors and therefore limit the capacity of women of color to make decisions, choices, take initiatives, assume responsibility, or take on leadership (Pinderhughes, 1983). Unfortunately, such behaviors do not foster a positive sense of self.

Oppression, victimization, and anger, are often central issues to women of color (Healy, 1991). Inequitable treatment can exacerbate power struggles (Pinderhughes, 1989). It then becomes a challenge for women of color with professional status to express their anger in a nonself-destructive manner. According to Pinderhughes (1989), effective interventions involve helping women become aware of other ways of being strong. Espín (Chapter 10, this volume) posits that empowering psychotherapeutic orientations can validate women of color's anger and facilitate the management of that anger as a source of strength in oppressive contexts. She identifies social action and other types of actions that attempt to alleviate oppression as productive expressions of anger. Women of color with professional status may use coping skills such as linking professional aspirations with community needs, being the conscience of their organizations, and using their jobs to make changes as various means of expressing anger in a productive manner. Their presenting problems in mental health treatment often involves an overt or covert difficulty with expressing anger. Therefore, clinicians working with this population need to examine anger issues presented by their clients as well as their own anger. Similarly, Espín (Chapter 10, this volume) stresses that an empowering approach presupposes that clinicians are able to deal with their own anger as well as with anger directed toward them.

MENTAL HEALTH PROBLEMS AND TREATMENT ISSUES

The constant stress encountered by women of color with professional status can deteriorate into mental health problems. While the covert anger discussed above can promote a sense of powerlessness even adaptive behaviors can have a taxing effect on women of color with professional status. While autonomy facilitates going it alone, such strength can also create isolation (Pinderhughes, 1989). The different coping reactions that women develop at work can add further stress and become dysfunctional. Some of the most common mental health problems that women of color with professional status experience are conflicts in self-esteem, depression, stress reactions, anxiety, psychosomatic disorders, and addiction.

Common Mental Health Problems

Conflicted Self-Esteem

Conflicted self-esteem is not a psychiatric disorder in itself, however, we believe that as a symptom or reaction to a stressful and oppressive situation, it can become a mental health problem for professional women. The special racist and sexist discrimination that professional women experience at work and the barriers that preceded them can lead to conflicts in their self esteem. When ethnic minorities in professional settings do not fully understand the origins of some form of discrimination, they may develop a tendency to explore their own personal attributes (such as their organizational politics, appearance or speech, etc.) or blame themselves before exploring the racial implications of the situation (Lykes, 1983). This is often reinforced by institutions that are reluctant to acknowledge their own racist practices. The situation is particularly trying for women of color who must consider the multiple determinants of a discriminatory incident (i.e., race, gender, or both; Smith & Steward, 1983). Consequently, such questioning can be exhausting and greatly diminishing of self-confidence (Dickens & Dickens, 1982). The dilemmas and contradictions in status that many women of color in professional settings face can threaten their inner security (Carey, 1990) and challenge their self-esteem.

Women of color with professional status tend to experience conflict in their self-esteem. For example, Chan (1987) found that in a nonclinical group of Asian American professional women, all of the members expressed feelings of sexual objectification and the accompanying feelings of distrust, worthlessness, and internalized self-blame. Additionally, some women of color with conflicted self esteem may feel like impostors. The impostor phenomenon stipulates that when the woman succeeds, she does not internalize a sense of success and feels that she has fooled everyone, and experiences anxiety and guilt (Clance & Imes, 1978). For women of color, the impostor phenomenon tends to be compounded by negative societal attributions directed at women with professional status. Another type of impostor phenomenon involves dissociation from one's skill or talent. This occurs when being smart is responded to negatively, perhaps by significant others and/or the mainstream society. Penalized for her success she may attribute it to something other than her own ability, perhaps luck or circumstances. Many women of color suffering from the impostor phenomenon procrastinate in the face of taking professional responsibilities or panic at a promotion (Greene, 1992, 1994). They fear being found out at the next professional stage, as is illustrated below.

Rhonda, an African American administrator, was vice president of a small college. When the college presidency became vacant she was invited to apply. This invitation triggered anxiety in Rhonda, who felt that her previous achievements were product of being in the right place at the right time. In discussing her feelings with a friend, she stated, "I have been fooling everyone except myself. I am an impostor."

Depression

Low self-esteem is a common component of depression. Women of color's professional achievements usually involve some distancing from their communities of origin. The distance from their own ethnoracial group and the lack of full acceptance from the majority group may contribute to the development of depression. In the general population, professional women have a higher incidence of depression and suicide than women who are not professionals (McGrath et al., 1990), particularly women physicians (Carlson & Miller, 1981) and women chemists (Browne, 1987; Li, 1969). Although we did not find empirical literature on suicide among women of color with professional status, clinical reports suggest that depression and self-destructive tendencies may be a significant problem among this population.

Professional women in the general population encounter complexities that can lead to depression. Notwithstanding the advantages of their professional status, career women struggle with a variety of conflicts and stressors that may increase their risk to depression (McGrath et al., 1990). Professional women tend to have difficulty reconciling their achievement with their affiliative needs (Post, 1987). McGrath and her associates (1990) state that among women in the dominant group, being self-reliant, a characteristic central to professional advancement, may lead to difficulties in establishing intimate relationships, thus leading to loneliness and isolation. They further observe that many professional women may be rejected by men because their competence may be threatening to their male self-esteem. Conversely, professional women may question the impact of a high-powered position on their marital prospects and their ability to mother their offspring adequately. We believe that many of these issues arise for women of color with professional status.

Different therapeutic orientations have been employed to treat professional women with depression. The interpersonal therapy (IPT) approach is an effective therapeutic orientation for depressed women, given the special emphasis in women's lives on the role of relationships (McGrath et al., 1990). IPT is a focused, short-term, time-limited therapy that emphasizes the current interpersonal relations of the depressed patient while recognizing the role of genetic, biochemical, developmental, and personality factors in causation of and vulnerability to depression (Klerman, Weissman,

Rounsaville, & Chevron, 1984). With its emphasis on contextual factors, IPT is highly relevant for some women of color (Comas-Díaz, 1988). Additionally, the IPT techniques such as interpersonal inventory, decision analysis, and communication analysis can help clarify some women of color's definitions of self in context.

Stress and Anxiety

The constant exposure to pressure on women of color with professional status can culminate in stress and anxiety (Denton, 1990). Some women may use adaptively the excessive energy generated by anxiety to continue their fast pace. However, anxiety can become paralyzing and this may be the time for the busy professional woman to seek help. Many women of color can benefit from learning stress management techniques. Mastering such techniques can be empowering and congruent with their history of self-reliance. The therapist can help them to reorganize their priorities, learn to delegate authority, and to make a commitment to taking time off for themselves (Conarton & Silverman, 1988) before they become paralyzed with anxiety. However, the clinician needs to be cognizant that such techniques need to be congruent with women's cultural and economic realities.

Psychosomatization

Somatization and psychosomatization are another mental health problem that some women of color with professional status may experience. As Conarton and Silverman (1988) state, highly achieving women do not seek therapy because they are too busy. Instead, they may drive themselves to physical illness, and the illness provides the opportunity to stop, get off the merry-go-round, and examine their lives.

For some people of color, somatization is a form of expressing emotional discomfort. As an illustration, depression is expressed through vegetative symptoms among some Chinese (loss of appetite, energy, libido) (Kleinman, 1980) and through metaphors of clouds, rain, and mist among some Japanese (Marsella, 1977). Therefore, psychosomatization may be a symptom that for the professional woman is a culturally congruent response to stress.

Addictive Behaviors

Addictive behaviors can be a potential mental health problem among women of color. Given ethnic minorities' disturbingly high abuse of substances such as alcohol (Spiegler, Tate, Aitken, & Christian, 1985) as a coping strategy for escaping an oppressed situation, the clinician working with professional women needs to assess their substance use and/or abuse.

Alcoholism among women of color may be a significant problem. Among American Indian women, the use of alcohol and drugs often seems to represent a self-medication response to stress and emotional disturbance (LaFromboise, Heyle, & Ozer 1990). Although African American women tend to be abstainers, when they drink they appear to be heavy drinkers (Gary & Gary, 1985). Similarly, Latinas report to be either abstainers or light drinkers (Caetano, 1989), but Latinas with higher income and education level are more likely to use alcohol (National Coalition of Hispanic Health and Human Services Organizations, 1988). Alcoholism among some Latinas may be a closet issue, given the cultural values that tend to inhibit women from acknowledging their use of alcohol (Comas-Díaz, 1986).

Some professional contexts promote alcohol use as a means of conducting business, making it difficult for some individuals to avoid alcohol use. Thus, the clinician working with women of color with professional status needs to be familiar with alcohol and substance abuse prevention and treatment. Additionally, culturally relevant assessment and treatment interventions of addictive behaviors need also to be included in the treatment. An example of such intervention is the "future past" technique developed by Comas-Díaz (1986) for the treatment of alcoholic Latinas (see p. 190, this volume, for elaboration).

Eating disorders among professional women constitute another mental health problem. It has been assumed that eating disorders among women of color occur rarely (Root, 1990). Eating and eating disorders are culturally defined and contextualized. Eating special foods may constitute part of woman of color's identification with her ethnoracial group. Similarly, different cultures have different norms about physical size and attractiveness based on body type. However, it has been suggested that eating disorders are increasing among African American women (Hsu, 1987; Pumariega, Edwards, & Mitchell, 1984). According to Root (1990), women of color may develop eating disorders to counteract negative societal images depicting them as fat, powerless, asexual, exotic, hysterical, and stupid. Restrictive dieting, a precipitant of eating disorders, appears to be a strategy many women use to increase self-esteem, credibility in the workforce, and to contend with conflicting gender-role proscriptions (Root, 1990). Women of color may view dieting as a means of deemphasizing differences and/or of having a professional image. Eating disorders also involve an issue of control. For some women of color with professional status, determining what they eat, how much and when may be the only remaining area in which they feel they can exercise some control. Consider the following example.

Irene, an African American engineer, was working in a consulting organization conducting business with African countries. She had been promoted and was in charge of managing an important department within her organization. Irene developed an eating disorder soon after she was promoted. In 6 months she gained 75 pounds. During the initial interview with the therapist, she stated,

"My life is overcontrolled. I feel that my supervisors are always monitoring me because as a Black woman they are unsure of my competence. I have too much stress and pressure. The only area where I can let myself go is in eating."

Medication Issues

The prescription and use of psychopharmacology substances among women of color in general, and in particular for those with professional status, is a complex matter (Jacobsen, Chapter 12, this volume). There are several cultural values that may encourage the use of psychotropic drugs among women of color. For example, many women initiate their help-seeking behavior by visiting a regular physician. For some women of color, their cultural background stigmatizes their seeking a mental health treatment, while, visiting a physician for emotional problems would be an accepted behavior. Some professional women may feel more comfortable in relation to issues of self-reliance by conceptualizing mental health as physical health, and are therefore more amenable to medication and less so to psychotherapy. Those who opt for traditional mental health treatment may face different dilemmas. People of color have been disproportionately prescribed medication over psychotherapy (see Chapter 12, this volume, for elaboration). The institutionalized racism prevalent in medicine, coupled with individuals' racism and sexism could in some situations lead a physician (male or female) to prescribe medications because they assume the patient would not benefit from psychotherapy.

Within this context, women of color with professional status may still face another aspect of institutionalized racism within the field of medicine (Comas-Díaz & Jacobsen, in press). The APA Task Force on Women and Depression asserts that underprescribing antidepressants because of lack of education among clinicians can be a health hazard for those women who need this type of treatment (McGrath et al., 1990). Women of color may be at risk of not being properly evaluated and diagnosed, and thus, may not be considered for psychopharmacological treatment. The interested reader can see Jacobsen's discussion of women of color and psychopharmacology (Chapter 12, this volume).

Similar to their nonprofessional sisters, professional women of color have been exposed to risk factors conducive to mental health problems, particularly depression. Some of these risk factors include female roles, poverty, and victimization, among others. Although occupational status and prestige are important predictors of mental health, job related stress can be a risk factor in depression for professional women (McGrath et al., 1990). In addition to the female susceptibility to occupational stress, women of color confront the complex effects of inter- and intraracial sexism. For instance, the much debated dynamic between Anita Hill and Clarence Thomas illustrated that for women of color with professional status, sexual harassment takes on a different tone and expression.

Treatment Implications

Regardless of the mental problems that the professional woman faces, treatment needs to aim at reinforcing and restoring her sense of competence, self-reliance, and balanced functioning. As suggested previously, empowering women of color can provide a blueprint for addressing their conflictive self-esteem. Specifically, empowering women of color involves the teaching of culturally assertive responses (Comas-Díaz & Duncan, 1985), conflict management skills, and supporting their seeking appropriate support systems (Vasquez, Chapter 4, this volume). Professional women are highly resourceful and the clinician can tap into their resources in order to help them cope with their mental health problems.

Regardless of theoretical orientation, the clinician working with women of color with professional status needs to incorporate elements of managing the stress of discrimination. This issue transcends therapeutic theoretical orientations. It implies that the clinician needs to be aware of and sensitive to labor market conditions (Jenkins, 1985) and dynamics, as well as ethnocultural factors surrounding women of color's presence in the professional arena. Along these lines, the clinician may need to encourage women to talk openly about the sexist and racist discrimination during mental health treatment.

For women of color, dwelling on perceived discrimination in the workplace often promotes feelings of powerlessness, preventing them from adopting a creative, problem-solving mind-set (Wiltz, 1991). Treatment may need to incorporate the building of skills to deal with discrimination. The clinician could recommend the client to look for traditional and nontraditional role models. As an illustration, the clinician can have the client ask her mother or maternal figure about her life and how she dealt with racism and sexism (Greene, 1990; Wiltz, 1991). Another illustration of specific strategies for helping women deal with the discrimination in the professional arena involves strategies for avoiding the discouragement of the glass ceiling. Wiltz (1991) discusses several strategies ranging from developing more realistic professional expectations to maintaining emotional and spiritual balance.

Another illustration of the management of work-related issues involves being able to teach the client coping skills for survival in the professional market. As an example, LaFromboise (1989) developed a professional skills training manual for American Indian women. The main goal of the training is to help American Indian women achieve a balance of traditional and contemporary leadership strengths and roles. The manual includes comprehensive workshops designed to help women develop the skills necessary to succeed in the White professional world. Some of these areas include self-esteem, assertiveness, career planning, and financial management. If clinicians do not have expertise in some of these areas, they may want to refer the client to appropriate professionals for conjoint treatment.

Another aspect of managing the stress caused by discrimination involves the encouragement of the utilization of support systems. Many women of color with professional status need to network, connect, and bond with other women of color with professional status (Denton, 1990; LaFromboise et al., 1990; Lykes, 1983). Sometimes the clinician can refer the client to a support group for professional women. If the geographical area where the client lives does not have such a resource, the clinician can encourage her to connect with or develop a network at a state or national level. Professional and trade organizations can aid her to identify potential support.

The diverse theoretical therapeutic orientations offer the clinician a repertoire of options for treating women of color with professional status. For example, cognitive and behavioral techniques can enable professional women to learn to respect their own needs. Many professional women often fulfill the needs of others, including supervisors, clients and coworkers, to the exclusion of their own needs (McGrath et al., 1990). This self-sacrifice dictum may be central to many women of color, who may have difficulties being assertive on behalf of themselves.

Following a cognitive–behavioral orientation, Lemkau and Landau (1986) addressed the self-denying syndrome among professional women. They used cognitive restructuring, self-monitoring of daily activities, role playing, and skills training in conflict resolution to help women assert their own needs. However, McGrath and her colleagues (1990) suggest that the training must additionally include building skills for dealing with reactions of coworkers and significant others when a woman rightfully places her needs above those of others. This warning is particularly relevant for clinicians working with women of color who have an extended and contextual self definition (see Comas-Díaz, Chapter 11, this volume).

For women of color, the cognitive–behavioral approach needs to incorporate an examination of the cultural context of such frameworks. For example, due to their collective definition of self, many women of color may not believe that the subordination of their needs is pathological in itself. A way of translating this concept into their cultural values may be to suggest that taking care of themselves is an effective way of taking care of significant others. As an illustration, the interested reader can examine Lewis' discussion (Chapter 8, this volume) of the use of cognitive–behavioral approaches with women of color.

Another psychotherapeutic approach relevant for professional women, particularly those who experience difficulties establishing rewarding intimate relationships, is the one based on self-in-relation theory (Surrey, 1991; McGrath et al., 1990). This approach emphasizes the centrality of interpersonal connectedness in women's lives (Kaplan, 1991; Surrey, 1991). According to this approach, depression among women is related to the experience of emotional loss, inhibition of action and assertiveness, plus anger and low self-esteem, which are focused on during treatment (Kaplan, 1991). This approach is relevant to professional women because it draws upon their intellectual skills to understand and resolve long-standing conflicts and fosters empowerment, and respect for their own relational abilities. For a fuller discussion of the applicability of the self-in-relation theory to women of color see (Comas-Díaz) analysis of the integrative approach to mental health treatment for women of color (Chapter 11).

Notwithstanding the therapeutic approach used, the clinician working with women of color with professional status needs to include a feminist perspective in treatment. The emphasis on empowerment is particularly relevant to professional women. Oliva Espín (Chapter 10, this volume) discusses this approach with women of color. Furthermore, mental health treatment of women with professional status requires a comprehensive perspective. For instance, Comas-Díaz (Chapter 11) discusses an integrative mental health treatment approach to the special needs of women of color. The integrative approach offers a reconciliation of traditional therapeutic orientations with women of color 's dual and sometimes multiple minority group membership within an empowerment framework. The following is a full case illustrating several of the issues discussed in this chapter.

CASE ILLUSTRATION

Presenting Complaint and Identifying Data

Carmina was a 32-year-old married Latina woman. She worked as an attorney in a private firm. She had a 16-year-old daughter from a previous common-law marriage. She had no children from her current marriage. Her husband, also an attorney, was an European American, born and raised in New York City. Carmina presented to mental health treatment stating that she was afraid of running her body down. By this she meant that she had been working so hard and doing so many things that her body was not keeping up with her. She was experiencing general tiredness and sleeping difficulties, for which she had consulted several physicians. Her internist, finding no physical basis for her symptoms, advised her to learn how to manage stress. She then gave Carmina the name of a Latina mental health therapist with expertise in working with women of color with professional status.

During the first session, Carmina appeared somewhat resistant to mental health treatment. Her self-image involved being self-reliant, strong, perseverant, and needing to have things under control. Being in a mental health treatment situation was incongruent with such self-image. However, she was able to identify stress at work as a major source for her symptoms.

Assessment: The Influence of Ethnic, Racial, Gender, and Class Variables

Given Carmina's clinical presentation, the clinician decided to complete a comprehensive assessment. Such assessment revealed the influence of racial, ethnic, gender, and class variables on the client's life.

Carmina was a Black Puerto Rican woman. Being a Black Puerto Rican is not uncommon (Comas-Díaz, in press). The Puerto Rican population is the result of the confluence of Taíno Indians, Mediterranean Europeans (mostly Spaniards), and Africans (Fernández Méndez, 1970). Her father was a Black Puerto Rican and her mother was *trigueña* (olive-skinned brunette). Although all of her siblings were dark, Carmina was the darkest, and was called *prieta* (a pejorative term designating a Black female).

Carmina was born and raised in New York City, except for a few periods of time of no more than 6 months each, when she lived in Puerto Rico with her maternal grandparents, to whom she very close. Carmina was the oldest of three siblings. Her sister was 30 years old and her brother was 28 years old. The family was Catholic until the mother converted to Pentecostalism when Carmina was 12 years old. This conversion created conflict between her mother and her grandmother, who was a devout Catholic. Carmina remained a Catholic.

Carmina's family was from a low socioeconomic background. Her father was a taxi driver and her mother worked in a factory. Carmina appeared to be her father's favorite; since he was a fan of the opera, he had named her after one of his favorite pieces (*Carmina Burana*). Being true to her name, Carmina (from the Latin meaning "song") had a beautiful voice and enjoyed singing.

As the elder offspring, Carmina grew up with sex-role expectations of being responsible for her younger siblings. She was the little mother, taking over some of the parenting tasks while her mother was away working at the factory. Carmina and her siblings grew up in the barrio, where a non-kin extended family was available to them. Notwithstanding the availability of her non-kin relations, Carmina was the parental child. She grew up combining gender roles in that she was both instrumental and expressive.

Carmina finished vocational-secretarial courses during high school. She did so well in school that one of her high school teachers became her mentor and urged her to complete both general and the secretarial courses. Through the guidance of her teacher, she was able to successfully apply for a full scholarship and was accepted at an Ivy League university. After 2 years of college, she dropped out because her mother had stopped working because of a car accident. Carmina worked full time as a secretary, financially helping her family. During this period of time, she met a Black Puerto Rican man who had been recently translocated from Puerto Rico, with whom she began a romantic relationship. This relationship was not approved of by her family because they wanted Carmina to "*adelantar la raza*" (literally to "advance the race," meaning to have lighter skinned children by selecting a light-skinned or White partner). Her common-law marriage of 2 years resulted in the birth of a daughter. However, Carmina and her common-law husband separated, mainly due to differences in achievement orientation: She wanted to complete a college education, but he was unsupportive of that goal.

Carmina returned to school and completed her bachelor's degree in political science. Afterwards, she worked for the city government at an entry-level position. The experiences in this job helped her to make the decision to go back to school and become a lawyer. Carmina obtained another full scholarship and entered law school at an Ivy League university. Although she was studying full time, she had to work part time to help her family financially. She dropped out of school for a year in order to work full time and subsidize her brother's university studies, given that her family had always been supportive of her academic achievement. After a year of working full time, she returned to law school and completed her degree. Carmina was the first person in her family to complete a graduate degree.

Carmina met her second husband during law school. As indicated previously, he was a European American man from an upper-class background. After they married, he legally adopted Carmina's daughter. Although they were an interethnic and interracial couple, the main overt area of conflict for Carmina was their differing socioeconomic backgrounds. Partly due to her husband's affluence and to her professional status, Carmina was living an upper-middle-class lifestyle. This created a conflict in her and was expressed in unrealistic expectations she had about her husband. Some of these expectations revolved around her concept of manhood, which was tied up with a working class orientation. For instance, she would get upset when her husband exhibited upper-class behaviors, such as hiring people for doing physical repair work around the house. She expected him to do the physical work himself, just like her father did. Carmina was experiencing survival guilt and was projecting such guilt onto her husband. For instance, she would frequently accuse her husband of not understanding her because he was not a person of color, which often had the effect of cutting off communication. Moreover, she demanded inordinate loyalty from her husband. She recognized that her husband was very sensitive to gender and racial issues—his caseload of *pro bono* legal work was comprised of ethnic minority clients. Carmina admitted, however, that her overly sensitive interpretations of many racial incidents acted as a barrier for her intimacy needs within her marriage. It appeared that she was venting at home legitimate anger over race- and gender-related issues she faced at work, thus alienating her husband, who was her main supporter. This process was accentuated when her husband became partner at his law firm. During that time Carmina was still an associate in her place of employment and was informed that she was not partner material. She then began to develop the physical symptoms that led her to seek treatment.

Work-Related Issues

Fueled by the Civil Rights and feminist movements, Carmina had developed high expectations and professional ambition; she believed that a good education and hard work was all she needed to get ahead. She behaved accordingly, working extremely hard, being overly responsible and believing that she understood the politics of race and gender. For instance, she did recognize that the corporate reality for many women of color involves paying their dues and slow progress.

Carmina had dealt successfully with the qualification question: the belief of many dominant group members that people of color with professional status have made solely it because of affirmative action policies, and not because of their merits. She had worked hard and was able to see the fruits of such work. Initially, she received excellent evaluations and was informed that she was capable of becoming a partner. She enjoyed high visibility and her work performance in different projects was very well received by her supervisors.

Although there was no blatant discrimination, the behavior of some of her colleagues toward Carmina appeared to be racially motivated. Such behavior intensified after she successfully completed a major project. She interpreted several incidents involving her coworkers as occurring because of her race and ethnicity. Feeling that she had proved her competence and earned enough organizational credits, she decided to report her colleagues' behavior.

Carmina identified herself as a doer and as "taking the bull by its horns." After the firm's management appeared to be unresponsive to her complaints, she decided to take things into her own hands. Capitalizing on her gender and her mixed racial and ethnic background Carmina established a coalition of women and people of color in her agency. The coalition became very successful, developing strong ties between the firm and the community at large. It enhanced the firm's image in the public interest. Indeed, due to the coalition's work, the firm won an award for its contribution to the community.

The work in the coalition enhanced Carmina's visibility in the agency. However, at the beginning of her fourth year she received a lukewarm evaluation. After she requested more feedback, she was informed that she lacked the capacity to be partner material. Carmina was devastated, and became very angry at the evaluation. When she expressed her anger by openly discussing the situation at a staff meeting, she became the target of more retaliation. She was told she was difficult and was not being a team player. This series of incidents marked the beginning of a vicious cycle which Carmina became professionally frustrated and found herself in a stalemate. She then stopped expressing her anger. Her pent-up feelings of anger and rage metamorphosed into an emotional disorder.

Coping Style

Carmina had many personal and professional strengths. She was bright, hard working, responsible, persistent, determined, strong, creative, and resourceful. She was also adept at some of the corporate politics and had an effective interpersonal style. Being aware of the interaction between her gender, ethnicity, and race, she had worked overtime and behaved according to the firm's expectations of a professional woman of color. For instance, although she joked about being a superwoman, it appeared that she was really trying to be one. When she faced racism and sexism in the workplace, she opted for acting as the conscience of the organization by becoming the spokesperson for diversity issues at her firm. She was also able to redefine success by linking professional aspirations with the needs of the ethnic minority community's needs.

But this previously functional coping style became dysfunctional. For example, Pinderhughes (1986) asserts that strength, hard work, persistence, determination, adaptability, and creativity are critical strategies for managing the oppressive societal strain on women of color. However, under stress, adaptability can slip into inconsistency, strength into abuse, persistence into stubbornness, and hard work into overdriven dedication (Pinderhughes, 1986). Under stress, Carmina's behavior was characterized by stubbornness, rigidity, and overdriven dedication. Furthermore, Carmina had difficulties expressing her frustration and anger. Although she had been aware of the source of her anger, particularly the one generated by racial issues, she was afraid of continuing to express her negative feelings in the workplace, fearing more retaliation. Instead, she projected these feelings onto her husband. Carmina did not use the support system her marital relationship could have been, and began to alienate her husband. Additionally, she appeared to be internalizing some of her anger, and began to drink alcohol heavily, although she denied her drinking problem, stating that she was not behaving like her alcoholic grandfather, who used to become violent when he drank. Carmina's drinking became such a family problem that her daughter left the house, moving in with her aunt.

Self-Esteem

Carmina was impressive in her appearance. Physically she was quite striking. She had an imposing presence and projected self-assurance. She had been extremely successful in the professional arena, particularly considering her background. Notwithstanding her accomplishments, Carmina had conflicted self-esteem. Dealing with her multiple sources of identity—including but not limited to gender, racial, ethnic, and class variables—took an emotional toll on her. She was ambivalent toward the Puerto Rican community, as well as toward mainstream society. Being a Black Puerto Rican woman meant coping with being an outsider and having conflicted needs related to a sense of belonging (Comas-Díaz, in press).

In a poignant article describing the experiences of Black Puerto Rican women, Jorge (1979) argued that they are oppressed because of their race, ethnicity, and gender. Jorge further described the series of oppressions that Black Puerto Rican women experience throughout their lives. She stated that during childhood and adolescence, confined to the boundaries of the barrio, the family often reaffirms the greater Puerto Rican community's claims of the inferiority of the Black *Puertorriqueña*'s race. This reaffirmation continues throughout adulthood and permeates her life, affecting her self-esteem, selection of romantic partners, access to the mainstream society, and vocational/ professional performance.

Carmina's multiple identity resulted in her feeling like an outsider. Being discriminated against from within her own ethnic group because of her race and gender, she began to identify with African Americans during her adolescence. Indeed, many Black Puerto Ricans in the United States tend to assimilate into society as African Americans (Seda Bonilla, 1970). Carmina's family reacted very negatively to this identification. Therefore, she decided not to risk being ostracized by them and by the Puerto Rican community at large. Carmina stopped seeing her African American friends. This situation reinforced her sense of marginality. She reported that as an adolescent, she felt like an outsider among Puerto Ricans, Anglos, and African Americans as well.

Carmina had experienced several "traumatas" in her life that left an indelible effect on her self-esteem. The term refers to the series of little traumas, events that when coupled with general life stresses and reduced environmental and psychological resources can bring the individual to the traumatic stress flashpoint (Puig, 1991). To the message that she was inferior because of gender, race, and ethnicity, was added class discrimination. As discussed previously, she was sensitive to class issues, particularly regarding the traumatic experiences she had when she was in college and in law school. Often, in the Ivy League environment, she was the only student from a low socioeconomic class background, becoming the target of subtle and not so subtle classist innuendos. Personally, she also felt like an outsider because she could not relate to the experiences of her elitist classmates. Furthermore, Carmina recalled feeling like an outsider when her fellow students and professors automatically questioned her competence because she was a woman of color. She appeared to have internalized the experience of being an outsider.

As a child, growing in the barrio, Carmina was further exposed to the traumata of living in the ghetto. Of particular significance was the death of Carmina's 10-year-old male cousin, who was her same age. He was killed by a car in an accident that occurred when a police car was chasing a suspect. This cousin had been Carmina's favorite, and his death underscored the unpredictability and danger of living in the barrio. She recalled this incident as the loss of her innocence.

Treatment

Carmina's mental health treatment was divided into two major phases. The first phase addressed immediate work stress issues and the development of functional coping skills. The major goal was to restore Carmina's sense of self-mastery. The second treatment phase addressed Carmina's self-esteem, with the goal of increasing it. An integrative approach to mental health treatment was utilized (see Comas-Díaz, Chapter 11, this volume, for a detailed discussion of this approach).

The first treatment phase involved the development of a stress management program tailored to Carmina's gender, racial, and ethnocultural issues. After a family session with Carmina's husband and daughter, the drinking problem was addressed. Previously, Carmina had denied any substance abuse. In addition to the stress management, Carmina was asked to attend Alcoholics Anonymous (AA) meetings for adjunct treatment. She was referred to an AA group for professional women. She was also referred for couples treatment, but she refused to follow through. Carmina stated that she was already compromising by agreeing to attend AA meetings in addition to individual treatment.

The initial therapeutic work concentrated on the examination and reassessment of her expectations, given that work pressure coupled with her expectations had created an internal pressure cooker. Cognitive–behavioral techniques were utilized in alleviating the pressure. These techniques challenged Carmina's dysfunctional assumptions and helped her develop more functional ones. For example, some of these included the concept of being powerful but vulnerable, of being imperfect but great, and many others. The realities of racism and sexism in the workplace were given focused attention during this therapeutic phase. Within this context, the cognitive–behavioral approach was also used to help Carmina deal with her anger in a non-self-defeating way. The therapist incorporated a cultural component into the therapeutic task of expressing anger. This component challenged the Puerto Rican cultural value that one should avoid expressing anger directly. Although Carmina was an assertive woman within professional situations, she manifested difficulties expressing negative feelings in the context of relationships with significant others. Indeed, the expression and management of anger became an ongoing therapeutic issue.

The mental health treatment also helped Carmina deal with the glass ceiling. She was encouraged to get support from a national professional women's organization. Characteristic of Carmina's modus operandi, she began to achieve leadership positions in the national professional organization she joined as well as in her women's organization. However, while involved in these activities, had neglected taking care of herself. Therefore, treatment also focused on helping her design ways of taking care of herself that were congruent with her self-identification. Utilizing a decisional analysis, the clinician helped Carmina reorganize her priorities, and make a commitment to devote time to herself. An example of this task was Carmina's long-standing interest in taking singing lessons, but felt that she did not deserve them. Given that this was a very important issue for Carmina, it was reframed and presented to her as an example of effectively managing her stress, by taking better care of herself.

The second phase in treatment addressed Carmina's self-esteem. Although she was aware of her conflicted self-esteem, she was unaware of negative assumptions about herself that were dysfunctional. Additionally, she had a series of self-defeating behaviors that were interfering with her well-being. For example, she was both a workholic and a perfectionist. As a workholic, she had learned to derive her self-esteem from keeping busy and being productive. Pervasive racist and sexist questioning of her abilities seemed to reinforce this dynamic. However, her workholic and perfectionist tendencies had interfered with her relationship with significant others, particularly her daughter. As a perfectionist, Carmina did not appear to be satisfied with herself. She was very critical of herself and of others, placing stress on her professional and interpersonal relationships. Her functional coping mechanisms became dysfunctional under severe stress.

Therapeutic work involved helping Carmina realize the negative consequences of her behavior. An integrative approach comprising interpersonal, systems, psychodynamic, and cognitive–behavioral orientations was utilized in this treatment phase. Given Carmina's refusal to attend couples treatment, the clinician also utilized the approach of conducting family therapy with one person (see Boyd-Franklin & García-Preto, Chapter 9, this volume) to deal with the client's family and marital issues. Within this framework, Carmina was able to successfully address her anger toward her family of origin, particularly toward her mother. For cultural reasons she could not confront her mother directly. Thus, she was guided in the construction of analog situations, such as writing letters to her mother that she never sent and role playing (playing both herself and her mother) in to work through her anger. Of particular significance was the fact that Carmina initiated a dialogue with her daughter regarding sexism and racism and the reality of being a Black Puerto Rican woman. Within this context, she was able to include her mother, who in the interest of educating her granddaughter was able to discuss these topics. Although Carmina still could not discuss parenting in the context of multiple racial and gender discrimination directly with her mother, it was therapeutic for Carmina to communicate vicariously with her through her own daughter.

Another aspect in Carmina's self-esteem that was addressed was her internalized colonization. By reconstructing her reality, she became aware that she had internalized racism, sexism, and classism. The treatment took Carmina through the process of decolonization on four fronts: gender, color, ethnicity, and class. By examining her individual, family, and group legacies, she was able to identify her role in the generations of her family, reclaim her sense of identity, begin to integrate disparate parts of herself, and, finally, to accept herself. This was a painful, yet therapeutic process for her.

During this period, Carmina examined the priorities in her life and decided to stop fighting the racism and sexism at work. She realized that she did not have the stamina for pursuing the partner track and that she had bumped into the glass ceiling. After serious consideration, she decided to establish her own business and developed her own work agenda. Although she devoted a significant amount of time to her business, she felt that she was more in control. She reported having more satisfactory relations with her significant others and spending more time on relaxation and self-actualization. In other words, she was no longer deriving her self-esteem solely from her professional work.

Treatment Termination and Follow-Up

After Carmina's transition to her new position was completed, she and the clinician decided to terminate treatment. They agreed on a follow-up visit to monitor Carmina's progress.

At follow-up (a year after treatment termination) Carmina was pleased that she had decided to move into private business. She was professionally successful, and most importantly, she felt content in both her work and personal life. She was heading a law firm specializing in women's legal issues. At the time of the follow-up, she was the president of her state bar association, and as a pet project she had developed a mentor program for people of color and women lawyers. She reported that she was still attending AA meetings because, although she was not drinking, she was still struggling with self-defeating behaviors.

CONCLUSIONS

This chapter has presented the mental health needs, coping styles, and treatment issues of many women of color with professional status. These women encounter a series of conflicts trying to manage their lives as professionals in a White male-dominated culture. The effects of the double discriminatory bind of racism and sexism in the workplace—resulting in tokenism and its dynamics of visibility, performance pressure, and retaliation—all contribute to the added stress they face. The special coping responses to stress, such as becoming the conscience of the organization, linking their professional needs with those of the ethnic community's, and others, can be both functional and dysfunctional. Although professional women of color have extraordinary strength and stamina—the product of historical resistance and resilience, which is evidenced by their attainment of their professional positions—they also develop vulnerability to mental health problems. The cultural paradox of stated opportunity for minorities and the hidden pitfalls they will face places women of color with professional status at risk for developing mental health problems, specifically depression, anxiety and other stress-related reactions, psychosomatic disorders, and addictive behaviors. Clinicians working with this population need to utilize a gender- and race-relevant orientation with an empowering and integrative approach to treatment. Special attention needs to be given to self-esteem, work-related issues such as racism, sexism, and the glass ceiling phenomenon. Mental health goals need to aim at developing functional coping skills, as well as restoring women of color's sense of mastery.

ACKNOWLEDGMENTS

The authors would like to acknowledge the comments made by Pamela T. Reid, Gwendolyn Keita, and Laura S. Brown on earlier versions of this work.

REFERENCES

Alexander, K. L. (1990, July 25). Both racism and sexism block the path to management for minority women. *Wall Street Journal*, p. B1.

Allen, P. G. (1986). *The sacred hoop: Recovering the feminism in American Indian traditions*. Boston: Beacon Press.

Almeida, R. V. (1993). Unexamined assumptions and service delivery systems: Feminist theory and racial exclusions. *Journal of Feminist Family Therapy, 5*(1), 3–23.

Almquist, E. (1989). The experience of minority women in the United States. In J. Freeman (Ed.), *Women: A feminist perspective* (4th ed., pp. 414–445). Mountain View, CA: Mayfield.

Amaro, H., Russo, N. F., & Johnson, J. (1987). Family and work predictors of psychological well-being among Hispanic women professionals. *Psychology of Women Quarterly, 11*(4), 505–521.

American Association for the Advancement of Science. (1992). Women in science. *Science, 255*(13), 1365–1388.

American Association for the Advancement of Science. (1993). Women in science '93: Gender and the culture of science. *Science, 260*, 383–430.

Barber, J., & Watson, R. E. (1991). *Sisterhood betrayed: Women in the workplace and the all about Eve complex*. New York: St. Martin's Press.

Barret, S. E. (1990). Paths toward diversity: An intrapsychic perspective. *Women and Therapy, 9*, 41–52.

Bell, E. (1990). The bicultural life experience of career-oriented black women. *Journal of Organizational Behavior, 11*, 459–477.

Bernardez-Bonesatti, T. (1978). Women and anger: Conflicts with aggression in contemporary women. *Journal of the American Medical Women's Association, 33*, 215–219.

Binion, V. J. (1990). Psychological androgyny: A Black female perspective. *Sex Roles, 22*, 487–507.

Boyd, J. (1990). Ethnic and cultural diversity: Keys to power. In L. S. Brown & M. P. P. Root (Eds.), *Diversity and complexity in feminist therapy* (pp. 151–167). New York: Haworth.

Browne, M. W. (1987, August, 4). Women in chemistry: Higher suicide risk seen. *New York Times*, p. C9.

Caetano, R. (1989). Drinking patterns and alcohol problems in a national survey of U.S. Hispanics. In D. Spiegel, D. Tate, S. Aiken, & C. Christian (Eds.), *Alcohol use among U.S. minorities* (Research Monograph No. 18). Rockville, MD: National Institute on Alcohol Abuse and Alcoholism.

Carey, P. M. (1990). Beyond superwoman: On being a successful black administrator. *Journal of National Association for Women Deans, Administrators, and Counselors, 53,* 15–19.

Carlson, G. A., & Miller, D. C. (1981). Suicide, affective disorder, and women physicians. *American Journal of Psychiatry, 138,* 1330–1335.

Carter, S. T. (1991). *Reflections of an affirmative action baby.* New York: Basic Books.

Castro, J. (1990, Fall). Get set: Here they come! *Time* [Special Issue, *Women: The road ahead*], *136,* 50–52.

Chan, C. S. (1987). Asian American women: Psychological responses to sexual exploitation and cultural stereotypes. *Women and Therapy, 6,* 33–38.

Chow, E. N. (1989). The feminist movement: Where are all the Asian American women? In Asian Women United of California (Ed.), *Making waves: An anthology of writings by and about Asian American women.* Boston: Beacon Press.

Cidylo, L. (1990, August). Women and psychotherapy: A new look. *Psychiatric Times: Medicine and Behavior,* 25–27, 30–32.

Clance, P. R., & Imes, S. A. (1978). The impostor phenomenon in high achieving women: Dynamics and the therapeutic intervention. *Psychotherapy: Theory, Research, and Practice, 15,* 241–247.

Comas-Díaz, L. (1986) Puerto Rican alcoholic women: Treatment considerations. *Alcoholism Treatment Quarterly, 3*(1), 47–57.

Comas-Díaz, L. (1988). Feminist therapy with Hispanic/Latina Women: Myth or reality? *Women and Therapy, 6,* 39–61.

Comas-Díaz, L. (1989). Culturally relevant issues and treatment implications for Hispanics. In D. R. Koslow & E. Salett (Eds.), *Crossing cultures in mental health* (pp. 31–48). Washington, DC: Society for International Education Training and Research (SIETAR).

Comas-Díaz, L. (1991). Feminism and diversity in psychology: The case of women of color. *Psychology of Women Quarterly, 15,* 597–609.

Comas-Díaz, L. (in press). LatiNegra: Mental health issues of African Latinas. *Journal of Feminist Family Therapy.*

Comas-Díaz, L., & Duncan, J. W. (1985). The cultural context: A factor in assertiveness training with mainland Puerto Rican women. *Psychology of Women Quarterly, 9,* 463–475.

Comas-Díaz, L., & Jacobsen, F. M. (1991). Ethnocultural transference and countertransference in the therapeutic dyad. *American Journal of Orthopsychiatry, 61*(3), 392–402.

Comas-Díaz, L., & Jacobsen, F. M. (in press). Psychopharmacology for women of color: An empowering approach. *Women and Therapy.*

Conarton, S., & Silverman, L. K. (1988). Feminine development through the life cycle. In M. A. Dutton Douglas & L. E. Walker (Eds.), *Feminist psychothera-*

pies: Integration of therapeutic and feminist systems (pp. 37–67). Norwood, NJ: Ablex.

Denton, T. C. (1990). Bonding and supportive relationships among black professional women: Rituals of restoration. *Journal of Organizational Behavior, 11,* 447–457.

Dickens, F., & Dickens, J. B. (1982). *The Black manager: Making it in the corporate world.* New York: AMACOM.

Dumas, R. (1980). Dilemmas of black females in leadership. In L. Rodgers-Rose (Ed.), *The black woman* (pp. 201–215). Newbury Park, CA: Sage.

Epstein, C. F. (1973). Positive effects of the multiple negative: Explaining the success of Black professional women. In J. Huber (Ed.), *Changing women in a changing society.* Chicago: University of Chicago Press.

Epstein, C. F. (1987). Multiple demands and multiple roles: The conditions of successful management. In F. J. Crosby (Ed.), *Spouse, worker, parent: On gender and multiple roles* (pp. 23–25). New Haven, CT: Yale University Press.

Espín, O. M. (1986). Cultural and historical influences on sexuality in Hispanic/ Latin women. In J. Cole (Ed.), *All American women* (pp. 272–284). New York: Free Press.

Espín, O. M., & Gawalek, M. A. (1992). Women's diversity: Ethnicity, race, class and gender in theories of feminist psychology. In L. S. Brown & M. Ballou (Eds.), *Personality and psychopathology: Feminist reappraisals* (pp. 88–107). New York: Guilford Press.

Fernández Méndez, E. (1970). *La identidad y la cultura* [Identity and culture]. San Juan, Puerto Rico: Instituto de Cultura Puertorriqueña.

Farrant, P. A. & Williams, L. E. (Eds.). (1990). Black women in higher education [Special issue]. *Journal of National Association of Women Deans, Administrators and Counselors, 53.*

Fox, J. (1991, July/August). How to gain recognition: Learn to stand out in the business crowd. *Amtrak Express,* pp. 14–18.

Gary, L. E., & Gary, R. B. (1985). Treatment needs of Black alcoholic women. In F. L. Brisbane & M. Womble (Eds.), *Treatment of Black alcoholics.* New York: Haworth Press.

Giddings, P. (1984). *When and where I enter: The impact of Black women on race and sex in America.* New York: Bantam Books.

Gilkes, C. T. (1982). Successful rebellious professionals: The Black woman's professional identity and community commitment. *Psychology of Women Quarterly, 6,* 289–311.

Graves, S. B. (1990). A case of double jeopardy? Black women in higher education. *Journal of the National Association for Women Deans, Administrators, and Counselors, 53,* 3–8.

Green, R. (1976). The Pocahontas perplex: The image of Indian women in American culture. *Massachusetts Review, 14,* 698–714.

Greene, B. (1990) Sturdy bridges: The role of African American mothers in the socialization of African American children. *Women and Therapy, 10,* 205–225.

Greene, B. (1992). Still here: A psychodynamic perspective on psychotherapy with African American women. In J. Chrisler & D. Howard (Eds.), *New directions in feminist psychology: Practice, theory and research* (pp. 13–25). New York: Springer.

Greene, B. (1994). Diversity and difference: The issue of race in feminist therapy. In M. P. Mirkin (Ed.), *Women in context: Toward a feminist reconstruction of psychotherapy* (pp. 333–351). New York: Guilford Press.

Greider, W. (1991, September 5). The politics of diversion: Blame it on the Blacks. *Rolling Stone*, pp. 32–33, 96.

Harragan, B. L. (1977). *Games mother never taught you: Corporate gamemanship for women.* New York: Warner Books.

Healey, S. (1991, Summer). The therapeutic value in challenging clients' racism. *Interchange, 9,* 8.

Henry, W. A. (1990, April 9). Beyond the melting pot. *Time, 135*(15), 28–31.

Hernton, C. C. (1965). *Sex and racism in America.* New York: Grove Press.

Hines, P. M., & Boyd-Franklin, N. (1982). Black families. In M. McGoldrick, J. K. Pearce, & J. Giordano (Eds.), *Ethnicity and family therapy* (pp. 84–107). New York: Guilford Press.

hooks, b. (1981). *Black women and feminism.* Boston MA. South End Press.

Horner, M. (1972). The motive to avoid success and changing aspirations of college women. In J. Bardwick (Ed.), *Readings on the psychology of women* (pp. 62–67). New York: Harper & Row.

Hsu, L. K. (1987). Are the eating disorders becoming more common in Blacks? *International Journal of Eating Disorders, 6,* 113–124.

Jenkins, I. M. (1985). The integration of psychotherapy-vocational interventions: Relevance for Black women. *Psychotherapy, 22,* 394–397.

Jorge, A. (1979). The Black Puerto Rican woman in contemporary American society. In E. Acosta-Belén (Ed.). *The Puerto Rican woman* (pp. 134–141). New York: Praeger.

Kanter, E. R. (1977). *Men and women of the corporation.* New York: Basic Books.

Kaplan, A. (1991). The self in relation: Implications for depression in women. In J. V. Jordan, A. G. Kaplan, J. B. Miller, I. P. Stiver, & J. L. Surrey, *Women's growth in connection: Writings from the Stone Center* (pp. 206–222). New York: Guilford Press.

Kaufman, D. R. (1989). Professional women: How real are the recent gains? In J. Freeman (Ed.), *Women: A feminist perspective* (4th ed., pp. 329–346). Mountain View, CA: Mayfield.

Kleinman, A. (1980). *Patients and healers in the context of culture: An exploration of the borderland between anthropology, medicine, and psychiatry.* Berkeley: University of California Press.

Klerman, G. L., Weissman, M. M., Rounsaville, B. J., & Chevron, E. S. (1984). *Interpersonal psychotherapy of depression.* New York: Basic Books.

LaFromboise, T. D. (1989). *Circles of women: Professional skills training with American Indian women.* Newton, MA: Women's Educational Equity Act Publishing Center.

LaFromboise, T. D., Heyle, A. M., & Ozer, E. J. (1990). Changing and diverse roles of women in American Indian cultures. *Sex Roles, 22,* 455–476.

La Rue, L. (1970). The black movement and women's liberation. *Black Scholar, 1,* 17–20.

Leggon, C. B. (1980). Black female professionals: Dilemmas and contradictions of status. In L. Rodgers-Rose (Ed.), *The Black woman.* Beverly Hills, CA: Sage.

Lemkau, J. P., & Landau, C. (1986). The "selfless syndrome": Assessment and treatment considerations. *Psychotherapy, 23,* 227–233.

Lerner, G. (1973). *Black women in White America: A documentary history.* New York: Random House.

Lerner, H. G. (1988). *Women in therapy.* New York: Harper & Row.

Levinson, W., Tolle, S. W., & Lewis, C. (1989). Women in academic medicine: Combining career and family. *New England Journal of Medicine, 321,* 1511–1517.

Li, F. P. (1969). Suicide among chemists. *Archives of Environmental Health, 19,* 518–520.

Lott, B. (1991). Social psychology: Humanistic roots and feminist future. *Psychology of Women Quarterly, 15,* 505–519.

Loo, C. (1988, August). *Socio-cultural barriers to the achievement of Asian American women.* Paper presented at the 96th annual convention of the American Psychological Association, Atlanta, GA.

Loo, C. (Chair). (1989, August). *Anger and the legacy of minorities.* Symposium at the 97th annual convention of the American Psychological Association, New Orleans.

Lykes, M. B. (1983). Discrimination and coping in the lives of black women: Analyses of oral history data. *Journal of Social Issues, 39,* 79–100.

Marsella, A. J. (1977). Depressive experience and disorder across cultures. In H. Triandis & Draguns (Eds.), *Handbook of cross-cultural psychology: Vol. 5. Culture and psychopathology.* Boston: Allyn & Bacon.

Mathias, B. (1991, March 5). Sabotaging women: When the workplace becomes a battlefield. *Washington Post,* p. B5.

Mays, V., & Comas-Díaz, L. (1988). Feminist therapies with ethnic minority populations: A closer look at Blacks and Hispanics. In M. A. Dutton-Douglas & L. E. Walker (Eds.), *Feminist psychotherapies: Integration of therapeutic and feminist systems* (pp. 228–251). Norwood, NJ: Ablex.

McCombs, H. G. (1986). The application of an individual/collective model to the psychology of Black women. In D. Howard (Ed.), *The dynamics of feminist therapy.* New York: Haworth Press.

McGoldrick, M., & García-Preto, N. (1984). Ethnic intermarriage: Implications for therapy. *Family Process, 23,* 347–364.

McGoldrick, M., García-Preto, N., Hines, P. M., & Lee, E. (1989). Ethnicity and women. In M. McGoldrick, C. M. Anderson, & F. Walsh (Eds.), *Women in families: A framework for family therapy* (pp. 169–199). New York: W. W. Norton.

McGoldrick, M., Pearce, J. K., & Giordano, J. (Eds.). (1982). *Ethnicity and family therapy.* New York: Guilford Press.

McGrath, E., Keita, G. P., Strickland, B. R., & Russo, N. F. (Eds.). (1990). *Women and depression: Risk factors and treatment issues.* Washington, DC: American Psychological Association.

McKenzie-Mohr, D., & Zanna, M. P. (1990). Treating women as sexual objects: Look to the (gender schematic) male who has viewed pornography. *Personality and Social Psychology Bulletin, 16,* 296–308.

Melia, J., & Lyttle, P. (1986). *Why Jenny can't lead: Understanding the male dominant system.* Saguache, CO: Operational Politics.

Miller, J. B. (1986). *What do we mean by relationships?* (Work in progress No. 22). Wellesley, MA: Stone Center.

Morrison, A. M., & Von Glinow, M. A. (1990). Women and minorities in management. *American Psychologist, 45,* 200–208.

Moses (1991, July). Ties that bind can limit minority valedictorians. *APA Monitor, 22,* 47.

Nieva, V., & Gutek, B. (1981). *Women and work: A psychological perspective.* New York: Praeger.

National Coalition of Hispanic Health and Human Services Organizations. (1988). *Delivering preventive health care to Hispanics: A manual for providers.* Washington, DC: Author.

Painton, P. (1991, October 28). Women power. *Time, 138*(17), 24–26.

Peterson, S. (1990). Challenges for Black women faculty. *Journal of National Association for Women, Deans, Administrations, and Counselors, 53,* 33–36.

Person, E. S. (1982). Women working: Fears of failure, deviance, and success. *Journal of the American Academy of Psychoanalysis, 10,* 67–84.

Pinderhughes, E. (1983). Empowerment of our clients and for ourselves. *Social Casework, 64,* 331–338.

Pinderhughes, E. (1986). Minority woman: A nodal point in the functioning of the social system. In M. Ault-Riche (Ed.), *Women and family therapy.* Rockville, MD: Aspen Systems.

Pinderhughes, E. (1989). *Understanding race, ethnicity, and power: The key to efficacy in clinical practice.* New York: Free Press.

Post, R. D. (1982). Dependency conflicts in high-achieving women: Towards an integration. *Psychotherapy, 19,* 82–87.

Puig, A. (1991). A traumatic-stress model for EPAs. *EPA Digest, 12*(1), 22, 53–54.

Pumariega, A. J., Edwards, P., & Mitchell, C. B. (1984). Anorexia nervosa in Black adolescents. *Journal of the American Academy of Child Psychiatry, 23,* 111–114.

Reid, P. T. (1988). Racism and sexism: Comparisons and conflicts. In P. A. Katz & D. A. Taylor (Eds.), *Eliminating racism* (pp. 203–221). New York: Plenum.

Reid, P. T., & Comas-Díaz, L. (1990). Gender and ethnicity: Perspectives on dual status. *Sex Roles, 22,* 397–408.

Rigdon, J. E. (1991, July 10). Exploding myth: Asian American youth suffer a rising toll from heavy pressures. *Wall Street Journal,* pp. A1, A8.

Robinson, C. R. (1983). Black women: A tradition of self-reliant strength. In J. H. Robbins & R. J. Siegel (Eds.), *Women changing therapy: New assessment, values, and strategies in feminist therapy.* New York: Haworth Press.

Romero, G. J., & Garza, R. T. (1986). Attributions for the occupational success/failure of ethnic minority and nonminority women. *Sex Roles, 14,* 445–452.

Root, M. P. P. (1990). Disordered eating in women of color. *Sex Roles, 22,* 525–536.

Rueschemeyer, D. (1972). Doctors and lawyers: A comment on the theory of professions. In E. Friedson & J. Lorber (Eds.), *Medical men and their work.* Chicago: Aldine-Atherton.

Sanders, K. W., & Mellow, G. O. (1990). Permanent diversity: The deferred vision of higher education. *Journal of the National Association for Women Deans, Administrators, and Counselors, 53,* 9–13.

Schwartz, F. N. (1989). Management women and the new facts of life. *Harvard Business Review, 89,* 65–76.

Seda Bonilla, E. (1970). *Requiem por una cultura* [Requiem for a culture]. Río Piedras, Puerto Rico: Editorial Edil.

Smith, A., & Steward, A. J. (1983). Approaches to studying racism and sexism in black women's lives. *Journal of Social Issues, 39,* 1–15.

Snipp, C. M. (1990). A portrait of American Indian women and their labor force experiences. In S. E. Rix (Ed.), *The American woman, 1990–91: A status report* (pp. 265–272). New York: W. W. Norton.

Spiegler, D. L., Tate, D. A., Aitken, S. S., & Christian, C. M. (Eds.). (1985). *Alcohol use among U.S. ethnic minorities.* Rockville, MD: U.S. Department of Health and Human Services, Alcohol, Drug Abuse, and Mental Health Administration.

Stevens, W. (1950). *Famous women of America.* New York: Dood, Meade.

Surrey, J. L. (1991). The "self-in-relation": A theory of women's development. In J. V. Jordan, A. G. Kaplan, J. B. Miller, I. P. Stiver, & J. L. Surrey, *Women's growth in connection: Writings from the Stone Center* (pp. 51–66). New York: Guilford Press.

Trochet, G. I. (1991). Can parenthood and medical practice co-exist? *Medical Economics, 68,* 90–94.

Trotman, F. K. (1984). Psychotherapy of Black women and the dual effects of racism and sexism. In C. M. Brody (Ed.), *Women therapists working with women: New theory and process of feminist therapy* (pp. 96–108). New York: Springer.

True, R. H. (1990). Psychotherapeutic issues with Asian American women. *Sex Roles, 22,* 477–486.

Vobejda, B. (1991a, September 20). Racial pay closes for women. *Washington Post,* pp. A1, A8.

Vobejda, B. (1991b, November 11). 25% of Black women may never marry. *Washington Post,* pp. A1, A12.

Watts-Jones, D. (1990). Towards a stress scale for African-American women. *Psychology of Women Quarterly, 14,* 271–275.

Watson, V. M. (1989, November). Minorities and the legacy of anger. *APA Monitor,* 30–31.

Weems, R. (1991, May). Can we be friends? *Essence, 38,* 128–127.

Weitz, R., & Gordon, L. (1993). Images of Black women among Anglo college students. *Sex Roles, 28,* 19–34.

Williams, L. E. (1990). The challenges before Black women in higher education. *Journal of the National Association for Women Deans, Administrators, and Counselors, 53,* 1–2.

Wiltz, T. (1991, May). Glass-ceiling survival. *Essence, 35,* 37.

Woo, D. (1985). The socioeconomic status of Asian American women in the labor force: An alternative view. *Sociological Perspectives, 28,* 307–338.

Woo, D. (1989). The gap between striving and achieving: The case of Asian American women. In Asian Women United of California (Eds.), *Making waves: An anthology of writings by and about Asian American women.* Boston: Beacon Press.

Wyche, K. F., & Graves, S. B. (1992). Minority women in academia: Access and barriers to professional participation. *Psychology of Women Quarterly, 16,* 429–437.

14

Lesbian Women of Color: Triple Jeopardy

Beverly Greene

The professional literature on mental health has in recent years significantly expanded its inquiry into the roles of culture, ethnicity, gender, and sexual orientation in mental health, and the delivery of psychological services to women. This inquiry has included closer scrutiny into the impact of racism, sexism, heterocentric bias, and the factors associated with them on the psychological development of women of color, and thus on the process of assessment and treatment. The literature of professional psychology in these areas has slowly begun to reflect the appropriate exploration of the effects of membership in institutionally oppressed and disparaged groups on the development of both psychological resilience and psychological vulnerability, and has done so from a wide range of perspectives (Greene, 1990a). Lesbian women of color, however, often still find themselves and their concerns invisible in the scholarly research of both women of color and of lesbians.

This chapter includes African American, Black American of Caribbean descent, Latina, Asian American, Native American, and Indian women in the designation "women of color." Those who consider that their primary romantic/sexual attractions are to women are considered lesbian. Hence, women from the aforementioned ethnic minority groups who consider themselves lesbians will be the group referred to in this chapter as lesbian women of color. Clearly, there are lesbians from other ethnic minority groups who could also be considered lesbian women of color and to whom many of the statements made in this chapter could apply. The observations made here, however, are limited in their generalizability to the groups mentioned. The absence of specific mention of the others is not intended to suggest that their concerns are of lesser significance; rather, I have limited this discussion to those groups about whom there are clinical, empirical, or anecdotal studies available.

The vast majority of clinical and empirical research on or with lesbians is conducted with overwhelmingly White, middle-class respondents (Amaro, 1978; Chan, 1989, 1992; Gock, 1985, 1992; Greene, in press,; Mays & Cochran, 1988; Mays, Cochran & Rhue, in press; Morales, 1989; Tremble, Schneider, & Appathurai, 1989; Wooden, Kawasaki, & Mayeda, 1983). Similarly, the scant research on women of color rarely if ever acknowledges that not all of the groups' members are heterosexual. Hence, there is no exploration of the complex interaction between sexual orientation and ethnic and gender identity development. Nor does the literature take into account the realistic social and psychological tasks and stressors that are a component of lesbian identity formation for women who are members of visible ethnic minority groups. An exploration of the vicissitudes of racism, sexism, homophobia, same-gender socialization, and their effects on the couple relationships of lesbians of color is another important but neglected area of scrutiny.

Empirical and clinical research on lesbians and on women of color rarely states that their generalizability is limited to heterosexual women of color and lesbians who are White. This practice can inadvertently lead readers of these studies to assume that findings that are applicable to women in these groups are equally applicable to lesbians of color, or that the concerns of lesbians of color do not warrant specific attention in the mental health literature. Such narrow clinical and research perspectives leave us with a limited understanding of the diversity of women of color and of lesbians as a group. Another more serious consequence of such omissions is that practitioners are left ill-equipped to address, in culturally sensitive and literate ways, the clinical needs of lesbians who are also stigmatized by their racial or ethnic identity.

A note of caution: broad descriptions of cultural practices or values in this chapter should not be applied with uniformity to all lesbian women of color or to all lesbians in any specific cultural or ethnic group. There are significant differences between the experiences and realities of lesbians of color and their White counterparts, but there is also great diversity within groups of lesbians from specific cultures and races. Clients should not be made to fit arbitrarily into preconceived notions of what all of the women of a group must be like. For example, lesbians who are Latina come from many different countries, with different languages and often many different cultural norms. Asian lesbians come from similarly diverse geographical regions and cultural backgrounds and speak different languages, as do their Indian and Native American counterparts. In these examples, the group's label conceals many different subgroups and distinct cultures. Furthermore, within each subgroup, distinctive differences may be found between lesbians from rural and urban environments as well as between lesbians from various socioeconomic and educational backgrounds within an ethnic culture.

Just as the experience of sexism is "colored" by the lens of race and ethnicity for women of color, so is the experience of heterosexism similarly filtered for lesbian women of color. This chapter provides practitioners with a framework from which to begin looking at lesbians and women of color from a more diverse perspective and at lesbians of color with greater cultural sensitivity. Its aim is to assist in sensitizing practitioners to cultural factors bearing significantly on the ways that lesbian women of color perceive the world, the unique tasks and stressors they must manage on a routine basis, and mental health and therapy issues. It is necessary, however, for practitioners to explore every client's plight with an understanding of the client's own unique perspective of her cultural heritage, sexual orientation, and the respective significance of these in her life.

THE CONDITIONS OF TRIPLE JEOPARDY

The underpinnings of traditional approaches to psychology are riddled with androcentric, heterocentric, and ethnocentric biases (Garnets & Kimmel, 1991; Glassgold, 1992; Greene, 1993a), thus reinforcing the triple discrimination lesbians of color face in the world at large. Heterocentric thinking often leads both professional and lay persons to make a range of inaccurate and unexamined but commonly held assumptions about lesbians. These assumptions are maintained to varying extents within ethnic minority groups as much as they are in the dominant culture. Among many commonly accepted and fallacious notions is that women who are lesbians either want to be men, are "mannish" in appearance (Taylor, 1983), are unattractive or less attractive than heterosexual women (Dew, 1985), are less extroverted (Kite, 1994), are unable to get a man, have had traumatic relationships with men which presumably "turned" them against men, or are defective females (Christian, 1985; Collins, 1990; Greene, 1994; Kite, 1994). Members of ethnic minority groups, like their counterparts in the dominant culture, believe that sexual attraction to men is embedded in the definition of what it means to be a normal woman. Acceptance of this assumption often leads to a range of equally inaccurate conclusions. One is that reproductive sexuality is the only form of sexual expression that is psychologically normal and morally correct (Garnets & Kimmel, 1991; Glassgold, 1992). Another incorrect assumption is that there is a direct relationship between sexual orientation and a woman's conformity or lack thereof to traditional gender roles and physical appearance within the culture (Kite & Deaux, 1987; Newman, 1989; Whitley, 1987). The mistaken conclusions that follow are twofold. One is that women who do not conform to traditional gender-role stereotypes must be lesbian. The equally mistaken corollary to this is that those who do conform to such stereotypes must be heterosexual. These assumptions are used in many cultures to threaten women with the stigma of being labeled lesbian if they fail to adhere to traditional gender-role stereotypes in which males are dominant and females are submissive (Collins, 1990; Gomez & Smith, 1990; Smith, 1982).

The fear of being labeled a lesbian can be used to prevent women who fear it, whether they are lesbian or not, from seeking nontraditional roles or engaging in nontraditional behaviors. Shockley (1979) suggests that the fear of being labeled lesbian has been strong enough to have deterred Black women writers from examining lesbian themes in their writing. In an atmosphere of tenacious homophobia within ethnic minority groups as well as within the dominant culture, some scholars who are also women of color feel that simply writing about or acknowledging such themes will raise questions about their own sexual orientation (Clarke, 1991). In a patriarchal society, in which male dominance and female subordination has been viewed as normative, threats of being labeled lesbian, fears of that label, and its realistic negative social consequences may be used in the service of maintaining inequitable patterns in the distribution of power.

ASSESSMENT OF RELEVANT CULTURAL FACTORS

A range of factors should be considered in determining the impact of ethnic identity, gender, lesbian sexual orientation, and the ongoing dynamic interaction of these with one another in the course of a woman's development. An understanding of the meaning and the reality of being a woman of color who is lesbian requires a careful exploration and understanding of these factors. These factors include the nature and importance of the culture's traditional gender-role stereotypes and their relative fluidity or rigidity, the role and importance of family and community, and the role of religion/spirituality in the culture. Other important factors include the role of racial and ethnic stereotypes, the prevalence of sexism within their minority culture, racism and ethnic discrimination from the larger culture, and the contribution of these to the ethnosexual mythology applied to these women.

For members of some oppressed groups, specifically African Americans and Native Americans, reproductive sexuality is given even greater importance than it is given by other groups because it is the way of continuing the group's presence in the world, when that presence has been historically endangered by racist, genocidal practices. Hence, sexual practice that is not reproductive may be viewed by persons of color as yet another instrument of an oppressive system designed to limit the growth of these groups or to eliminate them altogether. Kanuha (1990) refers to such beliefs as "fears of extinction" (p. 176) and posits that they are used in the service of scapegoating lesbians of color as if they were responsible for threats to the group's survival. It is interesting to note that such fears do not attend to the reality that a lesbian sexual orientation is not synonymous with a disinclination toward having children, particularly among lesbians of color. This does not mean that fears of extinction among persons of color are unwarranted, rather that it is the institutional racism of the dominant culture that places the survival of persons of color at risk, not lesbians or heterosexual women of color who choose not to reproduce. Nonetheless, the internalization of this view can make it more difficult for a lesbian of color to accept affirmatively her sexual orientation. When this internalization occurs, addressing it must be considered a part of the therapeutic work.

In therapy with lesbian clients of color the family context, the role and expectations of parents in the lives of their children are important factors to consider. For example, the extent to which the parents or family of origin may continue to control or influence children, even when they are adults, and the importance of the family as a source of economic and emotional support warrants understanding (Mays & Cochran, 1988). Other factors to consider include the importance of procreation and the continuation of the family line, the importance of ties to the ethnic community, the degree of acculturation or assimilation of the individual client, significant differences between the degree of acculturation of family members and the individual, and the history of discrimination or oppression that the particular group has experienced from individuals and institutions of the dominant culture. When examining the history of discrimination of an ethnic group, it is imperative that group members' own understandings of their oppression and their strategies for coping with discrimination be incorporated into any analysis. A cursory review of only the dominant culture's perspectives on lesbians or women carries the danger of perpetuating ethnocentric, heterocentric, and androcentric biases.

Another important dimension that must be considered is that of sexuality. Sexuality and its meaning is contextual. Therefore what it means to be a lesbian will be related to the meaning assigned to both gender and sexuality in the individual's culture. Espín (1984) suggests that in most cultures a range of sexual behaviors is tolerated, and that that range varies from culture to culture. It is important for the clinician to determine where the client's behavior fits within the spectrum for her particular culture (Espín, 1984). The therapist must also explore the range of sexuality that is sanctioned, in what forms it may be expressed and by whom, as well as the consequences for those who deviate from or conform to such norms. In exploring the range of sexuality tolerated by the woman's culture it is helpful to determine if there are sexual practices that are formally forbidden but tolerated as long as they are not discussed and not labeled.

It is also important to determine the ethnosexual mythology that has been part of a woman of color's upbringing and its relationship to her understanding of a lesbian sexual orientation. This mythology may include the sexual myths the dominant culture has generated and holds about women of color. Such myths and stereotypes often represent a complex combination of racial and sexual stereotypes designed to objectify women of color, set them apart from their idealized White counterparts, and facilitate their sexual exploitation and control (Collins, 1990; Greene, 1993a; hooks, 1981). The symbolism of these sterotypes and its interaction with stereotypes held about lesbians are important areas of inquiry.

CULTURAL FACTORS IN THE LIVES OF LESBIANS OF COLOR

Immigration and Acculturation

Espín (1987) suggests that the time of and reasons for immigration are important factors in the treatment of Latina lesbians in the United States. In my experience, these factors are also relevant for Black lesbians from the West Indies and Caribbean islands, as well as for other lesbians of color who are members of immigrant groups. In her discussion, Espín (1987) addresses the effect of separation from one's homeland. Such separation often involved leaving significant family members behind (or even perhaps having been left behind for a time) as well as other major changes in the family's lifestyle. A mourning process associated with this type of loss may be normative. Even when entire families immigrate, many persons of color continue to have intense attachment to their birthplace or homeland, often for many years after leaving. Lesbian women of color are no exception. Departures from the country they consider home may be painful in ways that a therapist who is born and raised in the United States, particularly if she or he is a member of the dominant culture, may have difficulty appreciating. Furthermore, just because immigration is voluntary—such as when the client is escaping an oppressive political regime, seeking a place where she may have greater freedom to be open as a lesbian, or seeking work that is unobtainable in her native country—this does not eradicate significant ties to the homeland itself.

If immigration is recent, the lesbian woman of color may have a significant dependence on her family members and members of her ethnic community for emotional and perhaps economic support. This may complicate issues involved in "coming out" or being open about a lesbian sexual orientation. It is particularly problematic if the family, community, and/or traditional cultural values are perceived or selectively interpreted as rejecting lesbian sexual orientation. New immigrants, if not acculturated, may not yet have contact with a broader lesbian community, or even with lesbians of their own communities. Chan (1989, 1992) writes that the latter tend to be invisible, if they exist at all in Asian and some other ethnic minority communities (Garnets & Kimmel, 1991; Pamela H., 1989). Some lesbians from the West Indies and other Caribbean islands have left their native lands because they believe that their sexual orientation will be easier to be open about in the heterogeneity of the United States than it is on small islands with smaller interconnected communities. In such a setting anonymity is nearly impossible and discovery is difficult to avoid. Silvera's (1991) essay effectively describes the shroud of secrecy around the existence of lesbians in her native home, Jamaica, as well as the contempt with which they are regarded.

Language

Espín (1984) writes that a bilingual woman's first language may be laden with affective meanings that are not captured in translating the words themselves. Since a language reflects a culture's values, it may contain few or no words for lesbian that are not negative, if the culture views lesbian sexual orientations negatively. Espín (1984) suggests that shifts between first (native) and second languages may represent attempts at distancing and estrangement around certain topics in therapy. Espín (1984) observes that a lesbian's second language may be used to express feelings or impulses that are culturally forbidden and that many women would not dare verbalize in their native tongue, which allows them to distance themselves from these feelings. Sexuality is considerably laden with cultural values and as such if a client shifts from speaking in one language to the other during discussions of this material may be revealing. It is also worth noting that in cultures where English is spoken fluently by the majority of the population, such as India, some Caribbean islands, and for Native Americans, the second language is not always processed or understood similarly, nor do the same words necessarily have the meaning they do in mainstream America (Tafoya & Rowell, 1988).

Family and Gender Roles

Lesbian women of color (and their heterosexual counterparts) see the family as the primary social unit and as a major source of emotional and material support. The family and the ethnic community provide women of color with an additional and important support, functioning as a refuge and buffer against racism in the dominant culture. Lesbians feel separation and rejection by family and community keenly, and many women will not jeopardize their connections to their families and communities by forming alliances with the broader lesbian community or even by simply divulging the fact that they are lesbians. These observations are true for Latina, African American/Caribbean, Asian American, Indian, South Asian, and Native American lesbians (Allen, 1984, 1986; Amaro, 1978; Boyd-Franklin, 1990; Espín, 1984, 1987; Gock, 1992; Greene, 1986, 1993a; Hidalgo & Hidalgo-Christensen, 1976; Icard, 1986; Mays & Cochran, 1988; Morales, 1989, 1992; Moses & Hawkins, 1982; Vasquez, 1979). The boundaries of the family in many ethnic cultures go beyond that of the nuclear family in Western culture; they extend to persons who are not related by blood but are experienced as though they were. These persons are considered extended family. The complex networks of interdependence and support in these families that include lesbian members should not be seen as undifferentiated by a culturally naive therapist.

I will discuss characteristic features of negotiating a lesbian sexual orientation within the family and the ethnic community, complicated by the strong family ties that are common in most ethnic cultures. Lesbian women of color tend to perceive that their ethnic communities not only reject lesbian sexual orientations and are antagonistic to women who overtly label themselves as lesbian, but also that they are more tenaciously antagonistic than the dominant culture (Allen, 1984, 1986; Chan, 1987; Croom, 1993; Espín, 1987; Folayan, 1992; Greene, 1990b, 1993a, in press; Mays & Cochran, 1988; Morales, 1989; Namjoshi, 1992; Poussaint, 1990; Ratti, 1993; Weston, 1991). The perception that antagonism toward lesbians is greater in the ethnic than in the dominant culture is based only on anecdotal reports of lesbians of color about their respective communities. There are no empirical studies to date that systematically assess attitudes toward lesbian sexual orientation in any of these groups.

It is also important to distinguish same-gender sexual behavior that may be known and accepted within a culture from a lesbian identity. Chan (personal communication, November 1992), Espín (1984), Comas-Díaz (personal communication, January 1993) and Jayakar (Chapter 6, this volume) note that same-gender sexual behavior is known to occur in India, Asian, and Latin cultures between males, but that it is not accompanied by a self-identification as homosexual. It is noteworthy that in same-gender sexual behavior between Latino men, it is the role of the passive or female identified recipient that is devalued.

In many cultures same-gender sexual behavior between women may not be defined or adopted by those who engage in such behavior or relationships as lesbian sexual orientation. This may be particularly so in cultures where lesbians are not tolerated, but the behavior is tolerated as long as it is not accompanied by such a label. There may be a sense that the stigmatized identity would only result from adopting the label; such relationships or behavior can be engaged in in other ways. This type of strategy may also represent a culturally prescribed way of managing a potential conflict indirectly rather than in direct confrontation with it. This phenomenon can be problematic for the clinician in attempts to determine whether the avoidance of the label has its origins in culturally prescribed methods of managing potential conflicts, in culturally distinct or different concepts about what constitutes a lesbian identity, in a reflection of internalized homophobia, or in all of these elements. Attention to the client's personal history and a familiarity with her cultural norms will be crucial to making such determinations accurately. In many cultures, openly adopting the identity of lesbian or declaring a sexual preference for persons of the same gender is what is most problematic for and unacceptable to family members and heterosexual ethnic peers.

LESBIAN WOMEN OF COLOR: DISTINCT POPULATIONS

African American Lesbians

The legacy of sexual racism plays a role in the response of many African Americans to lesbians in their families and as visible members of their communities. Generally, the African American community is perceived by many of its lesbian members as extremely homophobic and rejecting of lesbians (Croom, 1993; Mays & Cochran, 1988). This rejection increases the pressure on lesbians to remain in the closet and hence invisible in their communities (Clarke, 1983; Collins, 1990; Croom, 1993; Gomez & Smith, 1990; Greene, 1993b, in press; Icard, 1986; Mays & Cochran, 1988; Mays, Cochran, & Rhue, in press; Poussaint, 1990; Smith, 1982).

Gender roles in African American families have been somewhat more flexible than in those of their White and many of their ethnic minority counterparts. This flexibility is explained in part as a derivative of the value of interdependence among group members and the more egalitarian nature of many precolonial African tribes. It is also a function of the need to adapt to racism in the United States. The question then is, how did this homophobia—and particularly that directed toward lesbian sexuality—develop?

African Americans are a diverse group of persons, whose cultural origins I have elaborated on in Chapter 1 of this volume. Their ancestors were unwilling participants in their immigration, as they were the primary objects of the U.S. slave trade (Greene, 1992, 1993a, 1993b, in press). The roles of African American women, as women, were as pieces of property; forced sexual relationships with African males and White slavemasters were the norm for them. African American women of Caribbean but not Latin descent come from diverse backgrounds in Caribbean islands that were colonized by Great Britain and France, their cultural values and practices may be significantly different from those of African Americans, reflecting the culture of the country responsible for their colonization.

Ethnosexual stereotypes about African American women have their roots in images created by a White society struggling to reconcile a range of contradictions. An elaboration of those contradictions is beyond the scope of this chapter (they are discussed in detail in Chapter 1). hooks (1981) proposes that the image of women as castrating was promulgated by psychoanalysis in the 1950s to stigmatize any woman who wanted to work outside the home or cross the gender-role barriers of a patriarchal culture. Because the history of racism had not conferred on African American women the feminine role of homemaker nearly to the degree White women held this role, these women were already working outside the home in greater proportion than White women. Popular images of these women as castrating, therefore, developed as part of an arrangement of social power in which African American men and women were subordinate to Whites, and women were subordinate to men. Hence, today's stereotypes are riddled with a legacy of ethnosexual myths that depict African American women as not sufficiently subordinate to African American men, inherently sexually promiscuous, morally loose, independent, strong, assertive, matriarchal, and castrating masculinized females when compared to their White counterparts (Christian, 1985; Clarke, 1983; Collins, 1990; Greene, 1986, 1990a, 1990b, 1993a; hooks, 1981; Icard, 1989; Silvera, 1991). African American women clearly did not fit the traditional stereotypes of women as fragile, weak, and dependent, since they were never allowed to be that way. They came to be defined as all of the things that normal women were not supposed to be. Stereotypes that depict lesbians as masculinized women poignantly intersect with stereotypes of African American and African Caribbean women in this regard. They suggest that both lesbians and African American women are defective females who want to be or act like men and are sexually promiscuous. It is important to understand the history of institutional racism and the significant role it has had in the development of a legacy of myths and distortions regarding the sexuality of lesbians from these groups.

Additionally, racism and sexism come together in attempts to present African American women as the cause of failures in family functioning, suggesting that a lack of male dominance and female subordination has prevented African Americans from being truly emancipated. Males in the culture are encouraged to believe that strong women are responsible for their oppression, and not racist institutions. Many African American women, including those who are lesbians, have internalized these myths. When internalized, such distortions of the sexuality of African American women which is treated as if it were depraved, can intensify the negative psychological effects on African American lesbians and further compromise their ability to obtain support from the larger African American community (Clarke, 1983; Collins, 1990).

The African American family has functioned as a necessary and important protective barrier, a survival tool against and refuge from the racism of the dominant culture. Villarosa (quoted in Brownworth, 1993) observes that the status of the African American family and community as central tools for survival and a safe haven makes the process of "coming out" for African American lesbians significantly different from that of their White counterparts:

> It is harder for us to consider being rejected by our families . . . all we have is our families, our community. When the whole world is racist and against you, your family and your community are the only people who accept you and love you even though you are black. So you don't know what will happen if you lose them . . . and many black lesbians (and gay men) are afraid that's what will happen. (p. 18)

Because of the strength of family ties lesbian family members may not be automatically rejected, although there is an undisputed rejection of a lesbian sexual orientation. Villarosa observes that in African American families they do not throw a lesbian out because of the importance of family members to one another, rather, they "keep you around to talk you out of it" (Brownworth, 1993, p. 18).

A clinician should not infer from this "tolerance" that the family approves of its member being a lesbian (Acosta, 1979). Tolerance is usually contingent on silence about one's lesbian sexual orientation. Serious conflicts between family members may in fact erupt if a family member openly discloses, labels herself, or discusses being a lesbian.

Homophobia among African Americans and many African Caribbeans can be explained as a function of many different determinants. One is the significant presence of Western Christian religiosity, which is often an exaggerated expression of the strong religion spiritual orientation of these cultures. In this context, selective interpretations of biblical scripture are used to reinforce homophobic attitudes (Claybourne, 1978; Greene, in press; Icard, 1986; Moses & Hawkins, 1982). Silvera (1991) writes that when she was 27 years old her grandmother discovered that she was a lesbian, sat her down with bible in hand, and explained that "this was a ting only people of mixed blood was involved in" (p. 16).

Clarke (1983), Silvera (1991), and Smith (1982) cite heterosexual privilege as another determinant of homophobia among African American women. Because of the rampant sexism in both the dominant and African American cultures, and racism in the dominant culture, African American women often find themselves at the bottom of the racial and gender hierarchies heap. Hence, being heterosexual is the only privileged status they may possess.

Internalized racism may be seen as another determinant of homophobia among African Americans and African Caribbeans. For those who have internalized negative stereotypes of people of African and Caribbean descent as they are constructed and held by the dominant culture, the notion that one mistake is a negative reflection on all African Americans is a common idea (Greene, in press; Poussaint, 1990).

Sexuality has always been an emotionally charged issue, intensified by pejorative ethnosexual myths and stereotypes about African American men and women (Wyatt, Strayer, & Lobitz, 1976). One reaction to negative stereotypes previously mentioned is that of avoiding any behavior that might conform to or resemble those stereotypes. Hence there may be an exaggerated need to demonstrate "normalcy" and fit into the dominant culture's depiction of what people are supposed to be (Clarke, 1983; deMonteflores, 1986; Gomez, 1983; Greene, 1986, in press; Wyatt et al., 1976). As a result, acceptance of a lesbian sexual orientation can be thought of as contradicting the dominant culture's ideal. Hence lesbians may be experienced by persons who strongly identify with the dominant culture as an embarrassment to them (Poussaint, 1990). Indeed, the only names for lesbians in the African American community are derogatory: "funny women" or "bulldagger women" (Jeffries, 1992, p. 44; Omosupe, 1991). Silvera (1991) writes of her childhood in Jamaica,

> the words used to describe many of these women would be "Man royal" and/or "Sodomite." Dread words. So dread that women dare not use these words to name themselves. The act of loving someone from the same sex was sinful, abnormal—something to hide. (pp. 15–16)

She explains that the word "sodomite," derived from the Old Testament, is peculiar to Jamaica in its use to describe lesbians as well as any strong, independent woman. She continues, "Things are different now in Jamaica. Now all you have to do is not respond to a man's call to you and dem call you sodomite or lesbian" (p. 17).

Clarke (1983) and Jeffries (1992) observe that there was a period of quiet tolerance for gay men and lesbians in some poor African American communities in the 1940s, through the 1950s. Clark explains this as "seizing the opportunity to spite the White man" by tolerating members of a group that the dominant culture devalues. Jeffries attributes this "tolerance" to the empathy of African Americans as oppressed people for the plight of another oppressed group. The recent heightened visibility of lesbians in the dominant culture in general and the higher visibility of African American lesbians in African American communities may ultimately remove the denial of lesbian orientation that has heretofore been required for "tolerance."

Bell and Weinberg (1978), Bass-Hass (1968), Croom, (1993), Mays and Cochran (1988), and Mays et al. (in press) are among the few studies made up exclusively or that include significant numbers of African American lesbian respondents. Among the findings of these studies are that African American lesbians are more likely to maintain strong involvements with their families; more likely to have children; and to depend to a greater extent on family members or other African American lesbians for support than their White counterparts. The findings also indicate that they are likely to have more continued contact with men and with heterosexual peers than their White counterparts. The studies found a greater likelihood that African American lesbians will experience tension and loneliness but are less likely to seek professional help. This may contribute to a delay in the seeking of help during a crisis or a condition and may leave African American lesbians more vulnerable to negative psychological outcomes.

Despite the acknowledged homophobia in the African American community, African American lesbians claim a strong attachment to their cultural heritage and to their communities, and cite their identity as African Americans as primary (Acosta, 1979; Croom, 1993; Mays et al., in press). They also cite a sense of conflicting loyalties between the African American community and the mainstream lesbian community, particularly when confronted with homophobia in the African American community (Dyne, 1980; Greene, 1990b, in press; Icard, 1986; Mays & Cochran, 1988).

Native American Lesbians

Allen (1986) writes, "The lesbian is to the American Indian what the Indian is to the American—invisible" (p. 245). In her brilliant treatise on the role of women in American Native traditions, Allen explains that the written history of Native Americans is a selective one. Those portions of this written history that would establish (1) that the primary social order of native cultures were gynocentric prior to 1800, and (2) that in such systems women held important positions and had the authority to make decisions on all tribal levels—that essentially contradicted a Western, patriarchal worldview—were almost completely deleted. The existence and tolerance of Native American lesbians, who in fact played an integral part of tribal life, had to be obliterated to serve patriarchal interests, resulting in their contemporary invisibility (Allen, 1984, 1986; Tafoya, 1992).

Allen (1986) and Williams (1986) note that in precolonial Native American tribes, physical anatomy was not inextricably linked to gender roles and that mixed, third gender, or alternative gender roles were at one time accepted and integrated into tribal life. LaFromboise et al. (Chapter 2, this volume) examine important differences between Western and Native communities' understandings of the world, as well as important differences within the immense numbers of different tribes. Tafoya (1992) suggests that Native people may have a more "sophisticated taxonomy which addresses spirituality and function rather than appearance" (p. 254) and that these elements are understood as they appear situationally in relation to something else, not as absolute entities in and of themselves. Within such a paradigm, dichotomous or mutually exclusive categories such as male and female or lesbian and heterosexual may not accurately capture the Native person's understanding of sexuality and gender (Allen, 1984, 1986; Tafoya, 1992).

While there were divisions of roles by gender, they were divided in ways allowing men and women to assume them irrespective of their gender. For example, women who would be considered lesbians by today's standards would have assumed roles usually occupied by men and would have been considered men in some tribes (Allen, 1986). Persons whom we might consider androgynous or lesbian by today's standards were valued and in some tribes were accorded special respect and honor (Allen, 1986; Grahn, 1984; Weinrich & Williams, 1991). They were also often viewed as people who combined aspects of masculine and feminine styles in one person spiritually, reflected in the roles they assumed (Weinrich & Williams, 1991). Allen (1986) observes that in gynocratic systems, people assume roles within the social order by virtue of the realities of the human constitution, rather than on "denial based social fictions" (p. 3) that force people into arbitrary categories determined by powerful and privileged persons within that society.

Jacobs (cited in Grahn, 1984) found 88 tribes whose documented cultural characteristics mention gayness, and 22 of those include specific references to lesbians, with specific names for lesbians in each tribe (Allen, 1986). The 11 tribes who denied, to White anthropologists, the existence of lesbians were observed to come from territories where the most intense and severe puritanical influence from Whites was felt. Allen (1986), Tafoya (1992), and Williams (1986) observe that from the outset Native American people learned not discuss matters of gender and sexuality with European settlers since the latter groups viewed tribal customs and rituals with contempt, quickly seeking to eradicate them.

It is important to understand the devastating effect of the colonization of Native Americans on tribal life, values, and practices and its role in current attitudes toward lesbians. The degree of acceptance of a gay or lesbian sexual orientation may also be a function of the religious group that was involved in colonizing a particular tribe (V. L. Sears, personal communication, May 1992). Allen (1986) asserts that colonization resulted in a shift from a gynocentric, egalitarian, ritual-based social system to a secular system that more closely resembles European patriarchy. In the course of this shift, women, lesbians, and leaders who observed tribal customs and rituals have suffered the most severe losses of power, status, and leadership (Allen, 1984, 1986; Tafoya, 1992). Colonizers who came from patriarchal cultures could not tolerate groups who allowed women to be powerful and sought to "discredit" the status of women, as well as the tolerance for lesbians and gay men by the deliberate destruction of both records and lives (Allen, 1986). Williams (1986) writes that the stark homophobia of White recorders of tribal life, reflected in their negative judgments of same-gender sexual relationships, stands in stark contrast to the recorded history of easy acceptance of lesbians and gay men among Native Americans themselves. The colonizers' ultimate goal was to present patriarchy as the best alternative (Allen, 1986). This trend is linked to the growth of homophobia, once a rare phenomenon in many tribes. Allen (1986) cites highly acculturated and Christianized Native Americans as those who are most likely to express "fear and loathing" for lesbians, as for any other aspects of traditional tribal life (p. 199).

Tafoya (1992) suggests that the concept of "two-spirited people" (p. 256) is more relevant to Native American people than English-defined categories of lesbian or heterosexual. A two-spirited person possesses a male and female spirit, regardless of his or her biological gender. In this paradigm, an individual's sexuality is viewed on a continuum, and a wide range of sexual behaviors are deemed acceptable. The dichotomous notions of heterosexuality and homosexuality are of little use in such a continuum model, where less stigma is attached to women whose behavior is "masculine" or to men whose behavior is "feminine" (Tafoya, 1992).

In Blumstein and Schwarz's (cited in Tafoya & Rowell, 1988) research with over 200 interracial same-sex couples, a higher rate of bisexual behavior was found among Native American respondents than among any other ethnic group in the United States. Additional findings reveal that self-identified Native American lesbians had higher reported rates of heterosexual experiences than their other ethnic counterparts (Tafoya, 1992). In this context, a Native American lesbian might assume more masculine or feminine behavior depending on her partner and the context (Tafoya & Rowell, 1988). This observation supports the assumption of a more fluid concept of gender relations and sexual expression among Native American people than in both their White and other ethnic counterparts.

Despite these findings, contemporary Native Americans, particularly those who reside on reservations, are less accepting of lesbian sexual orientation than their ancestors. This is explained as a function of colonization, genocide, internalized oppression, and a loss of contact with traditional values (Allen, 1986; V. L. Sears, personal communication, May 1992; Tafoya, 1992; Williams, 1986). Hence, Native American lesbians may experience more pressure to be closeted if they live on reservations than not, prompting many to move to larger, urban areas (V. L. Sears, personal communication, May 1992; Williams, 1986). Obliteration of Native American history and lingering fears about acknowledging practices that were once ridiculed and severely punished result in the continued invisibility of Native American lesbians on reservations. Tafoya (1992) notes that many younger lesbians may even assume that they must leave the reservation to find other lesbians.

Family and community assume as significant a level of importance to Native American lesbians as they do for their other ethnic counterparts, and for similar reasons. This country's legacy of pervasive, disparaging media depictions of Native Americans are often as deeply embedded in the psyche of lesbians in the mainstream as they are in that of the rest of the dominant culture. Hence, the mainstream lesbian community, while it provides a safer place to explore a nontraditional sexual orientation, is not free of the same racism that Native American lesbians experience in other parts of society. The move away from the reservation into the lesbian community may result in the experience of loss of culture and support from family and Native American community. This loss is significant and can precipitate feelings of isolation and depression (V. L. Sears, personal communication, May 1992). Tafoya and Rowell (1988) note that ethnic identity may be primary to Native American lesbians. They may be less likely to present themselves to Native American counseling agencies, out of fear that their sexual orientation will be viewed more negatively by other Native Americans (the same is often true of Asian lesbians, as discussed below).

Tafoya and Rowell (1988) suggest that family therapies are most useful in reintegrating a lesbian member back into the family, and thus they support the culturally syntonic value of reestablishing connectiveness. While there may not be great pressure to marry, the family is often most concerned that a lesbian sexual orientation is synonymous with being childless. Motherhood is an important role for Native American women, since children are seen as the future of the tribe. However, given the higher rates of heterosexual relations of Native American women, this may be less of a realistic concern for them than for their other lesbians of color (Tafoya & Rowell, 1988). Sears (personal communication, May 1992) reports that it is not uncommon for lesbians, including those on reservations, to have children.

Despite these findings, clinicians may encounter Native American lesbians who know nothing of these traditions or concepts and may believe, as do many lesbians on first acknowledging their sexual orientation, that there is no one else like them (Ratti, 1993; Tafoya, 1992).

Asian American Lesbians

Asian American lesbians come from a number of different ethnic groups, which makes any generalizations about them potentially inaccurate. For the purposes of this discussion, the category of Asian American lesbians will comprise lesbians of Japanese or Chinese ancestry only, because it is with these groups that most research has been done.

A salient feature of Asian American families is the expectation of obedience to one's parents and their demand for conformity. This is consistent with the respect accorded elders, and the sharp delineation of gender roles (Bradshaw, 1990, and Chapter 3, this volume; Chan, 1989, 1992; Garnets & Kimmel, 1991; Gock, 1985; H., 1989). Women are expected to derive status from their roles of dutiful daughter and ultimately wife and mother, passively deferring to men, to whom they are deemed inferior (Chan, 1992; H., 1989).

Pamela H. (1989) observes that for Asian women a problem in the development of an identity as a lesbian lies in their devalued identity as women in the culture. In her analysis, women are discouraged from developing any sense of basic self-worth or identity beyond their preordained roles in the family.

In the role of mother, they are responsible for socializing children appropriately, and are thus considered responsible by family and peers if children do not conform. Hence mothers, perhaps more than other family members, are apt to be blamed if a daughter strays from the predetermined path and declares that she is a lesbian (C. Chan, personal communication, November 1992).

Heterosexual marital relationships are seen as somewhat inevitable, not as something that occurs been two people, but rather between two families for the good of the families. It may be difficult in this context for family members to view a lesbian family member as anything but selfish, in that she has deliberately made her own sexual preference and therefore her own feelings the most important variable in selecting a mate and planning her life.

The development of any sexual identity is also complicated by the taboo against open discussions about sex, which is considered a shameful topic (Chan, 1992; H., 1989). Discussions about sexuality, when they occur, focus on its biological aspects and do not explore nontraditional sexual orientations (H., 1989). Chan (personal communication, November 1992) notes that sex is presumed to be unimportant to women. Asian women are depicted in stereotyped media images in the United States as "passive, quiet, servile" (H., 1989, p. 286) and either "exotically sexy or totally asexual" (p. 293). These images contribute to the ethnosexual mythology that members of the dominant culture hold about Asian women and that some Asian women internalize themselves. Racism in the mainstream lesbian community may be expressed in the expectations of other lesbians that Asian American lesbians actually fit those stereotypes. (Gock, 1992, has reported that this racism is also reflected in the practices of bars, dances, discos, and the like in the mainstream lesbian community, who require more types of identification from Asian American lesbians than from their White counterparts.)

Pamela H. (1989) appropriately reminds us that the media images of lesbians in American films are usually dominated by White women. The tendency for Asian parents to view lesbian sexual orientation as a "Western concept" (p. 284), a product of too much assimilation or a function of losing touch with Asian heritage, may have some of its origins in the invisibility of Asian lesbians in American media depictions of lesbians (Pamela H., 1989). Pamela H. further notes that many Asian parents may be quite "oblivious" to the existence of Asian lesbians and notes that there is no word for "lesbian" in most Asian languages. A declaration of a lesbian sexual orientation may be regarded as an act of open rebellion as well as a blatant rejection of Asian heritage. The declaration of the desire for same-gender relationships may also be regarded as a temporary disorder that the parents hope or just assume their daughter will outgrow. At the other extreme, a lesbian daughter may be thought of by parents as a source of shame to the entire family (Chan, 1992; Pamela H., 1989). Lesbian sexual orientation is viewed as volitional and is presumed to represent a conscious desire to tarnish the family honor. Parents may express the feeling that they can no longer face friends or community.

Because lesbians are incorrectly presumed to be disinterested in becoming parents, a daughter's open disclosure that she is lesbian may be interpreted as a rejection of the role of mother and therefore of her most important role culturally (Chan, 1992; Garnets & Kimmel, 1991; Wooden et al., 1983).

Openly adopting a lesbian sexual orientation will generally be met with disapproval, although individual reactions will of course vary (C. Chan, personal communication, November 1992). The maintenance of outward roles and conformity is an important and distinctive cultural expectation. The fear of negative reactions to disclosure contributes significantly to the pressure to remain closeted within the Asian American community or move away from it to avoid discovery. Chan (1989) noted that over 75% of Asian American lesbians (and gay men) surveyed expressed concerns about revealing their sexual orientation to other Asians because of what they perceived as the potential for rejection and stigmatization. This may have relevant implications for choice of therapist. More research is required to determine if Asian American or other lesbians of color deem sexual orientation or a familiarity with such issues a more important variable in therapist selection than the race or ethnicity of the therapist. If lesbians of color experience members of their own ethnic group as more homophobic than members of the dominant culture, this assumption may also apply to their perception of therapists who are members of the same ethnic group. Croom (1993) provides some support for this notion in her study on African American lesbians. Chan (1992) notes that invisibility leads to the absence of Asian American lesbians who might serve as role models for young women struggling with questions about their sexual identity.

Asian American lesbians, like their other ethnic counterparts, frequently report feeling a pressure to choose between these two communities and subsequently declare the aspect of their identity that is primary. In her 1989 study of Asian American gay men and lesbians, Chan found that most respondents saw their primary identification as a gay man or lesbian rather than Asian American. This study noted however that the primacy of sexual orientation and ethnicity shifts during development, depending on which stages of ethnic-identity development and sexual-orientation identity formation the individual fits at that time. Identification may also vary depending on the need at the time. Gock (1992) proposes a detailed descriptive analysis of the identity integration process of Asian Pacific American lesbians and gay men. Lee (1991) writes of her rejection of her cultural identity,

> For most of my life, I belonged to the "don't wanna be" tribe, being ashamed and embarrassed of my Asian back ground, rejecting it. . . . My father tried his best to jam "Chineseness" down my throat, . . . (he) warned, "If you marry a White we'll cut you out of our will." . . . With my father's wish for my awareness of cultural identity came his expectation that I grow up to be a "nice Chinese girl." This meant I should be a submissive . . . obedient, morally impeccable puppet who would spend the rest of her life deferring to and selflessly appeasing her husband. . . . He wanted me to become all that was against my nature, and so I rebelled with a fury, rejecting and denying everything remotely associated with Chinese culture. . . . Becoming a lesbian challenged everything in my upbringing and confirmed the fact that I was not a nice, ladylike pamperer of men. (pp. 116, 117)

Similar intricate and complex conflicts of loyalty are also observed in lesbians of color from other ethnic groups.

Unlike gay and lesbian members of other ethnic groups, who report feeling more discrimination for their race than sexual orientation, the Asian

American gay male sample in this study reported experiencing more discrimination because they were gay than because they were Asian (Chan, 1989). This finding underscores the importance of exploring subtle gender differences in the experience and meaning of certain phenomena, even within the same culture.

Pamela H. (1989) writes that the persistent invisibility of lesbians within Asian American communities is slowly changing, with the development in the early 1980s of Asian American lesbian support and social groups within those communities. Such groups have developed in part in reaction to experiences of invisibility and racial discrimination in the broader lesbian communities, which are predominantly White and often offer little contact with other ethnic lesbians (Noda, Tsui, & Wong, 1979).

Indian and South Asian American Lesbians

Lesbians who identify with the cultures of Bhutan, Bangladesh, India, the Maldives, Nepal, Pakistan, and Sri Lanka are considered South Asian. Although they find themselves confronted with psychological tasks that are similar to other visibly ethnic lesbians (Ratti, 1993), they are virtually absent in the psychological literature. The lesbians of these cultures and countries are markedly heterogeneous. They do not necessarily identify with African American lesbians or other women of color, nor do they necessarily consider themselves persons of color at all. Vaid (cited in Meera, 1993) observes that many Indians view Great Britain as their mother country and for that reason may more closely identify with Whites. Hence clinicians must consider the psychological demands made of lesbians who may be viewed as women of color because of their skin color, but who do not experience themselves as ethnic minorities in the same way that lesbians of color who have been raised in the United States may. They must also consider the conundrum of identifications, alliances, and expectations lesbians of color often have of one another based on assumptions about the meaning of skin color as well as sexual orientation in different parts of the world (see Jayakar, Chapter 6, this volume).

Bearing some similarity to broader Asian cultures, gender roles in Indian and South Asian societies are clearly delineated, in a patriarchal social organization. Strict obedience to parents, even among adult children, is expected, as is conformity to social expectations. Among those expectations is that of marriage, which is still frequently arranged by parents or families, and having children. The pressure to marry and have children is quite explicit and may be quite intense. As it is in most patriarchal societies, women are considered inferior and of less importance than men.

Ratti (1993) and Jayakar (Chapter 6, this volume) observe India and South Asia as lands of contradiction. Jayakar notes in particular that the open discussion or expression of sexuality is taboo, in the same land that produced the Kama Sutra, the world's first literary classic on sexual matters

(AIDS Bhedbar Virodhi Andolan [AIDS BVA], 1993; Ratti, 1993). This makes the discussion of lesbian sexual orientation even less likely and more difficult. Despite a history of sexual behavior between women, reflected in art, literature, sculpture, and painting, as well as sexual and emotional involvement that is self-identified as lesbian, contemporary mainstream Indians view lesbians in much the same way as their other ethnic counterparts, as a social or psychological aberration (AIDS BVA, 1993); as a Western phenomenon or disease that is alien to Indian culture (Bannerji, 1993; Heske, Khayal, & Utsa, 1986; Ratti, 1993).

Generally, the existence of lesbians is not acknowledged in these cultures, but this was not always the case. Heske et al. (1986) write that a history of tolerance of same-gender sexual behavior, particularly in India, was punished and then suppressed by British colonization. Utsa (in Heske et al., 1986) notes that despite (or because of) the patriarchal context of Indian society, there is significant emotional bonding and warmth between women. It would be natural, in a society that is segregated on the basis of gender in many arenas, that women who develop in great proximity to one another, and apart from men, would have more opportunities for close and intimate relationships among them.

The imposition of British morals and values influenced the creation of repressive Indian laws in 1861 (based on British law) that forbid homosexual behavior (Heske et al., 1986). As of 1986 homosexuality was still a legal offense under Section 377 of the Indian penal code, punishable with prison sentences ranging from 10 years to life (Heske et al., 1986). Kim (1993) observes that gay men and lesbians in India do not make themselves as visible as their White counterparts in the United States, out of a pragmatic fear of the backlash of homophobia that would accompany it.

Ratti (1993) notes that the intense pressure for women to marry—usually in arranged marriages—and raise a family makes it extremely difficult for women who are lesbians to build a life with another woman. This forces many into unhappy heterosexual marriages. Some of these women have secret liaisons with women lovers but maintain a heterosexual marriage. Another significant factor mitigating against such relationships is the economic dependence of women in India. Leaving the country and moving to the United States or Great Britain is often an alternative only for a well-educated or financially secure minority (Heske et al., 1986). Of course some women come to the United States to study, but they are usually not from the poorer classes or rural areas. Hence, many Indian lesbians encountered in treatment settings in the United States are from more economically or educationally privileged backgrounds.

Ratti (1993) estimates that there are 80 million gay men and lesbians in India (based on an estimate of 10% of the general population). But these large numbers of lesbians in India are spread over a vast country. There are no organized, vocal lesbian movements or communities within the country, and few if any magazines or clubs similar to those in the United States. Heske et al. (1986) observes that with the exception of small isolated groups who meet individually and informally, it is difficult to know who is lesbian and who is not and thus even to meet other lesbians. Isolation is therefore a significant issue.

In the United States, Indian and South Asian lesbians report that while the broader lesbian community affords them the opportunity to meet other lesbians in a less stigmatized environment, there remains a significant sense of isolation and invisibility (Bannerji, 1993; Heske et al., 1986; Ratti, 1993). Ratti (1993) attributes this invisibility to scarcity and neglect of the concerns of Indian and South Asian lesbians in the lesbian movement in the United States as well as the expectation that lesbians fit a generic lesbian mold, one that is usually articulated from a majority perspective. This expectation overlooks important cultural differences, which Indian lesbians are left to negotiate. Heske et al. (1986) write that for some Indian lesbians, public displays of affection between lesbians in the United States and the transitory nature of some relationships is at variance with their culture's emphasis on public propriety and longstanding monogamy. Utsa (in Heske et al., 1986) states, "I come from a culture where people have very deep, long-standing bonds with each other. . . . For me to look at relationships and friendships in such a short-term fashion is very hard" (p. 143).

Jayakar (Chapter 6, this volume) notes that Indian women are social-ized to deny directly both their sexuality and any sexual knowledge. The clinician may not assume that Indian lesbians would be any more comfort-able with direct discussions of sexual matters than their heterosexual coun-terparts, even in the private context of therapy. Such discussions must be handled with particular sensitivity.

Another challenge confronting lesbians in these groups is that of racism and ethnocentrism in the broader lesbian community in the United States. Khayal (in Heske et al., 1986) characterizes White women as narrow minded in their concepts of lesbianism in other societies. Heske (in Heske et al., 1986) offers an example in reporting her own surprise in finding that an Indian woman dressed in traditional Indian clothing who she had recently met was a lesbian, and that there was a large population of Indian women who were lesbian as well. This phenomenon may also be a reflec-tion of the invisibility of Indian lesbians in India and the absence of their images in the popular media depictions of lesbians in the United States. Each phenomenon may then circularly reinforce the other.

Like lesbians from other groups discussed here, Indian American lesbians are faced with marginalization and racism in the broader lesbian community (Bannerji, 1993; Heske et al., 1986; Khush, 1993; Ratti, 1993). Reports of being treated like strange, exotic creatures are not uncommon, nor are episodes of discrimination in bars, clubs, dances, meetings, and collectives (Bannerji, 1993; Heske et al., 1993). Bannerji (1993) writes:

Much of the experience of racism is constructed through gender. As a child
and adolescent, I not only yearned to be a White girl, . . . I also saw White
femaleness through White men's eyes. . . . The first women to whom I was
attracted reflected the White male gaze I had obediently eroticized. I found
nothing sensual about my own body nor the bodies of black and Indian girls
around me. (p. 61)

She continues and comments on the parallels between her invisibility as a
woman in a patriarchal society and as an Indian lesbian in the broader
U.S. lesbian community: "Just as men had silenced me in the solidarity
committees and meetings of the left, so too I found White lesbians talking
for me and about me as though I was not present" (Bannerji, 1993, p. 60).

Shah (1993) posits that South Asian lesbians have to define themselves
because of the extreme lack of awareness of them in both South Asian
patriarchal societies and in Western lesbian communities. In the absence
of the word "lesbian" in their native languages, they have developed their
own names for themselves. The Sanskrit word "*anamika*" (p. 114), which
means "nameless" was taken by a lesbian collective in 1985 and was used to
address the lack of names in South Asian languages for lesbian relationships
(Shah, 1993). Other names have been developed out of various South Asian
languages by lesbians of those cultures who wish to name themselves in
affirmative ways.

Like their ethnic counterparts, the relationships between Indian and
South Asian lesbians and their families is intense and complex. While there
is a strong commitment to family, and family bonds may override the
family's homophobia, Parmar (cited in Khush, 1993) notes that "coming
out" carries the realistic risk of being rejected, to the extreme of being
completely shunned.

Latina Lesbians

Espín (1984) and others (Amaro, 1978; Hidalgo & Hidalgo-Christensen,
1976; Morales, 1989; Vasquez, 1979) report that gender roles are well
established within Latino families and culture. Women are generally expected to be overtly submissive, virtuous (virginal), respectful of elders,
and willing to defer to men, who are considered superior to women (Espín,
1984; Morales, 1989). While women are encouraged to maintain emotional
and physical closeness to other women, such behavior is not presumed to
be lesbian (Amaro, 1978; Espín, 1984; Hidalgo & Hidalgo-Christensen,
1976). Closeness with female friends is encouraged, particularly during
adolescence, and may serve as a way of protecting the virginity of young
women by diminishing their contact with males. The open discussion of
sex and sexuality between women is not culturally sanctioned, and women
are expected to be sexually naive (Espín, 1984). Comas-Díaz (personal
communication, January 1993) suggests that there is a known tolerance

for same-gender sexual behavior among males, as long as it is not overtly labeled as the person's preferred behavior. This avoidance of adopting a stigmatized identity is explained as a function of the cultural importance of saving face, a key component of maintaining dignity and commanding respect. Being indirect is the culturally prescribed way of managing conflict, since in that way participants do not lose face. Espín (1987) contends that in labeling themselves lesbian, Latina women force a culture that denies the sexuality of women to confront it. Furthermore, it implies not only a woman's conscious participation in sexual behavior—behavior that is taboo and that is not performed out of duty to her husband but out of her own desire—but also a confrontation of others with the fact that she engages in forbidden behavior. This stance not only violates the taboo against engaging in such behavior but also challenges the cultural directive to be indirect or avoidant in the face of conflict.

According to Trujillo (1991), the majority of Chicano heterosexuals view Chicana lesbians as a threat to the established order of male dominance in Chicano communities. Their existence is viewed as having the potential of raising the consciousness of Chicana women, causing them to question the premises of male dominance and female subordination.

Espín (1984), Hidalgo and Hidalgo-Christensen (1976), and Morales (1992) suggest that disapproval in Latino communities is more intense than the homophobia in the dominant "Anglo" community. They further suggest that a powerful form of heterosexist oppression takes place within Latin cultures leaving many lesbian members feeling a pressure to remain closeted. Declaring a lesbian sexual orientation may be experienced as an act of treason against the culture and family. Espín (1984, 1987) and Hidalgo (1984) note that a lesbian family member may maintain a place in the family and be quietly tolerated, but this does not constitute acceptance of her lesbian sexual orientation. It is more likely that such tolerance reflects the family's denial. Generally, only masculine looking females ("butch") would be perceived as lesbian and challenged.

The extent to which Latina lesbians will present themselves as gender-role stereotyped in their own relationships, or the degree to which they will observe stereotypes learned in a culture where gender roles are somewhat rigid, will be a function of their level of acculturation, as well as of the extent to which their own families engage in traditional gender roles (Morales, 1989). Despite the anti-lesbian sentiment of their ethnic communities and families, Espín (1987) and Hidalgo (1984) found that there was a deep attachment among Latina lesbians to those communities. Gutierrez (1992) writes:

> It isn't easy to be part of a gay and lesbian culture whose rites and institutions too often consider us to be peripheral or an acquired taste. . . . Our families may reject us but we belong to them nonetheless. . . . The same is true for our friends, neighborhoods, etc. . . . We must not abandon them, . . . they

are ours. . . . Even if it is impossible to stay, they remain ours for as long as we claim them. (p. 242)

MENTAL HEALTH ISSUES

Lesbian women of color exist within a tangle of multiply devalued identities, surrounded by the oppression and discrimination that accompany institutionalized racism, sexism, and heterosexism. Unlike their White counterparts, lesbians of color bear the additional task involved in integrating major features of their identity when they are conspicuously devalued. Unlike their ethnic identities, their sexual orientation and sometimes their gender may be devalued by those closest to them in their families.

Women of color usually receive positive cultural mirroring during development, generally but not exclusively through their families. This helps to buffer the demeaning messages and distorted, stereotyped images of themselves created and maintained by the dominant culture. Those who do not receive positive cultural mirroring are at risk for internalizing society's racism.

Lesbians of color also learn a range of negative stereotypes about lesbian sexual orientation long before they know that they are lesbian themselves. With the exception of Native Americans, other ethnic groups have either no words in their language for lesbian or only words and names that are degrading. The unquestioned internalization of pernicious attitudes about lesbians, gleaned from loved and trusted figures, complicates the process of lesbian identity development and self-acceptance for women of color in ways that are not as complex for their White counterparts (Gock, 1992).

Regardless of the specific ethnic group to which they belong, lesbian women of color must manage the dominant culture's racism, sexism, and heterosexism, as well as that of their own ethnic group. Although most lesbians of color experience their ethnic communities as being of great practical and emotional significance, the homophobia in these communities makes lesbian members more vulnerable, perhaps more inclined to remain closeted, and therefore invisible to them (Chan, 1992; Espín, 1984; Greene, 1993, in press; Mays & Cochran, 1988; Morales, 1989; Moses & Hawkins, 1982). This increases their psychological vulnerability. How important these ties may be to an individual client may vary depending on the degree of her attachment to her cultural background and the degree of acculturation (Falco, 1991). Appropriate, intense ties to ethnic community and family may complicate the "coming out" process for lesbians of color in ways that it may not for their White counterparts. Decisions about coming out to family members are already fraught with anxiety for most women who are lesbians, but for lesbians of color there is often more to lose. Lesbians of color cannot presume acceptance by the broader lesbian community if their families reject them, and they risk giving up an important source of support if this feared rejection occurs.

Just as the oppression created by heterosexism produces greater stressors for lesbians than for heterosexual women, the combined effects of racism, sexism, and heterosexism for lesbians of color intensify and complicate the stressors for them (Morgan & Eliason, 1992). While we may assume that the stress of coming out is intense for lesbians of color, because they must manage multiple oppressions, we must also assume that they may bring unique resources and resiliences to this task. Lesbians of color, unlike their White counterparts, have often been forced to learn useful coping mechanisms against racism and discrimination, long before they ever realized that they were lesbians. When confronted with managing other devalued aspects of their identities they may call on the mechanisms used against racism to assist them. Psychotherapy can be useful in developing an awareness of these resources in the client and assisting her in their effective use. Problems occur when previously learned coping mechanisms are maladaptive or self-destructive, hence clients in this category are perhaps more vulnerable to the development of serious pathology. Other variables include not simply the mere presence of other stressors, but their intensity and the amount of attention they require on an ongoing basis. There is no empirical data with significant numbers of lesbians of color to justify more than clinical speculations in this area, but it might be safe to say that it is somewhat more difficult for lesbians of color to be out than for their White counterparts. Further research is needed.

The quiet toleration observed in many ethnic minority families for a lesbian member is generally marked by denial and the need to view lesbian sexual orientations as something whose origins exist outside the culture. Tremble et al. (1989) suggests that attributing lesbian sexual orientation to some outside source may in fact enable some families to accept a family member while removing themselves or that family member from any perceived sense of responsibility. Hence the ubiquitous notion that a lesbian sexual orientation is a Western or White man's disease that is "caught" or chosen. Thus a rationale for rejecting lesbian sexual orientation can be developed by presenting it as if it and ethnic identity were mutually exclusive (Chan, 1992; Espín, 1987; Greene, 1994, in press; Hidalgo, 1984; Mays & Cochran, 1988; Morales, 1989, 1992; Tremble et al., 1989). The woman who is lesbian is then presented with the notion that if she were true to her ethnic heritage she would have no part in such a lifestyle.

Many people of color believe that only heterosexual orientation is natural or normal and, by correlation, that a woman of color who is lesbian has "chosen" her sexual orientation. Thus follows the assumption that she could choose to be heterosexual if she wanted to do so. Some family members may assert that the choice a lesbian family member makes to acknowledge this aspect of her identity is done deliberately to hurt them. When treating a family member of a lesbian of color it is important to be familiar with these stereotypes, to assist them in understanding that a lesbian relative does not consciously choose her sexual orientation any more than a heterosexual woman does, and to advise them that their support is important to her.

Members of ethnic minority communities as well as White lesbians often choose to view identity as if it were a singular entity. Strong identification with one's ethnic group and alternately sexual orientation are often perceived as if they were mutually exclusive of each other as well as other aspects of identity. Hence, being lesbian is often viewed by ethnic heterosexual peers as a repudiation of one's ethnicity. Similarly, lesbians from the dominant culture often lack an appreciation for the ongoing work required to cope adaptively with racism and, concomitantly the strength and importance of ethnic ties. This can leave lesbians of color feeling poorly understood, as well as guilt ridden about which community to devote their resources to.

Lesbians of color find themselves confronted with racial stereotypes and discrimination in the broader lesbian community. With the exception of large cities, most minority communities are not large enough to maintain a distinct or formal lesbian community of their own (Tremble et al., 1989). Hence, interactions with members of the mainstream lesbian community become important outlets for social support and for meeting others. However, lesbians of color commonly report discriminatory treatment in lesbian bars, clubs, and social and political gatherings and in individuals within the lesbian community (Chan, 1992; Dyne, 1980; Garnets & Kimmel, 1991; Greene, 1994, in press; Gutierrez & Dworkin, 1992; Mays & Cochran, 1988; Morales, 1989). They describe feeling an intense sense of conflicting loyalties to two communities, in both of which they are marginalized by the requirement to conceal or minimize important aspects of their identities in order to be accepted.

Lesbians of color frequently experience a sense of never being part of any group completely, leaving them at greater risk for isolation, feelings of estrangement, and increased psychological vulnerability. When in the midst of groups like themselves there may be a tendency to idealize the group. What often follows is the expectation of a level of similarity, acceptance, being liked, and being understood in ways that never quite live up to the fantasy. Hence, a client may experience a disturbing sense of aloneness or disappointment, or a heightened sense of not fitting in any setting when idealized environments fail to meet all of their expectations, or when their expectations are unrealistic. While the variance within these groups may be as wide as the variance between them and other groups, that variance may be concealed by similarities. Similarities in experiences and characteristics between people are important, but they do not warrant the assumption that they will automatically result in a person's being perfectly understood on all levels.

Some clients with more serious preexisting psychopathology may tend to idealize people who are like them and devalue people who are not like them, rather than make judgments on a person-to-person basis. In some clients this may reflect a particular stage of lesbian–ethnic minority identity development. However, it may also represent the client's own deeply rooted sense of self-hate. In any case such a stance actually increases her difficulty getting support from the outside world by restricting the range of people from whom it may be obtained. This difficulty then fuels or confirms a self-fulfilling fear of being unable to get support or of being unworthy. More seriously disturbed clients may rapidly alternate between idealization and devaluation of the group, a particular aspect of themselves about which they feel conflicted, and, if known, that same aspect of the therapist. Ethnicity, gender, and sexual orientation are overdetermined characteristics for idealizing and devaluing stances; such behavior thus may be most acute during the early stages of coming out or at other times of crisis.

Relationship Issues for Lesbian Women of Color

Lesbian women of color find themselves in relationships that are largely unsupported outside of the lesbian community. Differences within the lesbian community on preferences for some relationship structures over others are pertinent, but beyond the scope of this chapter. What is clear, however, is that these women may encounter unique challenges in relationships with partners who have the same gender socialization, in a culture that has few open, healthy models of such relationships. That same environment conspicuously devalues their person and devalues their relationships on many levels as well. While lesbian women of color may be accustomed to obtaining family support for their struggles with racism and perhaps sexism they may not presume the appropriate support of family for their romantic relationships or for their appropriate distress if that relationship is troubled. On seeking professional assistance they may find few if any therapists who have training in addressing the many nuances of nontraditional relationships.

Lesbians of color are found in relationships with women who are not of their own ethnic group to a significantly greater degree than are their White counterparts (Croom, 1993; Mays & Cochran, 1988; Tafoya & Rowell, 1988), a phenomenon that has been attributed in part to the fact that there are larger numbers of White lesbians to choose from (Tafoya & Rowell, 1988). While heterosexual interracial relationships bring unique challenges and often lack support on both sides of families and communities, for lesbians of color, they provide yet another challenge in a process that is already fraught with difficulty.

An interracial lesbian couple may be more publicly visible, as a couple, than two women of the same ethnic group. This brings realities of racism that the White partner may have never encountered before. Clunis and Green (1988) observe that because women have tried to avoid racism does not mean that it disappears from their relationships. Lesbians of color have usually developed a variety of coping strategies in addressing racism, and often wear a protective psychological armor (Sears, 1987). Because it is a ubiquitous reality and stressor for them they learn to prioritize their responses to it. A White partner may never have had to do this and may be less prepared (Clunis & Green, 1988). The latter may either fail to notice slights that are racist in origin and experience her partner's anger as inappropriate, may overreact (experience her partner as underreactive), or may take on a protective role that her partner does not require or desire, and may even find patronizing.

A White partner may also feel guilty about racism and may be unaware of the distinction she must make between her personal behavior in the relationship and the racism in the outside world. In the latter case she may attempt to compensate her partner personally for the racism she faces in the world, a task that she cannot do successfully and that will ultimately leave her feeling angry and frustrated. In such relationships neither the lesbian of color nor her White partner can realistically assume that a White partner is free of racism because of her political beliefs or intentions (Clunis & Green, 1988; Garcia, Kennedy, Pearlman, & Perez, 1987). The lesbian of color in such relationships may also need to be aware of her own jealousy or resentment of her lover's privileged status in the dominant culture and in the lesbian community. Both partners may be perceived as lacking loyalty to their own cultures and may even feel ashamed of their involvement with a person who is not of the same race (Clunis & Green, 1988; Falco, 1991; Greene, in press). This complicates both the resolution of issues within the relationship and intensifies the complex web of loyalties and estrangements for lesbian women of color.

While racial issues and cultural differences may contribute to realistic challenges to lesbian relationships, they do not account for all of the problems within them. Racial and cultural differences are often scapegoated as the problem, allowing the couple to avoid looking at more threatening issues. Differences that are most visible lend themselves to be seen as the cause of problems, particularly when simple explanations are desired. At times racial differences may be the cause of significant difficulties, but other problems may be experienced as if they were about racial or ethnic differences when they have more complex origins within the relationship.

Choices of partners and feelings about those choices may reflect conflicts about intimacy and other interpersonal issues. They may also reflect conflicts about racial and ethnic identity. These conflicts may be expressed by lesbian women of color who choose or are attracted to White women exclusively, or who devalue lesbians of color as unsuitable partners.

Lesbians of color who experience themselves as racially or culturally deficient or ambiguous may presume that a partner who is a member of their own ethnic group will somehow compensate for their perceived deficiency or that such a choice will demonstrate their cultural loyalty.

There may also be a tendency for a lesbian of color in a relationship with a lesbian from a different minority ethnic group to presume a level of similarity of experience or worldview that is not present. While many of their experiences in the dominant culture as oppressed women of color and lesbians may be similar, their respective views on their roles in a relationship, maintaining a household, and the role of other family members in their lives can be very different.

Some lesbians of color may be appropriately sensitive to what Sears (personal communication, May 1992) refers to as "pony stealing" and Clunis and Green (1988, p. 140) as "ethnic chasing," while Lee (1991, p. 117) describes certain White lesbians as "Asianophiles." These terms are used to identify White women who seek out lesbians of color as partners to assuage their own guilt about being White, to compensate for their lack of a strong ethnic identity, or to prove their liberal attitudes. The ethnosexual stereotypes of lesbians of color as less sexually inhibited than their White counterparts may serve as another determinant of this behavior. An ethnic chaser may seek, usually unconsciously, to gain from proximity to a lesbian of color whatever they perceive to be lacking in themselves. As these attempts at self-repair are doomed to fail, the partner who is not a woman of color may respond by feeling angry, resentful, and somehow betrayed by her partner. In treatment settings it is helpful to assist women in such relationships to clarify their expectations about being in any relationship. Beyond this general assessment, the kinds of assumptions held about ethnic or White women in an intimate relationship should be explored.

Exclusive choices in this realm may also reflect a woman's tendency to idealize people who are like her and devalue those who are not, or the reverse. When this is the case, the reality often does not live up to the fantasy, resulting in disappointment and self-denigration. It is important to remember that many of these decisions are made without conscious awareness of them and, most importantly, that they may have many different determinants.

A therapist should not presume that participation in an interracial lesbian relationship is an automatic expression of cultural or racial self-hate in the woman of color. Nor should he or she presume that a relationship between two lesbians of color is necessarily anchored in loyalty or respect for that culture, or in any of the aforementioned problematic premises. What is of significance is that the therapist be aware of a wide range of clinical possibilities and explore them accordingly.

TREATMENT IMPLICATIONS: COUNTERTRANSFERENCE ISSUES

Lesbian sexual orientation, racial differences, and the social conflicts that surround these matters are issues about which most people have intense feelings. Psychotherapists are no exception. The sensitive treatment of lesbian women of color in psychotherapy brings those provocative issues together in a profound way, and creates a range of challenges for even the most experienced psychotherapist.

Initially, the therapist must be culturally literate, familiar with the broader characteristics of the client's culture as well as the special strengths and vulnerabilities of clients who are lesbians. A majority of graduate training programs do not routinely offer training in these areas; therefore, therapists must be willing to seek that training elsewhere. This may be accomplished by combining attendance in special workshops or classes with individual or group supervision with clinicians who have training in these respective areas. Failure to do so can result in less than adequate treatment to clients (Greene, 1994, in press).

The interaction between culture, gender, and sexual orientation is not static. Rather, it is dynamic, encompassing major dimensions around which people organize their assumptions about who they are in the world. In therapy, unraveling these issues, their interactions, and the mechanisms developed to adapt to them is complex, to say the least. The therapist who has not taken the time to explore the manifestations of these dilemmas fully will find it difficult if not impossible to unravel them successfully. This process must also include the therapist's personal examination of her or his own feelings and responses to women of color and to lesbians, as well as her or his own sexual orientation, gender, and ethnicity. Therapists must also be aware of the stereotypes and beliefs about women of color and lesbians that they have internalized without question. These variables may, if unexamined, predispose the therapist to make a range of inaccurate assumptions about clients and their experiences.

Heterosexual female therapists who are insecure in their own feelings about sexual orientation, or who expect lesbian clients of color to be preoccupied with sexual matters, may be predisposed to have greater expectations of eroticized transferences from lesbian clients of color. In this example, if the therapist has a personal need to see such transferences, she may tend to overlook or minimize issues that are of greater importance to the client. For some heterosexual therapists such transference reactions are frightening and may be perceived as a threat to the therapist's own sexual orientation, particularly if the therapist is insecure about it. If therapists fear that such transference reactions will occur, they may tend to overlook them, avoid appropriate explorations of material that might expose such feelings in the client, or avoid addressing the client's direct expressions of such material. Heterosexual therapists who are insecure about their own sexual orientation may also find themselves "leaking" personal information to the client, particularly in the midst of eroticized transference reactions, presumably to let clients know that they are not lesbian. The therapist may find that this occurs despite the fact that she does not ordinarily disclose such information without judicious consideration of how it would be helpful to the client to do so, or despite being generally neutral about such matters.

Most therapists struggle with the delicate balance involved in urging a client who is a lesbian of color to assume greater personal responsibility for her actions, when appropriate, without seeming insensitive to the realistic barriers that are a result of the many levels of discrimination she faces. The therapist errs, however, if feeling sorry for or admiring the client leads him or her to avoid setting appropriate limits in treatment or to fail to direct the client's attention to her own role in her dilemma. Such a therapist may feel uncomfortable when the situation warrants more than support and validation for the client's struggles.

Therapists who are White and heterosexual, regardless of gender, may inadvertently find themselves bending over backward to accommodate the client who is a lesbian of color, failing to maintain appropriate boundaries or behaving in ways that they would not with other clients. Such behavior may be evoked in the therapist if the client makes him or her feel guilty, angry, uncomfortable or incompetent. There may be a need to compensate the client in some way for the therapist's feeling of inadequacy. Therapists may also feel guilty about their memberships in dominant and oppressive groups and may seek to compensate the client by being indulgent. Of course this is never helpful to the client, since it is motivated by the therapist's guilt rather than his or her genuine concern for the client's welfare (Greene, 1994).

Judith White (personal communication, February 1993) observes that sexual behavior, like any other behavior, constitutes a vehicle for communicating feelings and as such warrants exploration in therapy. It is not unusual for the lesbian of color to express reluctance or refusal to explore this area in any detail, if at all, with a heterosexual therapist. They may be even less likely to agree to discuss such matters with a heterosexual therapist who is a member of the client's ethnic group. Such reluctance is understandable, since many lesbian clients have accurately experienced such inquiries as voyeuristic on the part of homophobic therapists. It is also noted that lesbian clients of color may perceive therapists who are members of their ethnic group and whom they presume are heterosexual as potentially more homophobic than a therapist from the dominant culture (Croom, 1993; Gock, 1992; Tafoya, 1992).

It is important to be sensitive to the client's feelings about making such disclosures, but that does not mean that the material should go unexplored. It is the therapist's responsibility to earn the client's trust and assist her in understanding the importance of such inquiries. It may be helpful to assist the client in understanding by whom she feels sexually excited and why. If the therapist, however, feels uncomfortable with this material, he or she may respond to the client's reluctance by avoiding any further exploration of it. The therapist may believe this is respecting the client's feelings, but avoidance may just as likely be contrary to a client's interests as in them. For example, the therapist may be avoiding what he or she thinks the material will elicit from the client, or may not want to challenge any of the client's assumptions or perceptions. This may arise out of some irrational fear of what the client will do in response, worrying that, for example, the client will discontinue therapy. The therapist may fear that the client's departure from therapy would reflect badly on the therapist, confirming the therapist's fears of incompetence. Hence, the therapist's insecurity about treating lesbians of color and anxiety that they may terminate treatment can cripple his or her ability to challenge and explore clients' feelings appropriately.

Similarly, a White heterosexual therapist may have difficulty understanding and accepting the realistic barriers imposed by racism and homophobia in the client's life, just as a male therapist may not fully understand the role of sexism in a woman's life. This does not mean that all White heterosexual or male therapists are destined to respond in this way, but rather that this is a potential occurrence. This dilemma may be responded to by attempting to move too quickly past communications about discrimination by avoiding, dismissing, or minimizing their importance. While clients may unconsciously use realistic problems associated with racism, sexism, and heterosexism to avoid an exploration of material that is even more painful, the realistic magnitude of life stressors associated with these dimensions cannot be underestimated. They warrant the same respectful attention in therapy as intrapsychic explorations (Greene, 1994).

The therapist who is also a lesbian of color may be predisposed to certain countertransference dilemmas. The most obvious is observed in the therapist who is overidentified with the client, and as a result tends to overlook or minimize psychopathology. The therapist may attribute all of the client's problems to the barriers that result from institutional oppression, and may unconsciously avoid an exploration of other significant aspects of the client's personal life. A therapist who harbors a fear of overidentification or loss of her own boundaries tends to avoid any identification with the client, which can impair the therapist's capacity for empathy.

The therapist who is a lesbian or lesbian of color may face other countertransference issues related to the maintenance of therapeutic boundaries. Most therapists are faced with the challenge of maintaining appropriate distance without seeming aloof and disinterested in the client's dilemma. This is complicated by the tendency for some clients with multiple minority status similar or identical to that of the therapist to harbor idealized expectations of the therapist and of therapy. There may be a tendency to presume that the therapist "knows" exactly how she feels because she is the "same." In this fantasized view of the therapist, the client may presume that the therapist will not need to ask detailed questions about sensitive issues or explore intrapsychic parameters of realistic problems related to ethnicity, gender, sexual orientation, or the discrimination that accompanies them.

While such assumptions may be flattering to the therapist initially, one must be careful not to reinforce these erroneous beliefs. Doing so often serves the purpose of blocking or cutting off communication and exploration rather than facilitating it. Furthermore, acting on these beliefs predisposes the therapist to substitute intellectual discussions of social phenomena for therapeutic inquiries. The latter practice should not be confused with validating the client's accurate perception of discriminatory barriers.

Lesbian women of color are often vulnerable to isolation and estrangement. Therapists who are members of these groups are no exception. Therapists who are lesbians of color must be sure that they have developed supportive networks of peers and colleagues and adequate social and emotional support in their own lives, lest they inadvertently seek to gratify these needs, turning to clients with whom they share these important human dimensions. Many aspects of the psychotherapy process can facilitate a client's wish for a personal relationship with the therapist. In this scenario, lesbian of color clients and therapists share significant and realistic experiences, and are members of groups that are much smaller than the mainstream. In this context it can be tempting for the therapist to view clients as potential social acquaintances, friends, or even lovers. This is a natural phenomenon when people share important attributes or life experiences, and particularly when they are members of minority groups in hostile environments. If, however the therapist succumbs to the temptation to develop a dual relationship with the client, she engages in the unethical practice of abdicating her primary role and responsibility to respond to the needs of the client as a therapist, adopting instead the easier social role. Similarly, therapists who discuss their ambivalence about maintaining the boundaries of the relationship or their own desire for a personal relationship with a client risk being seductive. Discussions of this sort should take place in the therapist's own therapy or supervision. While such behavior gratifies the therapist's personal needs, there is no evidence to suggest that it is ever helpful to the client. In fact, most evidence suggests the contrary (Gartrell, 1993). Furthermore, client requests or even demands for such contacts or relationships do not relieve therapists of responsibility for the negative effects of granting such requests. The failure to maintain boundaries in this area appropriately can effectively undermine the client's treatment.

SUMMARY

Many lesbian women of color in the United States come from ethnic groups who were at some point in history colonized or captured by invaders from countries with patriarchal values. For all of these women, the original values and practices of their cultures were altered by this contact; some were almost obliterated. As a result, many people took on the patriarchal values of their colonizers and others became more intensely patriarchal than they were prior to contact. In these systems, women who are not subordinate to men and who challenge or do not rigidly adhere to traditional gender roles must be discredited, making lesbian sexuality an affront. Men of color are expected to treat women in accordance with these values. Openly acknowledging or tolerating lesbians of color may be perceived as a failure to keep the women in their culture subordinate. Hence there are complex roots to homophobia in the groups discussed earlier, and in lesbians of color themselves.

In this context, there is the potential for negative effects on the health and psychological well-being of lesbian women of color. Mental health practitioners must make themselves aware of the distinct combinations of stressors and psychological demands impinging on lesbians of color, particularly the potential for isolation, anger, and frustration. Aside from being culturally literate, the practitioner must develop a sense of the unique experience of the client with respect to the importance of their ethnic identity, gender, and sexual orientation and their need to establish priorities in an often confusing and painful maze of loyalties and estrangements.

ACKNOWLEDGMENT

The author thanks Nancy Boyd-Franklin, Connie Chan, Lillian Comas-Díaz, Vickie Sears, and Judith White for their helpful comments and discussions during the preparation of this chapter. This work is dedicated to the memory of Dr. E. Kitch Childs (1937–1993) and Audre Lorde (1934–1992).

REFERENCES

Acosta, E. (1979, October). Affinity for Black heritage: Seeking lifestyle within a community. *The Blade, 11,* A-1, A-25.

AIDS Bhedbar Virodhi Andolan. (1993). Homosexuality in India: Culture and heritage. In R. Ratti (Ed.), *A lotus of another color* (pp. 21–33). Boston: Alyson.

Allen, P. G. (1984). Beloved women: The lesbian in American Indian culture. In T. Darty & S. Potter (Eds.), *Women identified women* (pp. 83–96). Palo Alto, CA: Mayfield.

Allen, P. G. (1986). *The sacred hoop: Recovering the feminine in American Indian traditions.* Boston: Beacon Press.

Amaro, H. (1978). *Coming out: Hispanic lesbians, their families and communities.* Paper presented at the National Coalition of Hispanic Mental Health and Human Services Organization, Austin, TX.

Bannerji, K. (1993). No apologies. In R. Ratti (Ed.), *A lotus of another color* (pp. 59–64). Boston: Alyson

Bass-Hass, R. (1968). The lesbian dyad: Basic issues and value systems. *Journal of Sex Research, 4,* 126.

Bell, A., & Weinberg, M. (1978). *Homosexualities: A study of human diversity among men and women.* New York: Simon & Schuster.

Boyd-Franklin, N. (1990). *Black families in therapy: A multisystems approach*. New York: Guilford Press.

Bradshaw, C. (1990). A Japanese view of dependency: What can Amae psychology contribute to feminist theory and therapy? *Women and Therapy, 9*, 67–86.

Brownworth, V. A. (1993, June). Linda Villarosa speaks out. *Deneuve, 3*(3), 16–19, 56.

Chan, C. (1987). Asian lesbians: Psychological issues in the "coming out" process. *Asian American Psychological Association Journal, 12*, 16–18.

Chan, C. (1989). Issues of identity development among Asian American lesbians and gay men. *Journal of Counseling and Development, 68*(1), 16–20.

Chan, C. (1992). Cultural considerations in counseling Asian American lesbians and gay men. In S. Dworkin & F. Gutierrez (Eds.), *Counseling gay men and lesbians* (pp. 115–124). Alexandria, VA: American Association for Counseling and Development.

Christian, B. (1985). *Black feminist criticism: Perspectives on Black women writers*. New York: Pergamon.

Clarke, C. (1983). The failure to transform: Homophobia in the Black community. In B. Smith (Ed.), *Home girls: A Black feminist anthology* (pp. 197–208). New York: Kitchen Table–Women of Color Press.

Clarke, C. (1991). Saying the least said, telling the least told: The voices of Black lesbian writers. In M. Silvera (Ed.), *Piece of my heart: A lesbian of color anthology* (pp. 171–179). Toronto, Ontario: Sister Vision Press.

Claybourne, J. (1978). Blacks and gay liberation. In K. Jay & A. Young (Eds.), *Lavender culture* (pp. 458–465). New York: Jove/Harcourt Brace Jovanovich.

Clunis, M., & Green, G. D. (1988). *Lesbian couples*. Seattle, WA: Seal Press.

Collins, P. H. (1990). Homophobia and Black lesbians. In *Black feminist thought: Knowledge, consciousness, and the politics of empowerment* (pp. 192–196). Boston: Unwin Hyman.

Croom, G. (1993). *The effects of a consolidated versus non-consolidated identity on expectations of African American lesbians selecting mates: A pilot study*. Unpublished doctoral dissertation, Illinois School of Professional Psychology, Chicago, IL.

deMonteflores, C. (1986). Notes on the management of difference. In T. Stein & C. Cohen (Eds.), *Contemporary perspectives on psychotherapy with lesbians and gay men* (pp. 73–101). New York: Plenum.

Dew, M. A. (1985). The effects of attitudes on inferences of homosexuality and perceived physical attractiveness in women. *Sex Roles, 12*, 143–155.

Dyne, L. (1980, September). Is D.C. becoming the gay capitol of America? *Washingtonian*, pp. 96–101, 133–141.

Espín, O. (1984). Cultural and historical influences on sexuality in Hispanic/Latina women: Implications for psychotherapy. In C. Vance (Ed.), *Pleasure and danger: Exploring female sexuality* (pp. 149–163). London: Routledge & Kegan Paul.

Espín, O. (1987). Issues of identity in the psychology of Latina lesbians. In Boston Lesbian Psychologies Collective (Eds.), *Lesbian psychologies: Explorations and challenges* (pp. 35–51). Urbana, IL: University of Illinois Press.

Falco, K. L. (1991). *Psychotherapy with lesbian clients*. New York: Brunner/Mazel.

Folayan, A. (1992). African American issues: The soul of it. In B. Berzon (Ed.), *Positively gay* (pp. 235–239). Berkeley, CA: Celestial Arts.

Garcia, N., Kennedy, C., Pearlman, S. F., & Perez, J. (1987). The impact of race and culture differences: Challenges to intimacy in lesbian relationships. In

Boston Lesbian Psychologies Collective (Eds.), *Lesbian psychologies: Explorations and challenges* (pp. 142–160). Urbana, IL: University of Illinois Press.

Garnets, L., & Kimmel, D. (1991). Lesbian and gay male dimensions in the psychological study of human diversity. In J. Goodchilds (Ed.), *Psychological perspectives on human diversity in America* (pp. 137–192). Washington, DC: American Psychological Association.

Gartrell, N. (1993). Boundaries in lesbian therapy relationships. *Women and Therapy, 12,* 29–50.

Glassgold, J. (1992). New directions in dynamic theories of lesbianism: From psychoanalysis to social constructionism. In J. Chrisler & D. Howard (Eds.), *New directions in feminist psychology: Practice, theory and research* (pp. 154– 163). New York: Springer.

Gock, T. S. (1985, August). *Psychotherapy with Asian Pacific gay men: Psychological issues, treatment approach and therapeutic guidelines.* Paper presented at the meeting of the Asian American Psychological Association, Los Angeles, CA.

Gock, T. S. (1992). Asian-Pacific islander issues: Identity integration and pride. In B. Berzon (Ed.), *Positively gay* (pp. 247–252). Berkeley, CA: Celestial Arts.

Gomez, J. (1983). A cultural legacy denied and discovered: Black lesbians in fiction by women. In B. Smith (Ed.), *Home girls: A Black feminist anthology* (pp. 120–121). New York: Kitchen Table–Women of Color Press.

Gomez, J., & Smith, B. (1990). Taking the home out of homophobia: Black lesbian health. In E. C. White (Ed.), *The Black women's health book: Speaking for ourselves* (pp. 198–213). Seattle, WA: Seal Press.

Grahn, J. (1984). *Another mother tongue: Gay words, gay worlds.* Boston: Beacon Press.

Greene, B. (1986). When the therapist is White and the patient is Black: Considerations for psychotherapy in the feminist heterosexual and lesbian communities. *Women and Therapy, 5,* 41–66.

Greene, B. (1990a). Sturdy bridges: The role of African American mothers in the socialization of African American children. *Women and Therapy, 10*(1/2), 205–225.

Greene, B. (1990b). African American lesbians: The role of family, culture and racism. *BG Magazine,* pp. 6, 26.

Greene, B. (1993a). Psychotherapy with African-American women: Integrating feminist and psychodynamic models. *Journal of Training and Practice in Professional Psychology, 7*(1), 49–66.

Greene, B. (1993b). Stereotypes of African American sexuality: A commentary. In S. Rathus, J. Nevid, & L. Rathus-Fichner (Eds.), *Human sexuality in a world of diversity* (p. 257). Boston: Allyn & Bacon.

Greene, B. (in press). African American lesbians: Triple jeopardy. In A. Brown-Collins (Ed.), *The psychology of African American women.* New York: Guilford Press.

Greene, B. (1994, April). Ethnic minority lesbians and gay men: Mental health and treatment issues. *Journal of Consulting and Clinical Psychology, 62*(2).

Gutierrez, E. (1992). Latino issues: Gay and lesbian Latinos claiming La Raza. In B. Berzon (Ed.), *Positively gay* (pp. 240–246). Berkeley, CA: Celestial Arts.

Gutierrez, F., & Dworkin, S. (1992). Gay, lesbian, and African American: Managing the integration of identities. In S. Dworkin & F. Gutierrez (Eds.), *Counsel-*

ing gay men and lesbians (pp. 141–156). Alexandria, VA: American Association of Counseling and Development.

H., Pamela. (1989). Asian American lesbians: An emerging voice in the Asian American community. In Asian Women United of California (Eds.), *Making waves: An anthology of writings by and about Asian American women* (pp. 282–290). Boston: Beacon Press.

Heske, S., Khayal, & Utsa (1986). There are, always have been, always will be lesbians in India. *Conditions: 13. International focus*, 1, 135–146.

Hidalgo, H., & Hidalgo-Christensen, E. (1976). The Puerto-Rican lesbian and the Puerto-Rican community. *Journal of Homosexuality*, 2, 109–121.

Hidalgo, H. (1984). The Puerto Rican lesbian in the United States. In T. Darty & S. Potter (Eds.), *Woman identified women* (pp. 105–150). Palo Alto, CA: Mayfield.

hooks, b. (1981). *Ain't I a woman: Black women and feminism*. Boston: South End Press.

Icard, L. (1986). Black gay men and conflicting social identities: Sexual orientation versus racial identity. *Journal of Social Work and Human Sexuality*, 4(1/2), 83–93.

Jeffries, I. (1992, February 23). Strange fruits at the purple manor: Looking back on "the life" in Harlem. *NYQ*, 17, 40–45.

Kanuha, V. (1990). Compounding the triple jeopardy: Battering in lesbian of color relationships. *Women and Therapy*, 9(1/2), 169–183.

Khush. (1993). Fighting back: An interview with Pratibha Parmar. In R. Ratti (Ed.), *A lotus of another color* (pp. 34–40). Boston: Alyson.

Kim, (1993). They aren't that primitive back home. In R. Ratti (Ed.), *A lotus of another color* (pp. 92–97). Boston: Alyson.

Kite, M. (1994). When perceptions meet reality: Individual differences in reactions to lesbians and gay men. In B. Greene & G. Herek (Eds.), *Lesbian and gay psychology: Theory, research, and clinical applications*. Newbury Park, CA: Sage.

Kite, M., & Deaux, K. (1987). Gender belief systems: Homosexuality and the implicit inversion theory. *Psychology of Women Quarterly*, 11, 83–96.

Lee, C. A. (1991). An Asian lesbian's struggle. In M. Silvera (Ed.), *Piece of my heart: A lesbian of color anthology* (pp. 115–118). Toronto, Ontario: Sister Vision Press.

Mays, V., & Cochran, S. (1988). The Black women's relationship project: A national survey of Black lesbians. In M. Shernoff & W. Scott (Eds.), *The sourcebook on lesbian/gay health care* (2nd ed., pp. 54–62). Washington, DC: National Lesbian and Gay Health Foundation.

Mays, V., Cochran, S., & Rhue, S. (in press). The impact of perceived discrimination on the intimate relationships of Black lesbians. *Journal of Homosexuality*.

Meera. (1993). Working together: An interview with Urvashi Vaid. In R. Ratti (Ed.), *A lotus of another color* (pp. 103–112). Boston: Alyson.

Morales, E. (1989). Ethnic minority families and minority gays and lesbians. *Marriage and Family Review*, 14(3/4), 217–239.

Morales, E. (1992). Latino gays and Latina lesbians. In S. Dworkin & F. Gutierrez (Eds.), *Counseling gay men and lesbians: Journey to the end of the rainbow* (pp. 125–139). Alexandria, VA: American Association for Counseling and Development.

Morgan, K., & Eliason, M. (1992). The role of psychotherapy in Caucasian lesbians' lives. *Women and Therapy*, *13*, 27–52.

Moses, A. E., & Hawkins, R. (1982). *Counseling lesbian women and gay men: A life issues approach.* St. Louis, MO: C. V. Mosby.

Namjoshi, S. (1992, June 14). *Flesh and paper: An interview* [Television program]. New York: WNET.

Newman, B. S. (1989). The relative importance of gender role attitudes to male and female attitudes toward lesbians. *Sex Roles*, *21*, 451–465.

Noda, B., Tsui, K., & Wong, Z. (1979, Spring). Coming out: We are here in the Asian community: A dialogue with 3 Asian women. *Bridge: An Asian American perspective.*

Omosupe, K. (1991). Black/lesbian/bulldagger. *differences: A Journal of Feminist and Cultural Studies*, *2*(2), 101–111.

Poussaint, A. (1990, September). An honest look at Black gays and lesbians. *Ebony*, pp. 124, 126, 130–131.

Ratti, R. (1993). Introduction. In R. Ratti (Ed.), *A lotus of another color: An unfolding of the South Asian gay and lesbian experience* (pp. 11–17). Boston: Alyson.

Sears, V. L. (1987). *Cross-cultural ethnic relationships.* Unpublished manuscript.

Shockley, A. (1979). The Black lesbian in American literature: An overview. In L. Bethel & B. Smith (Eds.), *Conditions: 5. The Black women's issue*, *2*(2), 133–144.

Shah, N. (1993). Sexuality, identity, and the uses of history. In R. Ratti (Ed.), *A lotus of another color* (pp. 113–132). Boston: Alyson.

Silvera, M. (1991). Man royals and sodomites: Some thoughts on the invisibility of Afro-Caribbean lesbians. In M. Silvera (Ed.), *Piece of my heart: A lesbian of color anthology* (pp. 14–26). Toronto, Ontario: Sister Vision Press.

Smith, B. (1982). Toward a Black feminist criticism. In G. Hull, P. Scott, & B. Smith (Eds.), *All the women are white, all the blacks are men, but some of us are brave* (pp. 157–175). Old Westbury, NY: Feminist Press.

Smith, B., & Smith, B. (1981). Across the kitchen table: A sister to sister dialogue. In C. Moraga & G. Anzaldúa (Eds.), *This bridge called my back: Writings by radical women of color* (pp. 113–127). Watertown, MA: Persephone Press.

Tafoya, T. (1992). Native gay and lesbian issues: The two spirited. In B. Berzon (Ed.), *Positively gay* (pp. 253–260). Berkeley, CA: Celestial Arts.

Tafoya, T., & Rowell, R. (1988). Counseling Native American lesbians and gays. In M. Shernoff & W. A. Scott (Eds.), *The sourcebook on lesbian/gay health care* (pp. 63–67). Washington, DC: National Lesbian and Gay Health Foundation.

Taylor, A. T. (1983). Conceptions of masculinity and femininity as a basis for stereotypes of male and female homosexuals. *Journal of Homosexuality*, *9*, 37–53.

Tremble, B., Schneider, M., & Appathurai, C. (1989). Growing up gay or lesbian in a multicultural context. *Journal of Homosexuality*, *17*, 253–267.

Trujillo, C. (Ed.). (1991). *Chicana lesbians: The girls our mothers warned us about.* Berkeley, CA: Third Woman Press.

Vasquez, E. (1979). Homosexuality in the context of the Mexican American culture. In D. Kukel (Ed.), *Sexual issues in social work: Emerging concerns in education and practice* (pp. 131–147). Honolulu: University of Hawaii School of Social Work.

Weinrich, J., & Williams, W. L. (1991). Strange customs, familiar lives: Homosexuality in other cultures. In J. Gonsiorek & J. Weinrich (Eds.), *Homosexuality: Research findings for public policy* (pp. 44–59). Newbury Park, CA: Sage.

Weston, K. (1991). *Families we choose: Lesbians, gays and kinship*. New York: Columbia University Press.

Whitley, B. E., Jr. (1987). The relation of sex role orientation to heterosexual attitudes toward homosexuality. *Sex Roles, 17*, 103–113.

Williams, W. L. (1986). *The spirit and the flesh: Sexual diversity in American Indian culture*. Boston: Beacon Press.

Wooden, W. S., Kawasaki, H., & Mayeda, R. (1983). Lifestyles and identity maintenance among gay Japanese-American males. *Alternative Lifestyles, 5*, 236–243.

Wyatt, G., Strayer, R., & Lobitz, W. C. (1976). Issues in the treatment of sexually dysfunctioning couples of African American descent. *Psychotherapy, 13*, 44–50.

15

Women of Color
in Battering Relationships

Valli Kanuha

The contemporary understanding of violence against women is largely attributable to the political analysis and activism of the "second wave" of the feminist movement, dating from the 1960s through the present. From women's consciousness raising groups to crisis hotlines for rape and sexual assault victims, followed by the first shelter for battered women in 1970, the women's movement has been credited with bringing the problem of violence against women out of the private domain and into the public arena, challenging academic, health, judicial, and other major social institutions to respond.

Indeed, it was the groundbreaking work of feminist scholars and activists in the last decade that has illuminated the prevalence of violence against women in its many covert and overt manifestations. It is now well established that violence against women in the home is commonplace, and statistics indicate a very troubling picture (National Network of Women's Funds [NNWF], 1992):

- An estimated 3 to 4 million American women are battered each year by their husbands.
- Wife beating results in more injuries that require medical treatment than rape, auto accidents, and muggings combined.
- Thirty percent of female homicide victims are killed by husbands or boyfriends.
- In one hospital emergency room, 20% of pregnant women had been battered. These women had twice as many miscarriages as nonbattered women.

While feminist-based political organizing to end violence against women has catalyzed public attention to sexist violence in contemporary society, these social movements have frequently been criticized for (and, in fact, self-critical of) their Eurocentricism. This has made for the exclusion of women of color perspectives and experiences in theory development, service delivery models, and research (Burns, 1986; Schecter, 1982). The appraisal of both the antiviolence and feminist movements as primarily reliant on the perspectives of White women has been put forward by feminist women of color from the 1960s through the present (Hull, Scott, & Smith, 1982; Moraga & Anzaldúa, 1983). This chapter attempts to contribute to an expanded analysis of violence against women by examining the complex and understudied relationships between race/ethnicity and gender as they affect women of color who experience violence by their partners in the context of their intimate, domestic relationships.[1]

For the purposes of this discussion, the term "women of color" refers to women who are not of European American descent, but those women of Asian and Pacific Island, African American or African-Caribbean, Latina, or Native American origins.[2] While there are many other groups of women to whom the term "women of color" applies, this chapter focuses on the racial/ethnic groups described above, which reflect both the experiences of the author and the majority of written work available on battered women of color.

It is important as an introductory note for readers to understand that the issues discussed herein represent broad categories that have different but very important implications for battered women of color in the United States. Generalizations are by necessity made about the applicability of these factors to diverse groups of women, the danger of which is that universal statements such as, "Asian battered women do . . ." or "the experience of Latina battered women . . ." may be construed as the very stereotypes the author is attempting to dispel. Each of the particular racial/ethnic groups discussed in this chapter are as culturally diverse and independent within their own ethnic groups as they are from the racial groups with which they are being compared. The complex interaction of many factors, in addition to race/ethnicity, affects the interpretation of any individual or collective experience of women of color who are battered. Therefore, any inferences or generalizations must be understood as approximations necessary for framing the discussion, but by no means always true of specific individuals in the given group or the group as a whole.

This chapter presents an overview of the relevant issues for battered women of color, with an emphasis on the interface of racial/ethnic identity with social, cultural, and economic factors as they affect (1) the incidence of battering, (2) models of domestic violence etiology, and (3) intervention strategies developed to address violence against African American, Asian/Pacific Islander, Latina/Hispanic, Native American, or indigenous women. I will begin with a critique of the primary sources on battered women, followed by a review of available work that addresses the perspectives of violence against women of color. Finally, clinical implications and recommendations for mental health practitioners who work with battered women of color are discussed.

CRITIQUE OF THE LITERATURE ON DOMESTIC VIOLENCE AGAINST WOMEN

The three primary categories of study regarding battered women are: (1) incidence rates of domestic violence, (2) the etiology or "causes" of battering, and (3) intervention strategies to address violence against women in the home. This section addresses separately each of these three categories of study, focusing on the predominant theories about and clinical interventions in domestic violence that have been developed over the last 20 years. While not intended as an exhaustive review of the literature, this section critically examines the existing empirical and nonacademic literature to elucidate the shortcomings and gaps in our current knowledge base regarding women of color who are battered in their primary relationships.

For mental health practitioners, feminist and nonfeminist alike, it is important first to understand the political context in which violence against women as a social and mental health problem was brought to light in the 1970s. Dobash and Dobash (1992) and Schecter (1982) provide particularly cogent descriptions of the feminist foundations of the battered women's movement, and the influence of social activism on the subsequent development of social policy, services, and research addressing domestic violence both in the United States and internationally. The primary contribution of the feminist antiviolence movement has been the consistent emphasis on the social construction of violence against women in the context of gender-based role expectations, attitudes, and behaviors. While the analysis and social change strategies of feminist activists were sometimes at odds with the more "objective" needs of social scientists to analyze the dynamics of this complex human phenomenon, researchers from most academic disciplines and their activist counterparts now agree upon one critical notion: that domestic violence does exist in a social and cultural context, and is not solely a mental health problem resulting from individual pathology (Bograd, 1984; Schecter, 1987; Thorne-Finch, 1992; Yllo & Bograd, 1988).

Incidence of Domestic Violence

There are three primary sources of incidence data on battered women. They are: (1) statistical reports, primarily from law enforcement, health, or criminal justice institutions; (2) survey-based research from both men and women about violence in the home; and (3) self-report interviews or surveys of battered women and/or batterers, most of which are located in domestic violence programs such as shelters or abuser's treatment services.

Incidence Reports from Public Sources

Government- or public-agency-sponsored statistical reports, such as the FBI Uniform Crime Reports of the U.S. Department of Justice, national surveys administered by the National Opinion Research Center, and the U.S. Census Bureau have two inherent biases that are problematic in terms of elucidating battering in non-White populations. First, due to socioeconomic factors, it is well documented that non-Whites, the poor, and other groups of disenfranchised people are the predominant users of public services such as emergency rooms, community health clinics, and other social welfare programs. Therefore they are more likely to be over-represented in indices of negative social conditions such as poverty, crime, disease, and child abuse, from which inferences about social deviance including domestic violence are often made (Cooper, 1986).

A second limitation of statistical reports is that African Americans, Latinos, and Native Americans (both men and women) are also overrepresented in all parts of the criminal justice system (police arrests, indictments, criminal trials, incarceration rates, etc.) disproportionate to their numbers in the U.S. population (Mann & LaPoint, 1987). Therefore, especially with regard to domestic violence and violent behavior in general, statistical reports are sometimes used to generalize that the aforementioned racial groups are more or differently violent than their White counterparts. While such an inference may and should warrant further examination, we must consider the limitations of statistical reports as the basis for sound theory building about domestic violence especially with regard to non-White populations.

Survey-Based Research of Family Violence

The most prolific survey-based research about domestic violence was conducted by Gelles (1974), Straus, Gelles, and Steinmetz (1980), and Straus and Gelles (1986). In these hallmark studies of domestic violence, however, consideration of race as an intervening variable for battered women was primarily limited to African American populations. While the findings of Straus et al. (1980) suggest that African American men may be significantly more violent toward their wives than White men, a number of researchers cite differences in family income as an explanation (Cazenave & Straus, 1979; Fagan, Stewart, & Hansen, 1983). Others have criticized this survey research as biased with regard to race, class, and gender factors because it did not include single-parent families, noncohabiting couples, families with children under age 3, or respondents who were illiterate—all categories in which people of color are represented (Asbury, 1987; Fagan et al., 1983; Lockhart, 1987).

Self-Report Surveys

The most common sources of both incidence data and descriptive studies of battered women are self-reports from battered women and/or their abusers. The first printed works on battered women by Pizzey (1974) in Britain and Martin (1981) in the United States were based on interviews with battered women. These authors were the first to assert that violence in the home did indeed occur in millions of households around the world, and that the primary victims of abuse were women and children. While both emphasized that battering occurred among all women "regardless of race, class, and other factors," neither author specifically mentioned the effect of race as a differential factor for women of color in violent homes.

Other empirical studies of battered women and/or their abusers are based on interviews or questionnaires conducted in social service agencies or domestic violence programs (Blackman, 1989; Langley & Levy, 1977; Pagelow, 1981; Roy, 1977; Walker, 1979). All of these studies highlight the prevalence of domestic violence against women, but very few include proportionate samples of non-White battered women in their analyses.

There are few descriptive or comparative research studies that specifically explore the effects of domestic violence on women who are of African American, Asian American, Native American, or Latina/Hispanic descent. Torres (1987) compared a sample of Hispanic battered women to European American battered women in shelters and found that the severity and frequency of violence was similar for both groups of women; however, no conlusions could be made about the overall incidence of battering in Hispanic populations. Gondolf, Fisher, and McFerron (1988) studied 5,708 residents of Texas battered women's shelters and found few differences in the kinds and extent of abuse in European American, Hispanic, and African American samples, while Lewis (1987) confirmed earlier reports that wife abuse is no more likely in Black couples than White couples when social class is controlled. On the contrary, Lockhart and White (1989) reported that among African American and White women in battering relationships, middle-class Black women experienced more violence than their White counterparts. Finally, in the only survey of the literature on battering and African American couples, Coley and Beckett (1988) found that most study samples were small, anecdotal in nature, and not designed to measure accurately the incidence of battering in African American families.

Etiology of Domestic Violence

While there is now more widespread acknowledgment of both the existence and the prevalence of domestic violence, researchers and clinicians alike are not always in agreement about the etiology of battering. Among the public at large, the most commonly asked question related to the etiology of domestic violence is, "Why do women allow themselves to be battered in the first place, and why do they stay in violent relationships?" For feminist researchers and clinicians, however, the more salient concern is, "Why are men violent toward women in their intimate relationships?"

The following section briefly describes the three major theories of the etiology of violence against women in intimate relationships, which are: (1) the sociobiological model, (2) the social constructionist or sociocultural model, and (3) the psychological model. All three are interrelated, but distinguished by their emphasis on and methodological approach to various aspects of the study of battered women and batterers.

Sociobiological Model of Battering

The first explanatory model of domestic violence, the sociobiological approach, has its roots in early Darwinism and studies of the physiological bases of all types of human behavior. Of most relevance to sociobiologists interested in domestic violence are studies of the genetic or biological roots of aggressive behavior, including related factors such as testosterone levels, territoriality, and kinship ties (Konner, 1982; Thorne-Finch, 1992).

Social Constructionist or Sociocultural Model of Violence

The social constructionist or sociocultural model of human behavior was applied to domestic violence as an outgrowth of the feminist analysis of battering as a socially constructed system of male control. Primarily developed by feminist activists and progressive sociologists, this model views spousal battering as a complex process that sanctions both heterosexuality and gender-bound behavior as well as the passive and active countenance of all forms of male control of women (Dobash & Dobash, 1979; Schecter, 1982; Yllo & Bograd, 1988).

Psychological Model of Violence

Of most relevance and interest to mental health clinicians is the third model of etiology regarding domestic violence, the psychological perspective. This model of etiology emphasizes the emotional, psychodynamic, and internally interpreted experiences that affect the propensity for men to batter and for women to be battered. This view explains violence as a manifestation of both individual psychopathology and learned behavior, with roots in early childhood abuse, family dysfunction, drug abuse, or disorders of personality, thought, or impulse control (Thorne-Finch, 1992).

Intergenerational violence, in which batterers and battered women report having witnessed or experienced violence in their families of origin, is widely accepted by clinicians and researchers alike as a viable explanation for partner abuse (Browne, 1987; Okun, 1986). A related aspect of the intergenerational model of domestic violence is the influence of social learning theory, which emphasizes the reinforcement of and opportunity for violence as learned behavior (Gelles, 1983).

Critique of Models of Etiology

All three models of etiology have limitations and strengths in clarifying the complexity of domestic violence for women of color. The emphasis of the biological perspective on internal, individual drives and physiological processes does not adequately consider the social, economic, and historical conditions in which women and men experience violence and control. The social constructionist theory has been criticized for insufficiently analyzing the intrapsychic and biophysical aspects of human nature that may predispose individuals to be violent against their partners.

Of most interest to mental health clinicians, the psychological perspective is a favored remedy for domestic violence because it is perceived as a legitimate and viable solution to this pervasive social problem. In fact, over the last 20 years one of the predominant strategies for reducing violence against women is psychosocial support for battered women and treatment for batterers. However, although these programs have been in existence for almost 20 years, their effectiveness in reducing the rate of violence against women has not been well substantiated (Thorne-Finch, 1992).

The primary limitation of all three theories lies in the historically prejudicial process of theory development in the political, social, and biological sciences, which overlooks or misrepresents the experiences of women and people of color (Hill-Collins, 1990). Therefore, defining the causes of domestic violence without including samples of people of color in proportion to their representation not only in the general population, but in relation to the subpopulation of victims and perpetrators of domestic violence, skews our understanding about violence across all racial groups. In addition, there has long existed a gender bias in our analysis and study of human behavior, which for women of color is only compounded by the race factor in an analysis of battering (Bohan, 1992; Brown & Root, 1990).

Intervention Strategies to Address Domestic Violence

A review of the literature indicates that most of the strategies to alleviate battering of women in intimate relationships have been developed by feminist activists working in collaboration with progressive legal experts, mental health providers, and social scientists. These strategies include shelters and safe home networks for women and children; individual and systems advocacy; legal sanctions such as mandatory/probable cause arrest and orders for protection; social support and therapy; and batterer's treatment services.

The empirical literature is sparse with regard to the impact of various domestic violence intervention strategies with subsamples of battered women of color, while works examining programs or policies designed specifically for battered women of color are even more meager. In Coley and Beckett's (1988) literature review on African American battered women, studies suggest that the nature, extent, and type of help-seeking supports (such as social networks and extended family) may have a positive effect on Black women's perceptions of options to leave their batterers. No similar literature reviews exist for other groups of battered women of color. Hispanic battered women who were interviewed in shelters reported that they had more difficulty seeking help from social service or other providers due to the influence of family cohesiveness and of "keeping the family together" as values in some Latino cultural groups (Torres, 1987). Ho (1990) suggests that certain Asian American or Asian immigrant battered women are reluctant to use any services for battered women because of the perception that battering is a "private matter."

Most of the written work that addresses battering and women of color has been in the form of anecdotal accounts, cultural analyses, anthologies, or curricula developed by battered women's programs around the United States. White (1985) and Zambrano (1985) published the first books targeted specifically to empower battered women of African American and Latina descent. Battered women's activists drew from their own organizing and service delivery experiences to explore race, culture, and gender-role conflicts for battered women of color (Richie, 1985; Rios, 1985), while political scientists such as Davis (1985) focused on the historical legacy of institutional racism and sexism to challenge violence against women of color. Native American women organizing in the context of battered women's coalitions have called for indigenous women to reinstate traditional tribal values of respect for women and children by challenging domestic violence in Native American families (American Indian Women Against Domestic Violence, 1984). Burns (1986) edited a frequently cited but much too brief work, which is one of the few anthologies addressing the effects of battering on American Indian, Asian, African American, and Latina women within a historical, social, and racial context.

Over the last two decades, many battered women's programs have produced training manuals and curricula for service providers, addressing battering from a racial and cultural perspective as part of comprehensive, multicultural approaches to working with victims of domestic violence (Massachusetts Coalition of Battered Women's Service Groups, 1990; National Coalition Against Domestic Violence [NCADV], 1990; Richie, 1988).

Finally, continued and consistent leadership in the analysis of race, gender, and battering is usually found in the proceedings of national conferences and gatherings of battered women's activists and other feminist organizations, which have maintained a commitment to ongoing debate about this important issue (NCADV, 1990; NNWF, 1992; NNWF and Women and Foundations/Corporate Philanthropy, 1991; Walker, 1988).

SOCIOCULTURAL FACTORS THAT AFFECT BATTERED WOMEN OF COLOR

The following section describes the major factors that affect the individual and collective experiences of battered women of color differently from their White counterparts. These factors will highlight some of the reasons battered women of color have not and currently do not utilize either mental health or designated battered women's services as often as their European American battered women counterparts.

The Impact of Institutional Racism

Because most legal, social, and cultural institutions are controlled and dominated primarily by White males and/or White male perspectives, many battered women of color are reluctant to bring attention to themselves, their families, and by extension to their racial/ethnic communities for fear of further contributing to the stigmatization and stereotyping of people of color as pathological. For example, some African American women are reluctant to report being victimized by their partners as a protective measure against the historical, institutional racism to which African American families have been subjected (Rogers, Taylor, & McGee, no date). For battered women of color, this "detrimental sense of racial loyalty" (White, 1986) is translated not only into denial of the extent of violence perpetrated against them by their partners, but rationalization of that violence as an extension of living in a society that has been and is dehumanizing to both men and women of color.

Another effect of historical and institutional racism on all women of color, which is especially complicated for those who are battered, is the societal attribution and subsequent self-perception that women of color are stalwart and resilient in the face of all odds (White, 1986). This "superwoman" expectation, based on the notion that women of color (and *all* women) are the caregivers and matriarchs of the family and community, results in some battered women minimizing their own needs, and prioritizing the demands of the family and even their batterers over their own protection. The paradoxical truth of this public and self perception is evident; women of color are, in fact, not very powerful relative to the predominant White culture. However, their so-called "resilience" is actually built on centuries of resistance to the brutal and oppressed conditions under which most of them have had to live.

The importance of racism as a legacy for all people in the United States, and its negative impact on people of color cannot be underestimated in our analysis of woman abuse in African American, Asian American, Hispanic/Latino, or Native American communities. However, racism alone does not appear to be the single barrier with which battered women of color are faced. Socioeconomic class, geographic location, and sensitivity of professional caregivers to women who are both battered and non-White appear to be important cofactors that affect the real and perceived options that battered women of color may elect to employ.

The Racial/Ethnic Context of Heterosexism and Gendered Role Behaviors

While most feminist theory and research on gender roles has been generated in and with Western cultures and nationalities, there has been an emerging body of cross-cultural, feminist-based literature on the status of women (Mohanty, Russo, & Torres, 1991; Reinharz, 1992). While vastly different in nature and kind, the subordination of women vis à vis the socioeconomic hierarchy appears to be a cross-cultural phenomenon.

As stated earlier, while the particular effects of the social construction of gender-bound values, attitudes, and behaviors have been well documented by feminist theorists in the United States, the impact of intimate violence as a specific manifestation of both racism and sexism against battered women of color has been inadequately studied. However, there are a number of reports by women of color that illuminate our understanding of the impact male and female roles in racial/ethnic contexts have on women's perceptions of vulnerability in violent situations.

Buddhism and Confucian philosophy have had a significant influence on the role of some women in Asian American or Asian immigrant populations. For some Asian women—whether Chinese, Japanese, Taiwanese, Vietnamese, Korean, Laotian, or other—religious traditions have often inculcated in them roles subservient not only to their husbands, but to all males, including their sons, fathers, uncles, and grandfathers (Chow, 1989). While this may not inherently be a negative condition for Asian women, a controlling male partner, in combination with the deep-seated value of family loyalty, women's limited economic and social mobility, and related values such as shame and religious fatalism (e.g., in Japanese *shikataganai* means a situation cannot be helped) can persuade some Asian women to remain in battering situations (Ho, 1990; Lai, 1986). For Asian women who are refugees, new immigrants, or who are not yet legal residents of the United States, they are often more dependent on their male partners, even in a battering situation, as a means to preserve their legal status (Takagi, 1991). In addition, some Asian American women have limited fluency in English, may be employed in a menial or illegal capacity, or be isolated from extended family members or friends due to war and/or political repression in their homelands and therefore lack the necessary resources and support to confront their batterers (Kanuha, 1987; Rimonte, 1989).

For indigenous tribes in the Americas, matrilinear hierarchies were not uncommon prior to the arrival of White men in the 15th century (Allen, 1986b). The roles of males and females in indigenous cultures have often been gender-bound, but not necessarily with subordination as a requisite condition for females (Ammott & Matthei, 1991). However, the occurrence of domestic violence in Native American families, attributed by some Native American feminists to the European American invasion of indigenous tribal nations and the subsequent infusion of Christianity and alcohol in Native communities, has reinforced the opportunity and sanction for some batterers to use violence as a means of controlling their partners (Allen, 1986a). Similar to other colonized people, the dismantling of family and sociocultural systems in indigenous peoples due to White racism has been a contributing factor in the breakdown of traditional values such as family harmony and respect for women, which might counteract the incidence of violence in the home. A Chippewa woman in the Midwest expressed shame at her battering experience because she believed and understood that it was not in the tradition of her tribe for men to beat women; therefore, she interpreted the abuse in terms of self-blame that she somehow was not able to maintain that traditional value in her own marriage.

Similar to many Asian cultural groups, some Latina and Hispanic women ascribe the causes of domestic violence to the influence of organized religious doctrine, particularly Catholicism upon the attitudes and behaviors of men toward women (Rios, 1985). Gendered roles of men and women in Hispanic or Latino cultural groups often delineate the complex expectations and responsiblities of males as superior, gentlemanly, and honor-bound, and females as passive, compliant, and responsive to others' needs (Ginorio & Reno, 1986). As with all social roles, the requisite expectations and behaviors must be considered in a cultural context that is relevant to particular Latino cultural groups and communities. However, in the context of cultural loyalty, the vulnerability of the family, and other socially constructed expectations and psychogical factors, some batterers have more often misused these values to control Latinas in the sanctioned primacy and privacy of intimate relationships (Anzaldua, 1990).

A final but important aspect of domestic violence, that relates directly to heterosexism and gendered roles, is battering in intimate lesbian and gay relationships. Although male–female violence is more prevalent in domestic abuse situations, lesbian battering has emerged as a significant social problem over the last 10 years (Lobel, 1986; Renzetti, 1992). The issue of lesbian battering has forced clinicians and theorists alike to reexamine their analysis of domestic violence as a fundamentally male–female phenomenon. The existence of violence in lesbian relationships reinforces the prevalence and pervasiveness of the patriarchy, which defines women as subordinate within any institution specifically constructed to control women, such as marriage or any intimate, primary relationship. Therefore, even in same-sex relationships between women (or men), one partner's implicit sanction to dominate or control his or her partner is an objective and logical extension of the patriarchal definition of relationships, which unfortunately is not limited to heterosexual men and women.

While there is some published work on lesbian battering, the inclusion of perspectives on battered lesbians of color has been minimal (Kanuha, 1990). Some of the specific complications and differences that compound the "triple jeopardy" (as women, lesbians, and non-White) for battered lesbians of color are discussed later in this chapter.

CLINICAL CONSIDERATIONS WITH BATTERED WOMEN OF COLOR

As the preceding sections indicate, there are some key historical and theoretical factors that have important implications for clinical interventions with women of color who are battered in their intimate relationships. Unfortunately, current social science literature does not adequately address the variety of strategies employed with battered women of color, nor does it compare their effectiveness with those applied to interventions with European American battered women. This final section, based on a compilation of anecdotal reports and available literature, addresses the factors that enhance the accessibility and effectiveness of clinical interventions with battered women of color.

Important variations in the understanding or acceptance by women of color of concepts such as "women's rights," "feminism," and/or "violence in domestic relationships" is largely based on the degree of acculturation or assimilation to the values, principles, and practices espoused by Westerners or White European Americans who privilege the norms of mainstream America. Therefore, as the subsequent discussion clarifies, differences in the ability of battered women of color to analyze their overall status as women, acknowledge the culpability of their batterers, and, most importantly, take action to end the violence against them, may be partially explained by their degree of acculturation or assimilation to the norms and social roles of men and women in contemporary American culture.

As should be evident at this point, the application of the following list of clinical considerations with battered women of color should be dependent upon a combination of elements, including race, class, age, and other "identities." All of these variables must be integrated into a comprehensive assessment of any battered woman with whom a clinican intervenes.

Receptivity to Mental Health Intervention

Over the last 20 years, there has been a growing body of work addressing the specific mental health needs of Asian and Pacific American, African American, Latino, Native American, and other racial and ethnic groups in the United States (Letley & Pedersen, 1986; Marsella & Pedersen, 1981; Mays, 1985; Sue, 1981). Additionally, feminist clinicians have described the unique mental health perspectives of women of color, for whom the dual stigma of race and gender has resulted in poor or inadequate attention from social service and mental health practitioners (Brown, 1990).

While White, middle-class women are more likely to seek mental health assistance through private physicians or health insurance programs, the majority of women of color enter the mental health system through emergency rooms, community health clinics, or other collateral public social services such as the child welfare system (Perales & Young, 1988). This point illustrates the interrelationship of race and socioeconomic class for many women of color who are under- or unemployed and therefore relegated to using public or emergency health services for ongoing medical care. Because public health care is often inadequate and compromised by limited resources and staff, women of color and their families frequently do not receive the quality and level of mental health and social services they require and deserve.

In addition, while females are more frequent users of ongoing mental health services than males, this again is largely attributable to their gender-appropriate roles as more relational, process-oriented, and able to deal with their feelings (Bohan, 1992). An important fact, however, is that women of color initiate mental health intervention less often than White women, and usually under duress, in crisis, or as a last measure. As discussed earlier, this reluctance is tied to the paradoxical belief held by many women of color that they must care for their families first—and by extension their "race" first—by persevering under dire circumstances before considering or seeking help for themselves (Burns, 1986; White, 1986).

The receptivity of battered women of color to using mental health services is in part dependent on their degree of acculturation and assimilation to the American mental health system, and the cultural sensitivity of those services and practitioners. Second or third generation Asian/Pacific Islander and Latina battered women, for example, may be more familiar with mental health as an acceptable helping function for domestic violence than are immigrant women. On the other hand, many Native American women who have resided primarily on or near reservations where primary health care has been provided by the U.S. government-sponsored Indian Health Service may be ambivalent or suspicious about "mainstream" mental health practitioners, due to the legacy of racism and paternalism in many types of government programs that have been imposed upon indigenous peoples.

As victims of domestic violence, therefore, many women of color are already suspicious of mental health practitioners, expect to be inadequately served, may underestimate the extent and kind of assistance they require, and as a result may never consider seeking mental health care at all.

Views of Battered Women of Color Regarding Available and Accessible Options to Abuse

In comparative analyses and anecdotal reports, one of the most salient factors that emerges about battered women of color is their perception of available options to the violence perpetrated upon them. Coley and Beckett's (1988) literature review suggests a parallel between the use of mental health services and domestic violence services for African American women. They and others have observed that African American women often perceive helping professionals as insensitive to the racial and cultural contexts of their lives, and therefore, when battered, Black women may not view such services as real options (Asbury, 1987; Richie, 1985).

This sense of limited options for battered women of color in comparison to White battered women is primarily related to the inaccessibility and racial insensitivity of existing social, psychological, and domestic violence services. Ironically, anecdotal reports from many women of color suggest that maltreatment of their batterers, especially by the police, often discourages women from seeking help when the violence is at its height (Richie & Kanuha, 1993). When men of color are mandatorily arrested in certain jurisdictions, for example, they may return home with more bruises at the hands of police personnel than those they inflicted upon their women partners (E. Pence, personal communication, 1986).

Lack of culturally appropriate social services also contributes to the perception of limited options for battered women of color. For example, Latina or Asian women who have limited English language skills or who are fearful of the criminal justice system because of past experiences with political and military repression in their countries of origin, may view public services as a last resort ("Double Jeopardy," 1990; Rios, 1985). For battered lesbians of color, the dual stigma of both institutionalized racism and homophobia in many domestic violence and counseling services, with the concomitant belief of many mental health providers that domestic violence does not exist in lesbian relationships, results in their reluctance to seek help from helping professionals (Kanuha, 1990).

It is important to note that not only is it the self-perception of battered women of color that they have been ill served by the very programs designed to protect them from violence, it is the reality. Providers for battered women, mental health practitioners, and feminist researchers uniformly agree that they have not been sufficiently culturally sensitive to meet the diverse and complex needs of women of color who are battered (Counts, Brown, & Campbell, 1992; Schecter, 1987; Walker, 1985). While all battered women, regardless of race, class, or other factors, require accessible and compassionate assistance to escape violence, for battered women of color, help-seeking is significantly compromised if they are new immigrants, have had racist encounters with service providers, or must seek help outside their ethnic-specific communities for such a "private" problem (Nishioka, 1992).

A complicating factor for battered women of color in their perception of options to their violent situations is that some women (along with their batterers and their families) regard interventions for battering as part of a White feminist movement, designed not only to break up families, but as "antimale" in their philosophy and origins (Richie, 1985). Therefore, feminist mental health providers in particular must be sensitive to the alliances some battered women of color must establish with their batterers against mainstream domestic violence programs that are perceived to have a feminist perspective.

A final issue that requires more precise and in-depth study is whether or not various groups of women of color both perceive and utilize differently their options for protection against violence in their primary relationships. Cazenave and Straus (1979), Lockhart and White (1989), and others have suggested that social support networks for African American couples appear to reduce the incidence of battering. In one study of incarcerated African American battered women, Richie (1992) described a pattern she refers to as "gender entrapment," whereby African American battered women were entrapped in illicit criminal behavior by coercion and violence from intimate male partners, who were also involved in criminal activity. Richie attributed gender entrapment to a complex relationship between family expectations, gender roles, and race, all of which are powerfully reinforced by domestic violence against some African American women. This research suggests that the perception of options for this subset of battered African American women was compromised not by a single factor, but by the complex interaction between race/ethnicity, gender, family role expectations, and social conditions in the African American community. Ho (1990) and I (Kanuha, 1987) have reported that prior to immigration to the United States, incidents of sexual assault and domestic violence in Asian cultural groups were handled within the community by leaders or healers. However, with the recent influx of new immigrants not only from Asia, but from Central and South America and the Caribbean, the establishment of new or modified forms of social control, combining both indigenous and American values and strategies, are still in formation. These studies support that battered women of color may have difficulty seeking help due to the lack of or unfamiliarity with social support networks in their acculturated or assimilated settings.

Isolation and invisibility are important factors that affect the perceived and real options for all battered women. Battered women in geographically isolated areas, regardless of race/ethnicity, may be more likely to use informal helping sources (vs. battered women's programs or the police) for protection and relief due to both the paucity of available services and the "closed" systems of geographically remote areas. Similarly, for lesbians in violent relationships, isolation and invisibility sometimes force them to use existing options that they would not ordinarily consider. For example, a battered lesbian who resided in a small midwestern town and needed to escape her batterer sought refuge with her parents and decided to come out to them in order to gain their trust and support for leaving. For both these groups of battered women, however, the question of race and ethnicity complicates an already difficult situation, which may enhance or diminish their effective use of options to end the violence in their lives.

The existence of children in domestic violence situations with women of color is a further complication in their consideration of options. Many battered women report that concern for their children is paradoxically both a motivating factor in and a deterrent to leaving abusive situations (Schecter, 1987; Ho, 1990; Rios, 1985). For battered women of color in particular, leaving their battering situation when they have children often has very serious ramifications. For example, African American and Native American battered women are more likely to lose custody of their children when reporting their own victimization (Takagi, 1991). In one ethnographic study of 26 African American battered women who were incarcerated, 25% of the women had been charged with homicide or as accessories to the murder of their own children when the children had actually been killed by the women's battering male partners (Richie, 1992). For women of color, their already tenuous relationship to the public social service system—which has characterized them as "bad mothers"—and their fear of retribution from their racial/ethnic communities for "breaking up the family and community" considerably limits their options to enduring the violence.

The Focus of Mental Health Practitioners on "the Individual"

A well-established principle in addressing domestic violence is that the safety of the victim is primary and paramount in any intervention. Rooted in the ideology of the feminist battered women's movement, the most important initial strategy in battering situations has typically been to protect the victim and her children. In the last 10 years, however, clinical services for batterers, children, families, and couples have developed in response to the call from activists, criminal justice officials, and most importantly from battered women and batterers themselves for more comprehensive strategies to address violence in the home (Bograd, 1984; Thorne-Finch, 1992).

Although there are few if any documented studies of preferred treatment modalities for people of color who are victims or perpetrators of domestic violence, anecdotal reports from providers and consumers alike suggest that the narrow focus on the battered woman, to the exclusion of the needs of her family, and indeed her batterer, may in part be responsible for the reluctance of battered women of color to seek help from abusive situations (Ho, 1990; Rogers et al., no date). As stated earlier, suspicion of public helping institutions and social service professionals is based on a long-standing racist and coercive relationship between the White middle class as providers and people of color as service recipients. It may be that for some battered women of color the need to preserve the family unit in the face of a racist, genocidal society is in direct contradiction to the admonishment of battered women's advocates that they should take care of their own needs and "just leave him" (or her). Therefore, encouraging battered women of color to leave their batterers, if one considers the extenuating race and class factors that affect their interpretation of the violence and their options to end it, may be an inappropriate and simplistic intervention, and should not be employed without careful consideration of the woman's specific circumstance. This hypothesis is an important and challenging area of domestic violence theory building, which requires more study and examination.

Again, while this conflict between self and others' needs is similar to that experienced by White battered women, for battered women of color the strong connection to one's racial and ethnic heritage—including residing in their own racial communities, participating in cultural activities among their own people, and maintaining other cultural artifacts such as language and religion—mitigates their ability to seek traditional mental health help.

Differences in the organization of community life, including the relative importance of the extended family, the presence or absence of social support networks, and other culturally relevant social foundations comparing White and non-White populations suggest that the value and subsequent maintenance of those processes that encourage autonomy and individuation in European Americans (represented by the work of Erik Erikson, Lawrence Kohlberg, and other developmental stage theorists), does not necessarily have a parallel among African American, Asian American, Latino, or Native American cultures (Marsella & Pedersen, 1981). The emphasis on family, community-group cohesiveness, and a sense of the individual's place vis-à-vis the social context is highly valued, often over the needs of the personal or individual among many of the racial/ethnic groups discussed in this chapter. As a result, the dissonance resulting from the competing values and expectations of autonomy versus dependence sometimes contributes to the difficulty that some battered women of color have in seeking help for themselves, or on behalf of their children, their battering partner, or other extended family members.

In summary, the challenge to mental health professionals who work with battered women of color is to balance the complex needs to (1) find the woman immediate protection from violence; (2) protect her children from violence as well (without undermining her role as a mother); (3) get help for the batterer (while protecting him or her from racist, discretionary treatment in the health and criminal justice systems); and (4) help battered women of color in a manner that maintains harmony and cultural consistency with the values, beliefs, teachings, and practices of their particular racial/ethnic group.

CLINICAL CASE EXAMPLE

The following describes one clinical case intervention with a battered woman of color. It is, more accurately, a composite case, which protects identifying features of the clients and case histories while still presenting salient social and cultural issues that battered women of color with similar profiles have experienced.

Case Description

Maria was a 30-year-old woman of Cuban American heritage. She was college-educated, and was involved in a battering relationship with her very first intimate partner, another woman, also Latina. Both women were involved in social activities in their local gay community, and met at a cultural meeting for Latina lesbians. As one of the few Latina social and cultural organizations for lesbians, many Latina lesbians in the gay community met through this group. However, neither Maria or Susana were very open about their sexual orientation, either in their jobs or with their families.

The relationship was very intense from the beginning but began deteriorating very soon thereafter, with Maria's partner, Susana, incessantly calling her at work to find out if she was really there. Susana was also extremely jealous, and would berate Maria after they were in any social situation in which Susana felt Maria paid attention to anyone else. Susana began to criticize Maria's family, with whom Maria was very close (but who lived in another state), and would attempt to curb Maria's phone conversations with them. Susana began telling Maria that her family was "old-fashioned" and was not adapting to life in the United States because Maria always conversed in Spanish with them. Susana was a fourth-generation Chicana, raised in a middle-class family who had become assimilated into the class and social structure of California. Susana did not speak Spanish, and was interested in studying Yoruba culture, including *santería*, a religious/spiritual philosophy and practice.

Susana was offered a position out of state, and while Maria was happy in her position, she resigned to support Susana's wish to move. Within the first few weeks in their new locale, Susana became more agitated and anxious, which manifested itself in increasing dependence on Maria. Very soon, Susana forbade Maria from calling her family, accusing her of "telling them lies in Spanish," which she could not understand. Susana began restraining Maria when she would attempt to leave their apartment to go to work, telling Maria that she didn't believe Maria would actually come home at the end of the day.

Over a period of 2 months, Susana began to push, shove and eventually hit Maria. After one particularly violent episode, Susana threatened to kill herself out of intense shame for what she had done to Maria. Maria was too ashamed and isolated to do anything but what she had done since the relationship had begun, which was to reassure Susana that everything would be alright. Finally, after another incident where Susana slapped and punched Maria, then threw all of her clothes out of their apartment window, Maria called her parents and told them everything. Her family was equally shocked about both the violence and that Maria was a lesbian. After saying that homosexuality was not respectable in the Catholic church, they told her that their family still believed in supporting their children and that she should come home to stay with them. Maria left Susana 6 months after they had moved out of state, under the guise of a visit to her family. She never returned.

Susana continued to harrass Maria by phone, threatening to come and get her. Susana also told Maria and her family that she would place a bad luck spell on them if Maria did not come back. Maria's family sought help from their priest, Maria from a domestic violence program, and both efforts continued to support her break-up with Susana. Maria stated that of all the things she endured in the relationship, the two most painful incidents were Susana sending copies of their intimate love letters to Maria's parents, and calling her new employer to tell them that Maria was a lesbian.

Case Discussion

While there are some unique dimensions to this case, it is also a common profile that occurs thousands of times each day in the United States and internationally. The level and kind of violence experienced by Maria is found in the cases of most battered women, especially the elements of emotional and psychological coercion and harrassment.

However, this case illustrates the following unique factors for some battered women of color:

1. The cultural dimensions that affect the level and intensity of bonding among intimate partners who are both people of color complicate issues of mutual reliance and dependence, and particularly the sense of the "collective us" against the predominant, historically oppressive, White culture.

2. For lesbians, the isolation and invisibility that is enforced by societal homophobia is only exacerbated when intimate relationship violence is used to silence and further isolate the battered lesbian from any existing support systems. In Maria's case, the realistically perceived cost to her being "outed" on the job and with her parents only complicated her sense that she should remain with Susana in order to protect herself from further recrimination.

3. Maria's cultural ties to her Latina history (through her knowledge of Spanish and her close ties to her family) created dissonance with Susana's racial/ethnic identity, which was more assimilated into Western mainstream culture. This both intensified their intimate bond, and was the fodder for Susana's need to find any means with which to control Maria.

4. As a lesbian, Maria did not feel comfortable with the mainstream battered women's program she contacted, which served primarily heterosexual women. After having left Susana for almost 1 year, Maria found a gay/lesbian domestic violence program that served primarily European American clients. She attended a support group for battered lesbians, half of whom were lesbians of color.

RECOMMENDATIONS FOR CLINICAL AND ORGANIZATIONAL INTERVENTIONS WITH BATTERED WOMEN OF COLOR

Based on the preceding discussion, there are a number of concrete strategies that mental health clinicians should consider in designing accessible, sensitive, and culturally appropriate interventions with women of color who are in battering relationships. Again, these recommendations must be implemented as part of an overall assessment of protection, cultural relevance, and collateral supports that are accessible and available for battered women of color who are seeking assistance from a violent situation. The recommendations address both one-to-one clinical intervention strategies as well as organizational development activities that will enhance service delivery to battered women of color.

Individual Clinical Interventions with Battered Women of Color

Every clinician must seriously consider the intense, historical, and reality-based conflict that some battered women of color have about protecting themselves from violence versus protecting their family or community from judgment or further stigmatization as a result of institutionalized racism. Internal and external struggle about one's racial/ethnic identity is part of the core and daily existence for every person of color who lives in the United States. For women of color who are battered, that struggle is intensified by questions about the historical and cultural "traditions" that define family values, intimate relationships, and gender roles in the context of a battering relationship.

Practitioners must balance the issue of safety for the battered victim with the real and perceived experiences of battered women of color that the very institutions mandated to help them such as the police and courts themselves have a legacy of violence toward men and women of color. Mental health and social service providers must explore the viability of all options available to battered women of color, and respect the self-determination of each woman to choose the most appropriate interventions for herself.

Comprehensive approaches to battering that incorporate both individual and family work may be more appropriate for some battered women of color. Based on self-reports from both battered women and providers, individual, intrapsychic, and psychodynamic methods of therapy alone do not seem effective with battered women of color. However, incorporated with group work, educational sessions about the etiology of violence against women, focused and structured treatment with batterers, couples work, family therapy, and, most importantly, culturally specific healing regimens and ceremonies, individual therapy can be a helpful tool with battered women of color, their partners, and their families.

Depending on the degree and extent of acculturation to both the mental health system (values, expectations, costs, etc.) and domestic violence as a serious issue for which she can seek help, the clinician–client match may be enhanced with more or less divergence. In the case of a small or closed racial/ethnic community, for example, it is sometimes preferable for the practitioner to be an "outsider" in order to protect the identity and confidentiality of the woman. In one sexual assault program for Southeast Asian refugees, for example, some women requested American providers because all of the community caseworkers and translators were either friends or extended family members (Kanuha, 1987). Some battered lesbians prefer to see heterosexual therapists who are trained in domestic violence issues rather than lesbian therapists, due to the "closed" nature and subsequent overlapping relationships among some gay and lesbian communities.

More holistic, flexible, and multicultural interventions are preferable to traditional mental health strategies with some battered women of color. The mental health system's historical lack of relevance regarding the complexity and diversity of experiences for women of color has sometimes compromised effective help-seeking or help-giving in favor of traditional mental health service. Programs for Native American battered women are now more often integrating traditional herbs, foods, meditation, and ceremonies to complement psychoeducational "talk therapy" about violence.

Some African American battered women find that they must first deal with the legacy of racism and discrimination that has confounded their relationship to their batterers before they can discuss the violence they are experiencing. Battered lesbians of color are not only isolated from their racial/ethnic communities due to homophobia, but from their lesbian community due to the invisibility of battering as a problem among lesbians and gays. A multifaceted approach that includes protection plans, understanding societal and internalized homophobia, and seeking social support from lesbian, feminist, and minority groups has been effective with battered lesbians of color.

A related strategy involves seeking the assistance of other non-mental health providers who are trained in domestic violence and who represent the cultural milieu in which battered women of color are situated. Collateral work with religious or spiritual healers, community leaders, health providers, extended family members, and others should be considered. The key, of course, is to help the woman identify a wide range of helpers in her network, and to remain committed to working with her and them as necessary and appropriate.

Developing approaches, policies, resources, and skills in the area of child custody issues for battered women, especially as they effect battered women of color, would be helpful for clinicians who work with battered women and their children. As described earlier, mental health and child welfare agencies, without full knowledge of the complex dynamics involved in wife abuse cases, have inadvertently or purposely punished mothers in battering cases, including removing children from the home or their mother's care. For women of color, these decisions are more heavily weighted due to the prejudicial treatment of women of color in the criminal justice system and the subsequent difficulty many women of color have in getting their children back once they are removed by the state. Therefore, intervention with domestic violence situations involving battered women with children must proceed with an understanding of both battering and child welfare issues.

Development or awareness of appropriate services and options that are located both within and external to racial/ethnic geographic communities should be made available to provide the maximum balance of protection, confidentiality, and accessibility for battered women of color. As stated earlier, some women of color prefer to seek help outside the geographic bounds of their ethnic communities, while others feel safer with providers of similar backgrounds or in neighborhood-based services that are familiar to them. Due to the complexity of issues for women of color, more and diverse alternatives enhance their receptivity and opportunity to address an abusive situation.

Organization Development Activities to Enhance Service Delivery for Battered Women of Color

Employing staff who represent the predominant composition of racial, ethnic, and class backgrounds of battered women of color in the given community, and who are also trained in domestic violence issues will maximize outreach and accessibility to mental health services. This strategy is key to increasing the receptivity of nonmainstream cultural groups to any established social institution.

Mental health providers should develop culturally appropriate strategies within and external to their work sites that would enhance the accessibility and viability of those options for women of color who are battered. Suggestions include:

1. Providing non-English capability in services, including printed materials, translators, and other modifications in English-language-dominated settings can greatly increase accessibility.

2. Staff training on multicultural issues or domestic violence alone is not necessarily adequate to enhance clinical interventions with battered women or people of color. Developing an organizational plan that includes staff development and training as components in a long-term organizational strategy is most effective in securing the cultural competence of a practice or agency. These plans should at a minimum include assessment of staff and organizational needs, training, and modification of organizational policies on hiring, staff development, and facilities.

CONCLUSION

As is evident, our understanding of women of color who are battered requires reflection, analysis, and theory building that is intricate in nature and form. Future research considerations should include exploration of battering in biracial couples and the impact of violence on interracial families, comparative studies of programs and services targeted to men and women of color in battering relationships, and development of clinical mental health training programs to strengthen delivery of service to battered women of color.

In light of this very complex interface of race/ethnicity, gender, class, and other variables, however, the primary consideration for mental health practitioners is a simple and pragmatic one: Battered women, regardless of their race, want the violence to end. How we, as practioners, assist women in considering the range of options available to them requires sensitivity and patience about the oftentimes competing understandings women and society have about issues of both race and domestic violence. For women of African American, Asian/Pacific Islander, Latino, Native American, or other non-White descent, factors of race and class must be considered in any intervention in a domestic violence situation to provide the requisite and ethical support necessary for batterered women of color to traverse successfully these conflicting grounds.

NOTES

1. Violence against women exists in many contexts and forms, including sexual assault by strangers/acquaintances, incest, date rape/assault, sexual harrassment in the workplace, pornography, and prostitution. In order to limit the parameters of the current discussion, this chapter focuses on battered women who are abused in their partnered or domestic relationships (marriage, coupling, etc.). Battering or domestic violence in this context refers to the full range of sexual, physical, psychological, emotional, verbal, economic, spiritual, and other forms of abuse and coercion that are intended by batterers and perpetrators systematically to hurt and control women.

2. Contemporary references to non-European American racial and ethnic groups are constantly examined and modified for cultural, historical, and contextual relevance. The terms "Hispanic" and "Latino/Latina" refer to a diverse ethnic population who share a common language (primarily Spanish), national origin (Central and South America, the Carribbean, and/or historical roots in Spain or Portugal), and certain other traits, norms, and mores. Similarly, the terms "African American" and "Black" refer to Americans who share ethnic origins in the continent of Africa, the Carribean and other geographic locales from which they were indentured to the United States. While respecting regional and political preferences in the United States and internationally, in this text both terms for both groups are used interchangeably for the purposes of consistency. The author acknowledges the limitations of these terms of reference in this text.

REFERENCES

Allen, P. G. (1986a). Violence and the American Indian woman. In M. C. Burns (Ed.), *The speaking profits us: Violence in the lives of women of color* (pp. 5–7). Seattle, WA: Center for the Prevention of Sexual and Domestic Violence.

Allen, P. G. (1986b). *The sacred hoop: recovering the feminine in American Indian tradition.* Boston: Beacon Press.

American Indian Women Against Domestic Violence. (1984). *Position paper.* (Available from the Minnesota Coalition for Battered Women, 570 Ashbury St., St. Paul, MN 55104)

Ammott, T. L., & Matthei, J. A. (1991). *Race, gender and work.* Boston: South End Press.

Anzaldúa, G. (Ed.). (1990). *Making face, making soul—Haciendo caras: Creative and critical perspectives by feminists of color.* San Francisco: Aunt Lute Foundation.

Asbury, J. (1987). African American women in violent relationships: An explanation of cultural differences. In R. J. Hampton (Ed.), *Violence in the Black family: Correlates and consequences* (pp. 89–105). Lexington, MA: Lexington Books.

Blackman, J. (1989). *Intimate violence: A study of injustice.* New York: Columbia University Press.

Bograd, M. (1984). Family systems approaches to wife battering: A feminist critique. *American Journal of Orthopsychiatry, 54*(4), 558–568.

Bohan, J. S. (Ed.). (1992). *Seldom seen, rarely heard: Women's place in psychology.* Boston: South End Press.

Brown, L. S. (1990) The meaning of a multicultural perspective for theory-building in feminist therapy. In L. S. Brown & M. P. P. Root (Eds.), *Diversity and complexity in feminist therapy* (pp. 1–22). New York: Haworth Press.

Brown, L. S., & Root, M. P. P. (Eds.). (1990). *Diversity and complexity in feminist therapy.* New York: Haworth Press.

Browne, A. (1987). *When battered women kill.* New York: Free Press.

Burns, M. C. (Ed.). (1986). *The speaking profits us: Violence in the lives of women of color.* Seattle, WA: Center for the Prevention of Sexual and Domestic Violence.

Cazenave, N. A., & Straus, M. A. (1979). Race, class and network embeddedness and family violence: A search for potent support systems. *Journal of Comparative Family Studies, 10,* 281–300.

Chow, E. N. (1989). The feminist movement: Where are all the Asian American women? In Asian Women United of California (Ed.), *Making waves: An anthology of writings by and about Asian American women* (pp. 362–376). Boston: Beacon Press.

Coley, S. M., & Beckett, J. O. (1988). Black battered women: A review of the empirical literature. *Journal of Counseling and Development, 66,* 266–270.

Cooper, R. (1986). Race, disease and health. In T. Rathwell & D. Phillips (Eds.), *Health, race and ethnicity* (pp. 21–79). London: Croom Helm.

Counts, D. A., Brown, J. K., & Campbell, J. (Eds.). (1992). *Sanctions and sanctuary: Cultural perspectives on the beating of wives.* Boulder, CO: Westview Press.

Davis, A. Y. (1985). *Violence against women and the ongoing challenge to racism.* Latham, NY: Kitchen Table–Women of Color Press.

Dobash, R. E., & Dobash, R. (1979). *Violence against wives: A case against the patriarchy.* New York: Free Press.

Dobash, R. E., & Dobash, R. (1992). *Women, violence and social change.* London: Routledge.

Double jeopardy, double courage. (1990, September/October). *Ms. Magazine,* pp. 46–48.

Fagan, J. A., Stewart, D. K., & Hansen, K. V. (1983). Violent men or violent husbands? Background factors and situational correlates. In D. Finkelhor, R. J. Gelles, G. T. Hotaling, & M. S. Straus (Eds.), *The dark side of families: Current family violence research* (pp. 49–68). Newbury Park, CA: Sage.

Gelles, R. J. (1974). *The violent home: A study of physical aggression between husbands and wives*. Beverly Hills, CA: Sage.

Gelles, R. J. (1983). An exchange/social control theory. In D. Finkelhor, R. J. Gelles, G. T. Hotaling, & M. A. Straus (Eds.), *The dark side of families: Current family violence research* (pp. 151–165). Newbury Park, CA: Sage.

Ginorio, A., & Reno, J. (1986). Violence in the lives of Latina women. In M. C. Burns (Ed.), *The speaking profits us: Violence in the lives of women of color* (pp. 13–15). Seattle, WA: Center for the Prevention of Sexual and Domestic Violence.

Gondolf, E. W., Fisher, E., & McFerron, R. J. (1988). Racial differences among shelter residents: A comparison of Anglo, Black, and Hispanic battered women. *Journal of Family Violence, 3*(1), 39–51.

Hill-Collins, P. (1990). *Black feminist thought: Knowlege, consciousness and the politics of empowerment*. Boston: Unwin Hyman.

Ho, C. K. (1990). An analysis of domestic violence in Asian American communities: A multicultural approach to counseling. In L. S. Brown & M. P. P. Root (Eds.), *Diversity and complexity in feminist therapy* (pp. 129–150). New York: Haworth Press.

Hull, D., Scott, P., & Smith B. (1982). *All the women are white, all the Blacks are men, but some of us are brave: Black women's studies*. New York: Feminist Press.

Kanuha, V. (1987). Sexual assault in Southeast Asian communities: Issues in intervention. *Response, 10*(3), 3–4.

Kanuha, V. (1990). Compounding the triple jeopardy: Battering in lesbian of color relationships. *Women and Therapy, 9*, 169–184.

Konner, M. K. (1982). *The tangled wing: Biological constraints on the human spirit*. New York: Holt, Rinehart, & Winston.

Lai, T. (1986). Asian women: Resisting the violence. In M. C. Burns (Ed.), *The speaking profits us: Violence in the lives of women of color* (pp. 8–11). Seattle, WA: Center for the Prevention of Sexual and Domestic Violence.

Langley, R., & Levy, R. C. (1977). *Wifebeating: The silent crisis*. New York: Dutton Press.

Letley, H. P., & Pedersen, P. B. (Eds.). (1986). *Cross-cultural training for mental health professionals*. Springfield, IL: C. C. Thomas.

Lewis, B. G. (1987). Psychosocial factors related to wife abuse. *Journal of Family Violence, 2*(1), 1–10.

Lobel, K. (Ed.). (1986). *Naming the violence: Speaking out about lesbian battering*. Seattle, WA: Seal Press.

Lockhart, L. L. (1987). A reexamination of the effects of race and social class on the incidence of marital violence: A search for reliable differences. *Journal of Marriage and the Family, 49*(30), 603–610.

Lockhart, L., & White, B. W. (1989). Understanding marital violence in the Black community. *Journal of Interpersonal Violence, 49*, 421–436.

Mann, C. R., & LaPoint, V. (1987). Research issues relating to the causes of social deviance and violence among Black populations. In R. L. Hampton (Ed.), *Violence in the Black family: Correlates and consequences* (pp. 207–236). Lexington, MA: Lexington Books.

Marsella, A., & Pedersen, P. (Eds.). (1981). *Cross-cultural counseling and psychotherapy: Foundations, evolutions and cultural considerations*. Elmsford, NY: Pergamon Press.

Martin, D. (1981). *Battered wives.* San Francisco: Volcano Press.

Massachusetts Coalition of Battered Women Service Groups. (1990). *For shelter and beyond: Ending violence against battered women and their children.* (Available from the Massachusetts Coalition of Battered Women Service Groups, 107 South St., Boston, MA 02111)

Mays, V. M. (1985). The Black American and psychotherapy. *Psychotherapy: Theory, Research, Preactice, Training, 22,* 379–388.

Mohanty, C. T., Russo, A., & Torres, L. (Eds.). (1991). *Third world women and the politics of feminism.* Bloomington, IN: Indiana University Press.

Moraga, C., & Anzaldúa, G. (Eds.). (1983). *This bridge called my back: Writings by radical women of color.* Latham, NY: Kitchen Table–Women of Color Press.

National Coalition Against Domestic Violence. (1990, July). Women of color and domestic violence. In *Women of Color Institute Manual* from the proceedings of the National Coalition Against Domestic Violence Conference, Amherst, MA.

National Network of Women's Funds. (1992, April). *A wind of change: Funders working to end violence against women.* Conference highlights from the seventh annual conference of the National Network of Women's Funds, Chicago, IL. (Available from the National Network of Women's Funds, 1821 University Ave., Suite 409N, St. Paul, MN 55104)

National Network of Women's Funds and Women and Foundations/Corporate Philanthropy. (1991, Spring). *Violence against women supplement.* St. Paul, MN: Author.

Nishioka, J. (1992, November). Asian women and the cycle of abuse. *New Moon,* p. 3. (Available from the Asian Task Force Against Domestic Violence, P. O. Box 73, Boston, MA 02120)

Okun, L. (1986). *Woman abuse: Facts replacing myths.* Albany, NY: State University of New York Press.

Pagelow, M. A. (1981). *Woman-battering.* Newbury Park, CA: Sage.

Perales, C., & Young, L. (Eds.). (1988). *Too little too late: Dealing with the health needs of women in poverty.* New York: Harrington Press.

Pizzey, E. (1974). *Scream quietly or the neighbors will hear.* Hammondsworth, England: Penguin Press.

Reinharz, S. (1992). *Feminist methods in social research.* New York: Oxford University Press.

Renzetti, C. M. (1992). *Violent betrayal: Partner abuse in lesbian relationships.* Newbury Park, CA: Sage.

Richie, B. E. (1985). Battered black women: A challenge for the Black community. *Black Scholar, 16,* 40–44.

Richie, B. E. (1988). *Understanding family violence within U.S. refugee communities: A training manual.* Washington, DC: Refugee Women in Development.

Richie, B. E. (1992). *Gender entrapment: An exploratory study of the link between gender-identity development, violence against women, race/ethnicity and crime among African American battered women.* Unpublished doctoral dissertation, City University of New York, New York.

Richie, B. E. & Kanuha, V. (1993). Battered women of color in public health care systems: Racism, sexism and violence. In B. Blair & S. E. Cayleff (Eds.), *Wings of gauze: Women of color and the experience of health and illness* (pp. 288–299). Detroit: Wayne State University Press.

Rimonte, N. (1989). Domestic violence among Pacific Asians. In Asian Women United of California (Ed.), *Making waves: An anthology of writings by and about Asian American women* (pp. 327–336). Boston: Beacon Press.

Rios, E. (1985). *Double jeopardy: Cultural and systemic barriers faced by the Latina battered woman.* Unpublished manuscript.

Rogers, B., Taylor, M., & McGee, G. (no date). *Black women and family violence: A guide for service providers.* (Available from the Minnesota Coalition for Battered Women, 570 Ashbury St., St. Paul, MN 55104)

Roy, M. (Ed). (1977). *Battered women: A psychosociological study of domestic violence.* New York: Van Norstrand Reinhold.

Schecter, S. (1982). *Women and male violence: The visions and struggles of the battered women's movement.* Boston: South End Press.

Schecter, S. (1987). *Guidelines for mental health practitioners in domestic violence cases.* (Available from the National Coalition Against Domestic Violence, Box 15127, Washington, DC, 20003-0127)

Straus, M. A., & Gelles, R. J. (1986). Societal change and change in family violence from 1975 to 1985 as revealed by two national surveys. *Journal of Marriage and the Family, 48*(3), 465–479.

Straus, M. A., Gelles, R. J., & Steinmetz, S. (1980). *Behind closed doors: Violence in the American family.* Garden City, NY: Doubleday.

Sue, D. W. (1981). *Counseling the culturally different: Theory practice.* New York: Wiley.

Takagi, T. (1991, Spring). Women of color and violence against women. In National Network of Women's Funds and Foundations/Corporate Philanthropy (C. Moliner, Ed.), *Violence against women supplement* (pp. S1, S6). St. Paul, MN: National Network of Women's Fund and Foundations/Corporate Philanthropy.

Thorne-Finch, R. (1992). *Ending the silence: The origins and treatment of male violence against women.* Toronto: University of Toronto Press.

Torres, S. (1987). Hispanic American battered women: Why consider cultural differences? *Response, 10*(3), 20–21.

Walker, L. E. (1979). *The battered woman.* New York: Harper Colophon.

Walker, L. E. (1985). Feminist therapy with victim/survivors of interpersonal violence. In L. B. Rosewater & L. E. Walker (Eds.), *Handbook on feminist therapy: Women's issues in psychotherapy* (pp. 203–214). New York: Springer Press.

Walker, L. E. (1988, May). *Legal self-defense issues for battered women of color.* Paper presented at the Advanced Feminist Therapy Institute Conference, Seattle, WA.

White, E. C. (1985). *Chain, chain, change: For Black women dealing with physical and emotional abuse and exploring responses to it.* Seattle, WA: Seal Press.

White, E. C. (1986) Life is a song worth singing: Ending violence in the Black family. In M. Burns (Ed.), *The speaking profits us: Violence in the lives of women of color* (pp. 11–13). Seattle, WA: Center for the Prevention of Sexual and Domestic Violence.

Yllo, K., & Bograd, M. (Eds.). (1988). *Feminist perspectives on wife abuse.* Newbury Park, CA: Sage.

Zambrano, M. A. (1985). *Mejor sola que mal acompañada: Para la mujer golpeada* [For the Latina in an abusive relationship]. Seattle, WA: Seal Press.

16

Mixed-Race Women

Maria P. P. Root

No.
I'm not feeling Asian today.
Or American.

And, no, I am not

FilipinaThaiSamoanHawaiian
MexicanBrasilianBurmeseSiamese
PolynesianTahitianMalaysianMoroccan
EgyptianIndo-ChineseIndonesianMicronesian

I have no race,
no country.
Only a soul composed of wars
mixed pride
and
agony.

—VELINA HASU HOUSTON (1985)

America's preoccupation with race is peculiar; we confuse it with ethnicity and nationality and then we construct policy, theories, and social order on the basis of simplistic, dichotomous notions of these concepts. This confusion illustrates how "racial racism" has been translated into a cultural variation (Essed, 1991). Nowhere is this confusion and oppression more apparent than in reviewing the history and treatment of mixed-race people in our country. Questions such as, "What are you?" "Where are you from?" or "What nationality are you?" expose the ignorance of the public to the issues of race and ethnicity. Our national tendency to treat race and ethnicity, core aspects of an individual's identity, as simplistic, dichotomous, and nonoverlapping classification systems has resulted in various forms of oppression of people of color and multiracial people (e.g., dispossession, alienation, marginalization, invisibility). These consequences ultimately impact the construction of positive self-regard and psychological well-being.

455

In this chapter, mental health issues and therapy with multiracial persons, particularly multiracial women, are presented. A selective, brief history of antimiscegenist thinking is offered as a context within which to understand the additional developmental tasks and complicated processes that face the multiracial person. For additional background, the interested reader is referred to Forbes (1988), Root (1992), and Spickard (1989). Subsequently, the mental health issues and themes in therapy with mixed-race persons are presented. My analysis of these issues is predicated on the assumption that multiraciality poses no inherent type of stress that would result in psychological maladjustment; any distress related to being multiracial is likely to be a response to an environment that has internalized racist beliefs. Please note that these discussions represent hypotheses based on recent empirical work and clinical data. Few studies have even considered gender differences in the experience of multiraciality.

WHAT COLOR?

If we consider the mass of U.S. citizens multigenerationally a significant proportion of the American population is of mixed race, including people of color classified with a monoracial label: African American, Native American, Latino, Hawaiian, and Asian (Fernandez, 1992; Forbes, 1989; Spickard, 1992; Wilson, 1992). The first-generation biracial person is often labeled monoracially because of three pervasive assumptions: (1) races are distinct, scientifically derived categories; (2) a person's emotional stability is predicated on having a core, static, monoethnic and monoracial identity; and (3) there is a manufactured hierarchy of racial ancestry that guides the rules of hypodescent (assigned to the racial and/or ethnic group with lower perceived status by the higher status group). Of course, these assumptions are derived from neither universal nor factual truths, but rather a long-standing pseudoscientific literature that rationalizes discrimination (Spickard, 1992) and that has not been critically examined until quite recently.

The concept of races as discrete categories of color correlated with physical and psychological functioning lacks biological validation; it more accurately represents a sociopolitical defense to determine, in this country and in many other places, the distribution of resources. In fact, Spickard (1992) observes that there is more variability within a "race" than between races. Because of the vast amount of misinformation held by many persons about race—and the attributions made to a visual construct (that at times has questionnable reliability and validity)—the multiracial person's developmental process in the United States becomes unnaturally complicated (Root, 1990a).

The Legacy of Antimiscegenist Thought

Although more than 25 years have passed since the last state laws outlawing mixed-race marriages were taken off the books, strong sentiment persists against racial mixing. These laws were presumably enacted to protect the economic, social, and power privileges of the dominant European American group (see, e.g., Daniel, 1992). Prejudicial attitudes against miscegenation are manifested in a range of behavior, from overt forms of violence (e.g., cross-burning at places of residence, physical assaults, and name calling) to more covert expressions (e.g., concern over how the children of mixed-race unions will fare in their familial, social, and emotional lives), to discourage interracial unions.

Both antimiscegenist and supremacist thinking have guided research questions and clinical interpretation of symptomatology in multiracial people. These, combined with gender biases such as the unequal distribution of power to women, women being viewed as sex objects, and a woman's worth assessed through her physical appearance, have put the multiracial woman at a particular disadvantage. Until recently the base of data on mixed-race persons has largely consisted of anecdotal case studies of poorly adjusted persons interpreted by persons unfamiliar with their experience and in a historical context that has been antimiscegenist (e.g., Gist & Dworkin, 1972; Henriques, 1975). Mixed-race women (this is usually based on women with Black and White parentage) have been described as lacking impulse control, particularly in their sexual desire and other consummatory behaviors (Nakashima, 1992). Alternative hypotheses to account for individuals' maladjustment have not been demonstrated because of limited research methodology (Root, 1992) and biased theories.

Johnson (1992) succinctly summarizes the prevailing psychosocial hypotheses suggesting that mixed-race persons are at high risk for being psychologically maladjusted. The first hypothesis, that risk is created by the negative responses of the community to interracial unions and offspring of such unions, is consistent with theories about marginal persons (Park, 1928; Stonequist, 1937), social activist theories (Friere, 1970), and ecological theories (Miller, 1992; Stephan, 1992). The bicultural minority-group person encounters additional stress when one of her or his cultures is less valued by society than the other.

The second prevailing hypothesis is that a bicultural and/or biracial identity creates marginality, and thus, predicts emotional and social maladjustment. This hypothesis interprets differences in experience (which the biracial woman inevitably faces) as harmful, and ignores the ability of humans to synthesize divergent experiences. The tendency of ethnocentrism in personal and social scientific (Eurocentric) discourse predicts that behavior different from the norm in the dominant group will be interpreted as deviant. This propensity is oppressive, because it suggests that most mixed-race people should be maladjusted. On the contrary, the majority of contemporary studies, utilizing nonclinical populations, have demonstrated that mixed-race individuals are predominantly well-adjusted (e.g., Cauce et al., 1992; Hall, 1980; Johnson & Nagoshi, 1986; Stephan & Stephan, 1989, 1991; Stephan, 1991, 1992; Thorton, 1983).

The third hypothesis suggests that individuals who enter into mixed-race unions are deviant and influence the adjustment of offspring adversely. This hypothesis dismisses the validity of the choices individuals make to be together; determines that an entire group of people, the offspring, are "mistakes"; predicts that the mixed-race person will be a "bundle of confusion"; and assumes more variability between races than among races. These are fallacious generalizations, and this hypothesis is not founded in data (cf. Ho & Johnson, 1991; Spickard, 1989).

This chapter represents an attempt to conceptualize some of the issues multiracial persons face, from a normative perspective and with special attention to unique issues for multiracial women. The difficulties multiracial persons face are discussed within a social context that I find to be most consistent with ecological and social activist theories.

Multiracial Development

> The internalization of negative images of ourselves, our self-hatred, poor self-esteem, makes our own people the *Other*. We shun the white-looking Indian, the "high yellow" Black woman, the Asian with the white lover, the Native woman who brings her white girl friend to the Pow Wow, the Chicana who doesn't speak Spanish, the academic, the uneducated. Her difference makes her a person we can't trust. Para que sea "legal," she must pass the ethnic legitimacy test we have devised. And it is exactly your internalized whiteness that desperately wants boundary lines (this part of me is Mexican, this Indian) marked out and woe to any sister or any part of us that steps out of our assigned places. (Anzaldúa, 1990, p. 143)

At some core level, the variability in the visual appearance of the mixed-race person challenges the meaning of race and the order of the world predicated on it. Instead of being offered the ability to define oneself, which is essential to empowerment (Helms, 1990), and simultaneously claim membership to and identity with more than one racial or ethnic group (Duffy, 1978; Hall, 1992; Root, 1990a), the mixed-race individual is usually forced to "choose just one" identity for the sake of society's comfort level (Hall, 1992; Root, 1990a). As such, society contributes at a very basic level to the unique developmental tasks that lie ahead of the mixed-race person at this point in the history in the United States.

The multiracial person confronts similar issues throughout her or his lifetime, but with more depth and breadth of experience and meaning each time through. For example, color differences start out having neutral meaning; however, as the issue is resurrected each time, in picking friends and relating to peers, dating, partnering, and parenting, a meaning is established that springs out of an illogical social order that defines color as a social category. This section will briefly present some of the unique developmental tasks facing many multiracial people, particularly multiracial women. This context should add depth to a therapist's understanding of themes that may surface in therapy.

The acquisition of a racial label, a core part of one's identity, begins early. Jacobs (1992) suggests that multiracial identity development for the young child has three stages, with several central tasks. Within the three stages, four critical factors were observed in the process of identity development in young biracial (Black and White) children: development of "color constancy" (akin to developing "gender constancy"); internalization of a biracial label; racial ambivalence; and perceptual distortions of color as applied to self and family members. The first stage reflects the absence of a sense of color constancy and a racial label for self. Stage 2 (between ages 4 and 8½ years) reflects a qualitative change in the experience of self in relationship to the environment, as the child has both color constancy and a racial label for self. Unfortunately, this accomplishment is also accompanied by perceptual distortions about color, reflecting society's perceptions of color, which causes racial ambivalence. Stage 3 is observed in 12-year-old biracial children. In this stage, the child understands that color is a social status category and that her or his "color label" is derived from the social status of the groups to which her or his parents belong rather than to appearance and skin color; subsequently, she or he is able to challenge negative internalizations of self and family, allowing her or him to overcome perceptual distortions.

The beginning of dating and the importance of the peer reference group during adolescence poses additional challenges for the multiracial adolescent, particularly having to do with physical appearance and social acceptance. Physical appearance becomes a central part of social relationships with the initiation of dating. Historically, it has been a pivotal characteristic by which to infer the worth and personal characteristics of a woman and her social desirability; physical appearance has been a "ticket for upward social mobility" throughout history (Root, 1990b). Lighter skin, particularly for women, has been important in determining beauty and social class (Neal & Wilson, 1989). The ambiguity or "differentness" of physical appearance can be very painful if it is a central part of the sense of self-worth, particularly when the individual is perceived inconsistently by others. Dating selections are often made on physical appearance according to complex determinations of who is desirable. Boys hold the initiative more frequently in dating relationships. Although conventions have loosened, they more often do the initial choosing of dating partners and seem to be less constrained by the social order of color lines. Although appearance is also important to the multiracial male, it does not tend to play as central a role in evaluating self-worth as it has for females. Boys are valued for many qualities other than physical appearance (e.g., intelligence, athleticism, social status, etc.). However, it should be noted that physical appearance has not been studied in depth in the literature on multiracial people and that physical appearance and ambiguity for multiracial male adolescents and young adults can be a critical part of their social interactions.

Approval and acceptance from the peer group the person wants to belong to become extremely important. Whereas this is important for both genders, it still appears to play a more critical role in the definition of self and establishment of well-being in women. Historically, women have been socialized to define self in terms of relationships to others. The social reactions and interactions the multiracial female adolescent experiences are likely to have a significant impact on her definition of self and potential self-regard. And although this hypothesis has not been empirically tested with multiracial women, it is a viable one.

Multiracial heritage may also be a more salient issue for many adolescent girls because it gives them a double lower status in some environments—female status and ambiguous social status related to color—and may serve as a catalyst for their questioning the implicit social order. Deborah Johnson (personal communication, January 1991) observes that girls, by their tendency to develop socially and physically faster than boys during adolescence, may encounter these issues earlier and more acutely than boys during adolescence.

Gibbs (1989) suggests that the basic tasks for the biracial adolescent are similar to those put forth by Erikson (1959) for adolescents in general—to form a unique identity that simultaneously has a sense of stability or sameness within the individual and has a sense of "historical continuity." However, identity tasks of biracial adolescents are complicated by a need to integrate both a personal and a racial identity. Root (1990a) suggests these identities may not appear to coincide with each other or with phenotype and may appear to be different in different sociopolitial contexts and stages in life.

Whereas the challenges multiracial adolescents may face are complex, in general, it appears that they are able to resolve these challenges positively. Recent studies of nonclinical populations suggest that they have good functioning at social, emotional, and academic levels (e.g., Cauce et al., 1992). If adolescence is extended to college age, several other studies using nonclinical samples suggest that mixed-race individuals are neither more disturbed than their counterparts nor without significant social relationships (e.g., Duffy, 1978; Hall, 1980; Kich, 1982; Murphy-Shigematsu, 1987; Thornton, 1983). For those multiracial adolescents who are not functioning well, it is too simplistic to assume that it is due to their being multiracial.

The young adult continues to work cyclically on a resolution of a satisfactory self-identification that may change through the course of a lifetime mediated by social context, peer relationships, and sociopolitical implications (Root, 1990a). Results of Kich's (1982) research on the developmental processes for asserting a biracial identity in Eurasians in an American sample suggests three stages in this process. In the first stage, the

individual is acutely aware of differences between self- and other perception. In the second stage, there is a struggle for acceptance by the important
reference group. Atkinson, Morten, and Sue (1979) describe a similar stage
in the process of ethnic minority identity, in which the adolescent may go
so far as to reject the part of their racial background that is negatively
evaluated by the reference group from which they seek acceptance. In the
third stage, Kich suggests that there is acceptance of a bicultural and biracial
existence. How one gets to this last stage is a very individual journey (Hall,
1980; Kich, 1982; Murphy-Shigematsu, 1987; Thornton, 1983).

It may be important to make a distinction between the racial mixes
that have been empirically studied (e.g., Asian–White, White–Black, and
Black–Asian). Results of a pilot study I conducted in Honolulu in 1990
demonstrate that there are different attitudes toward the three mixed mentioned above. Different attitudes may significantly impact the experience
of multiraciality and some developmental processes. Thus, generalizations
must be cautiously extended. Several recent studies comparing two different mixtures of multiracial heritage have provided rich data on the similarities and differences of the experience (Cauce et al., 1992; Stephan & Stephan, 1989, 1991; Stephan, 1991).

The majority of research on identity development has been concentrated on children and adolescents. The same has been the case for understanding multiracial identity development. It will be important to extend
our study of identity development to the rest of the life cycle to understand
better how identity is influenced by the stage of life (Root, 1990a) and
context (Root, 1990a; Stephan, 1991) for multiracial persons. Understanding the multiracial person's experience may support the development of
more fluid models of identity, such as those suggested here and consistent
with the evolving literature on women's integrations of different identities
and roles such as mother, daughter, worker, and lover.

MAJOR THEMES IN TREATMENT

> Nothing is harder than identifying with an interracial identity, with a mestizo
> identity. One has to leave the permanent boundaries of a fixed self, literally
> "leave" oneself and see oneself through the eyes of *Other*. (Anzaldua, 1990,
> p. 145)

The major themes related to multiraciality usually bloom in adolescence, and later again in young adulthood. The salience of these themes
at these stages of development may simply be attributed to the nature of
adolescence: a time for determining and defining who one is in relationship
to family, peers, and the larger social environment; a time of self-consciousness intensified by comparison with others and an age-appropriate narcis-
sism; the beginning of dating frought with anguish about being noticed,

fear of rejection, and a desire to be included; an intense desire to be accepted; and last, but not least, a preoccupation with appearance (and a changing physical appearance). Themes and issues may be revisited in young adulthood with more breadth and depth, particularly for women, with the experiences of parenting and pregnancy. These events are additional catalysts for evaluating the significance and meaning of multiracial heritage, and a multigenerational heritage, in one's life and identity.

Some of the general themes related to being multiracial are introduced in this section: (1) uniqueness, (2) acceptance and belonging, (3) physical appearance, (4) sexuality; (5) self-esteem, and (6) identity. The possible ways they may surface in therapy are discussed briefly. A multiracial existence is at the core of the experiences that shape who the mixed-race person of the first generation is. Thus, it is an important context within which to consider the meaning of interpersonal style, perception of the environment, and manifestations of distress. Where one lives in the country, the contact one has with other multiracial persons, and the degree to which parents and relatives have been able to prepare the individual for the meaning and value of a multicultural existence will influence the prominence and resolution of these issues along the developmental lifespan of the individual (Root, 1992). The issues for men and women are similar, but hypothetically manifest themselves in the additional context of gender. Understanding the intersection of gender and multiraciality means confronting the fears and mythology associated with multiraciality that are oppressive.

The mixed-race woman seldom enters therapy overtly to resolve issues that have to do with her multiracial or multicultural heritage. However, the therapist's ability to understand the issues and themes related to this experience allows her or him to facilitate a relief of symptoms and/or strategize problem solving more quickly and in an appropriate context. A brief case summary is provided below as an example of how these issues and themes may be manifested in therapy. All identifying information has been changed; this case represents a composite of several clients.

Cherise was a 28-year-old, single, multiracial woman, the second of four children and second girl. Her mother was White and her father Black. She reported their relationship to be positive, though there were tumultuous times during her adolescent years when her parents separated for 2 years. Her father had recently been diagnosed as terminally ill.

She sought therapy to "sort out relationship issues." Cherise was in a 4-year relationship with a man whom she met in college. This was her first sexually active relationship. She ended the relationship because she felt that something was missing; he didn't understand her perspective on life. Since graduating from college she had had several relationships. She had usually been the one to end the relationship for various reasons: the man put her on a pedestal, their backgrounds were too different, his family make judgments about her background, he didn't understand her, and so on. She wanted to have children and was worried that at the rate she was going she would never find a permanent partner. Her mother suggested that Cherise might be expecting too much from a partner; her friends suggested that Cherise just hadn't found her match, or alternatively, that she thought she was too good for the men she met. She was worried that there was something wrong with her ability to commit and relate in relationships.

Meanwhile she reported withdrawing from social interactions, eating more, and avoiding the increased attention men appeared to be paying to her.

Uniqueness

Adolescence is marked by ambivalence about being different from one's peers. On the one hand the adolescent laments "being the only one who is . . ." and on the other hand often makes stereotypical attempts to be unique. In some ways the adolescent experience extends throughout the multiracial person's lifetime. The theme of uniqueness is a significant part of the multiracial person's experience; it interfaces with all the other themes to be discussed in this chapter. Whereas one might think that the multiracial person would derive a developmental benefit from her or his uniqueness, ironically it may pose an additional obstacle to establishing a positive self-esteem and identity. Additionally, many of the interpersonal styles and defenses established to assert one's way of being and perceiving the world may be pathologized if misunderstood (Bradshaw, 1992).

The multiracial woman may feel ambivalent about being special. Her uniqueness in the eyes of others is initially related to the ambiguity of her racial features, and subsequently, to her heritage; she is often regarded as an object (e.g., exotic) or a curiosity. This type of oppression perpetuates feeling "outside" of a group; she may feel hurt, angry, and/or incorporate this information into a negative sense of self-esteem (i.e., something is wrong with her). Conversely, many multiracials receive a great deal of attention and may feel deflated or less valued if something changes and their appearance or existence is no longer perceived as being so special. With either experience, a multiracial woman may feel alienated, anxious, depressed, and angry in response to events not apparently related to the personal problems she anticipates. Issues or feelings may appear more intense than the manifest issue warrants. A task in development is to understand if and how these feelings are related to the multiracial experience, how to interpret the feeling, and how to cope.

Women are particularly vulnerable to society's reactions to their ambiguous features. These reactions will echo the overvaluation placed on women's physical appearance that plays a critical role in the development of some unhealthy practices such as eating disorders, cosmetic dieting, and some elective cosmetic surgeries. Furthermore, if a woman's uniqueness is seen as exotic, some women internalize this perception and will behave in ways to fulfill society's expectations of the exotic woman. As such, this experience interferes with self-discovery and the declaration of who one is, apart from physical appearance.

In therapy, the experience of being the "only one" may manifest itself through the personalization of events and interactions that perpetuate feeling "different" or misperceived. Such a style may also originate in growing up in a family that was isolated by a community, isolated itself as a protective reaction against antimiscegenist responses, or was unable to provide proper socialization for coping with being multiracial. The repeated experience of being misunderstood may also contribute to the development of a style of communicating that attempts to provide a great deal of context in order to be better understood. However, this style can look compulsive and at times paranoid.

A lifetime of uniqueness may coincide with tremendous feelings of isolation and attendant depression and self-doubt. This observation is particularly relevant for women, who more than men derive validation from their shared experiences with significant people in their environment. Helping such a woman to connect her current feelings with her experiences of being multiracial can be particularly enlightening. Much benefit can be derived from a multiacial support group.

In contrast, the unique vantage point of some multiracial people has led to much questioning on their part of how the world works and given them more trust in their own perceptions than in those of others; this outlook does not necessarily result from a dysfunctional family, but from a dysfunctional society. This position at times may look as though the multiracial woman thinks that she is better than others or "entitled" in a way that appears narcissistic. It is important to consider that many multiracial women have grown up in communities and during a time in which the subtle governing rules of the social order are often illogical; many of them have also felt it necessary to be the representative or protector of their family and their parents, partly as a defense mechanism for their own insecurity. The style that emerges is "normative" for many multiracial persons (Bradshaw, 1992). Exploration of their emotional pain (hurt, anger, depression) needs to be explored in a larger social context. The therapist can play a significant role in listening to the individual's reality and helping the woman to determine how she wishes to feel or act differently. Some individuals may wish to decrease their sense of self-consciousness and responsibility to others.

In the case of Cherise, there are at least two clues that suggest that the theme of uniqueness was contributing to her depression, anxiety, and feelings of isolation: (1) more than one partner had not understood her world perspective; and (2) her friends observed that she hadn't met her match or that she thought she was better than the men she dated. This latter point illustrates how "specialness" may convey expectations. Cherise was particularly distressed because although her perspective tended to be different from that of other people around her, it did work for her. But she was not so sure that she trusted her perceptions of herself. Increasing self-doubt and depression indicated that she was feeling misperceived and isolated in her experiences.

Acceptance and Belonging

At the core of the need to belong and to be accepted is that of connection, how one interpersonally experiences and is experienced in the world. This connection or grounding in one's social environment provides a foundation for positive self-esteem and identity. Many mixed-race people grow up with countless experiences that illogically and unnecessarily set them apart from others. For example, most multiracials have experienced being stared at and asked insensitive questions about their physical appearance (e.g., "What are you?"), family experience, and cultural differences (e.g., "Where are you from?"). Connection is difficult when one is the object of curiosity, pity, or fear.

There are rules about belonging to any group. Some of them become painfully apparent when dating starts, which, for the biracial woman, is potentially all interracial. For example, one light-skinned Eurasian woman described her high-school dating experience as being "liked by everyone and dated by no one." She attributed her situation to being perceived as a person of color by Whites, not really Japanese enough by the parents of her Japanese classmates, and not a person of color by her African American friends. The multiracial woman needs strategies for coping with these situations.

Belonging can also be a broader experience than many monoracial women's experiences. Many respondents in Hall's (1980) dissertation suggested that whereas their biracial identity resulted in their not fitting in perfectly to any situation, except perhaps with other mixed-race persons (also reported in Williams, 1992), they had membership in multiple groups. Sometimes the multiracial person will focus on the fact of not fitting in and feel isolated and alienated. A therapist can be particularly helpful to the multiracial person by validating these feelings and experiences and exploring how "the cup is half full" rather than always "half empty" (i.e., the advantages and comfort they have in initially being part of different groups).

The history of race relations in the United States contributes to the concern and even preoccupation with "acceptance" that some multiracial people experience; society's efforts to preserve color lines put the multiracial woman in a peripheral position. Many communities of color have narrow criteria for group membership; sometimes the criteria have sociopolitical significance (e.g., is this person visibly a minority person?). Sometimes the criteria are very inclusive for political reasons (e.g., when numbers count). Sometimes the criteria repeat the elitist, senseless process of treating race as a scientific concept and confusing it with ethnicity (e.g., "full-blood" individuals being more valued than those with mixed blood). The criteria become painful, however, when differences are emphasized and similarities are dismissed, the former resulting in exclusion of the multiracial person. Subsequently, many mixed-race persons suffer in the communities to which they are socially assigned because they do not "look right," "think right," or "act right." Consequently, some multiracial people try extra hard to prove that they are African American, Native American, Asian American, or Latino because belonging and acceptance are so important. And because some multiracial people do not stereotypically look like people of color they may attempt to prove ethnic group membership to the extent of engaging in negative sterotypic behavior (e.g., Wilson, 1992) or emphasizing identification with the cultural practices of only one part of their ethnic heritage.

The implications for therapy are significant. The multiracial woman may manifest social anxiety, general anxiety, detachment, or depression when she does not feel connected. These are reactions of powerlessness and alienation that may be based in a reality that at times is very subtle. Feelings of being an "imposter" might arise as a signal that she feels pseudo- or conditional acceptance within a group. The experiences that give rise to this feeling may also give rise to a lack of confidence in herself or lack of trust in how she perceives her environment. The therapist can provide a sociopolitical perspective to both explore this experience and increase the client's self-confidence, and also affirm that being different is not bad or inferior. It is helpful for the therapist to acknowledge that there are very real barriers in the social environment for mixed-race people that may heighten feelings of alienation and isolation, increasing vulnerability to depression and anxiety. The strategies one employs to fit in might also make one too dependent on validation from outside of oneself. Lastly, the therapist might explore whether the multiracial woman is denouncing parts of her heritage in order to belong. The therapist must be aware of the difference between ethnicity and race and the limitations of both of these concepts.

To return to our case study, Cherise's anxiety over her relationships opened the door to her talking about how she often feels "alone in a crowd." This experience was related to the themes of both uniqueness and belonging. She often felt she didn't quite fit. These feelings were subsequently linked to her experience of truly having a different perspective that was probably related to her multiracial background. She described an experience in junior high that conveyed the rules of belonging. Cherise, like other girls was experimenting with her hair, clothes, and makeup. On several occasions she had been confronted with "What are you? Black or what?" A popular girl told her that she had to "make up her mind and stick to it" and else people wouldn't trust her. Thus, in a matter of seconds, she was handed the illogical belief system about race. It is supposed to be a constant identity and status. Since then she has "acted" Black, but worries about acceptance by the Black community because she might not be "legitimately" Black enough. The therapist started to support her identification as multiracial and multicultural—and encourage the notion that she could even feel differently on different days.

Physical Appearance

Perhaps the existence of the multiracial woman has been minimized because to acknowledge her existence is to confront a social order based on color and racism within and between groups. The spectrum of appearance when races are mixed blurs the lines that are asserted because even the same combination yields a continuum of color and other racial features (Hall, 1980, 1992; Williams, 1992). For example, Black Japanese can look stereotypically Black, Japanese, Filipino, Hawaiian, Polynesian, or Eurasian. Black Native American people can look Black, Indian, Polynesian, and so on. Furthermore, although physical appearance plays an important role in ethnic identification (Neal & Wilson, 1989), Hall (1980) found that it did not predict identity choices of individuals in her study of Black Japanese.

There are several unique experiences related to physical appearance that interact with other issues for many multiracial women. Three are discussed here. Sometimes a name does not match what people expect to see. For example, a young woman with a German surname looks very Asian. People ask her if this is a married name, adopted name, and so on. A second unique experience is that of being stared at countless numbers of times. This experience fosters a self-consciousness that can exceed the adolescent years and is more intense and often more self-critical than the average self-consciousness of teenagers and young adults. It can be translated into feeling that one is being judged and evaluated, which may have a basis in fact. With the popularity of cognitive therapy, the therapist is advised to apply cautiously techniques that challenge irrational self-statements. The therapist should seriously consider the possibility that the multiracial person's experience is very different and the person may have a reality base for feeling "constantly judged and evaluated."

The third experience, a "flexible look" that changes with age, hairstyle, clothes, lighting, makeup, and who is looking, adds to the complexity of the multiracial woman's experience. First, because some multiracial women can voluntarily change how they are perceived racially, they can manipulate the types of subjective feedback and experiences to which they are exposed. (Consequently, she has unique access to first-hand experience of more than one group of people.) However, the flexibility of this look is sometimes in the eyes of the beholder: any one peron may "see" her in a way that does not correspond with how she sees herself, or to how most others see her. The result is that *the multiracial woman (or man) has to learn to establish a consistent, internal identity that resides within her and is not necessarily reflected back in the environment* by Anzaldúa's (1990) "other." The flexible look and attendant social reactions also contribute to the self-consciousness that has been discussed and also specific self-criticism of various parts of the body related to racial features: eyes, nose, mouth, hair, and so on. A particularly difficult issue may have to do with hair, particularly for persons who are of African American or Asian American heritage. Hair can determine physical identification by others with a specific ethnic and racial group, and thus becomes a vehicle through which symbolic integration of a multiracial identity occurs. Asian people with lighter hair may wish for darker hair. Conversely, darker-haired Asian people may wish for lighter hair. The African American biracial person may feel tormented by hair that isn't kinky enough. Conversely, the adolescent or young adult may grapple with issues of loyalty and belonging if she wishes to do anything with her hair that moves it toward being straighter or wavy. Lastly, individuals may "play" with their flexible look beyond the adolescent years, when experimentation is considered normal. Some days they may strive to look Black, other days mixed, and other days they may strive for an ethnic look that is not part of their heritage. Such behavior does not necessarily indicate pathology or lack of a stable identity, but may instead reflect a valuing of different pieces of the person's identity (much as one may choose a different color or style of clothing to suit one's mood), or even a conscious or unconscious challenge to society's social order. In my clinical experience I find that women and teenage girls engage in this behavior more often than boys and men, since physical appearance and fashion have been made more of an issue for women than for men.

Successfully and sensitively working with a multiracial client requires that the therapist has explored and continues to explore how she or he has internalized rules of racial categorization and accompanying ethnic stereotypes. For example, if a White–Black woman looks as if she is trying to "pass for White" could it also be that at times she is trying to "pass for Black"? And might it be that she is not trying to "pass," but that perceptions of passing reflect the therapist's implicit rules for racial boundaries? The therapist's clarity and flexibility and personal work to avoid prejudicial tendencies will provide her or him with an opportunity to distinguish dysfunctional from normative behavior and to help empower the client.

Although the issue of physical appearance is prominent for both multiracial women and men, it is embedded in a social context that classifies physical appearance as the most significant asset a woman possesses. Together with striving for acceptance, struggling with identity, developing self-worth, and placing an external emphasis on physical appearance, some mixed-race women may be particularly vulnerable to developing eating disorders (Root, 1990b). The multiracial woman is in a particularly odd position, as physical appearance may be a double-edged sword. The unique integration of racial features may be quite aesthetically pleasing (the international modeling industry is increasingly capitalizing on "cosmopolitan" or "exotic" looking models). However, stares and questions in everyday life can transform this same physical attractiveness into a burden.

Themes having to do with physical appearance were prominent in Cherise's life, and subtly related to her experiences and choices of relationships. The confrontation she had with the girl in junior high school, mentioned earlier, had a profound effect on her. She learned that she was an "oddity" because of the flexibility of her racial appearance. Futhermore, she also felt anxious and powerless about trying to control the way people categorized her racially. Self-conscious about her appearance, she described her experience "as though people see in me what is most different from them." She had been accused of trying to pass for White; she laughed, asking, "When have you seen a chestnut colored White?" And she said, "What is the problem if I look kind of White? That is part of me too, but somehow I can only be one thing." The therapist supported a discussion of how situational context very much "colors" what a person sees in another person or themselves, and encouraged her to play with her racial and ethnic appearance to suit her mood, much like she had in junior high. Her personal belief system about racial classification and the meaning of these categories was explored. Cherise started to talk about how conscious she was of the color of the men she dated because she felt judged according to whom she chose to date.

Sexuality

The oppression of discrimination against multiracial women, compared to that of multiracial men, is especially great in the area of sexuality. The "exoticness" attributed to a multiracial woman is usually part of a male fantasy in which he seeks possession and dominance over the sexuality and sexual behavior of a type of woman with which he is unfamiliar. Nakashima (1992) suggests that the attractiveness of the multiracial woman is partially linked to the stereotype of her being an unusually sexual being. She observes that

> the most constant off-shoot of this biological–psychological profile of people of mixed race is the stereotype that they are sexually immoral and out of control. This is especially true of multiracial women—whether they be "half-breed" Indian, Mexican "mestiza," "mulatta," or "Eurasian"; . . . They are consistently imaged as extremely passionate and sexually promiscuous. (p. 168)

This fiction is portrayed in the pornography industry's stereotype of multiracial women. She further suggests that the mythology about the multiracial person's sexuality is perpetuated by oppressive stereotypes of American racial minorities as immoral, degenerate, and uncontrollable, particularly in their sexual impulses.

Multiracial women are especially vulnerable to internalizing the oppressive expectations of the exotic woman because of society's socialization of the importance of physical appearance, mixed messages about women's sexuality, and the oppressive beliefs about the sexuality of multiracial women. Accepting an "exotic" role may provide the permission to be sexual. Conversely, some mixed-race women may curtail the expression of their sexuality in order not to be stereotyped.

Lastly, the racially mixed woman may be more open to exploring sexual orientation. This openness often reflects the lifetime experience of flexibility in considering aspects of racial identity, which society teaches us to perceive as mutually exclusive categories, as it does heterosexual and homosexual identities. Because the integration of otherwise mutually exclusive identities is a given with respect to race, the racially mixed woman is often more open to exploring sexual identity as well.

Those racially mixed women whose historical experience has weakened their sense of uniqueness, led them to view their specialness solely in terms of their appearance, or left them hungering for social acceptance may be more likely to choose partners who objectify them (as exotic) and seek to "possess" them, often as a way of bolstering their own sense of self-worth. Such a relationship is likely to revolve around sexual relations that are fueled by fantasies loaded with racial and gender stereotypes. Ultimately, the racially mixed woman will still feel emotionally unfulfilled. While there may be many paths of experience that lead to this type of relationship, the therapist should consider whether a history of sexual abuse, rape, or emotional abuse may account for her vulnerability to these relationships, as these experiences also objectify an individual.

Cherise's sexuality was tied in with issues of self-esteem and physical appearance and had sometimes been a source of conflict on dates she had had with men. She felt that she had dated several men who were attracted to her "exoticness," who sometimes thought she was of Polynesian background. She found that many of these men had fantasies that she would be really different. In fact, Cherise described herself as having often held back expressing her sexual feelings for fear of contributing to these fantasies. Her recent avoidance of men was related to her feeling that she was tired of being treated like an object "to possess."

Self-Esteem

Contemporary studies of nonclinical samples of mixed-race persons show successful adjustment and positive self-regard (e.g., Hall, 1980; Johnson & Nagoshi, 1986). Nevertheless, some mixed-race people are in environments that make it difficult for them to feel good about themselves (Gibbs, 1987) because of negative messages and expectations regarding their multiracial heritage. Some multiracial people work very hard to excel at something to counter covert expectations that they are somehow inferior to monoracial persons. For example, one Latina Black woman said it was essential for her to prove that she was better than most of her peers so that she would get respect for herself and her family. She equated excellence with acceptance and desirability; excellence resulted in her being sought out by different groups of people. She observed in retrospect that while she was aware at the time that she wanted respect, she only later related it to striving for acceptance and belonging, a theme in her life as a mixed-race person.

The mixed-race person may try extremely hard to "be good" or be an exemplary citizen in order to combat overt or covert negative evaluations of their parents' interracial union or their multiracial heritage. Some multiracial people counter negative expectations with a defense that magnifies Park's (1928) suggestion that the multicultural person is the cosmopolitan of the world. This defense can appear narcissistic, since the individual believes that special things are expected of her or him. This foundation for self-esteem is fragile, and those who have it may feel devastated when they do not meet the expectations upon which they base their self-worth. For example, a 23-year-old woman sought therapy for profound depression. She had been reluctant to seek help because she felt she should be able to overcome the depression herself. The onset of depression followed her failing the bar exam for her state; since then she had been unable to seek work or study for the next exam. Although the therapist attempted to characterize her failure of the bar exam as normal (saying that a significant proportion of bright people fail it each time and that they should try to see whether test anxiety was a factor) the client could not think of herself as part of the norm. She was terribly afraid that her world would end if she failed a second time. In therapy it became apparent that her self-esteem had been predicated upon being perceived as exceptional, consistent with her destiny as a "special person," which was itself consistent with her completing law school at such a young age.

Much of a person's self-esteem comes from feeling special, valued, connected, and accepted. The mixed-race woman's evaluation of self may rest in how much she thinks others value her more than in how much she values herself. This mindset is initially reflected by the family and later by the larger social environment. It is critical that parents understand their own racist beliefs, so that cultural differences are respected and do not have negative impact on a child's self-esteem and self-concept. Mothers particularly have carried the responsibilities of the early socialization of their children. Parents need to provide primary interventions or innoculations against the dysfunctional attitudes of the social system toward women (i.e., historically women more often than men seem to base their self-esteem on whether or not they receive social approval). Parents should acknowledge the complex effects of physical appearance, provide direct education about the fantasies and stereotypes that people may have about multiracial people and interracial families, and teach a child psychological and verbal defenses that are empowering.

The majority of multiracial people I have studied seem to be well adjusted and feel good about themselves, despite some of the extra hardships of growing up. Cherise appeared to be no exception. A therapist with internalized oppressive beliefs about multiracial people might be ready to conclude that Cherise's difficulties in relationships might stem from low self-esteem. But that was not the case with this therapist, whose greatest concern was that Cherise's feelings of being misperceived, isolated, depressed, and anxious would start to change her image of herself in a negative direction of the stereotype of the tormented biracial woman.

Identity

The sense of identity is a feeling of belonging. The theme of identity emerges, if not overtly through issues of belonging, then through feelings related to exclusion: isolation, depression, anxiety, and anger. The person who identifies herself or himself as multiracial possesses both multiracial and multicultural heritage and identity. For example, a major difference between African Americans and multiracially identified African Americans is not a fundamental difference in racial heritage but rather that the latter group identify themselves as multicultural and feel a kinship with more than one group. Identity can be a political, social, cultural, and/or physical issue to resolve. And these aspects of identity are not necessarily congruent.

Socialization of a sense of ethnic identity is a unique feature of the lives of minority group members in American culture because this culture has made race such an issue. Miller and Miller (1990) observe the important role that parents of biracial children play. They reflect on the necessity to orient biracial children to a minority agenda or they will be "defenseless against a social reality" (p. 176). Because little data exists, we do not know the influence of parents on the ethnic identity choices of their children. Some researchers suggest that at least for children at earlier ages, mothers may play a very important role in the ethnic socialization of children (e.g., Johnson, 1990), much as they play in other aspects of children's lives and in the general socialization of children of color (e.g., Greene, 1990).

Wilson (1991) observes that racial and ethnic identity for an individual may be different from one another and different also from phenotypic identity. Ultimately, with people who do not know them, it is important that multiracial persons be able to self-proclaim their identities and change them situationally because their ethnic and cultural identities are not necessarily apparent to the observer (Root, 1990a). Multiple identities do not pose an inherent problem for the individual, except for when a complex identity is viewed as abnormal by onlookers. Forbes (1989) reminds us that we all have multiple identities, but that somehow we have assumed a dichotomous and rigid approach to race, often confusing it with ethnicity. For example, some of the "cousins" will likely be in the "black" community, some are active "Indians," while still others may lead a dual life, sometimes being one thing, sometimes another. They may, for example, attend a "black" church where they do not publicly announce any Indian identity, and yet they may be Indian when visiting relatives or attending a pow-wow function. (p. 42)

Duffy (1978) concluded that such a duality may be viewed as a "simultaneously dynamic ethnic identity."

No empirical data exist about the choices multiracial women make in their partners. Society's dichotomies about race, a tendency to try to preserve color lines, mistaken beliefs about miscegenation, and confusion of ethnicity with race would predict that the multiracial person's choice of partner has added complexity. A person's beginning to date and make long-term commitments may expose the covert racism of significant others and the larger social system. Virtually all dating or partnering may feel interracial or interethnic to the multiracial person.

Many scholars in the area of multiracial identity (e.g., Wilson, 1992; Forbes, 1988) feel that left to her or his own devices the multiracial individual would work out identity issues. However, social forces complicate matters. For example, the U.S. Census Bureau, employers, health insurance, and so on expect us to choose only one racial and ethnic identity. The dilemma for the multiracial person of Native American, Filipino, and Scottish heritage might be to (1) remember what she or he checked the last time (and determine if the situation requires consistency); (2) consider the social, emotional, and historical implications of checking "other"; (3) consider the political and economic implications of checking "other" (would it deprive constituency, such as Native Americans of the numbers it needs for adequate representation?); (4) void the form by checking more than one identity; (5) write in an identity that will be ignored.

Some strategies used by multiracial people to reinforce and proclaim their identity may be misunderstood. Many of them center around names that are an important conveyor of ethnic identity and connection with their ancestors. Many mixed-race persons do not receive names that connote the multiple heritages. Therefore, they may change their names or add to their names, so as to strengthen an internal sense of belonging and/or identity with an important reference group and to provide historical continuity (cf. Murphy-Shigematsu, 1987). Others use middle names or reclaim formal names if their first names or nicknames obscure their ethnic heritage.

Sometimes people will fabricate ethnic identities that are more consistent with their appearance in order to avoid questions and negative reactions. For example, an adolescent Black–White girl said she would tell people she was Egyptian because this made her more interesting and did not lead to intrusive questions about whether or not her parents were married or about her home life.

During the lifespan, there are experiences that sometimes facilitate clarification of identity (e.g., the birth of a child, the death of a parent, the choosing of a partner, the endings of relationships, or sociopolitical events). Sometimes the impact of these experiences results in a clarification of identity that appears to others to be a change in identity. Given society's belief that racial and ethnic identity are static, a change or clarification in racial or ethnic self-identification declared by a racially mixed person may be misinterpreted as pathological. The clarifications and changes observed in some multiracial persons might be akin to parents reevaluating a piece of their identity as children leave home, when they become grandparents, when their parents die, and so on.

The multiracial woman's resolution of her ethnic identity is a political process whether it is consciously or unconsciously determined because of confusion in the United States of race and ethnicity. It subsequently influences her choice of partners. However, the multiracial woman's experience leads to less rigidity along color lines than others have in choosing partners; her reality is that all dating and partnering is interracial at some level. It is no surprise that Williams (1992) found that many of her respondents wished to be partnered with someone who was mixed; the other respondents were divided in their choices.

Cherise's identity gradually became more flexible in a way that was congruent with her needs. She moved from identifying herself as monoculturally Black to multiracial and multicultural, which appeared to be a move of empowerment. The expansion of her racial and cultural identity provided her a better understanding of what was "missing" in her relationships. With a redefinition of her social and cultural identity she felt freer to challenge the dictums of color lines in relationships and freer to choose her partners. Therapy helped her to validate herself and defend herself as a multiracial woman. She was able to assimilate these skills quickly because her parents had given her tools to validate and defend herself as a Black woman. She also came to realize that no one person could fulfill all the needs she currently had; she was getting some of these needs met by reading articles on multiracial people and subscribing to a newsletter for multiracial people. By the end of therapy she appeared more physically relaxed, reported feeling more "congruent" with herself, and was hopeful about her future relationships.

SUMMARY

Therapy with multiracial people can prompt us to examine our assumptions about race and ethnicity and the degree to which we have internalized a pseudoscientific and oppressive belief system. In this chapter, the unique pressures and experiences of multiracial women, and mixed-race people in general, have been highlighted. A concern at this time is the trend toward considering "exotic" looks intriguing, which may bring attention to multiracial people in this country, but also may continue the oppressive fantasies and the treatment of multiracial women as objects. Oppression insidiously affects mental health.

Despite oppressive mythology about miscegenation and the reality of multiracial people, mixed-race people tend to integrate their diverse experiences in a positive manner. Difficulties that arise from being multiracial are usually the results of an oppressive, dysfunctional environment that is perpetuated by ignorance and fear and falsely based notions of racial and cultural superiority. The distress that the multiracial woman may exhibit can be congruent with symptoms observed in people growing up in dysfunctional homes. The therapist is advised to consider how the symptoms of growing up isolated from other multiracial individuals and families in a dysfunctional sociopolitical environment can mimic family dysfunction. Without this consideration the therapist may conceptualize distress in a way that invokes one of the nonrational hypotheses that have maintained the hostility toward miscegenation through several generations. Then, the individual's distress would be blamed on the family, ultimately the mother, and used to support illogical disparagement of interracial unions. In order to evaluate such biases, I have provided guidelines to assess the validity and generalizability of a growing body of literature for professional and lay audiences.

It is possible that the themes I have outlined in this chapter—uniqueness, belonging and acceptance, physical appearance, sexuality, self-esteem and identity—will be less prominent issues in the lives of multiracial women in the future. Whereas the majority of multiracial people in this country at this time are biracial, the emerging generation will be multiracial. The next generation may benefit from biracial parents who can serve as role models and be empathetic to additional challenges of integrating a multicultural heritage, an experience largely absent for biracial people. Hopefully, as the number of multiracial people increases this will pose a concrete challenge to the racism that currently exists between and within groups. Consciousness is already starting to be raised in a way that is influencing theories and policies that affect our lives.

REFERENCES

Atkinson, D., Morten, G., & Sue, D. W. (1979). *Counseling American minorities: A cross-cultural perspective*. Dubuque, IA: Brown.

Anzaldúa, G. (Ed.). (1990). *Making face, making soul—Haciendo caras: Creative and critical perspectives by feminists of color*. San Francisco: Aunt Lute Foundation.

Bradshaw, C. K. (1992). Beauty and the beast: On racial ambiguity. In M. P. P. Root (Ed.), *Racially mixed people in America*. Newbury Park, CA: Sage.

Cauce, A. M., Hiraga, Y., Mason, C., Aguilar, T., Ordonez, N., & Gonzales, N. (1992). Between a rock and a hard place: Social adjustment of biracial youth. In M. P. P. (Root (Ed.), *Racially mixed people in America*. Newbury Park, CA: Sage.

Daniel, G. R. (1992). Passers and pluralists: Subverting the racial divide. In M. P. P. Root (Ed.), *Racially mixed people in America*. Newbury Park, CA: Sage.

Duffy, L. K. (1978). *The interracial individual: Self concept, parental interaction, and ethnic identity*. Unpublished master's thesis, University of Hawaii, Honolulu.

Erikson, E. H. (1959). Identity and the life cycle. *Psychological Issues, 1*.

Essed, P. (1991). Understanding everyday racism: An interdisciplinary theory and analysis of the experiences of Black women (M. Vogel, Trans.). *Interchange, 8*, 5–7.

Fernandez, C. A. (1992). La Raza and the melting pot: A comparative look at multiethnicity. In M. P. P. Root (Ed.), *Racially mixed people in America*. Newbury Park, CA: Sage.

Forbes, J. D. (1988). *Black Africans and Native Americans*. Oxford, England: Basil Blackwell.

Forbes, J. D. (1989). The manipulation of race, caste and identity: Classifying Afroamericans, Native Americans and Red-Black people. *Journal of Ethnic Studies, 17*, 1–51.

Freire, P. (1970). *Cultural action for freedom*. Cambridge, MA: Harvard Educational Review Press.

Gibbs, J. T. (1987). Identity and marginality: Issues in the treatment of biracial adolescents. *American Journal of Orthopsychiatry, 57*, 265–278.

Gibbs, J. T. (1989). Biracial adolescents. In J. T. Gibbs & L. N. Huang (Eds.), *Children of color: Psychological interventions with minority youth*. San Francisco: Jossey-Bass.

Gist, N. P., & Dworkin, A. G. (Eds.). (1972). *The blending of races: Marginality and identity in world perspective*. New York: Wiley-Interscience.

Greene, B. A. (1990). What has gone before: The legacy of racism and sexism in the lives of Black mothers and daughters. In L. S. Brown & M. P. P. Root (Eds.), *Diversity and complexity in feminist therapy*. New York: Haworth Press.

Hall, C. C. I. (1980). *The ethnic identity of racially mixed people: A study of Black-Japanese*. Unpublished doctoral dissertation, University of California, Los Angeles.

Hall, C. C. I. (1992). Please choose one: The ethnic identity choices for biracial individuals. In M. P. P. Root (Ed.), *Racially mixed people in America*. Newbury Park, CA: Sage.

Helms, J. (1990). What's in a name change? *Focus, 4*, 1–2.

Henriques, F. (1975). *Children of conflict: A study of interracial sex and marriage*. New York: E. P. Dutton.

Ho, F. C., & Johnson, R. C. (1991). Intra-ethnic and inter-ethnic marriage and divorce in Hawaii. *Social Biology, 37*, 44–51.

Houston, V. H. (1985, December). Amerasian girl. *Pacific Citizen*.

Jacobs, J. H. (1977). *Black/White interracial families: Marital process and identity development in young children*. Unpublished doctoral dissertation, The Wright Institute, Berkeley, CA.

Jacobs, J. H. (1992). Identity development in biracial children. In M. P. P. Root (Ed.), *Racially mixed people in America*. Newbury Park, CA: Sage.

Johnson, D. (1990). *Racial preference and biculturality in biracial preschoolers.* Unpublished manuscript.

Johnson, R. C. (1992). Offspring of cross-race and cross-ethnic marriages in Hawaii. In M. P. P. Root (Ed.), *Racially mixed people in America.* Newbury Park, CA: Sage.

Johnson, R. C., & Nagoshi, C. (1986). The adjustment of offspring of within-group and interracial/intercultural marriages: A comparison of personality factor scores. *Journal of Marriage and the Family, 48,* 279–284.

Kich, G. K. (1982). *Eurasians: Ethnic/racial identity development of biracial Japanese/ White adults.* Unpublished doctoral dissertation, The Wright Institute, Berkeley, CA.

Miller, R. (1992). The color wheel and ethnic and racial identity. In M. P. P. Root (Ed.), *Racially mixed people in America.* Newbury Park, CA: Sage.

Miller, R., & Miller, B. (1990). Mothering the biracial child: Bridging the gaps between African-American and white parenting styles. *Women and Therapy, 10,* 169–180.

Murphy-Shigematsu, S. (1987). *The voices of Amerasians: Ethnicity, identity, and empowerment in interracial Japanese Americans.* Unpublished doctoral dissertation, Harvard University, Cambridge, MA.

Nakashima, C. (1992). An invisible monster: The creation and denial of mixed race people in America. In M. P. P. Root (Ed.), *Racially mixed people in America.* Newbury Park, CA: Sage.

Neal, A., & Wilson, M. L. (1989). The role of skin color and features in the Black community: Implications for Black women and therapy. *Clinical Psychology Review, 9,* 323–334.

Park, R. E. (1928). Human migration and the marginal man. *American Journal of Sociology, 33,* 881–893.

Root, M. P. P. (1990a). Resolving "other" status: Identity development of biracial individuals. In L. S. Brown & M. P. P. Root (Eds.), *Diversity and complexity in feminist therapy.* New York: Haworth Press.

Root, M. P. P. (1990b). Disordered eating in women of color. *Sex Roles, 22,* 525–536.

Root, M. P. P. (Ed.). (1992). *Racially mixed people in America.* Newbury Park, CA: Sage.

Spickard, P. R. (1989). *Mixed blood: Intermarriage and ethnic identity in twentieth-century America.* Madison, WI: University of Wisconsin Press.

Spickard, P. R. (1992). The illogic of American racial categories. In M. P. P. Root (Ed.), *Racially mixed people in America.* Newbury Park, CA: Sage.

Stephan, C. W. (1991). Ethnic identity among mixed-heritage people in Hawaii. *Symbolic Interaction, 14,* 261–277.

Stephan, C. W. (1992). The causes and consequences of ethnic identity. In M. P. P. Root (Ed.), *Racially mixed people in America.* Newbury Park, CA: Sage.

Stephan, C. W., & Stephan, W. G. (1989). After intermarriage: Ethnic identity among mixed-heritage Japanese-Americans and Hispanics. *Journal of Marriage and the Family, 51,* 507–519.

Stephan, W. G., & Stephan, C. W. (1991). Intermarriage: Effects on personality, adjustment and intergroup relations in two samples of students. *Journal of Marriage and the Family, 53,* 241–250.

Stonequist, E. V. (1937). *The marginal man: A study in personality and culture conflict.* New York: Russell & Russell.

Thorton, M. C. (1983). *A social history of a multiethnic identity: The case of Black Japanese Americans.* Unpublished doctoral dissertation, University of Michigan, Ann Arbor.

Williams, T. K. (1992). Prism lives: Identity of binational Amerasians. In M. P. P. Root (Ed.), *Racially mixed people in America.* Newbury Park, CA: Sage.

Wilson, T. (1991). People of mixed race descent. In Y. I. Song & E. C. Kim (Eds.), *American mosaic: Selected readings on America's multicultural heritage.* Sacramento, CA: Ethnicus—Center for Multicultural Studies.

Wilson, T. (1992). Blood quantum: Native American mixed bloods. In M. P. P. Root (Ed.), *Racially mixed people in America.* Newbury Park, CA: Sage.

17

Southeast Asian American Refugee Women

Liang Tien

Ba, a 37-year-old Vietnamese American, sought psychotherapeutic treatment at the recommendation of her family physician. She presented with headaches and muscle spasms in her back.

Lin, a 25-year-old Cambodian American, was referred to treatment by Child Protective Services (CPS). Her 5-month-old infant was diagnosed with "failure to thrive." CPS placed the infant in foster care, with the stipulation Lin receive mental health treatment.

These two women, both Southeast Asians and refugees in America, present with different complaints for psychotherapy. Their cultural backgrounds and personal histories are quite different, though they are both from Southeast Asia. What they do have in common are their political status as refugees and their experience of war and forced migration. This chapter examines the unique cultural backgrounds, as well as the factors of gender, forced migration, and relocation to the United States, as it applies to the psychotherapeutic treatment of Vietnamese and Cambodian women.

Southeast Asian American refugee women come from a number of different countries, each of which is home to many diverse ethnic groups. Each ethnic group maintains different cultural, political, and religious heritages; each deserves its own chapter. Because of considerations of space, I have chosen to focus on women from the two largest groups of Southeast Asian refugees in America: the Vietnamese and Cambodians. This chapter is not intended as an in-depth discussion of the cultural backgrounds of Southeast Asian American refugee women. I discuss only those cultural practices and political issues germane to psychotherapy by examining two composites of the many Vietnamese and Cambodian women I have had the opportunity to treat personally, either as the supervisor of a direct-service therapist, or as a consultant to treatment programs. Unless otherwise credited, this material is based on 6 years of first-hand experience working with refugees from Southeast Asia.

I begin this chapter with a definition of some key terms. Then I present a review and discussion of the impact of politics and war on these women's lives. This is followed by an examination of treatment considerations. I conclude with a discussion of possible responses to the presenting complaints detailed in the above section.

DEFINITION OF TERMS

Between April 1975 and September 1988 approximately 881,500 Southeast Asian refugees entered the United States; approximately 45%, or 396,700, were women (Office of Refugee Resettlement [ORR], 1988). The phrase "Southeast Asian American refugee women" designates a specific group of women. "Southeast Asian" refers to the geographic region that encompasses all the countries in the Asian subcontinent that are south of China and east of India. These include the countries of Indonesia, Malaysia, Thailand, Burma, Bhutan, and Bangladesh, as well as Vietnam, Kampuchea, and Laos. The phrase "Southeast Asian American" refers to individuals with ancestry from any of the above named countries who reside in the United States with the stated intent of permanent resettlement. The term "refugee" refers to legal entry status, as designated by the United States Department of State.

The Refugee Act of 1980 defines refugees as those persons outside of their homeland who are unwilling or unable to return home because of "persecution or a well-founded fear of persecution" (PL 96-212). To date, only citizens from three Southeast Asian countries—Vietnam, Kampuchea, and Laos—are eligible for refugee status in the United States. It should be noted, however, that not all individuals from these three countries are refugees.

The term "Indochina" is a French legacy. The three countries of Vietnam, Cambodia, and Laos are geographic neighbors. Separated by a mountain range, each developed distinct and diverse cultures. Their fate became interwoven when France claimed the region as a colony and named it Indochina. To the southwest of Vietnam is Cambodia, an independent state with a highly developed culture. The Cambodians had historically referred to themselves as Khmers, but when the Khmer Rouge came into power in 1975 the country was renamed the Republic of Kampuchea. Though renamed, this country is still commonly referred to as Cambodia; individuals from there are either Cambodians or Khmers.

To Cambodia's north and Vietnam's west is Laos. This mountainous region is a land populated by separate and distinct tribes. Two tribes, the

Hmong and the Mien, were closely identified with the United States during the Vietnam war. These tribes were recruited by the CIA to assist the United States in its war efforts bordering North Vietnam. As a result of their intimate involvement with the U.S. war effort in the region, they were forced to flee their homelands; they have mostly resettled in the United States.

HISTORY OF MIGRATION

The fall of Saigon came unexpectedly for Ba. She and her husband's family were not evacuated by the U.S. military when the Vietcong came in April of 1975. Because he had been in the South Vietnamese military, her husband was imprisoned in a reeducation camp. The family lost their business under the communists. She lost touch with her husband, and not being on good terms with his family, she decided to arrange for her own escape from Vietnam by boat. After a first attempt failed, she escaped with 100 other individuals in a small boat. They encountered pirates on their second day out, who conducted body searches and took all their valuables, food, water, and gasoline, leaving them drifting on the open seas in the hot sun. Ba fell ill, became delirious, and had vivid hallucinations of being raped repeatedly by the pirates. On the sixth day, a friendly fishing boat towed them to Thailand. The refugees were given food and water by a native villager and pointed to the nearest refugee camp. After her recovery, Ba was told by fellow boat members that those hallucinations were actual events, that they had in fact been boarded, and she and others had been raped. She applied to resettle in France, since she spoke the language, but was denied entry. She waited for 1½ years before being accepted for resettlement in the United States.

Lin was awakened by her frantic parents telling her to pack quickly. Soldiers had come to their house in Phnom Penh and said they had to leave immediately. The family hastily packed and then left the house. Joining the rest of the inhabitants of the city, they walked out to the countryside. After 2 days of walking, they were told by the Khmer Rouge soldiers to go further into the countryside, to build a house and to start farming. Not being farmers, Lin's family lived in a state of semi-starvation for the next 4 years. During these years, government officials periodically ordered her to leave home and go to different parts of the country to join work groups. It was always a question as to whether she would be able to find and rejoin her family after these work group assignments. One time she returned home to discover the government had taken her father away 3 weeks earlier. No one who was removed in such a manner had ever survived and returned home. After her father's death there was even less food, and both her sister and her mother died. Lin then joined her aunt's family. Gradually, members of that family died. After her aunt's death, Lin walked for 2 weeks across the jungle, swam across a river, and arrived at a border refugee camp. There she had food daily and was physically safe. After a year she met her husband. She became pregnant twice, but both children died. During their second year in camp, her husband's family located his uncle in the United States. The uncle started the paperwork to sponsor the family, and after 5 years in the camp, she and her husband's family left for resettlement in the United States.

The legacy of political unrest and war in Vietnam and Cambodia is partially illustrated by Ba and Lin. Vietnamese American women from northern and rural Vietnam grew up experiencing the realities of war on a daily basis. By day, French and later U.S. soldiers swept through the area looking for Vietcong soldiers and those villagers sympathetic to the Vietcong. By night, the Vietcong entered the villages, executing those villagers who were thought to be sympathetic to the French and, then the Americans. To escape this constant terror and threat, those who had the means moved south, many into urban Saigon. These moves were but the first of a life-long series of forced migrations for Vietnamese American refugee women, which eventually lead them to one's office for psychotherapy in the United States. Psychotherapists should inquire into and take a detailed history of their migration, and expect that these Vietnamese American refugee women have experienced unimaginable horrors.

The lives of Saigon residents were less affected by the war, until 1975 when the United States troops withdrew, taking with them all U.S. citizens, a few U.S.-employed Vietnamese, and their families. Those evacuated constituted the first wave of Southeast Asian refugees. Women who left in 1975 were, by comparison, better educated and from a higher economic class than those who were to come later. Theirs was the least traumatic and problematic migration and resettlement experience. The journey from Vietnam to the United States did not last longer than 2 weeks. Most of them were employed within a relatively short period of time (Kelly, 1977).

Refugee women who did not leave Vietnam until after April 1975 fared far worse. Like Ba, these individuals survived under difficult conditions. They made their decision to leave Vietnam privately. Then, they fled in secrecy, either by themselves, leaving family and kin behind, or with their nuclear families. The exodus typically started with payment in gold to a middleman, in order to secure a place on a boat. The coastal fishing boat owners packed the small vessels beyond capacity.

The United Nations estimated that 50% of those who left by boat did not survive the journey. Under the best conditions a boat could reach the first country of asylum within 3 or 4 days, well before running out of fuel, food, or water. When the conditions were less than optimal, the refugees drifted on the China Sea in small boats, exposed to storm, starvation, dehydration, and the rape and pillage of privates. The types of traumatic experience have obvious ramifications for the mental well-being of a woman who survives and resettles in the United States.

Unlike the Vietnamese, Cambodian women did not spend their developmental years surrounded by war, and their escape was not as obviously traumatic. However, far more devastating than the war, and even far more devastating than the experience of the Vietnamese described above, was the reign of terror under the Khmer Rouge in Cambodia.

War seeped into Cambodia in 1970 with the U.S. bombing of the Cambodian countryside. The political structure was destabilized, and Prince Norodom Sihanouk was overthrown by U.S.-backed Lon Nol in 1970. The Khmer Rouge, under the leadership of Pol Pot, gained power after the withdrawal of the U.S. military in 1975, ruling for the next 3 years and 8 months. Their regime conducted a vigorous campaign to eradicate all Western influence. Anyone with any relationships, training, or even knowledge of Western ways was suspect and targeted for execution. The urban population was sent into the countryside to live like the peasants and to survive through subsistence farming, which led to mass starvation and death from disease. Various sources estimate the death toll to be between 1 to 4 million (Kinzie, Fredrickson, Ben, Fleck, & Kawls, 1984; Mollica, Wyshak, & Lavelle, 1987; Szymusiak, 1986).

The reign of terror ended in December of 1979 with a Vietnamese invasion. Many Cambodians took advantage of the political chaos to escape into Thailand. This journey was a perilous one, and once across the Mekone river, they did not find an easy welcome from the Thai. The Thai/Cambodian border has been the cite of many refugee camps, the safest of which are those under the auspices of the United Nations, each holding hundreds of thousands of refugees. Limited food, primitive sanitation, and minimal medical care are common complaints. Individuals may stay in these camps as long as 7 to 10 years, either waiting to return home or for resettlement in a third country. Life, though safe, was a succession of endless days of waiting: first to file papers, then to hear about resettlement.

Because of the Khmer Rouge, the Khmer in the United States have witnessed atrocities and experienced traumas that are inconceivable to most psychotherapists. As a result psychotherapists, either out of ignorance or abhorrence, avoid probing into these life experiences. I encourage those therapists who consider treating refugee women as clients to evaluate their own capacity to bear witness to such disclosures critically before accepting these clients. In the course of treatment, these women will understandably avoid discussion of the horrors of war. Unless the therapist is able to tolerate and probe for these incidences, the client and therapist may collude to avoid doing this critical piece of work.

CULTURAL/FAMILY BACKGROUND

Ba was the second daughter of an intact well-to-do family from Saigon. She grew up primarily under the care of her nursemaid, with limited contact with her parents. Her mother was an emotionally distant woman prone to dispense physical punishment for slight offenses, while her father appeared stern, but always kept up with her progress in the all-French private school she attended. Her childhood was not personally affected by the war that raged around her, and after secondary school she obtained training in law for a year. She worked as a paralegal for a very short time before marriage. Her parents arranged for her marriage, which she entered with anticipation and dreams of romance. She found her husband to be distant and somewhat disinterested; some months after the marriage she discovered that he had entered into the marriage unwillingly. He had had a love affair with a woman of whom his family did not approve and with whom he continued relations.

Lin was the oldest daughter of an intact family of three children from Phnom Penh. Her father worked as a government official, while her mother took care of the family. Her father was seldom home, but her mother paid close attention to the children, using maids to help with other domestic tasks. Lin received her education at home with a private tutor under the watchful eyes of her mother. She remembers days filled with study, visiting her many cousins, and playing with her mother. The Khmer Rouge interrupted this family life.

The developmental years for Southeast Asian American refugee women were spent in their country of origin, where they were not a racial minority. They did not grow up with the sense of differentness that goes with being an identifiable minority, as is the case with U.S.-born Asian Americans. Therefore, minority status is not a primary developmental issue, and does not become a central concern until later in the long-term adjustment of Southeast Asian American refugees.

As with other groups of recent Asian American arrivals, resettlement in the United States demands rapid cultural shifts to accommodate to the host culture. For a full discussion of the acculturation of Asians, refer to Bradshaw's discussion of Asian American women (Chapter 3, this volume). Each Southeast Asian American refugee group comes with its own culture, uniquely different from every other. China claimed Vietnam for 2,000 years. Vietnamese culture is thus heavily influenced by the Confucian structure, and shares similarities with the other Confucian-based cultures of China, Korea, and Japan. Unlike Vietnam, Cambodia was more influenced by the culture and religion of India, and shares similarities with the other Hindu-based cultures of India, Thailand, and Burma. Geographically separated from the cultural centers of China and India by the mountains, the Hmong and Mien people of Laos were not as heavily influenced by either country's major metropolitan areas. For more specific knowledge of these rich cultures I encourage the reader to start with Bliatout (1980) for the Hmong from Laos, and Khoa et al. (1981) and Whitmore (1979) for general discussion of various Southeast Asian cultures.

There are some cultural practices that can be generalized across the groups to which psychotherapists who are not familiar with these cultures may be exposed. For example, it is uncommon for females to have an extensive Western education such as that received by Ba and Lin; arranged marriages still occur in Vietnam for families of higher economic status; the role of the woman is a domestic one, as in the case of both Ba's and Lin's mothers; the role of the male is primarily as a financial provider; fathers are distant from the domestic concerns of children.

ADJUSTMENT

Arrival and Initial Adjustment

After a long and weary flight Ba arrived at the airport in Seattle, Washington. She had located Seattle on the map in camp, so she knew it was very far north and very cold. Despite this, she found herself surprised by the cold, gray fog that met her outside of the airplane. After customs, she walked into the waiting area, wondering what to do next. Thankfully, she saw someone holding a sign with her name. She approached, pointing to the sign and then to herself.

Lin arrived in the United States in August with her husband, and his mother. They were greeted at the airport by her husband's uncle, his wife, and their two young children. Lin was awed by the immense size of the airport, intimidated by the loudness, impressed by the uncle's being wealthy enough to own a small bus that accommodated many passengers, frightened by the speed at which they traveled in the car, and amazed at the strange vegetation she saw.

In the first few weeks after arrival, the refugees need to adjust to many new things. Some are concrete and physical like the weather, some common to all travelers like jet lag, some unique to refugees, like the technical advances in home appliances. These expected stresses among new arrivals are more obvious than those that arise later on, which may at first seem trivial, but can lead to unforeseen consequences. The clinician must take these stressors into account in order to make an accurate assessment of any refugee woman in treatment.

The immediate adjustments occur on a concrete level. Southeast Asian American refugees usually arrive directly from the Philippines, thus it takes several days to change their circadian rhythms. They come from a tropical climate, and are not familiar with cold weather. Resettlement in most states necessitates learning how to dress for and live in the cold. Less dramatically, the new arrival has to adapt to a host of other differences, such as the noise of the streets, smells of air pollution, speed of cars, the restrictive enclosure of apartments, and the largeness of buildings. The therapists, and the refugees themselves, rarely mention these stressors, yet they constitute a pervasive part of the general level of stress for the refugees. The clinician assessing any refugee must not minimize these environmental stress factors. When physical annoyances are reduced for the client, some psychological energy is freed to cope with other problems.

The next challenge for the refugee is the mastery of the indoor/home environment. Despite introductions to the American home while in the Philippines orientation programs, many refugees report not knowing how to use appliances such as central heating, stoves, indoor plumbing, dishwashers, clothes washers, vacuum cleaners, and many others. Learning the use of these appliances falls on the woman, and thus may be a major source of stress.

Short-Term Adjustment

Finally finished with all the government agencies after 2 weeks, Ba enrolled in English as a Second Language (ESL) class. There she met other Vietnamese women, and decided to move in with one of them. Within 2 months after arrival she found herself living on public assistance, wondering what was going to happen when welfare ran out within the year.

After 2 weeks, Lin settled into a routine of going to ESL classes, continuing to live with her husband, her mother-in-law, and the uncle's family. She did not see her husband during the day, since she went to morning ESL classes and he went in the afternoon. The uncle and his wife both worked outside of the home. Her mother-in-law took care of the uncle's children, which left the housework and cooking to Lin. After a few months Lin became restless, dissatisfied, and mildly agitated.

After this short period, necessary for initial adjustment to the physical surroundings, there is a period of settling into a new daily routine and making plans for the immediate future. In the first few weeks, refugees fill out seemingly endless forms to receive refugee assistance, to register for social security, to obtain alien identification cards, to complete physical examinations, and to enroll in ESL classes. The Refugee Assistance Act of 1980 provides for a package of aid that includes refugee cash assistance, eligibility for public assistance, medicaid, vocational training, and ESL classes. The Act specifically stipulates that all available refugee assistance is also to be accessible to women. As of October 1993, the refugee assistance package provides these services for the first 6 months after arrival. The specter of being left destitute within a year of arrival in a strange land can generate a high level of anxiety.

The refugees I encountered, both as clients and as colleagues, reported crying almost nightly during the time between arrival and getting their first job. My clinical experience has been that refugees experience feelings of sadness, loneliness, and overwhelming hopelessness starting approximately 2 months after arrival. The immediate issue of needing to be gainfully employed in order to survive in this country is understandably stressful, as is the growing realization that they will be living in the United States for quite some time. Concurrent with this realization is the surfacing of the sadness over the loss of their previous relationships and their previous lives.

The cumulative stress of trauma, migration, and resettlement appears in both physical symptoms and emotional problems. Many Southeast Asian Americans consider headaches and nightmares a normal part of life in the United States because of their common occurrence in the community. As evidenced by the low numbers of refugees in mental health services, it would appear that the majority manage these difficulties without professional treatment. Furthermore, the more severe mental illnesses do not appear until after the first year of resettlement (Beiser, 1988; Owen, 1985).

Long-Term Adjustment

Being fluent in French, it was relatively easy for Ba to master English. She obtained a part-time job in the tenth month after arrival as a job placement counselor for a social service agency that works with refugees. After the first year she enrolled in the local community college. Upon receipt of her Associate in Arts degree, she went from part-time to full-time work as a job placement counselor. She has worked there for the last 10 years. Her sister joined her 1½ years after arrival, and shortly after that her parents joined them. Her husband and his family contacted her 3 years after arrival. They, too, had escaped, and were in the United States. Feeling it was her obligation to carry out her duties as a wife, she reunited with her husband and his family. Both Ba and her husband have worked steadily and are now financially comfortable. They have two children and live close to the husband's parents.

Lin struggled through ESL as best as she could, but never really mastered the language. She became pregnant 6 months after her arrival. With the money from the federal program Aid to Families with Dependent Children (AFDC) and her husband's sporadic income as an unskilled laborer, they decided to rent a small apartment of their own. She stopped going to ESL after 12 months. She spent time either at home or socializing with other Cambodian women nearby. She started to feel disconnected from her surroundings, and memories of childhood and the many deaths she had witnessed became intrusive. She did not give special attention to her pregnancy, or seek prenatal care. She did, at the insistence of her family, deliver at the hospital. The feeling of disconnectedness continued after the delivery of the child.

The struggle to build a new life is a long process. There are circumstances shared by Southeast Asian American refugee women that are different from other Asian immigrant groups. The following discussion focuses on three issues with implications for long-term adjustment that are unique to refugee women: the change of class status, the effect of the simultaneous arrival of the women with the men, and the psychological unpreparedness for migration.

The first two issues are interrelated. Previous Asian migrations followed a pattern of young males, usually from poor families, coming to the United States to make their fortunes. Once the men were established, the women would gradually follow (Chang, 1991; Cordova, 1983; Glenn, 1986; Takaki, 1989; Yung, 1986). By contrast, Southeast Asian refugee women arrived simultaneously with the men so they learned to maneuver in this country as quickly as their husbands. This kind of empowerment alters their economic status, family position, and relationship to the community. In addition, most of the refugees from Southeast Asia had been of a higher socioeconomic class in their country of origin; the women came together with the men; and departure for Southeast Asian refugees was not in response to economic hardship, but rather to political changes that put their lives and livelihood in jeopardy. For the Vietnamese, since it took a great deal of money to escape, those women with financial resources would spend all of their reserve to make it out of the country. Cambodians of the upper classes were likewise targeted for harsher treatment, thus had greater reason to escape their country. Needless to say, using whatever resources left them to escape the country results in arrival in the United States without assets, which significantly changes their economic status. Entering U.S. society at the bottom of the economic ladder means many changes in lifestyle, such as the higher probability that these women will become employed outside of the home.

Understandably, a source of secure income is of primary concern. Two issues are key to securing employment for refugees: English proficiency and transferability of skills. For some, like Ba, employment is inevitable and comes with time. Once the refugee masters the English language, gainful employment follows. For others, like Lin's husband, employment is seldom beyond the manual labor level. Many get caught in a cycle of needing more English and vocational training to secure better paying jobs, but not having the time or the resources to get further training because they have to work longer hours at these low-paying jobs to make ends meet. Although in this situation there is greater pressure to have the wife enter the workforce, if she doesn't learn English the husband may take on two lower-paying jobs to make ends meet. This pattern further reduces the family's chances of greater economic security and further increases the women's social isolation.

In addition to the language barrier, it is difficult to find employment for someone whose skills are not transferable from their country of origin to the host country—for example, the subsistence farmers relocated in urban areas where farming skills are of no use for employment. Sometimes the skills are transferable, but the credentials are not, as is the case with professionals such as physicians who retain all their skills and knowledge of medicine, but cannot practice medicine because the state will not recognize their license to practice in this country. As a result, highly trained individuals often find themselves underemployed; physicians work as nurse's aides or physician's assistants. Then there are those skills that somewhat unexpectedly transfer to employment: women's domestic skills in housecleaning, child care, and handicrafts. A specific example is the marketability of the Hmong women's needlework.

Regardless of whether it is the woman who becomes employed while the man is not or whether it is a two-income family, the power structure of the family shifts with the women's employment. I advise the psychotherapist to examine those power issues for employed refugee women. Most of the issues for these women are no different than for mainstream European American women in the same situation, except for one: The Southeast Asian American woman may consider employment as an evil necessary for survival in the United States. She may attribute all her problems to migration. In such a case, the psychotherapist needs to explore all the circumstances discussed above: namely, the economic situation before 1975, the cultural expectations of marriage, the conditions of escape, and the conditions of present employment. Only then can there be an attempt to reframe her domestic problems in terms of a power differential.

Thirdly, refugees are less psychologically prepared for migration than the previous Asian immigrant groups. Presumably, immigrants migrated voluntarily. There was time to prepare for the departure, and they arrived at the destination with some resources and, most significantly, a dream to fulfill. Refugees do not migrate voluntarily, escaping to save their lives, without even the opportunity to make their farewells. They often have no knowledge of the whereabouts of their loved ones, and sometimes arrive without minor children, whom they were forced to leave behind. Their journey has been life threatening and perilous; their lives violently disrupted.

Like Lin leaving Phnom Penh, refugees expect to return to their homeland and former life when the political situation changes, and are thus less prepared than immigrants to engage in making a life for themselves in their new environment. They come to this country to wait for the day they can return home, to pick up their lives where they left off. The conflict between desire to return versus acknowledgment of present circumstances intensifies once it becomes possible to return home, as is the case for the Cambodians since 1989. Very few Cambodians have chosen to repatriate voluntarily. The realization that their children are Americans, that they themselves have adapted and changed, that there would no longer be a home to go back to, can be poignantly painful. At some level, the work of psychotherapy is to help women like Ba and Lin mourn the loss of their homeland and to help them deal with their current lives in the United States.

Part of the grieving process may be the loss of their culture in their children. Integral to a Southeast Asian American refugee woman's identity is her function as mother. Women like Ba strive to transmit Vietnamese cultural values as they parent their children, which may clash with those the children bring back from school. This penetration of host culture values and customs into the home through the children is impossible to prevent.

Part of the acceptance of their new lives is the acceptance of inevitable changes in their children.

A final issue of resettlement is important for psychotherapy. American society has historically and does currently discriminate on the basis of an individual's skin color. As persons of color, Southeast Asian American refugee women are subject to racial discrimination in the general community, in the work place, and in their children's schools. Since they did not grow up on the receiving end of racially discriminatory practices, they are often slow to recognize and apt not to believe the very real pain caused by such practices. This is particularly the case when their children come into contact with such practices in school or in the community. The psychotherapist must educate her client in how to recognize racial discrimination when it occurs, and what her options are for dealing with it.

Finally, underneath issues related to Southeast Asian American refugee women's experience of war and forced migration lie issues unique to the individual. In Ba's background, there was psychological and physical abuse during her developmental years that must color her interpretation of the subsequent events in her life. The psychotherapist must balance all those issues unique to the client's family of origin with those of migration, cultural differences, and acculturational forces.

MENTAL HEALTH TREATMENT

Health-Seeking Behavior

When the headaches came almost daily, Ba sought treatment with an herbalist, who gave her medicine that made them tolerable. Then, while putting away some papers, she discovered her husband's correspondence with his previous girlfriend. They had continued their relationship, and had even met in the United States. When she discussed her situation with her relatives and her priest, they consoled her and told her to stay with her husband. She continues to live in the same house, but has been estranged from her husband for the last 2 years. Three months after the discovery of her husband's correspondence with his previous girlfriend Ba started to experience tightness in the chest and pains in her back. For these she sought the services of a Western physician.

Lin's mother and husband were concerned about her disinterest in her pregnancy. They talked to community leaders, and sought the service of a healer who performed a blessing for the unborn child. As a result of this service, Lin agreed to go to the hospital for the delivery. After the delivery, her friends and family noted her continued disinterest in everything, including her baby. She was urged to talk to a Buddhist priest. Finally, her husband talked to their welfare case worker, who told him to take Lin and the baby to the hospital.

When emotional distress or mental illness occurs, the first contact for assistance is usually not a Western-style psychotherapist, but a host of other caregivers, as noted in the case. Herbalists are sometimes consulted either before or at the same time as a Western physician when the problem is experienced as primarily physical in nature. Religious persons, shamans, and community elders are sought when the problem is experienced as primarily emotional (Rieu, 1979; Rocereto, 1981; Westermeyer, 1979).

The Southeast Asian American client usually arrives in Western psychotherapy through the intervention of some mainstream, Western professional or agency. Psychotherapy is a foreign concept to Southeast Asian Americans, so clients show up not knowing what to expect. Their specific pretherapy expectations are dependent on the method of referral to health professionals. In general, they usually expect to tell the psychotherapist their problems in the first session. In the second session they expect the therapist to tell them what to do to get rid of the problems. If treatment deviates from this, then from their point of view psychotherapy has failed. At that point the client may leave treatment and seek assistance elsewhere.

Initial Assessment

Ba called for an appointment with a private practitioner. Her family physician referred her to therapy for treatment of stress-induced headaches and muscle spasms in her back.

Lin's husband called the local mental health center for an appointment for her. He reported that Child Protective Services (CPS) had removed their 5-month-old baby because the hospital had diagnosed the baby with "failure to thrive." CPS had also ordered treatment for Lin.

As the psychotherapist considers these initial complaints, the first treatment decision is whether to accept the case. Of primary consideration is the profession's ethical guidelines regarding treating cross-cultural clients (American Psychological Association, 1990b). In addition to recognizing racial and cultural differences, psychologists must understand the impact of socioeconomic and political factors, race, ethnicity, and culture on the development of culturally diverse groups (American Psychological Association, 1990a). I recommend that the therapist review the ethical guidelines from their respective disciplines regarding these issues. Moreover, unless a therapist has received special training and/or experience in the treatment of refugees and the general Asian culture, the therapist should not accept the case for treatment.

Regardless of our personal assessments of our own abilities as therapists, it remains in the best interest of the client that he or she be apprised of the best treatment available within the constraints of the provider system. The issue of the optimal psychotherapist–client match has been the subject of study for some time. Ibrahim's (1985) summary of the findings suggests that therapists who differ from their clients in several ways have the least potential in effecting constructive changes, and those most similar have a greater chance of assisting and intervening appropriately. In general, it is best for Southeast Asian American clients to receive treatment from trained professionals with the same cultural background who speak the same language. When this type of client–therapist match is possible, the clients must be made aware of the resource, and a referral made. Should the client decline, I recommend that the therapist assess the nature of the client's refusal.

Though it is best to have a cultural and linguistic match between therapist and client, except for a very few places in the United States, this is not possible. This does not mean good treatment cannot occur between therapists and clients of different cultures and languages. Tyler, Sussewell, and Williams–McCoy (1985), in their Ethnic Validity Model, suggest that cross-cultural psychotherapy holds growth potentials for both the therapists and the clients. In this situation, various combinations of a trained mental health professional and a bilingual/bicultural non-mental-health professional must then be considered. The two polar choices of treatment personnel are, on the one extreme, a mainstream mental health professional who is not a specialist in cross-cultural counseling, and at the other, a culture-specific bilingual/bicultural individual who is not a trained mental health professional. Between these two lies the use of a bilingual/bicultural social service case worker or bilingual/bicultural paraprofessional under the supervision of a mental health professional.

In my experience, two primary problems arise when a mainstream mental health professional who is not a cross-cultural specialist provides the treatment: the language barrier and the unfamiliar cultural background. Psychotherapy is language bound; it is imperative to establish a dialogue if treatment is to occur. All refugees, as noted earlier, receive some ESL training; as a result they have some knowledge of English, but usually only a very basic one. Professionals can be seduced into believing that language is not a barrier when the client nods assent to the therapist's query, "Do you understand?," or when she or he can repeat what the therapist has just said. ESL students are proficient at repetition drills, and can often repeat phrases without comprehension. If there are no other better suited resources available, and the decision is to accept the client into treatment, then it is best to obtain a foreign language interpreter. For a more detailed discussion of the use of interpreters in a mental health setting see Gerber (1980), Marcos (1979), and Westermeyer (1990).

When engaging the services of an interpreter, the therapist must specify the capacity in which the interpreter is to function and the type of interpretation. The interpreter can function in one of three ways: (1) as language specialist, (2) as bilingual worker, or (3) as bicultural/bilingual cotherapist. Translation can be either sequential or simultaneous. A trained foreign language interpreter can do either, and usually works in the capacity of language specialist. They are neither specialists in the culture—tempting as it is to equate language proficiency with cultural literacy—nor mental health professionals; therefore, they cannot be relied upon to provide the therapist with cultural information necessary for diagnosis and assessment. This arrangement gives the therapist the highest degree of control over the therapy process when conducting therapy in two languages. Liabilities of this arrangement are the cost, the scarcity of trained language interpreters, and the lack of a reliable source for cultural information.

An alternative arrangement is to obtain the services of a volunteer who speaks both languages. The advantages in using an untrained interpreter–volunteer are that there is no cost involved for the provider, and that such individuals are more readily available. The major problem in using an untrained interpreter lies in the possibility of a breach of confidentiality in the client's community and in losing control of the actual therapy session (Acosta & Cristo, 1981; Marcos, 1979; Price, 1975). Under no circumstances is it acceptable to use the voluntary services of a family member, especially the services of the children. The use of children, spouse, and/or other family members not only defies the principle of confidentiality, it may alter the power structure of a family through the therapist's granting a particular family member power to speak for other family members. Even if the interpreter is not known to the client, the possibility of a breach of confidentiality with an untrained interpreter is high. The interpreter (regardless of how well-intentioned he or she may be) may inadvertently discuss some small detail of the situation with acquaintances in the community. Most Vietnamese and Cambodian communities are fairly small, so that such information is easily identifiable, regardless of whether names are used. This lack of guaranteed confidentiality may contribute to the client's reluctance to share information.

Regardless of who the interpreter is, it is easy to lose control of the actual therapy session with an untrained interpreter. Other therapists, myself included, have had the experience of asking a question then sitting through a long interchange between the client and the interpreter, ending with the interpreter's replying, "no." The flavor and the content of the long interchange is lost for use in the assessment. I have had untrained interpreters tell me that they did not interpret everything the client said because they were embarrassed for the client and did not want to relay all the "crazy talk." If the combination of a mainstream mental health professional and an untrained interpreter is the best available treatment option in the provider network, and a therapist finds herself or himself in such a situation, it is best to meet with the interpreter before the session to establish the ground rules.

As an alternative to working through a foreign language interpreter, the psychotherapist can work with a bilingual/bicultural social service worker (Acosta & Cristo, 1981). In many situations, the worker will be the social service case worker who has referred the client to the therapist and is already providing all necessary back-up services to manage the client's life situation. The advantages are several: (1) an existing relationship between the client and the worker; (2) the worker provides assistance by following through with the therapist's recommendations; (3) language interpretation is readily available, and (4) culturally relevant information necessary for the treatment process is accessible.

However, this situation can have serious liabilities. If the relationship between the client and the bilingual worker is less than positive, it is very difficult to sort out which symptoms are a result of the client's illness, which ones are the worker's negative projections, and which ones are simply behaviors expressed for the benefit of the bilingual worker. The client may experience pressure to behave in such a way as to stay in the worker's good graces in order to continue receiving services. On the other side, the worker may be tempted to act as therapist, selectively filtering information. The therapist should assess the professionalism of the case worker prior to engaging in a collaborative treatment relationship, and make inquiries into the worker's character and standing in the community.

The fourth option is to work with a bilingual/bicultural mental health case worker who is not a fully trained mental health professional. In this situation, the bilingual/bicultural caseworker provides treatment under the supervision of a trained professional. The caseworker is from the same ethnic group as the client, speaks the same language, and is knowledgeable of the culture. The advantage of this treatment arrangement is an optimal therapist–client match. The disadvantage is that treatment is dependent on an untrained novice. The worker can often be oblivious to the significance of symptoms of mental illness, though with time and close supervision these workers can become quite skilled in assessment and intervention. This situation is probably the best alternative to having a fully trained bilingual/bicultural mental health professional, but the supervisor must be sure to attend to the usual issues related to supervising novice therapists. In addition, the caseworker must explain the supervisory relationship to the client. This keeps the client informed of the nature of the treatment and the extent of confidentiality, while also protecting the caseworker.

The caseworker's knowledge of the culture is another consideration. If the supervisor recommends an intervention and the caseworker says, "I don't think I can do that," or "We don't do things like that," or "In my country we do it this way," then the supervisor should take these objections seriously. These may not be the resistance of a novice therapist, but rather valid consultation on the workings of another culture. I recommend establishing the treatment goal, then joining with the worker to develop culturally congruent strategies to achieve this goal.

Assessment and Diagnosis

Ba arrived at her first appointment on time and by herself. She spoke fluent English. On the mental status exam she presented with initial and terminal insomnia, nightmares, a decreased sexual desire, avoidance of open water, and general anxiety. For the previous 6 months, she had taken medication for muscle spasms in her upper and lower back. Ba revealed her marital difficulties in her second session.

Lin arrived at her first appointment accompanied by an 18-year-old Cambodian female, who acted as her interpreter. Lin, through the interpreter, reported that she experienced some marital conflict but was otherwise doing well. She suspected that her husband thought she was having an affair and that he had arranged for the removal of her infant as punishment. After the second session, the therapist received a call from the interpreter's supervisor, who said the interpreter did not think Lin was sick and did not therefore need treatment. Apparently, Lin had talked extensively to the interpreter while being transported to and from the sessions. The interpreter claimed that Lin just needed to talk to a friend, and that she herself would be this friend.

Once the psychotherapist decides to accept the client in treatment, issues of assessment, diagnosis, and treatment planning come into the forefront. This section includes a brief general discussion of assessment and diagnosis for Southeast Asian Americans, and two case formulations, one each for Ba and Lin.

Assessment methods vary with the presenting complaints, the client's level of acculturation, and their English proficiency. For a general discussion of assessment issues for Southeast Asian American refugees see Williams and Westermeyer (1986) and Owen (1985).

There are two bilingual instruments that are short and may be self-administered. For Vietnamese, there is the Vietnamese depression scale (Kinzie et al., 1982). For the measurement of anxiety there is the Hopkins Symptom Checklist–25: Cambodian version, Laotian version, and Vietnamese version (Mollica, Wyshak, de Marneffe, Khuon, & Lavelle, 1987).

A survey of mental health centers in the state of Washington in 1987 (DMH, 1987) found that 60% of Southeast Asian American refugees treated in the system received a diagnosis of depression. Two of the clinicians who diagnosed these clients stated that the diagnosis was the best fit between the client's symptomology and what insurance would cover. An appropriate, though seldom used, diagnosis for refugees is posttraumatic stress disorder (PTSD). In an extensive review of factors that affect depression in women produced from the work of the Women and Depression Task Force of the American Psychological Association (McGrath, Keita, Strickland, & Russo, 1990), there is strong evidence of a relationship between the diagnosis of depression and/or PTSD and the variables of victimization and poverty. For the refugee women from Southeast Asia, not only is victimization prevalent, but they all enter the United States at the bottom layer of the economy, which may contribute to the presentation of depressive symptomology.

Major depression and PTSD may appear similar on initial assessment. To differentiate between the two, the psychotherapist needs to inquire into the etiology of the symptoms, the history of mental illness in the family, and the personal history of the client. If clinical evidence supports both diagnoses, I recommend the diagnosis of PTSD. This diagnosis allows the client to feel less flawed and to interpret her symptoms as understandable reactions to extraordinary life events. It also allows the therapist to explore in depth the traumatic incidents in the client's past, which will eventually lead to the appropriate mourning of the life she lost to war and migration.

The problem of the language barrier is illustrated in the situation with Lin, whose assessment was complicated by it. She did not have sufficient command of English to conduct sessions in English. As discussed earlier, the liabilities of using an untrained foreign language interpreter are that the therapist loses control of the session. This is exemplified by Lin's situation, in which information was not getting from the client to the therapist because of the interpreter's refusal to transmit the messages. Whether the interpreter is a social service worker engaged by an agency, or a kind-hearted volunteer, I recommend that the psychotherapist meet with the interpreter and her supervisor, without the client, to explicate the function of an interpreter, define confidentiality, and discuss the risk of premature termination from treatment. I also recommend that the interpreter be considered an extension of the therapist and have no contact with the client without the presence of the therapist.

As with any client who possesses limited ability to self-report accurate information, regardless of whether it is because of the client's psychopathology or because of a language barrier, the psychotherapist must consider obtaining information from collaborating sources. With a signed consent for exchange of information, the psychotherapist could contact members of the woman's family, her welfare case worker, her sponsor, and her resettlement case worker.

Presented below is an example of a psychodynamically based case formulation for Ba. Developmentally, Ba grew up rich in material wealth, but poor in emotional resources from her parents. Though her mother was both physically and emotionally abusive, the emotional impact of the abuse may have been mitigated by the presence of her nursemaid. Ba was exemplary in fulfilling her roles of wife and mother. Within the context of the Vietnamese American culture, she had the option not to reunite with her husband. Her choice to do so was an indication of the depth of her commitment to her culture's role for females. The experiences during the exodus out of Vietnam influenced the intensity of all of her symptoms, but contributed directly to the nightmares, the general anxiety, and the avoidance of open water; all of which are symptoms of PTSD.

The case formulation for Ba shows that she was a working mother, raising two children in an unhappy marriage. The extended family network supported her endurance of the situation. Cultural conflicts occurred as she was exposed to the role of women in the United States, and she found herself less inclined to accept her marital condition. Her symptoms had been present for some time. Most likely, the symptoms were considered a weakness in her character, not a treatable illness. With the onset of severe physical discomfort, a culturally recognized, treatable illness, she was able to seek assistance.

Diagnostically, her symptoms supported both depression, and PTSD. The psychosomatic nature of her presentation was culture bound, and, though it could not be ignored, neither was it central in the cluster of psychological symptomology. Though she had a history of abuse from her mother, inquiry had to be made into the nature of her relationship with her nursemaid to accurately assess the conditions of her early years.

Unlike Ba, Lin was at risk of an erroneous assessment secondary to inadequate language interpretation. Assuming adequate linguistic access, a psychodynamically based case formulation for Lin is as follows. Developmentally, Lin grew up in a well-to-do family. Her early life was in a warm and protected environment, which was abruptly ended by the Khmer Rouge. She matured into early adulthood amidst prolonged threats to her personal survival. She witnessed the death of her siblings and mother, sustained major losses of every family member, and later, experienced a miscarriage and the death of her son. The lack of nurturance for her baby may have been a combination of an inability to function amidst intrusive thoughts of her past and an attempt to shield herself from sustaining yet another loss.

Generally, Lin was a welfare mother living within the network of her husband's extended family. She could not interact with the host country because of the language barrier. She could not master the English language due to the severe symptomology of her mental illness. And she could not get treatment for her mental illness because of her language barrier.

Diagnostically, there was very little information about her mental status or symptoms of mental illness to support any diagnosis. However, her history of living through the Pol Pot regime argued for the diagnosis of PTSD.

Treatment

Ba continued to discuss her marital difficulties in the third session, revealing a history of emotional abuse, but no physical abuse. She believed her husband's behavior was acceptable within his role, especially in light of the fact she had been repeatedly raped by the Thai pirates and was therefore not deserving of better treatment. The psychotherapist challenged her beliefs and encouraged her not to tolerate the abuse. Ba then became quiet and appeared introspective. She did not return for the fourth session and did not acknowledge or return the therapist's calls.

After Lin failed to show for her third appointment the psychotherapist contacted CPS, who reordered Lin back into treatment. The therapist sought consultation from a mental health professional who was a specialist in treatment of Southeast Asian American refugees. Following the suggestion of the specialist, she arranged for her own foreign language interpreter, contacted the client, and arranged for another appointment. This time Lin's husband accompanied her. The session included the therapist, the interpreter, and the couple. A mental status examination revealed that Lin was severely withdrawn, hiding in her room for major parts of the day, and was fearful of sleep because of nightmares. Periodically, she thought her baby was the product of a rape by a Khmer Rouge soldier when she was in one of the work camps. Lin was placed on appropriate psychotropic medications. Her treatment continued with the same therapist and the new interpreter. Her husband transported her to sessions. Through therapy, Lin slowly started to rebuild her life.

An early issue in treatment is that of engaging the client. Referring back to the previous section on health-seeking behaviors, Ba was at risk for premature termination. In the first two sessions she appeared to engage in therapy without problems. There did not seem to be a language barrier, since her command of the English language allowed for the conduct of the sessions without foreign language interpretation. However, despite her English proficiency, she held traditional Vietnamese values and in many ways behaved as a traditional Vietnamese woman. These values were reflected in her tolerance of a very unpleasant marital situation and her willingness to live with the trauma of her rape in silence. Examination in treatment of the war and the events of her escape may have elicited feelings of shame. These cultural beliefs and emotions were not acknowledged when the psychotherapist challenged her belief about her husband's role in their marriage, which may have contributed to her premature termination of treatment.

Regardless of length of time in treatment, the prognosis for the treatment of Ba's PTSD is good. The traumas were relatively short in duration, specific in location, and not witnessed by family members. She could be helped to reframe the experience as one specific to war and not apt to be repeated again. However, her premorbid personality traits may be less amenable to change. This included her belief in the dominance of males, her subservient role in the relationship with her husband, and her predisposition to tolerate emotional abuse after having grown up with it.

Unlike Ba, the risks for Lin's premature termination from treatment were apparent from the onset. Resolution of the language barrier was necessary for treatment. More reliable information surfaced when sessions were conducted with a proficient language interpreter. It was revealed that Lin had been experiencing severe symptoms of PTSD. Her inattention to her baby was secondary to her mental illness. Once some of the extreme symptoms were under control, Lin would most likely be able to care adequately for her child.

Prognosis for the treatment of Lin's PTSD was less favorable than that of Ba. The traumas were extensive and protracted. It was more difficult to encapsulate her experience as only concerning the war. However, with treatment, the debilitating nature of her illness may be reduced, enabling her to lead a more productive life.

Risks of Premature Termination of Treatment

As discussed earlier and illustrated in the cases of Ba and Lin, the risk for premature termination of treatment is high for this population. The issues of language barrier and differences in expectations of treatment are enumerated earlier in this chapter. Value conflicts based on cultural differences may be the most difficult issue to address in premature termination for cross-cultural clients. As illustrated in the situation with Ba, the specific cultural belief of male dominance held by Ba was different from that of her Western psychotherapist. This difference led to the therapist's suggestion that Ba not tolerate what the therapist termed abuse, a culturally inappropriate recommendation that contributed to Ba's premature termination. The therapist should have worked with Ba's belief in the value of male dominance, while also addressing the rape as an occurrence that was neither her fault, nor acceptable behavior on the part of men.

Therapists who are not trained in treatment with trauma victims and cross-cultural counseling may ignore the more obvious effects of the trauma and instead focus on behavior changes that are based on cultural values. Psychotherapists who do not monitor how their own values and beliefs guide their therapeutic interactions unintentionally become an overt agent of social control. In general, I recommend that our training institutions make courses in cross-cultural counseling a requirement for those individuals who are destined to practice in clinical settings.

In specific, I do not recommend that psychotherapists advise clients to change in ways that may result in the clients' alienation from their culture of origin. This does not mean therapists should not engage in the examination of cultural beliefs that guide both the client's and the therapist's actions. The cultural issues should always be clearly delineated for the client. As with any modification of behavior, the nature of the client's relationship with those around her will be altered. For individuals who are from either an ethnic or a racial minority group, changes made at the suggestion of therapists who are outside of the client's racial and cultural group may create greater distance between the client and his or her culture group. At times, behavioral changes may lead to alienation from the cultural group. Because of these possible effects, any choices for change need to be carefully examined.

At times it may appear that certain cultural beliefs place a client in either extremely stressful or life-threatening situations, such as physical abuse. I recommend that the therapist and the client make clear distinctions between the underlying cultural values and the client's dysfunctional application of these values. The client may need encouragement to explore more culturally appropriate ways to protect herself from those negative situations.

CONCLUSION

Treatment of Southeast Asian American refugee women needs to address their unique combination of the factors of culture, gender, forced migration, and relocation in the United States. The etiology of certain aspects of their mental illness is rooted in the refugee experience. Psychotherapists who find themselves with such clients may find it helpful to be sensitive to and probe for the following:

1. History of family of origin: explore the impact that politics and war has had on these women's lives.

2. History of migration: uncover the traumatic experiences of war and migration, and then explore how these experiences effect the family relationships.

3. Adjustment: explore the many adjustments made in daily living to accommodate life in the United States, and then applaud the client for the strength to make these changes, to tolerate the differences, and to survive. Recognition of these accomplishments by the therapist increases the refugee woman's sense of self-worth and her confidence in her ability to not only survive, but also to thrive, in the strange land of her host country.

4. Grieving: help the client to identify the loss of her childhood homeland, her previous identity in the country of origin, and to some extent, the person she was prior to migration.

5. Acceptance: explore her new identity as a Southeast Asian American woman with higher gender status and with Americanized children.

In addition to the exploration of certain specific issues, I recommend the following changes to the customary psychotherapeutic practice in the treatment of Southeast Asian American women:

1. Personnel: consider training and/or supervising a mental health paraprofessional from the same ethnic and linguistic background as the client to work directly with the client.

2. Focus of treatment: consider making those issues that are secondary to the war traumas as the initial focus of treatment. If the client elects to do so, then consider focusing on pre-morbid personality factors.

3. Cultural conflicts: explore all potential ramifications of behavior changes in the client's relationship to her ethnic community, prior to making any therapeutic recommendations. This precautionary act functions as a safeguard against the psychotherapist becoming an agent of social control.

Refugees share the memory of war traumas, forced migration, the loss of everything familiar, and the hardship of adjusting to a different culture. Southeast Asian American refugee women have faced the challenges of life with great courage. When one of these women comes to seek help, we psychotherapists need to applaud their achievements, witness their pain, and participate in their healing.

REFERENCES

Acosta, F. X., & Cristo, M. H. (1981). Development of a bilingual interpreter program: An alternative model for Spanish speaking services. *Professional Psychology, 12(4)*, 475–482.

American Psychological Association. (1990a). Ethical principles of psychologists (Amended June 2, 1989). *American Psychologist, 45(3)*, 390–395.

American Psychological Association, Board of Ethnic Minority Affairs, Task Force on the Delivery of Services to Ethnic Minority Populations. (1990b, March). *Guidelines for providers of psychological services to ethnic, linguistic, and culturally diverse populations.* Washington, DC: Author.

Beiser, M. (1988). Influences of time, ethnicity, and attachment on depression in Southeast Asian refugees. *American Journal of Psychiatry, 145(1)*, 46–51.

Bliatout, B. T. (1980). The Hmong from Laos. In J. F. McDermott, Jr., W. T. Tseng, & T. W. Maretzki (Eds.), *People and cultures of Hawaii: A psychocultural profiler* (pp. 217–224). Honolulu: The University Press of Hawaii.

Chang, S. (Ed.). (1991). *Entry denied: Exclusion and the Chinese community in America, 1882–1943.* Philadelphia: Temple University Press.

Cordova, F. (1983). *Filipinos, forgotten Asian Americans: A pictorial essay, 1763–circa 1963.* Dubuque, IA: Kendall/Hunt.

De, T. T. D. (1989). *Vietnamese women and sexual violence (centrum Gezondheidszorg Vluchtelingen Report No. 1).* (Available from Refugee Health Care Centre, Library and Documentation, P.O. Box 264, 2280 AG Rijswijk, The Netherlands)

Division of Mental Health. (1987). *Analysis of factors that affect mental health and utilization of mental health services by the refugee population in Washington state.* Olympia, WA: Department of Social and Health Services.

Freeman, J. M. (1989). *Hearts of sorrow: Vietnamese-American lives.* Stanford, CA: Stanford University Press.

Gerber, B. M. (1980). Interpreting for the hearing-impaired patients in mental health settings. *American Journal of Orthopsychiatry, 50*, 722–724.

Glenn, E. N. (1986). *Issei, Nisei, war bride: Three generations of Japanese American women in domestic service.* Philadelphia: Temple University Press.

Grant, B. (1979). *The boat people: A "age" investigation.* Harmondsworth, England: Penguin Books.

Ibrahim, F. A. (1985). Effective cross-cultural counseling and psychotherapy: A framework. *Counseling Psychologist, 13(4)*, 625–638.

Kelly, G. P. (1977). *From Vietnam to America: A chronicle of the Vietnamese Immigration to the United States.* Boulder, CO: Westview Press.

Khoa, L. X., Pham, D. T., Doeung, H. H., Chaw, K., Pham, P. G., Bounthinh, T., Van Deusen, J. M., & Miller, B. (1981). Southeast Asian social and cultural customs: Similarities and differences, Part 2. *Journal of Refugee Resettlement, 1*, 27–47.

Kinzie, J. D., Fredrickson, R. H., Ben, R., Fleck, J., & Karls, W. (1984). Posttraumatic stress disorder among survivors of Cambodian concentration camps. *American Journal of Psychiatry, 141*(5), 645–650.

Kinzie, J. D., Manson, S. M., Vinh, D. T., Tolan, N. T., Ahn, B., & Pho, T. N. (1982). Development and validation of a Vietnamese-language depression rating scale. *American Journal of Psychiatry, 139*, 1276–1281.

Marcos, L. R. (1979). Effects of interpreters on the evaluation of psychopathology in non-English-speaking patients. *American Journal of Psychiatry, 136*, 171–174.

McGrath, E., Keita, G. P., Strickland, B. R., & Russo, N. F. (Eds.). (1990). *Women and depression: Risk factors and treatment issues.* Washington, DC: American Psychological Association.

Mollica, R. F., Wyshak, G., de Marneffe, D., Khuon, F., & Lavelle, J. (1987). Indochinese versions of the Hopkins Symptom Checklist—25: A screening instrument for the psychiatric care of refugees. *American Journal of Psychiatry, 144*(4), 497–500.

Mollica, R. F., Wyshak, G., & Lavelle, J. (1987). The psychosocial impact of war trauma and torture on Southeast Asian refugees. *American Journal of Psychiatry, 144(12)*, 1567–1572.

Owen, T. C. (1985). *Southeast Asian mental health: Treatment, prevention, services, training, and research* (DHHS Publication No. ADM 85–1399). Washington, DC: U.S. Government Printing Office.

Office of Refugee Resettlement. (1988). *Report to the congress: Refugee resettlement Program.* Washington, DC: U.S. Government Printing Office.

Price, J. (1975). Foreign language interpreting in psychiatric practice. *Australian and New Zealand Journal of Psychiatry, 9*, 263–367.

Refugee Act of 1980. Public Law 96-212.

Rieu, L. T. (Ed.). (1979). *Modern and traditional medical practices of Vietnam: Vietnamese concepts of illness and treatment.* San Francisco: Indochinese Mental Health Project, International Institute of San Francisco.

Rocereto, L. (1981). Selected health beliefs of Vietnamese refugees. *Journal of School Health, 51*, 63–64.

Szymusiak, M. (1986). *The stones cry out: A Cambodian childhood, 1975–1980.* New York: Hill & Wang.

Takaki, R. (1989). *Strangers from a different shore: A history of Asian Americans.* New York: Penguin Books.

Tyler, F. B., Sussewell, D. R., & Williams-McCoy, J. (1985). Ethnic Validity in psychotherapy. *Psychotherapy, 22*(2 Suppl.), 311–320

Westermeyer, J. (1979). Folk explanations of mental illness in rural Laos. *American Journal of Psychiatry, 136*, 901–905.

Westermeyer, J. (1990). Working with an interpreter in psychiatric assessment and treatment. *Journal of Nervous and Mental Disease, 178*(12), 745–749.

Whitmore, J. K. (Ed.). (1979). *An introduction to Indochinese history, culture, language and life—For persons involved with the Indochinese Refugee Education and Resettle-*

ment Project in State of Michigan. Ann Arbor: Center for South and Southeast Asian Studies, University of Michigan.

Williams, C. L., & Westermeyer, J. (Eds.). (1986). *Refugee mental health in resettlement countries.* Washington, DC: Hemisphere.

Yung, J. (1986). *Chinese women of America: A pictorial history.* Seattle, WA: University of Washington Press.

INDEX

Abandonment, fear of, 133
Abuse, physical; *see* Battered women;
    Domestic violence
Acculturation, 6, 91–92, 103; *see also*
    Transculturation
  and adolescent pregnancy, 127
  of Indian women, 171
  and outmarrying, 96
  of younger generation, 260
Acculturation stress, 31, 35, 78, 180, 281
  and biculturism, 214
  and familism, 122–123
  in refugees, 482, 487, 489, 500
  and substance abuse, 47
Acrophobia, 307, 308, 309
Addictive behaviors, 348, 369–371, 382; *see*
    also Alcohol abuse; Substance abuse
Adolescents
  American Indian, depression in, 44–45
  Indian, and premarital sex, 174
  multiracial, 459–461
  pregnancy in, 126–127
Adoption, 59
  in African American families, 239, 249
  of Korean children, 77
  in Pacific Islands, 84
Adrenalin, 326
Advocacy, 132, 133, 136
  for battered women, 434, 444
Affect; *see* Emotions
Affirmative action, 267, 347, 353, 354, 355
African American men, 5, 15, 244,
    245–246, 247, 398
African American women, 10–63
  and African American men, 360–361
  and alcohol abuse, 189, 370
  battered, 435, 442
  as caretakers, 14, 21, 239–240
  and childbearing, 13, 14

and cultural tasks, 12
and eating disorders, 370
and education, 15–16, 26, 240, 246,
    247, 349
and extended family, 239–240, 244,
    246, 249–251
and lesbianism, 10, 392, 397–400
and marriage, 13, 15
and medical establishment, 320–321
and misogyny, 356
as the other, 296
psychological flexibility in, 23
and religion, 306
self-image in, 18
and sexuality, 16, 398, 399
and spirituality, 245
and therapy, 21, 24–27, 202,
    233–236, 243
working, 5, 17, 347, 349–349, 351, 355
African Americans/Blacks
  ancestry of, 11
  and "black rage," 202
  and Caribbean Blacks, 144, 145,
      157–158
  communication style, 13
  cultural characteristics of, 12
  and drug effects, 323
  and gender roles, 6, 11, 13, 17, 246
  geographical distribution of, 10
  and Hispanic culture, 239
  and myth of inferiority, 12
  and parent–child relationships,
      246–247
  population, 3, 10
  self-designation, 7
  and smoking, 324
  and social structures, 13
  and socioeconomic status, 240
Aging, 14, 344; *see also* Elderly women